ORAL PATHOLOGY
for the *Dental Hygienist*

Perfect your skills and prepare for certification with interactive practice on the enclosed CD!

The **Companion CD** located in the back of this book is your key to enhanced understanding of oral pathology and interactive practice for the National Board Dental Hygiene Exam!

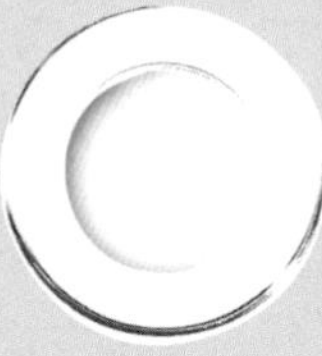

Prepare for professional success with…

- **More than 50 realistic case studies** that challenge you to apply your knowledge to clinical scenarios similar to those you'll encounter in practice.
- **Multiple choice questions** for each case that familiarize you with the testing format used on the National Board Dental Hygiene Exam and enable you to assess your understanding of key content.

Start using your companion CD now!

SL80379 JD/KB

ORAL PATHOLOGY for the *Dental Hygienist*

FIFTH EDITION

Olga A.C. Ibsen, RDH, MS

Adjunct Professor
Department of Oral and Maxillofacial Pathology, Radiology and Medicine
New York University
College of Dentistry
New York, New York
Adjunct Professor
University of Bridgeport
Bridgeport, Connecticut

Joan Andersen Phelan, DDS

Professor and Chair
Department of Oral and Maxillofacial Pathology, Radiology and Medicine
New York University
College of Dentistry
New York, New York

SAUNDERS

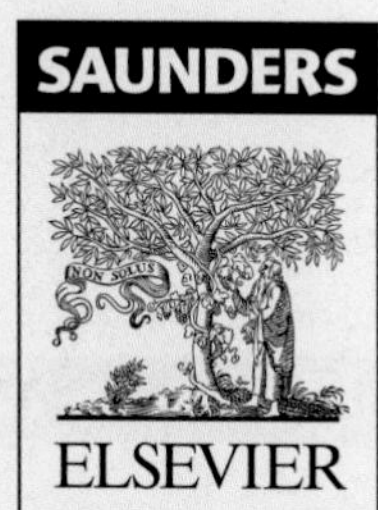

ELSEVIER

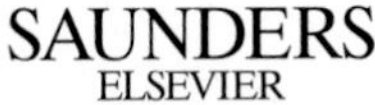

11830 Westline Industrial Drive
St. Louis, Missouri 63146

ORAL PATHOLOGY FOR THE DENTAL HYGIENIST, ED 5

ISBN-13: 978-1-4160-4991-3
ISBN-10: 1-4160-4991-6

Notice

Knowledge and best practice in this field are constantly changing. As new research and experience broaden our knowledge, changes in practice, treatment and drug therapy may become necessary or appropriate. Readers are advised to check the most current information provided (i) on procedures featured or (ii) by the manufacturer of each product to be administered, to verify the recommended dose or formula, the method and duration of administration, and contraindications. It is the responsibility of the practitioner, relying on their own experience and knowledge of the patient, to make diagnoses, to determine dosages and the best treatment for each individual patient, and to take all appropriate safety precautions. To the fullest extent of the law, neither the Publisher nor the Authors assume any liability for any injury and/or damage to persons or property arising out or related to any use of the material contained in this book.

The Publisher

Library of Congress Cataloging-in-Publication Data
Ibsen, Olga A.C.
Oral pathology for the dental hygienist / Olga A.C. Ibsen, Joan Andersen Phelan. -- 5th ed.
p. ; cm.
Includes bibliographical references and index.
ISBN-13: 978-1-4160-4991-3 (hardcover: alk. paper)
ISBN-10: 1-4160-4991-6 (hardcover: alk. paper) 1. Mouth--Diseases. 2. Dental hygienists. I. Phelan, Joan Andersen. II. Title.
[DNLM: 1. Mouth Diseases--pathology. 2. Tooth Diseases--pathology. 3. Dental Hygienists. WU 140 I14o 2009]
RK307.I27 2009
617.5'22--dc22

2008026617

ISBN-13: 978-1-4160-4991-3
ISBN-10: 1-4160-4991-6

Vice President and Publisher: Linda Duncan
Senior Editor: John Dolan
Developmental Editor: Courtney Sprehe
Publishing Services Manager: Julie Eddy
Senior Project Manager: Celeste Clingan
Design Direction: Charles Seibel

Printed in China

Last digit is the print number: 9 8 7 6 5 4 3 2

Dedication

To

Our Husbands

Lawrence and **Jerry**

For their years of support and encouragement of all our professional endeavors, especially each and every edition of *Oral Pathology for the Dental Hygienist*. They have assisted us in innumerable ways and we are most grateful to them. We appreciate their dedication to us! With our love,

Olga and *Joan*

Contributors

Margaret J. Fehrenbach, RDH, MS

Dental Hygiene Educational Consultant
Oral Biologist
Seattle, Washington
Inflammation and Repair; Immunity

Kenneth E. Fleisher, DDS

Assistant Professor, Department of Oral and Maxillofacial Surgery
New York University College of Dentistry
New York, New York
Attending, Department of Oral and Maxillofacial Surgery
Bellevue Hospital Center
Diplomate, American Board of Oral and Maxillofacial Surgery
New York, New York
Diseases Affecting the Temporomandibular Joint

Paul D. Freedman, DDS

Director, Section of Oral Pathology
New York Hospital Queens
Director, Oral Pathology Laboratory
Flushing, New York
Diplomate, American Board of Oral and Maxillofacial Pathology
Neoplasia

Joen M. Iannucci, DDS, MS

Professor of Clinical Dentistry
Director, Recruitment and Admissions, Sterilization Monitoring Service, Screening Clinic
The Ohio State University College of Dentistry
Columbus, Ohio
Developmental Disorders

Olga A.C. Ibsen, RDH, MS

Adjunct Professor, Department of Oral and Maxillofacial Pathology Radiology and Medicine
New York University College of Dentistry
New York, New York

Adjunct Professor
University of Bridgeport
Bridgeport, Connecticut
Introduction to Preliminary Diagnosis of Oral Lesions; Developmental Disorders; Nonneoplastic Diseases of Bone; Oral Manifestations of Systemic Diseases

Anne Cale Jones, DDS

Professor, Department of Pathology
The University of Texas Health Science Center at San Antonio
San Antonio, Texas
Diplomate, American Board or Oral and Maxillofacial Pathology
Neoplasia; Nonneoplastic Diseases of Bone

Joan Andersen Phelan, DDS

Professor and Chair, Department of Oral and Maxillofacial Pathology, Radiology and Medicine
New York University College of Dentistry
New York, New York
Diplomate, American Board of Oral and Maxillofacial Pathology
Inflammation and Repair; Immunity; Infectious Diseases; Neoplasia; Nonneoplastic Diseases of Bone; Oral Manifestations of Systemic Diseases

Heddie O. Sedano, DDS, Dr. Odont

Professor Emeritus University of Minnesota
Lecturer, Department of Oral Medicine and Orofacial Pain
School of Dentistry
UCLA
Los Angles, California
Lecturer, Department Pediatric Dentistry
San Diego Children's Hospital
San Diego, California
Diplomate, American Board of Oral and Maxillofacial Pathology
Genetics

Anthony Vernillo, DDS, PhD, MBE (Bioethics)

Professor, Department of Oral and Maxillofacial Pathology, Radiology, and Medicine
New York University College of Dentistry
New York, New York
Oral Manifestations of Systemic Diseases

Preface

Welcome to the fifth edition of *Oral Pathology for the Dental Hygienist.* We are delighted to have made some exciting changes in this edition, which we hope will contribute significantly to the teaching and learning process of oral pathology. Our goal has always been to facilitate teaching and learning and the fifth edition continues the two purposes set forth by the previous editions—to stand as both an excellent color atlas and invaluable resource text.

About This Edition

We received enthusiastic responses from faculty and students on the full-color clinical illustrations throughout the text in the fourth edition, and the fifth edition continues to offer an ideal combination of clinical photographs, radiographs, and discussion to help dental hygiene students and clinicians identify the appearance of variations of normal and disease states.

The fifth edition includes a variety of **learning features** to help students achieve the best possible outcomes in both the classroom and clinical setting. These features include:

- A **detailed vocabulary list** with definitions and pronunciations is presented at the beginning of each chapter. This list helps students learn essential new dental terminology so they can more effectively describe lesions and conditions in the classroom and in the clinical setting.
- Each chapter begins with a **list of objectives** that provides an overview of what is covered in the chapter. These objectives clearly define what the student is expected to learn and guide the faculty in test question preparation.
- Useful **synopsis tables** briefly outline the most critical information pertinent to each lesion, disease, or condition discussed in the chapter. This handy feature enables students to review all the disorders discussed in the chapter at a glance. This also serves as a quick reference for practicing hygienists in the clinical setting.
- **Review questions** at the end of each chapter help students test their knowledge of the chapter material and serve as good practice for taking the National Board Dental Hygiene Exam (NBDHE). All questions now have four answer selections, consistent with the national exam.
- An **extended list of references** appears at the end of each chapter which provided the student with additional study resources. References have been updated in this edition to reflect new research.
- A **comprehensive glossary** at the end of the text provides easy access to the definitions of all the highlighted words.

A **CD-ROM** containing over **50 case studies** is packaged with the text. These case studies present the material and concepts described in the text in a case-based format, which will help students master the important critical thinking skills they will need when working in the clinical setting as well as help them prepare for the NBDHE. By incorporating the case-based format, students are able to apply their knowledge to real-life situations. It's the next best thing to hands-on clinical practice. Not only is the CD an excellent preparation resource, it is also a great asset for class projects.

New to This Edition

In this edition, you will find a new section addressing the current concepts on **methamphetamine abuse** (Chapter 2) and new sections detailing **biophosphonate-associated osteonecrosis** and **acanthosis nigricans** (Chapter 9).

Each chapter has been thoroughly updated with new vocabulary, terminology and references. The glossary has been expanded to now include all of the bolded terminology within the chapters, making it an even more important reference.

All of the chapter review questions have been revised to offer four answer selections, which more clearly reflect the NBDHE design and format. This format change will assist faculty in preparing students for the NBDHE, course reviews, and curriculum examinations.

One of the biggest additions to the fifth edition is the **EVOLVE** site which includes a wealth of helpful information for both faculty and students. A complete listing of the material available on Evolve can be found on the **About EVOLVE** page following the preface.

From the Authors

We hope that this new edition, written specifically for dental hygienists, will continue to provide dental hygienists with the highest-standard oral pathology text. We strongly encourage instructors to continue to use the text in other courses, such as radiology, oral histology, and clinical courses. Dental hygienists have earned a reputation for excellence in identifying abnormal oral findings. The integration of oral pathology throughout the dental hygiene curriculum ensures more comprehensive patient care by the student and the dental hygiene practitioner.

Olga A.C. Ibsen, RDH, MS
Joan Andersen Phelan, DDS

About Evolve

An Evolve website, new to this edition, offers a variety of additional learning tools and greatly enhances the text for both students and instructors.

For the Student

Evolve Student Resources offers the following:

- **Pathology Identification Exercises.** These interactive identification exercises show photos of a variety of diseases/conditions. Students must identify the disease and move the correct label to the photo it describes. A great visual self-study tool, these exercises allow students to test their ability to identify diseases they may encounter in practice.
- **Practice Exam.** A 77-question practice exam, with questions taken from *Mosby's Comprehensive Review of Dental Hygiene,* ed 6, is designed to help students prepare for the National Board Dental Hygiene Examination (NBDHE) as well as course exams.
- **Dental Hygiene Forms.** A variety of forms the hygienist may encounter in practice are provided in a printable format. Forms provided include: a health history questionnaire, a head and neck physical examination documentation form, a prevention survey, an oral risk assessment worksheet, and a tobacco use assessment form.
- **Printable Versions of the Synopsis Tables.** The printable versions allow students to print out these helpful tables for inclusion with notes and make it easy to transport them from class to class.
- **Answers to Chapter Review Questions.** Answers to chapter review questions are now available on Evolve.
- **Weblinks.** Links to professional organizations, journals, additional image collections, smoking cessation, and meth mouth are provided to supplement the content of the textbook.

For the Instructor

Evolve Instructor Resources offers the following:

- **Testbank in ExamView.** A 400-question testbank divided by chapter is included along with rationales for all answer choices. The questions can be sorted by chapter or randomly, making the creation of quizzes and exams much easier for the instructor.
- **Image Collection.** This image collection includes every illustration from the book, making it easy for the instructor to incorporate a photo or drawing into a lecture or quiz.
- **PowerPoint Presentations.** Presentations created by the authors provide instructors with ready made lectures.

Acknowledgments

Through the years, many individuals have contributed to the success *of Oral Pathology for the Dental Hygienist.*

Our former editors at Elsevier have included Shirley Kuhn, who was with us through the first four editions, and Publisher, Penny Rudolph, who also guided us through the fourth edition. We sincerely appreciate their encouragement, support and direction.

This fifth edition was directed and supported by Senior Editor, John Dolan, Developmental Editor, Courtney Sprehe, Senior Project Manager, Celete Clingan, and Product Specialist, Cindy Ahlheim. They guided us through all the stages of production, and we thank them for their attention and encouragement to this outstanding product, especially their insight into the needs of the Evolve site.

We acknowledge Dr. William Forbes from Dover-Foxcroft, Maine, and Dr. Elias Kopti from Fargo, North Dakota, who provided detailed critiques of the first and second editions. It was Dr. Kopti who recommended that we include the valuable summaries at the end of each chapter. Students have found these summaries to be extremely helpful.

Also, contributing to this edition, we thank Lana Crawford, RDH, BS from Carrollton, Texas for recommending the inclusion of acanthosis nigricans in Chapter 9. Additionally, a special thanks to John Kacher, DDS from JKJ Pathology, The Woodlands, Texas for his careful review of the glossary.

We will always be grateful to our Oral Pathology teachers: Drs. Melvin Blake, Ernest Baden, Leon Eisenbud, Paul Freedman, Stanley Kerpel, Harry Lumerman, Michael Marder, James Sciubba, Philip Silverstein, Marshal Solomon, David Zegarelli, and Edward V. Zegarelli. Olga A.C. Ibsen is especially grateful to two individuals who influenced her personal and professional life: her dad, the late Dr. Joseph A. Cuttita, and her godfather, the late Dr. Edward V. Zegarelli. All of these individuals strongly influenced our passion for pathology!

Gloria Turner of the Diagnostic Pathology Laboratory at NYU College of Dentistry prepared most of the slides used for the color photomicrographs that enhance the fourth and fifth editions of *Oral Pathology for the Dental Hygienist.* We extend our sincere appreciation for her outstanding work. Additionally, color photomicrographs were also provided by the Oral Pathology Laboratory, Inc., Flushing, New York.

We are proud to present the fifth edition of *Oral Pathology for the Dental Hygienist.*

Olga A.C. Ibsen, RDH, MS
Joan Andersen Phelan, DDS

Acknowledgments

Contents

Introduction to Preliminary Diagnosis of Oral Lesions

chapter 1

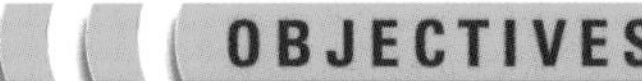

OBJECTIVES

After studying this chapter, the student will be able to:

1. Define each of the terms in the vocabulary list for this chapter.
2. List and define the eight diagnostic categories that contribute to the diagnostic process.
3. Name a diagnostic category and give an example of a lesion, anomaly, or condition for which this category greatly contributes to the diagnosis.
4. Describe the clinical appearance of Fordyce granules (spots), torus palatinus, mandibular tori, and lingual varicosities and identify them in the clinical setting or on a clinical photograph.
5. Describe the radiographic appearance and historical data (including the age, sex, and race of the patient) that are relevant to periapical cemento-osseous dysplasia (cementoma).
6. Define "variant of normal" and give three examples of these lesions involving the tongue.
7. List and describe the clinical characteristics and identify a clinical picture of median rhomboid glossitis, geographic tongue, ectopic geographic tongue, fissured tongue, and hairy tongue.
8. Describe the clinical and histologic differences between leukoedema and linea alba.

VOCABULARY

CLINICAL APPEARANCE OF SOFT TISSUE LESIONS

Bulla (adjective, bullous; plural, bullae) A circumscribed, elevated lesion that is more than 5 mm in diameter, usually contains serous fluid, and looks like a blister.

Lobule (adjective, lobulated) A segment or lobe that is a part of the whole; these lobes sometimes appear fused together (Figure 1-1).

Macule An area that is usually distinguished by a color different from that of the surrounding tissue; it is flat and does not protrude above the surfa[ce of the] normal tissue. A freckle is an example of a macule.

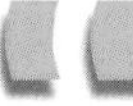

VOCABULARY (continued)

Papule A small, circumscribed lesion usually less than 1 cm in diameter that is elevated or protrudes above the surface of normal surrounding tissue.

Pedunculated Attached by a stemlike or stalklike base similar to that of a mushroom (Figure 1-2).

Pustules Variously sized circumscribed elevations containing pus.

Sessile Describing the base of a lesion that is flat or broad instead of stemlike (Figure 1-3).

Vesicle A small, elevated lesion less than 1 cm in diameter that contains serous fluid.

SOFT TISSUE CONSISTENCY

Nodule A palpable solid lesion up to 1 cm in diameter found in soft tissue; it can occur above, level with, or beneath the skin surface.

Palpation The evaluation of a lesion by feeling it with the fingers to determine the texture of the area; the descriptive terms for palpation are soft, firm, semifirm, and fluid filled; these terms also describe the consistency of a lesion.

COLOR OF LESION

Colors Red, pink, salmon, white, blue-black, gray, brown, and black are the colors used most frequently to describe oral lesions; they can be used to identify specific lesions and may also be incorporated into general descriptions.

Erythema An abnormal redness of the mucosa or gingiva.

Pallor Paleness of the skin or mucosal tissues.

SIZE OF LESION

Centimeter (cm) One hundredth of a meter; equivalent to a little less than ½ inch (0.393 of an inch) (Figure 1-4).

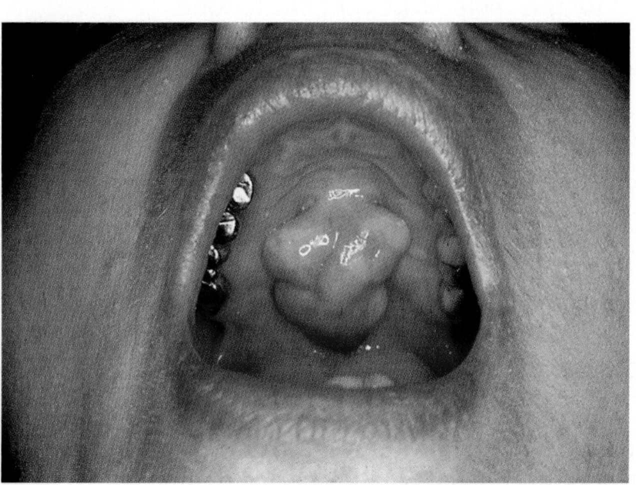

FIGURE 1-1 ■ Lobulated torus palatinus.

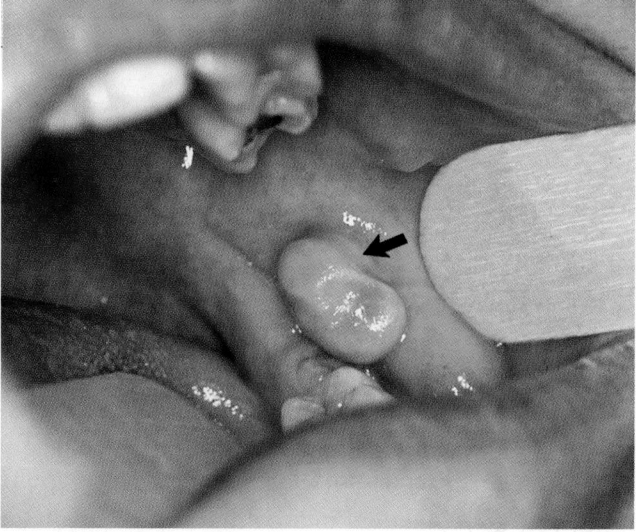

FIGURE 1-2 ■ Fibroma with a pedunculated base. *Arrow* points to the stemlike base.

VOCABULARY (continued)

Millimeter (mm) One thousandth of a meter (a meter is equivalent to 39.3 inches); the periodontal probe is of great assistance in documenting the size or diameter of a lesion that can be measured in millimeters (general terms such as small, medium, or large are sometimes used, but these terms are not as specific) (Figure 1-5).

SURFACE TEXTURE

Corrugated Wrinkled.

Fissure A cleft or groove, normal or otherwise, showing prominent depth.

Papillary Resembling small, nipple-shaped projections or elevations found in clusters.

Smooth, rough, folded Terms used to describe the surface texture of a lesion.

RADIOGRAPHIC TERMS USED TO DESCRIBE LESIONS IN BONE

Coalescence The process by which parts of a whole join together, or fuse, to make one.

Diffuse Describes a lesion with borders that are not well defined, making it impossible to detect the exact parameters of the lesion; this may make treatment more difficult and, depending on the biopsy results, more radical (Figure 1-6).

Multilocular Describes a lesion that extends beyond the confines of one distinct area and is defined as many lobes or parts that are somewhat fused together, making up the entire lesion; a multilocular radiolucency is sometimes described as resembling soap bubbles; an odontogenic keratocyst often presents as a multilocular, radiolucent lesion (Figure 1-7).

Radiolucent Describes the black or dark areas on a radiograph; radiant energy can pass through these structures; less dense tissue such as the pulp is seen as a radiolucent structure (Figure 1-8).

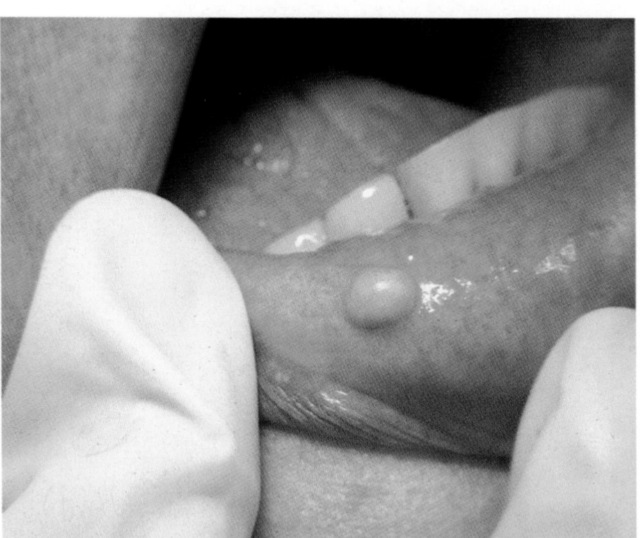

FIGURE 1-3 ■ Fibroma with a sessile base.

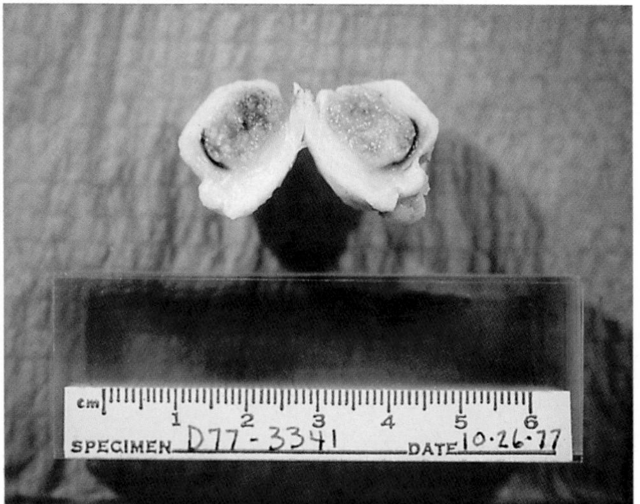

FIGURE 1-4 ■ A ruler measuring centimeters is used to measure all specimens submitted for microscopic examination.

VOCABULARY (continued)

Radiolucent and radiopaque Terms used to describe a mixture of light and dark areas within a lesion, usually denoting a stage in the development of the lesion; for example, in a stage I periapical cemento-osseous dysplasia (cementoma) (Figure 1-9, *A*), the lesion is radiolucent; in stage II it is radiolucent and radiopaque (Figure 1-9, *B*).

Radiopaque Describes the light or white area on a radiograph that results from the inability of radiant energy to pass through the structure; the denser the structure, the lighter or whiter it appears on the radiograph; this is illustrated in Figure 1-10.

Root resorption Observed radiographically when the apex of the tooth appears shortened or blunted and irregularly shaped; occurs as a response to stimuli, which can include a cyst, tumor, or trauma; Figure 1-11 illustrates resorption of the roots as a result of a rapid orthodontic procedure (see Figure 1-27); external resorption arises from tissues outside the tooth such as the periodontal ligament,

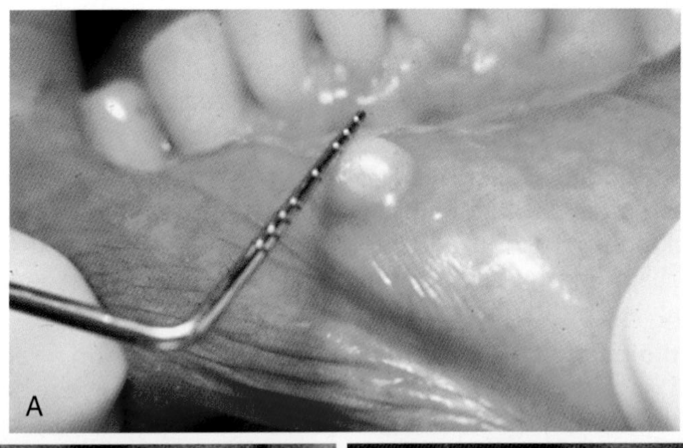

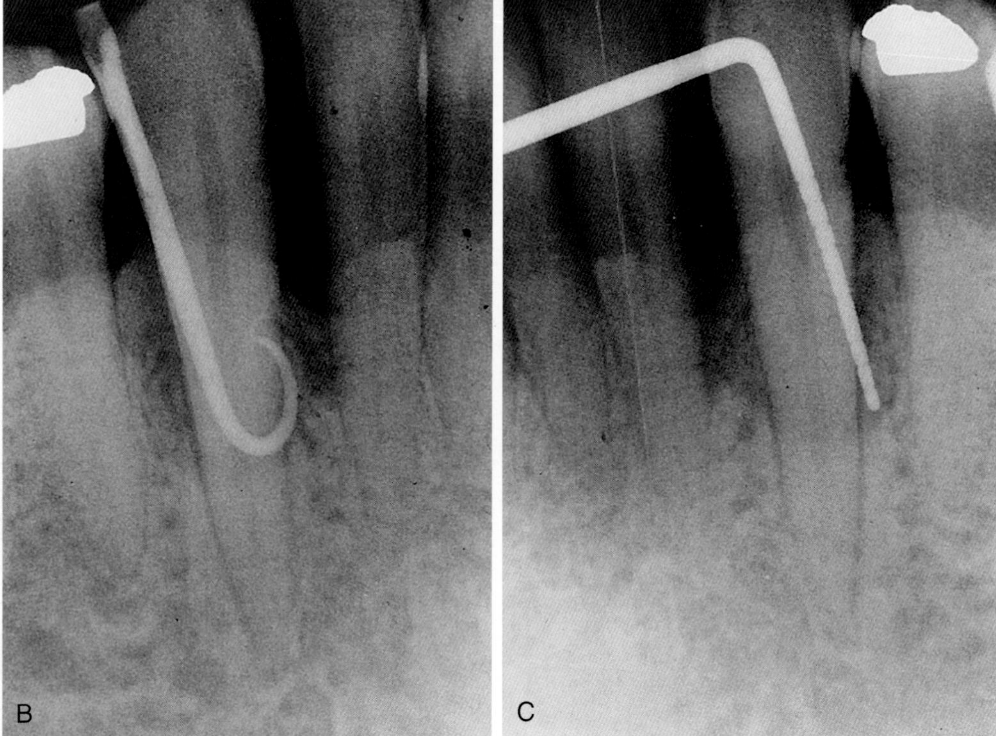

FIGURE 1-5 ■ **A,** Probe measuring the diameter of a fibroma with a sessile base. **B,** Gutta-percha point used to explore a radiographic defect. **C,** Periodontal probe placed before a radiograph is taken.

VOCABULARY (continued)

whereas internal resorption is triggered by pulpal tissue reaction from within the tooth; in the latter the pulpal area can be seen as a diffuse radiolucency beyond the confines of the normal pulp area.

Scalloping around the root A radiolucent lesion that extends between the roots, as seen in a traumatic bone cyst; this lesion appears to extend up the periodontal ligament (Figure 1-12).

Unilocular Having one compartment or unit that is well defined or outlined, as in a simple radicular cyst (Figure 1-13).

Well circumscribed Term used to describe a lesion with borders that are specifically defined and in which one can clearly see the exact margins and extent (Figure 1-14).

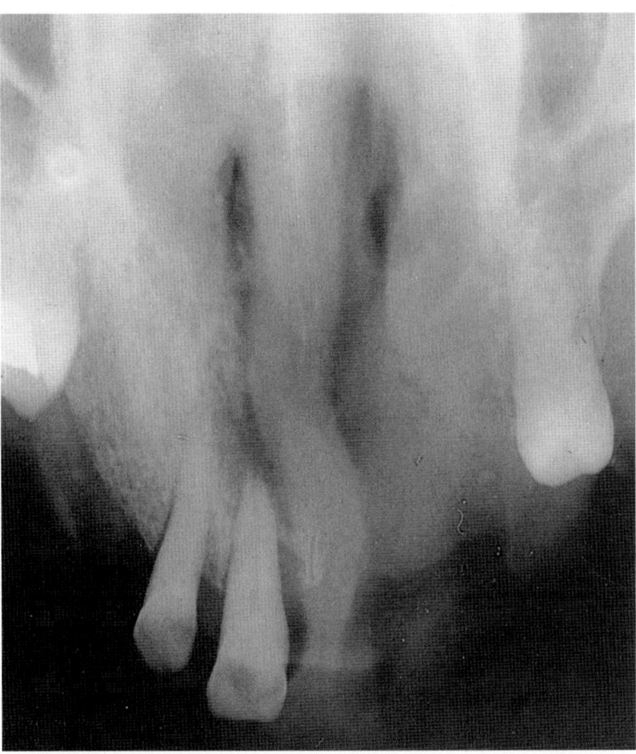

FIGURE 1-6 ■ Squamous cell carcinoma of the hard palate showing diffuse borders. (Courtesy Drs. Paul Freedman and Stanley Kerpel.)

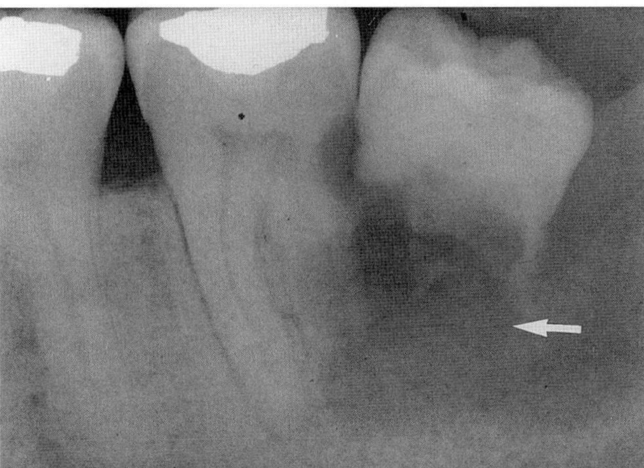

FIGURE 1-7 ■ Odontogenic keratocyst *(arrow),* illustrating a multilocular lesion. (Courtesy Dr. Victor M. Sternberg.)

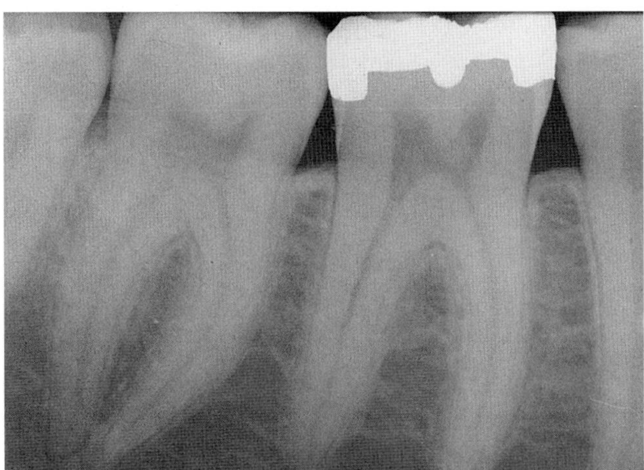

FIGURE 1-8 ■ Prominent pulp chambers, horns, and canals in mandibular molars.

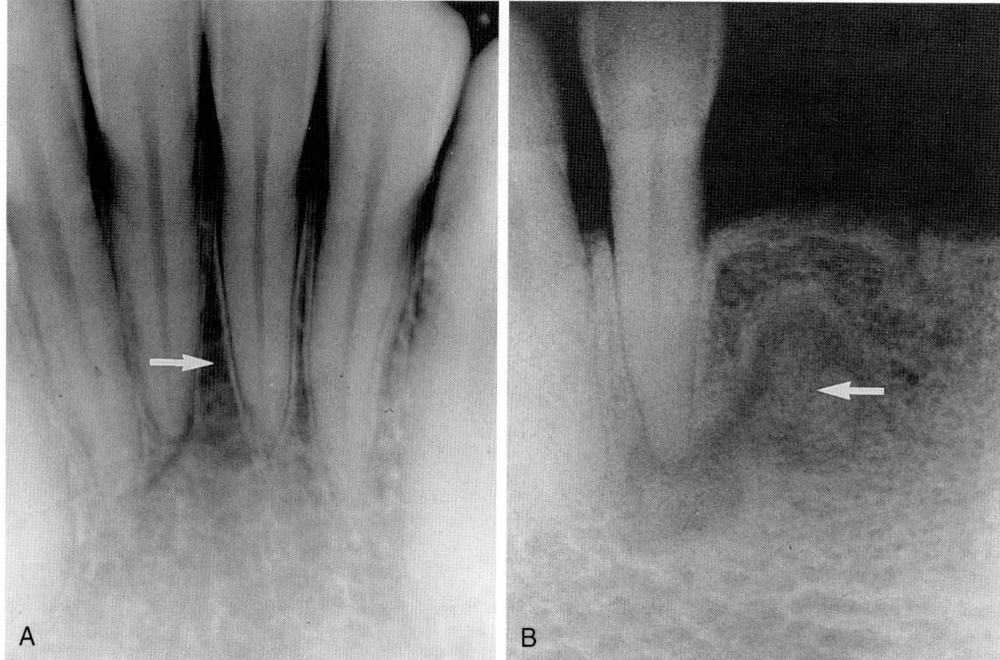

FIGURE 1-9 ■ **A,** Stage I periapical cemento-osseous dysplasia (cementoma). **B,** Stage II periapical cemento-osseous dysplasia (cementoma).

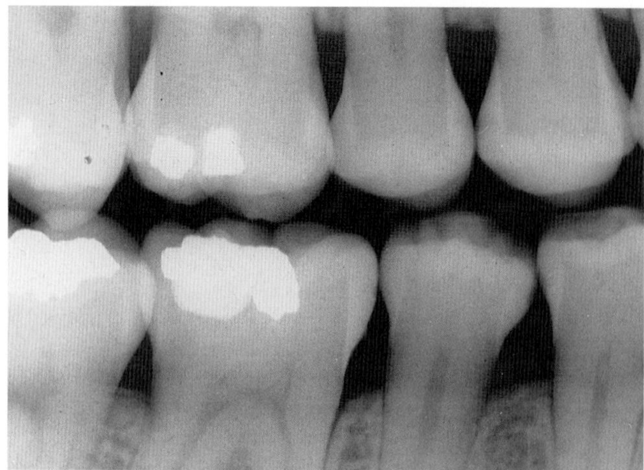

FIGURE 1-10 ■ Amalgam restorations on the occlusal surfaces of the maxillary and mandibular molars.

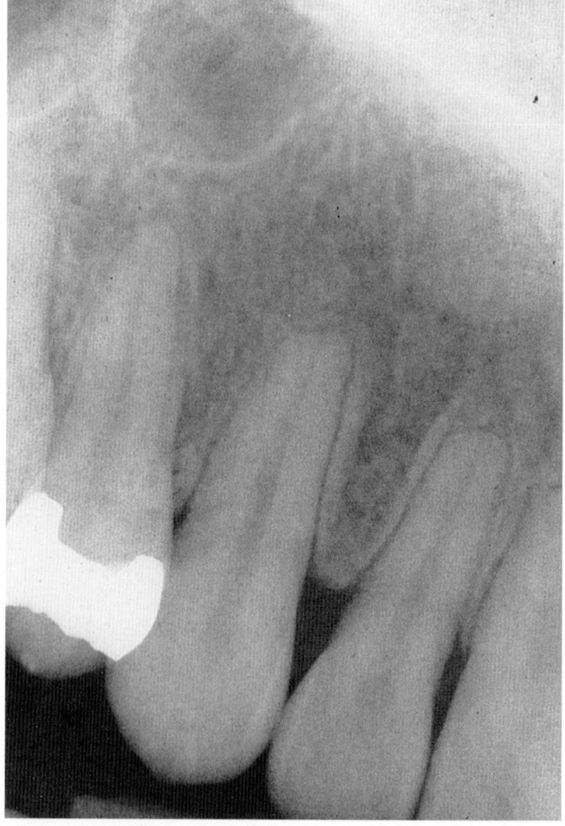

FIGURE 1-11 ■ Resorption of the roots on maxillary anteriors as a result of rapid orthodontic movement.

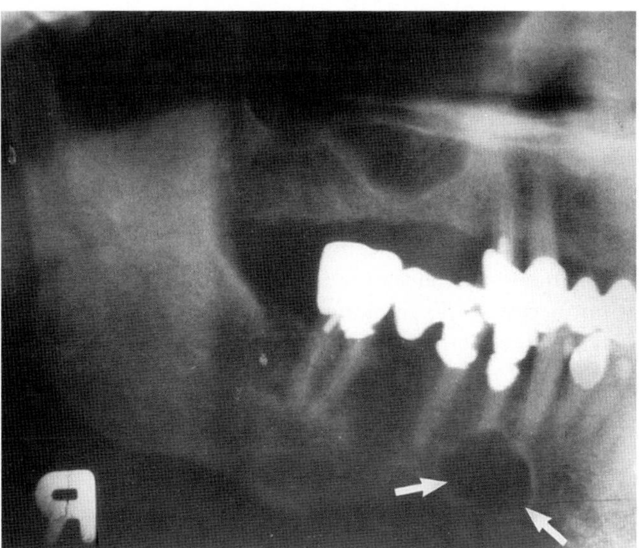

FIGURE 1-12 ■ Traumatic bone cyst around the roots. (Courtesy Drs. Paul Freedman and Stanley Kerpel.)

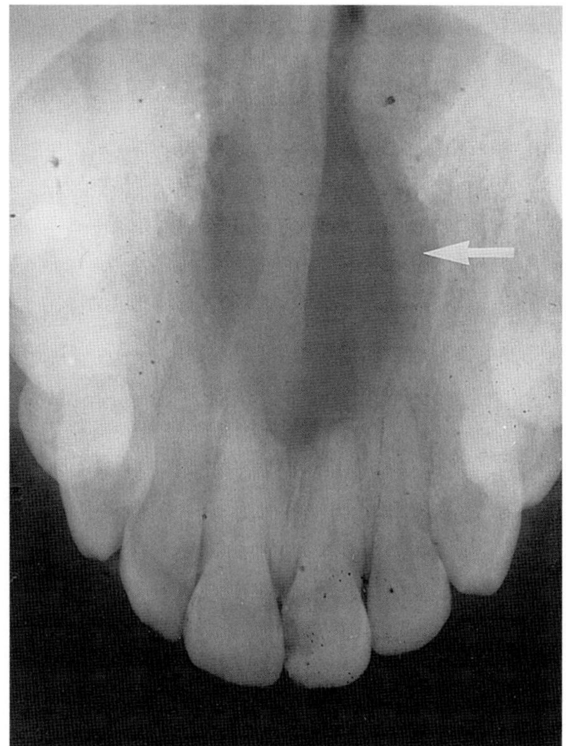

FIGURE 1-14 ■ Well-circumscribed median palatal cyst.

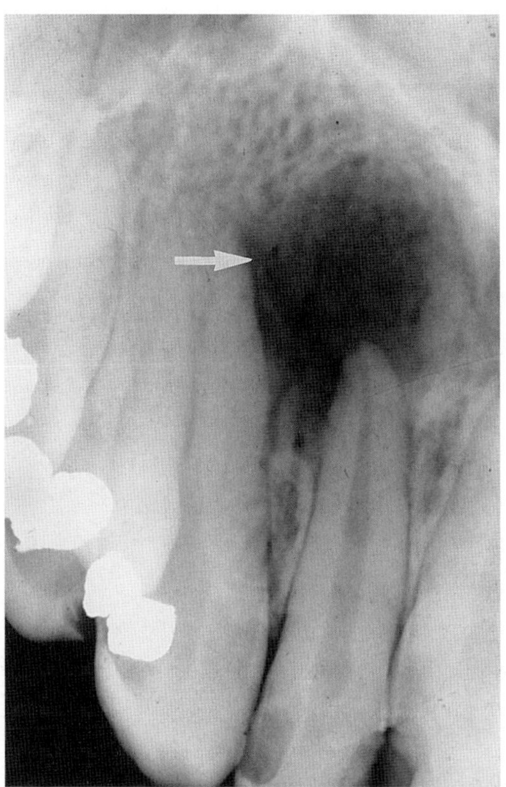

FIGURE 1-13 ■ Radicular cyst at the apex of the maxillary lateral incisor, illustrating a unilocular lesion.

To understand the material in this text, it is imperative that the reader approach it in a systematic manner. Significant time is spent in the dental hygiene curriculum identifying and describing normal structures. Before one can identify the abnormal condition, it is necessary to have a solid understanding of the basic and dental sciences such as human anatomy and physiology, histology, and dental anatomy. Once one has a solid understanding of normal structures and those that are variants of normal, findings that deviate from normal and pathologic conditions are recognized more easily. The preliminary evaluation and description of these lesions are within the scope of dental hygiene practice and are truly among the most challenging experiences in clinical practice.

In the first part of this chapter the definitions of commonly used terms that describe the clinical and radiographic features of a lesion, including terms used for normal, variants of normal, and pathologic conditions discussed throughout this text, are presented. The reader is encouraged to use these terms in the clinical setting so that they become part of an everyday professional vocabulary, thereby facilitating communication between the hygienist and other dental practitioners in the clinical setting.

The second part of this chapter focuses on the eight diagnostic categories that provide a systematic approach to the preliminary evaluation of oral lesions. Each area is described, and the strength of that area in the diagnostic process is illustrated using specific examples of lesions.

The final part of the chapter includes conditions that are considered variants of normal and those that are benign conditions of unknown cause. Most are diagnosed from their distinct clinical appearance and history.

THE DIAGNOSTIC PROCESS

MAKING A DIAGNOSIS

How is a diagnosis made? What are the essential components? The answers to these questions begin with data collection. The process of diagnosis requires gathering information that is relevant to the patient and the lesion being evaluated; this information comes from various sources.

Certain distinct diagnostic categories should be thought of as pieces in a puzzle, with each piece playing a significant role in the final diagnosis. The eight categories that contribute segments of information leading to the definitive or final diagnosis are (1) clinical, (2) radiographic, (3) historical, (4) laboratory, (5) microscopic, (6) surgical, (7) therapeutic, and (8) differential findings. It is important to note that usually one area alone does not provide sufficient information to make a diagnosis; the strength of the diagnosis is often derived from one or two areas. As the reader becomes more aware of the diseases and conditions discussed in this text, it will be most helpful to use the diagnostic categories as a guide to the evaluation of a lesion.

Clinical Diagnosis

Clinical diagnosis suggests that the strength of the diagnosis comes from the clinical appearance of the lesion. By observing the area in a well-illuminated clinical setting and palpating it if necessary, the clinician can establish a diagnosis for some lesions on the basis of color, shape, location, and history of the lesion. When a diagnosis can be made on the basis of these unique clinical features, biopsy or surgical intervention is not necessary. Examples of lesions that can be clinically diagnosed are Fordyce granules (Figure 1-15), torus palatinus (Figure 1-16), mandibular tori (Figure 1-17), melanin pigmentation (Figure 1-18), retrocuspid papillae (Figure 1-19), and lingual varicosities. These lesions are described later in this chapter.

Other benign conditions of unknown cause that are recognized by their distinct clinical appearance include fissured tongue (Figure 1-20), median rhomboid glossitis (Figure 1-21), geographic tongue (Figure 1-22), and hairy tongue (Figure 1-23). These conditions are also discussed later in this chapter.

Sometimes the diagnostic process requires historical information in addition to the clinical findings. For example, an amalgam tattoo (focal argyrosis) can be observed as a blue-to-gray patch on the gingiva or mucosa where an amalgam restoration is or has been located (Figure 1-24). Although this condition is usually easily observed and a clinical diagnosis made, any history involving the area can still be very helpful in confirming the clinical impression. The patient in Figure 1-24 had root canal therapy and a

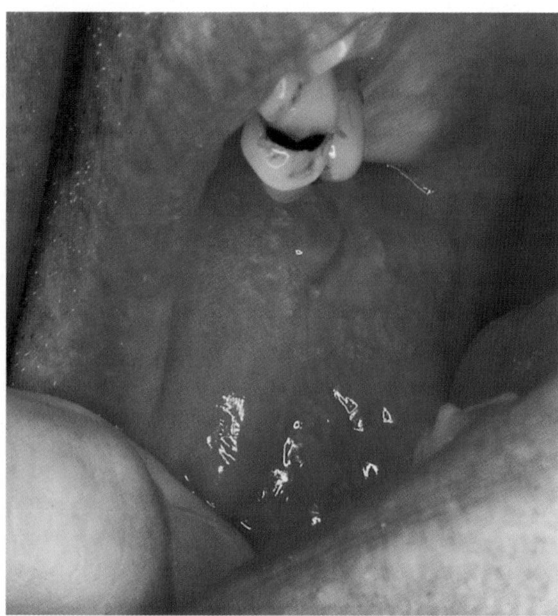

FIGURE 1-15 ■ Fordyce granules.

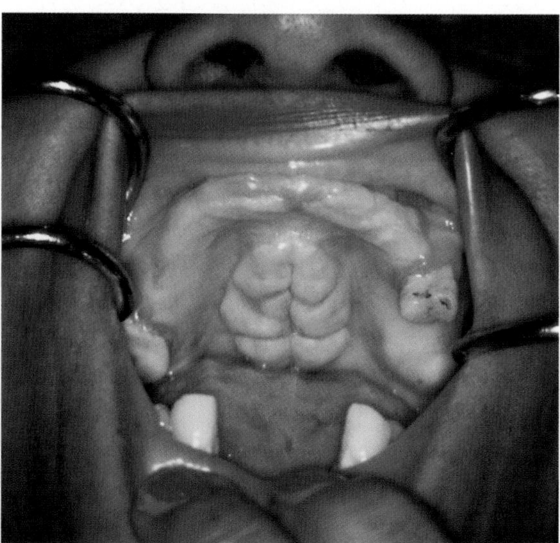

FIGURE 1-16 ■ Lobulated torus palatinus. (Courtesy Dr. Edward V. Zegarelli.)

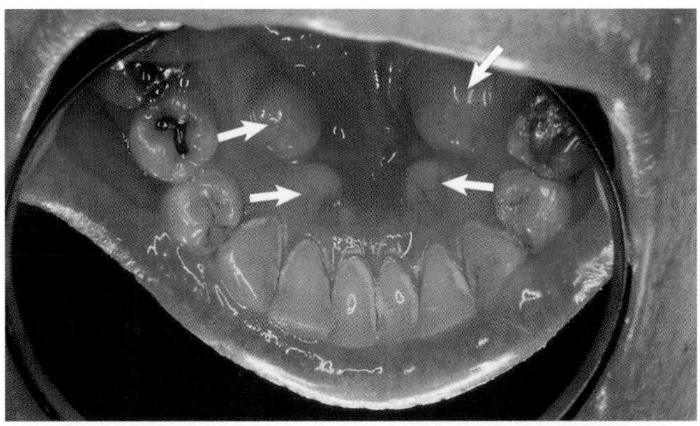

FIGURE 1-17 ■ Arrows point to mandibular tori.

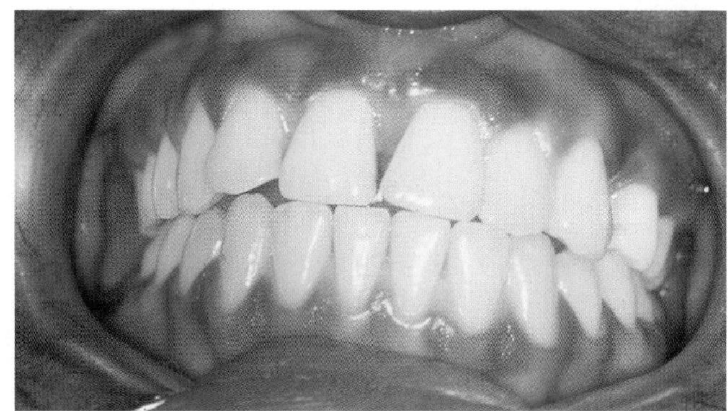

FIGURE 1-18 ■ Melanin pigmentation.

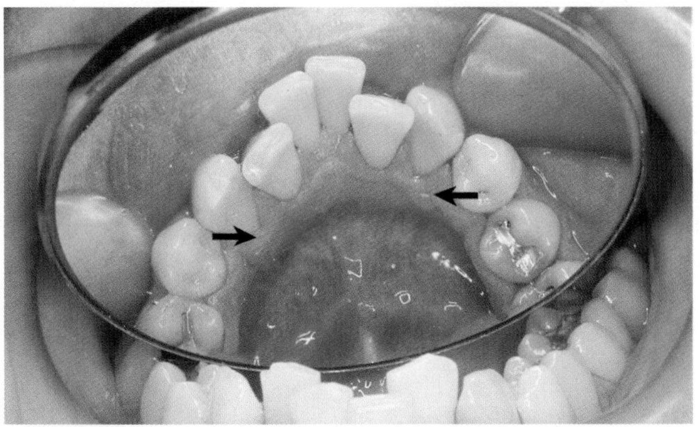

FIGURE 1-19 ■ *Arrows* point to the retrocuspid papillae on the gingival margin of the lingual aspect of the mandibular cuspids.

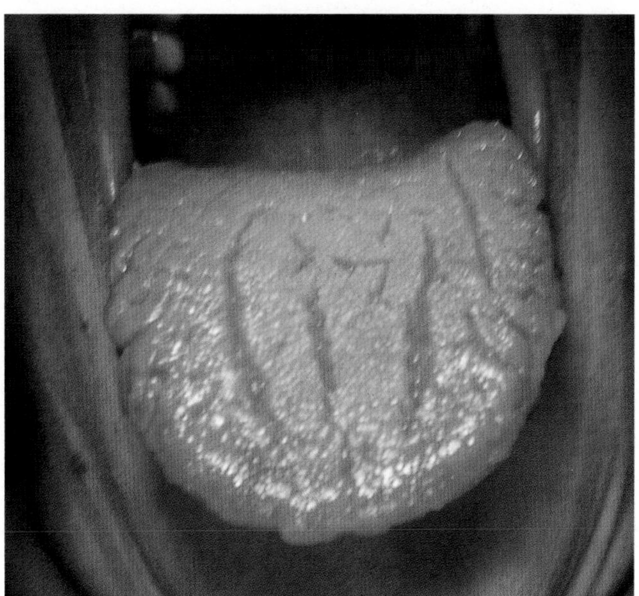

FIGURE 1-20 ■ Fissured tongue.

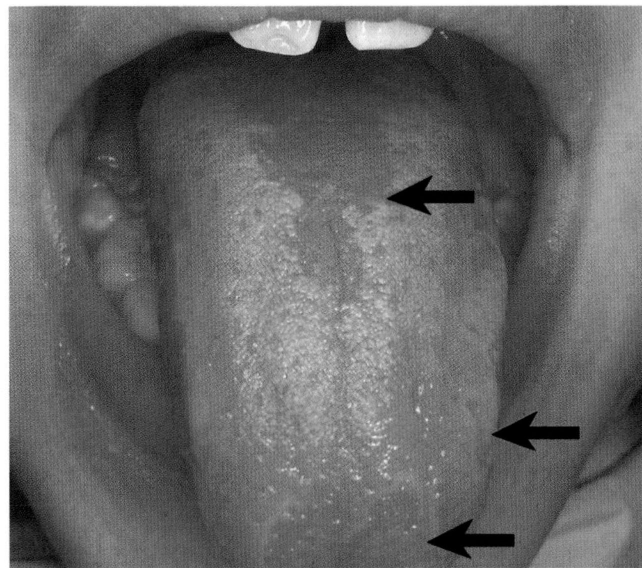

FIGURE 1-21 ■ Median rhomboid glossitis *(top arrow)* and geographic tongue *(bottom arrows).*

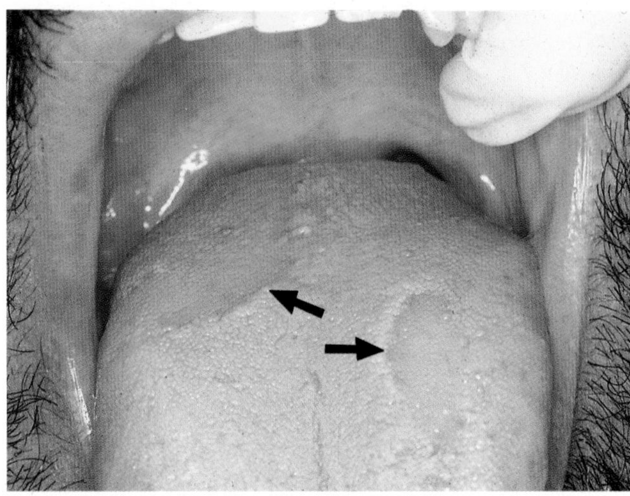

FIGURE 1-22 ■ Geographic tongue. *Arrows* point to areas of depapillation.

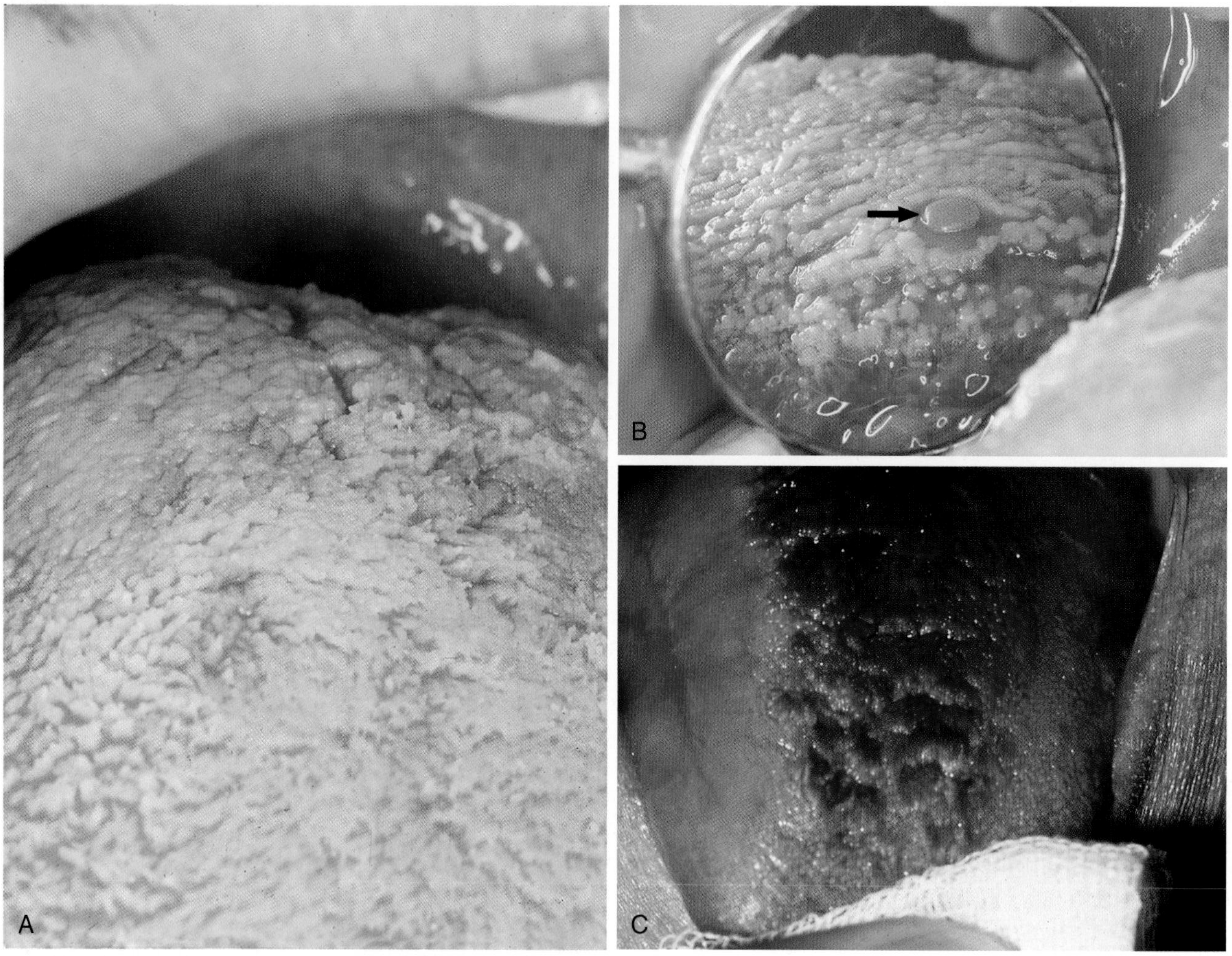

FIGURE 1-23 ■ **A,** White hairy tongue. **B,** White hairy tongue showing a circumvallate papilla *(arrow)*. **C,** Black hairy tongue.

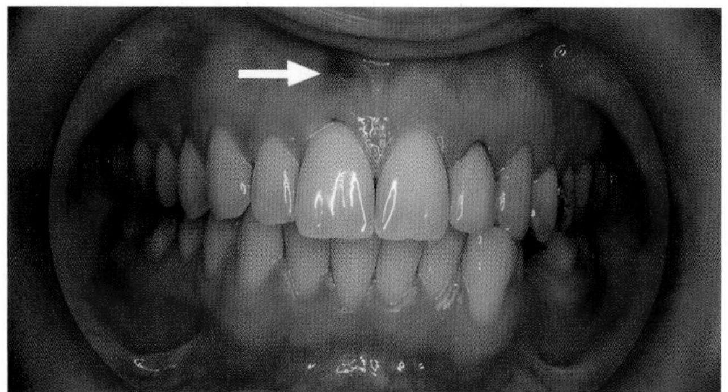

FIGURE 1-24 ■ *Arrow* points to an amalgam tattoo at the apical area of the patient's maxillary right central incisor. This patient had a root canal procedure on a deciduous tooth. No other amalgam restoration is in the area; therefore it was helpful to know the patient's past dental history to confirm this diagnosis.

retrograde amalgam on a deciduous tooth. The amalgam tattoo is observed in the apical area of the permanent central incisor; no evidence of an amalgam restoration exists in the entire anterior area. The history helped confirm the clinical diagnosis.

Radiographic Diagnosis

In a radiographic diagnosis the radiograph provides sufficient information to establish the diagnosis. Although additional clinical and historical information may contribute, the diagnosis is obtained from the radiograph. Conditions for which the radiograph provides the most significant information include periapical pathosis (Figure 1-25), internal resorption (Figure 1-26), external resorption (Figure 1-27), heavy interproximal calculus (Figure 1-28), dental caries (Figure 1-29), compound odontoma (Figure 1-30), complex odontoma (Figure 1-31), supernumerary teeth (Figure 1-32), impacted or unerupted teeth (Figure 1-33), and calcified pulp (Figure 1-34). Normal anatomic landmarks are also easily

Text continued on p. 14

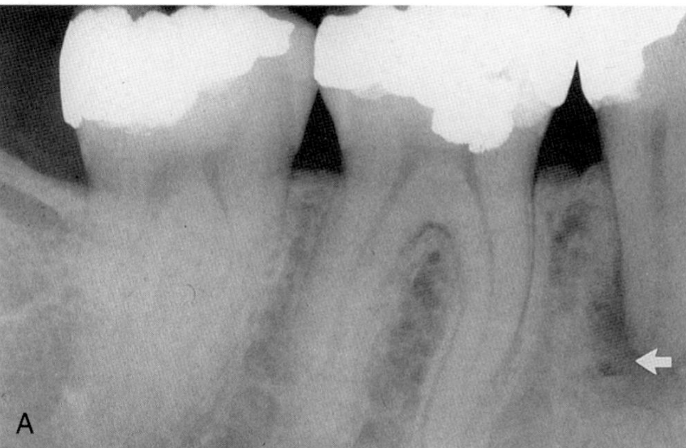

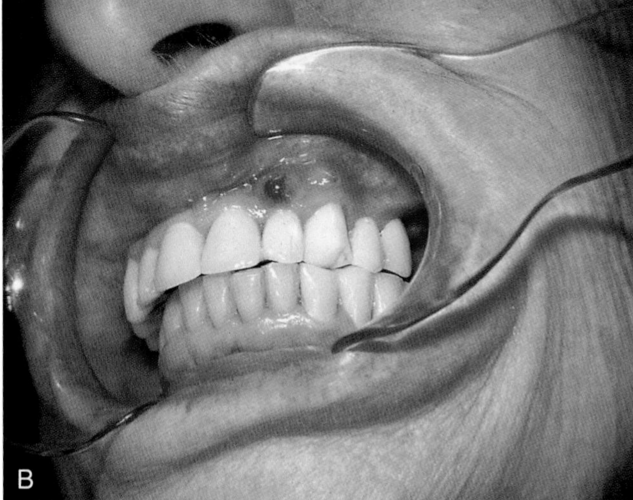

FIGURE 1-25 ■ **A,** Periapical pathosis (PAP); a radiolucency is seen at the apex of the mandibular second premolar. **B,** In another patient a fistula is seen on the maxillary lateral incisor. A fistula is usually an indication of PAP. When a fistula is observed clinically, a radiograph is necessary for diagnostic and treatment purposes.

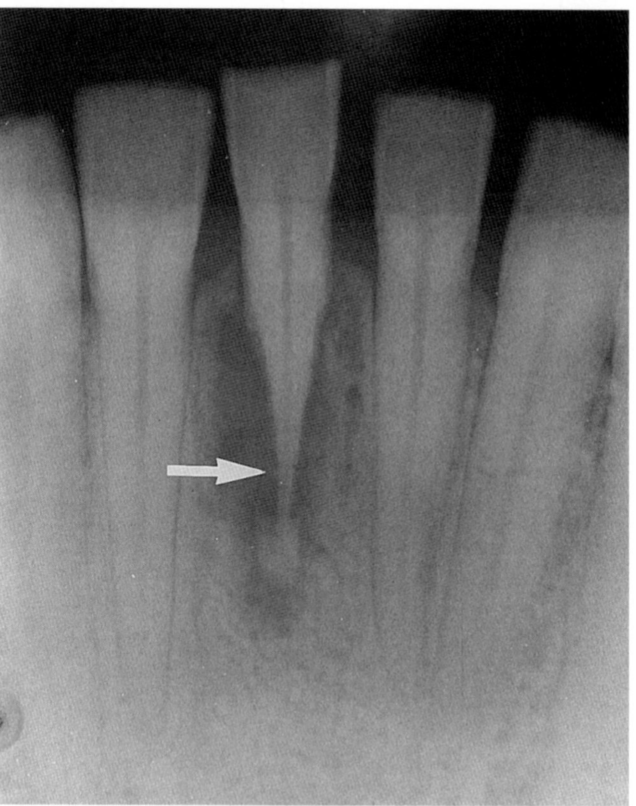

FIGURE 1-27 ■ External resorption on a mandibular central incisor. (Courtesy Dr. Gerald P. Curatola.)

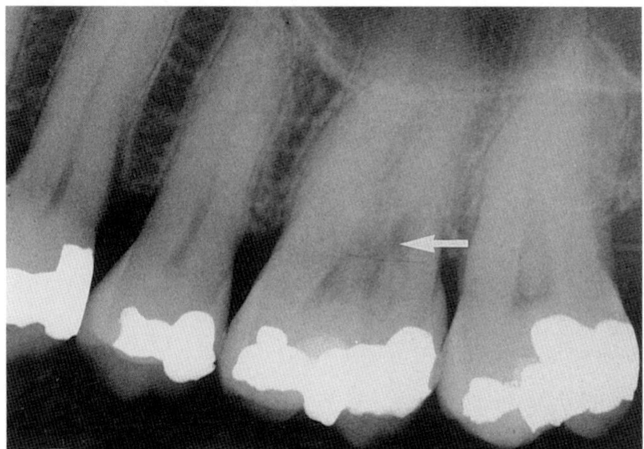

FIGURE 1-26 ■ *Arrow* points to the area of internal resorption on the maxillary first molar.

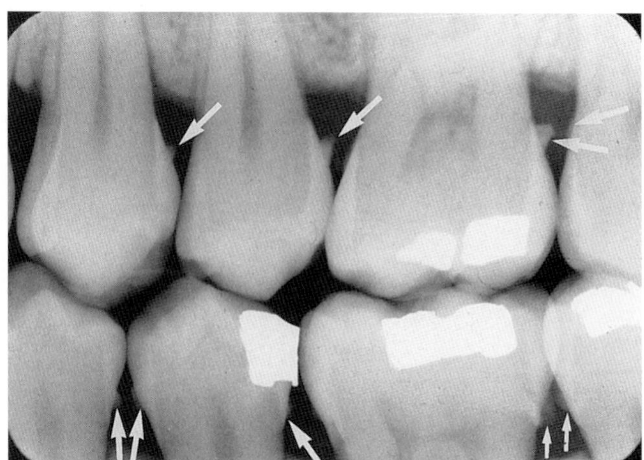

FIGURE 1-28 ■ Heavy interproximal calculus.

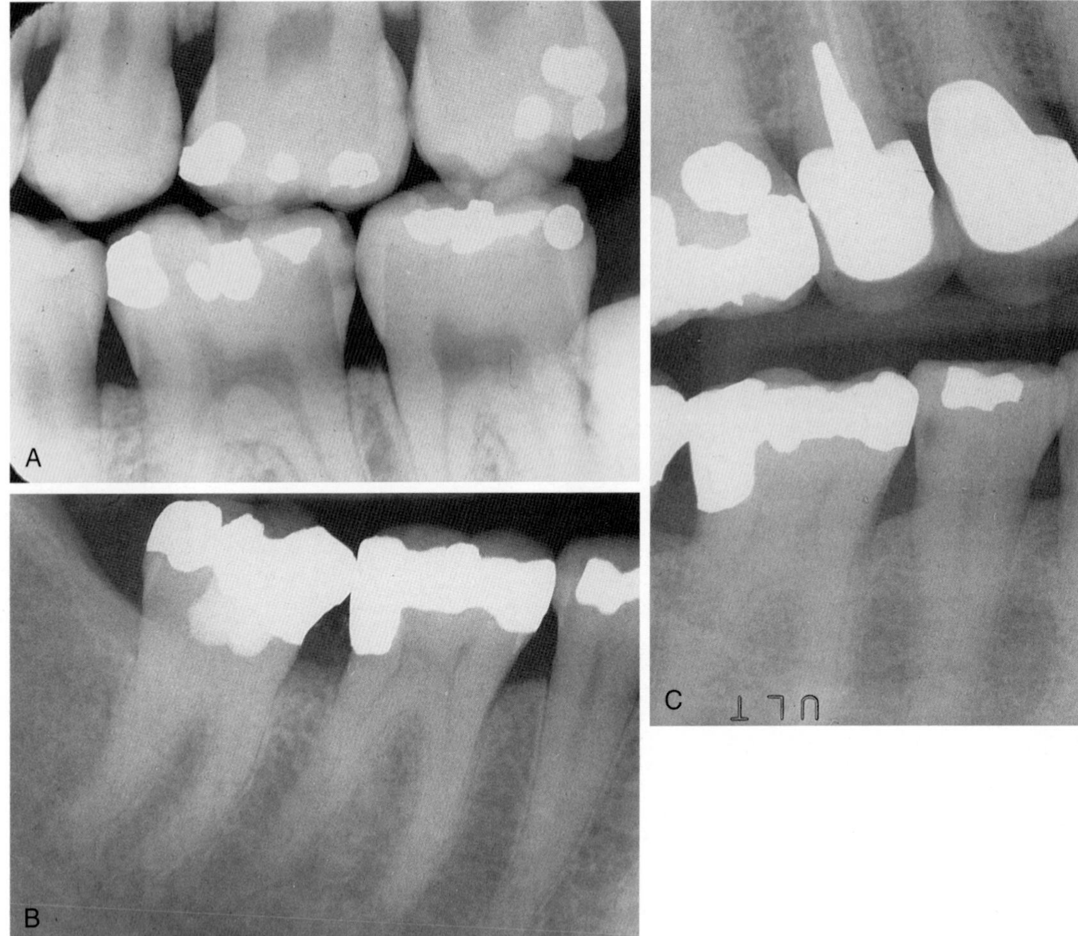

FIGURE 1-29 ■ **A,** Dental caries. The reader should observe the interproximal radiolucencies. Clinical examination is necessary to confirm the involvement of some of the areas. **B,** Periapical radiograph taken September 1989. A subtle carious area can be seen on the distal aspect of the mandibular second premolar. **C,** The patient in **B** was seen in June 1990. During the scaling procedure a defect on the distal aspect of the mandibular second premolar was detected. This vertical bitewing radiograph was taken. The reader should note the definite radiolucent, carious area on the distal aspect of the mandibular second premolar. This example emphasizes the need for careful clinical and radiographic evaluation. (**B** and **C** courtesy Dr. Victor M. Sternberg.)

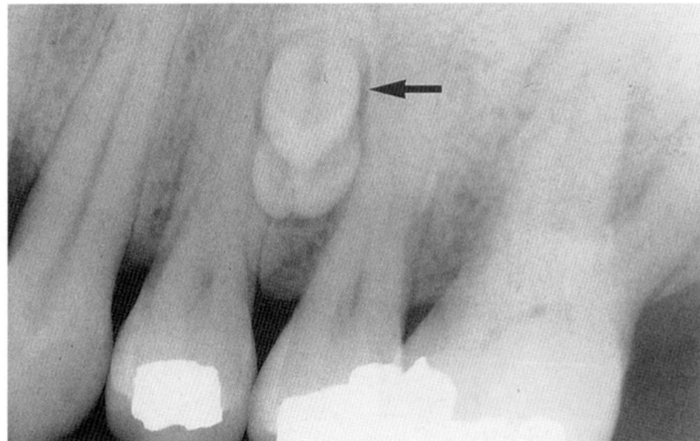

FIGURE 1-30 ■ *Arrow* points to compound odontoma.

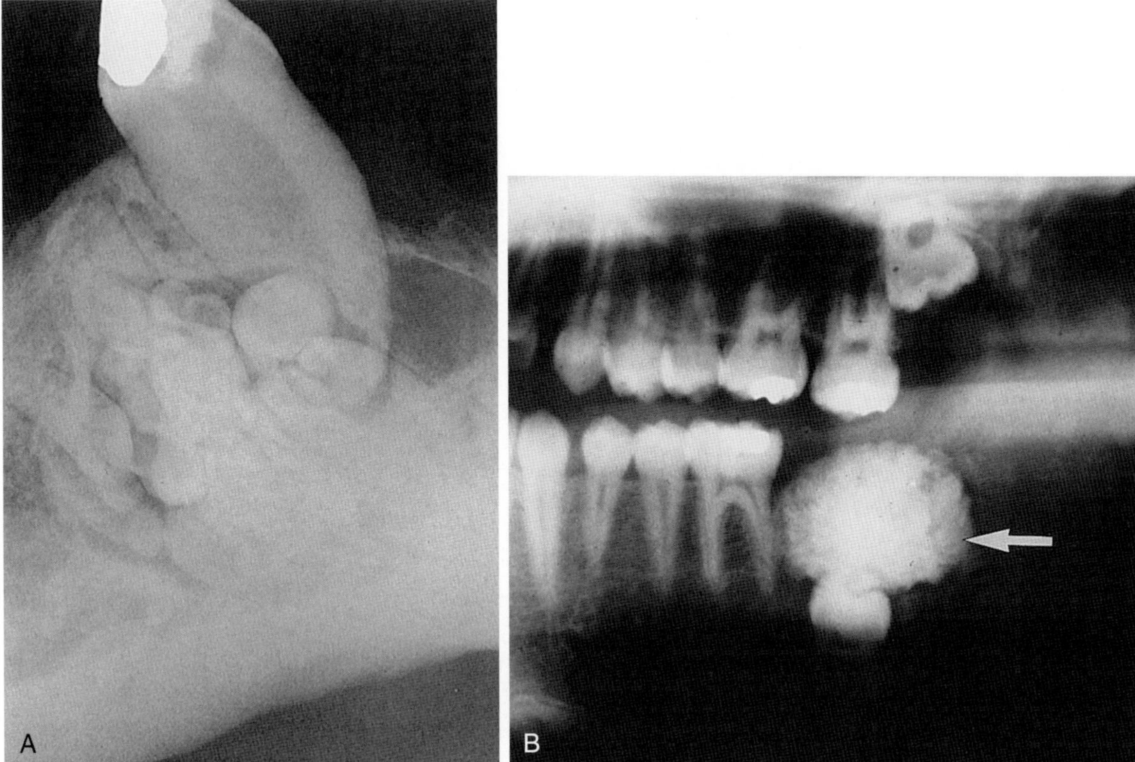

FIGURE 1-31 ■ **A,** Complex odontoma rather easily diagnosed from the radiograph alone. **B,** Complex odontoma not diagnosed from the radiograph alone. (**B** courtesy Drs. Paul Freedman and Stanley Kerpel.)

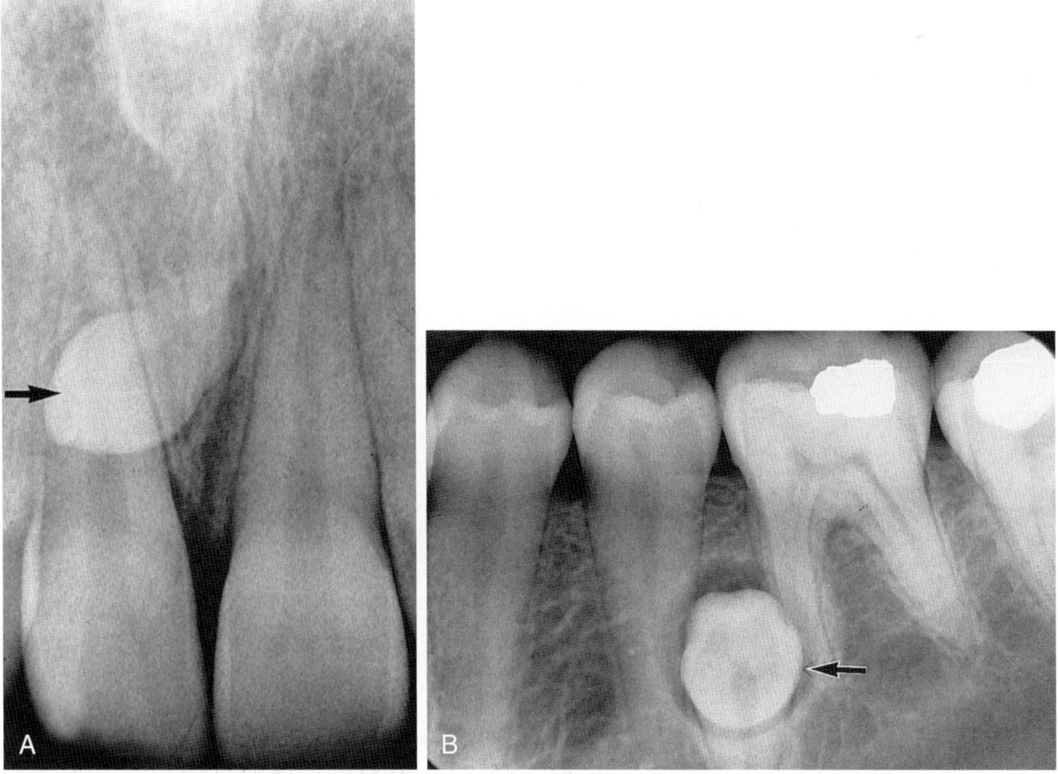

FIGURE 1-32 ■ **A,** Mesiodens. A supernumerary tooth is located between the maxillary central incisors. **B,** A radiograph showing a supernumerary mandibular premolar *(arrow)* surrounded by a radiolucent area diagnosed as a dentigerous cyst. Clinically this area was thought to be a mandibular torus (until the radiograph was taken).

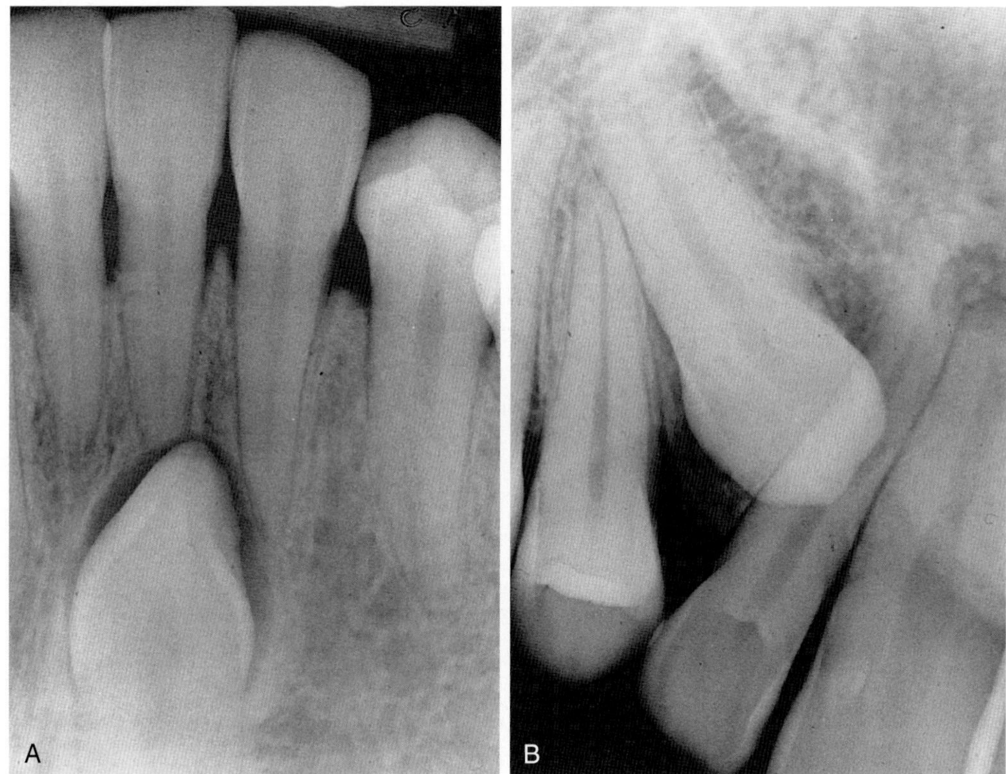

FIGURE 1-33 ■ **A,** Impacted mandibular cuspid. **B,** Impacted maxillary cuspid.

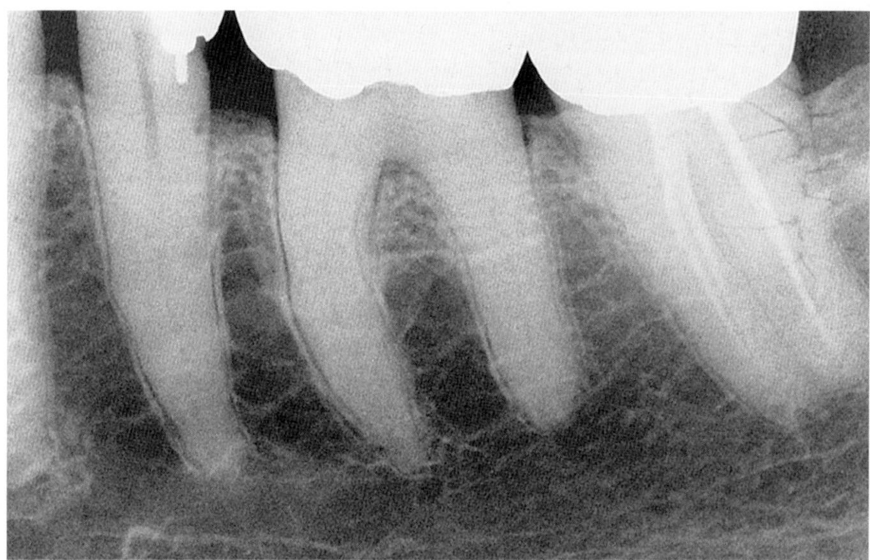

FIGURE 1-34 ■ Calcified pulp in the mandibular first molar.

observed radiographically. In some cases the radiograph may show very distinct and well-defined structures such as the nutrient canals seen in Figure 1-35, *A* and *B* and the mixed dentition seen in Figure 1-35, *C*. Unusual radiographic findings are illustrated in Figure 1-36.

Historical Diagnosis

Historical data constitute an important component in every diagnosis; occasionally when historical data are combined with observation of the clinical appearance of the lesion, the

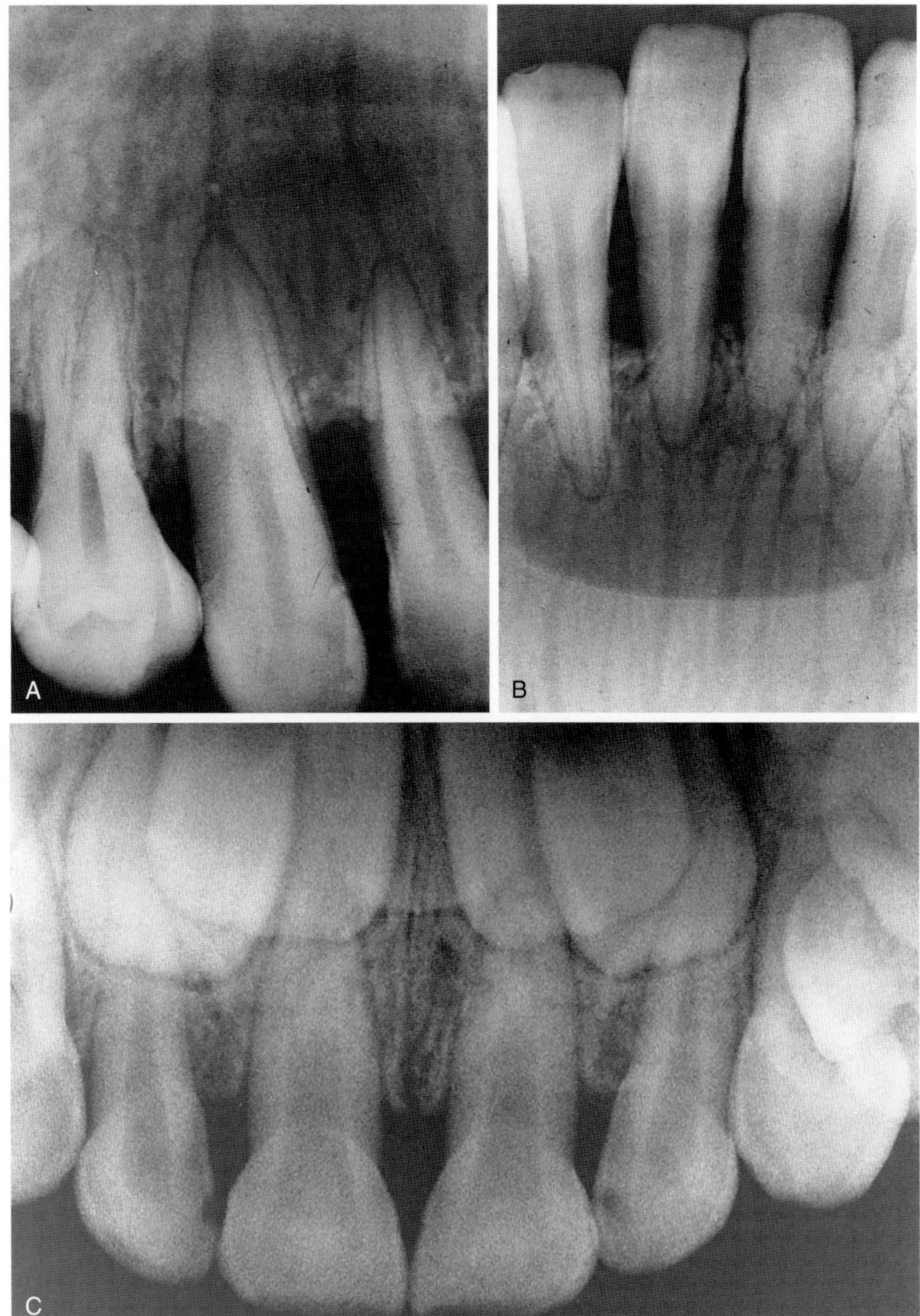

FIGURE 1-35 ■ **A,** Nutrient canals in the anterior maxillary arch. **B,** Nutrient canals in the mandibular anterior area. **C,** The mixed dentition of a 5-year-old child is observed in this radiograph.

historical information constitutes the most important contribution to the diagnostic process. Personal history, family history, past and present medical and dental histories, history of drug ingestion, and history of the presenting disease or lesion can provide information necessary for the final diagnosis. Thorough medical and dental histories must be a part of every patient's permanent record. The clinician should review these documents carefully and update them with the patient at each visit. Pathologic conditions in which the family history contributes a significant role in the diagnosis include amelogenesis imperfecta (Figure 1-37), dentinogenesis imperfecta (Figure 1-38), and many other genetic disorders. In addition,

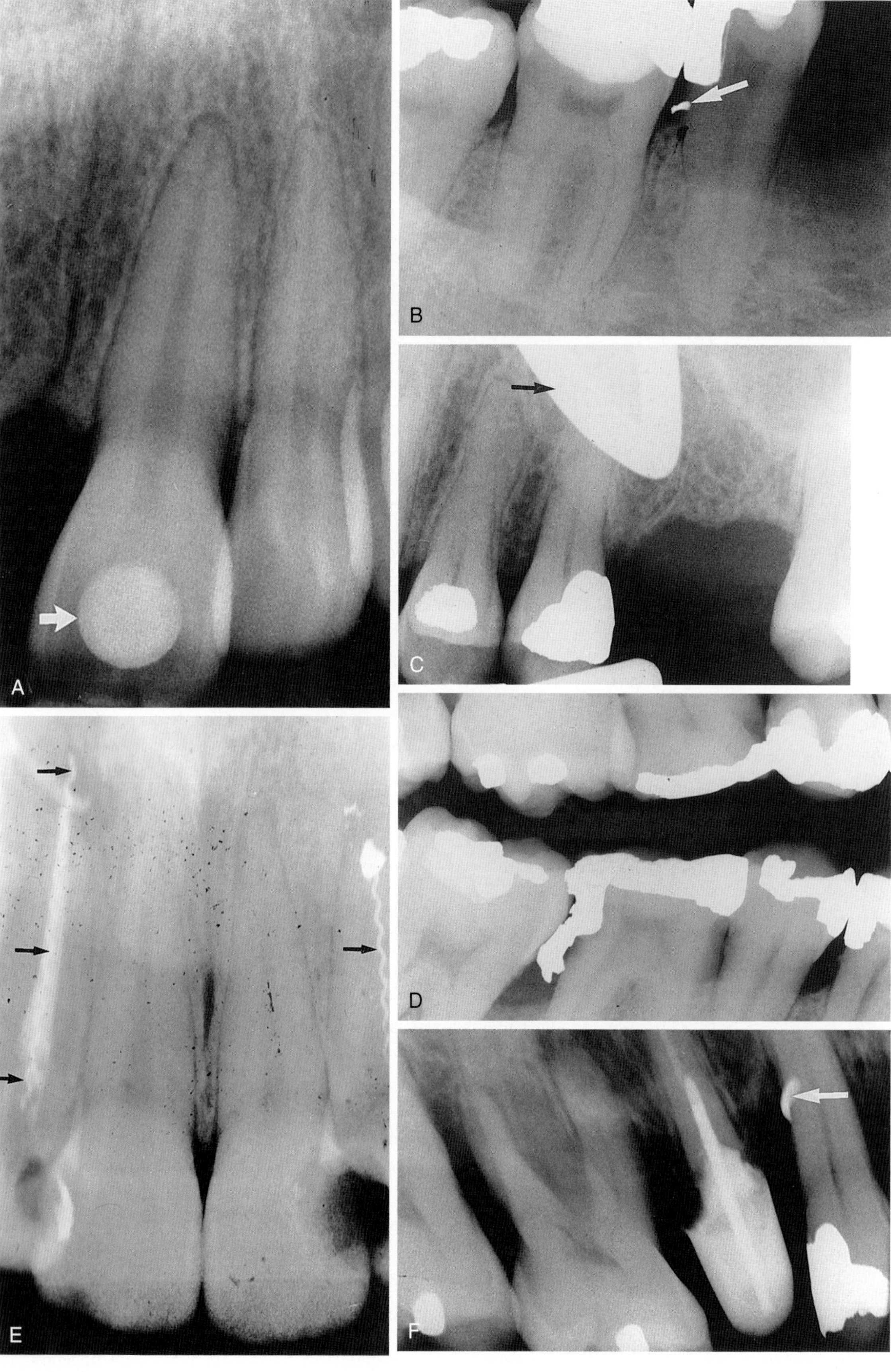
A
B
C
D
E
F

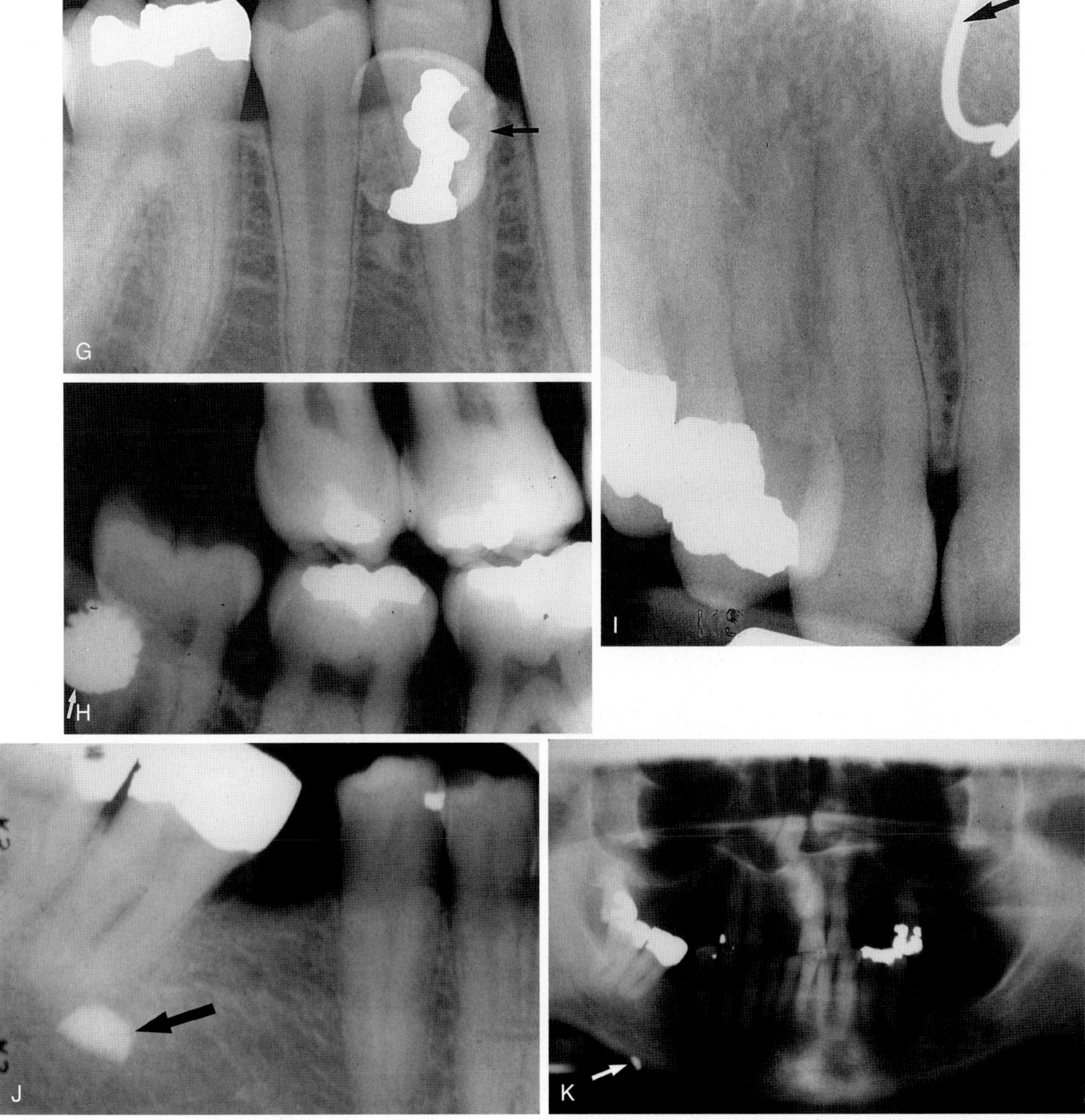

FIGURE 1-36 ■ **A,** *Arrow* points to a 7-carat cubic zirconia (a round stone) that was glued to this patient's maxillary left central incisor. **B,** The radiopaque area on the distal aspect of the mandibular second premolar *(arrow)* is an amalgam fragment. There was a subtle clinical amalgam tattoo in the interproximal papilla that was not detected or charted on initial examination, which included a full-mouth series of radiographs and incomplete scaling. When the radiographs were viewed after the patient was dismissed, the radiopaque area was thought to be the tip of a broken instrument. Further evaluation of the instruments used at that appointment ruled out the possibility of a broken instrument. When the patient returned for an additional appointment 2 weeks later, another radiograph, using the same long cone and precision Rinn instruments, was taken of the area. The radiopaque fragment remained in the exact same place. Clinically a very close look at the interproximal papilla in the area then revealed a subtle bluish-black area. The dentist surgically slit the papilla on the buccal aspect and revealed the amalgam particle. **C,** This patient wore wide-framed eyeglasses during the radiographic procedure. The arrow points to a U-shaped radiopacity from the eyeglass frame. **D,** This radiograph reveals an obvious radiopaque overhang from the amalgam restoration on the distal aspect of the mandibular first molar. **E,** Instruments from a root canal procedure were broken in these two maxillary lateral incisors *(arrows).* **F,** The broken tip of a curet *(arrow)* is observed as a radiopaque area on the distal aspect of the maxillary first premolar. **G,** *Arrow* points to a retained deciduous tooth with an amalgam restoration. **H,** *Arrow* points to a radiopaque area that identifies a retained shotgun pellet on the distal aspect of the mandibular third molar. **I,** *Arrow* points to a radiopaque circular area that is a nose ring. **J,** Periapical radiograph showing a radiopaque area at the apex of the mesial root of the mandibular second molar. This object was a retained piece of shrapnel. **K,** Panoramic radiograph of the same patient showing the same object. This radiograph gives a more accurate view of the location of the object. It was found to be in the soft tissue in the area and not within bone.

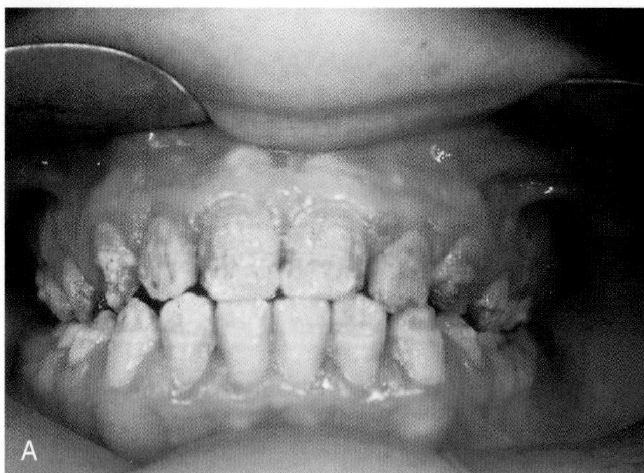

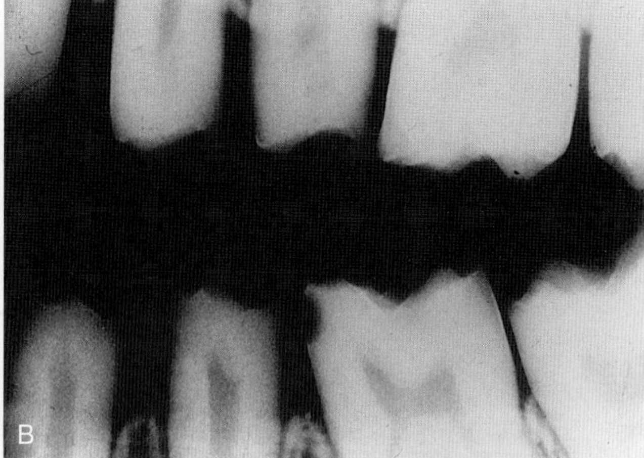

FIGURE 1-37 ■ **A,** One of the clinical appearances of amelogenesis imperfecta. **B,** The radiographic aspect of amelogenesis imperfecta. (Courtesy Dr. Edward V. Zegarelli.)

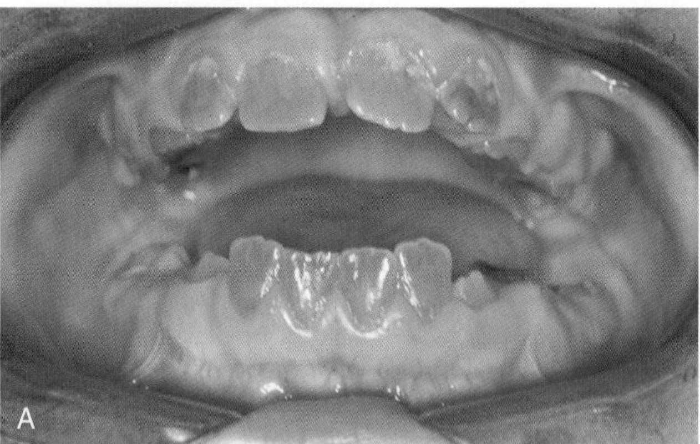

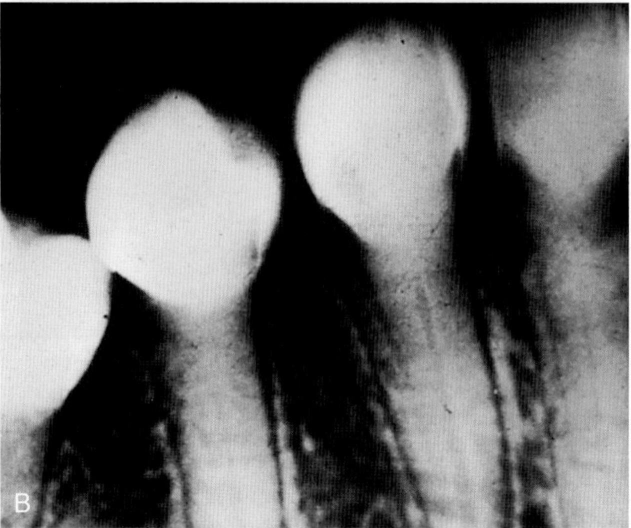

FIGURE 1-38 ■ **A,** Clinical appearance of dentinogenesis imperfecta. **B,** Radiographic appearance of dentinogenesis imperfecta. (Courtesy Dr. Edward V. Zegarelli.)

clinical findings and radiographs also provide significant assistance to the diagnostic process of these conditions.

A patient's medical or dental status, including drug history, can also contribute significant information to a diagnosis. For example, a history of ulcerative colitis may contribute to the diagnosis of oral ulcers (Figure 1-39, *A*), which could be related to this medical condition. Another example of the value of this type of information is the patient in Figure 1-39, *B*, who experienced gingival enlargement; drug history revealed that the patient was taking a calcium channel blocker.

A history of a skin graft from the hip to the ridge and mucobuccal fold area in the anterior mandible in a patient can provide significant information relevant to the diagnosis of a white- or brown-pigmented area on the mandibular anterior ridge and vestibule (Figure 1-40).

Periapical cemento-osseous dysplasia (cementoma) is another lesion in which the patient's personal history contributes significantly. It is found most frequently in black women in the third decade of life. Other characteristics of the lesion reveal that it is asymptomatic and that the teeth involved are vital (see Figure 1-19).

Laboratory Diagnosis

Clinical laboratory tests, including blood chemistries and urinalysis, can provide information that contributes to a diagnosis. An elevated serum alkaline phosphatase level is significant in the diagnosis of Paget's disease. This feature, in addition to a distinctive radiographic appearance that includes a "cotton-wool effect" (Figure 1-41) and hypercementosis, provides conclusive information for a definitive diagnosis. Laboratory cultures are also helpful in determining the diagnosis of oral infections.

Microscopic Diagnosis

Microscopic examination is of particular importance in the diagnostic process and therefore, although it is a form of laboratory diagnosis, it is discussed separately from laboratory diagnosis. The microscopic examination of the biopsy specimen taken from the lesion in question contributes significant

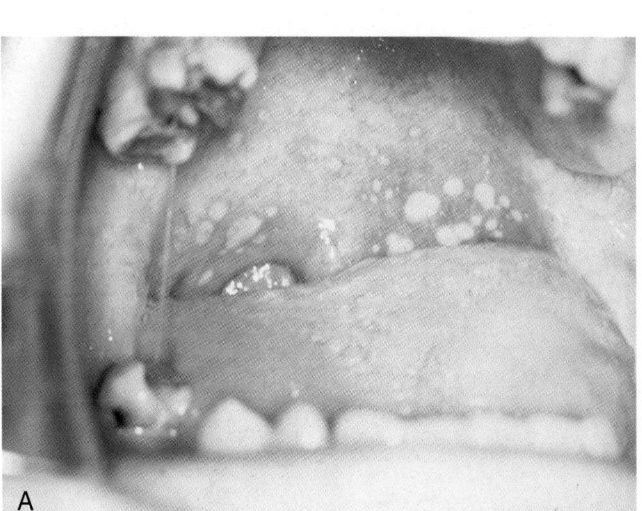

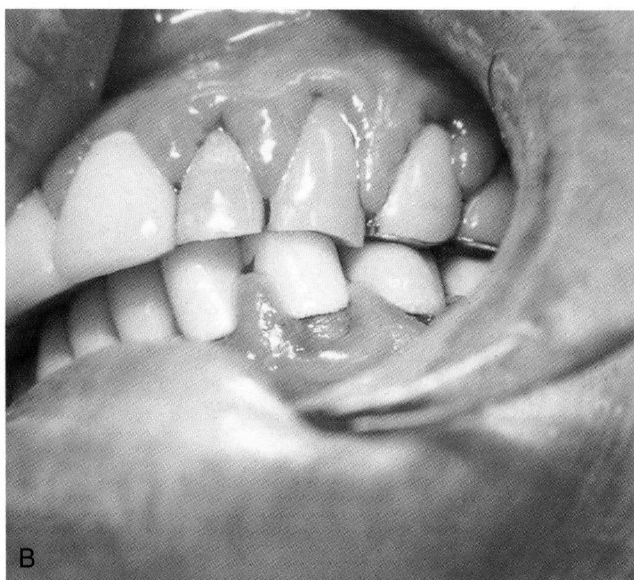

FIGURE 1-39 ■ **A,** Oral ulcers on the soft palate associated with ulcerative colitis. **B,** Gingival enlargement seen in a patient taking nifedipine, a calcium channel blocker. (**A** courtesy Dr. Edward V. Zegarelli.)

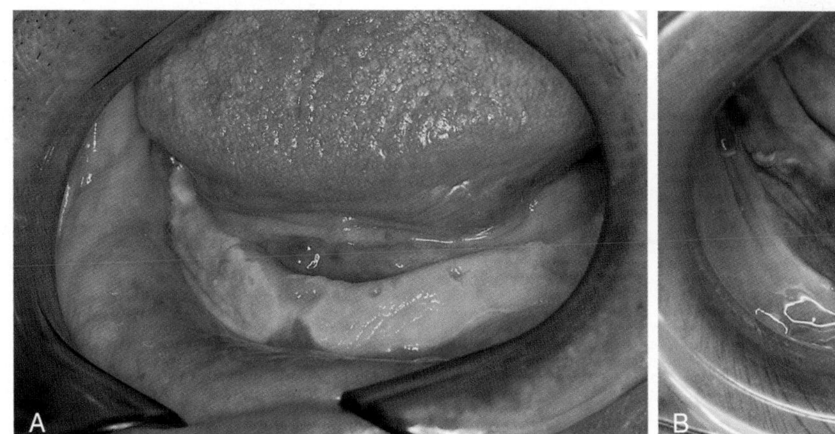

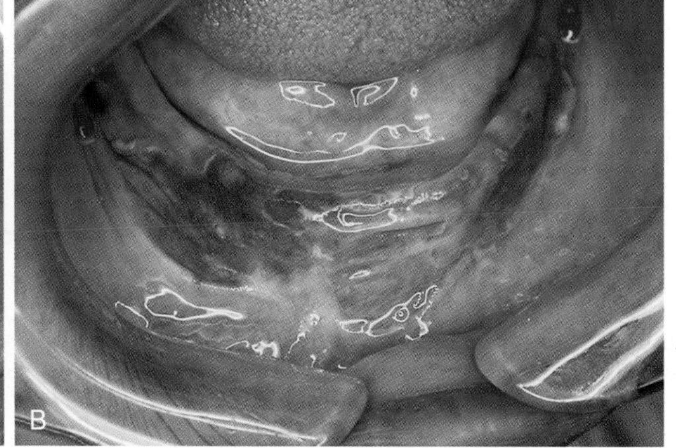

FIGURE 1-40 ■ Skin grafts performed to enhance the mandibular ridge in a white **(A)** and a black patient **(B)**. Without the patients' past medical and dental histories, it would be difficult to diagnose this anomaly of melanosis accurately.

information. This procedure is often the main component of the definitive diagnosis. However, the skill of the practitioner performing the biopsy is of equal importance. It is most important that an adequate tissue sample be removed for microscopic evaluation. If other diagnostic information such as clinical features or history of the lesion indicates the strong possibility of malignancy and the biopsy report does not concur, a second biopsy should be performed.

A procedure called the **brush test** can be used to obtain information from oral mucosal epithelium. This test was formerly referred to as a brush biopsy. This technique uses a circular brush to obtain cells from the full thickness of the epithelium, including cells from the keratin layer through the basal layer. Microscopic examination of the individual cells is used to assess whether normal, abnormal, or dysplastic cells are present. The results of this test may help determine if a scalpel biopsy is needed to establish a definitive diagnosis. Scalpel biopsy is considered the gold standard procedure used to provide the microscopic analysis that will establish the definitive diagnosis of a lesion.

A white lesion (Figure 1-42, *A*) cannot be diagnosed based on its clinical appearance alone. The microscopic appearance

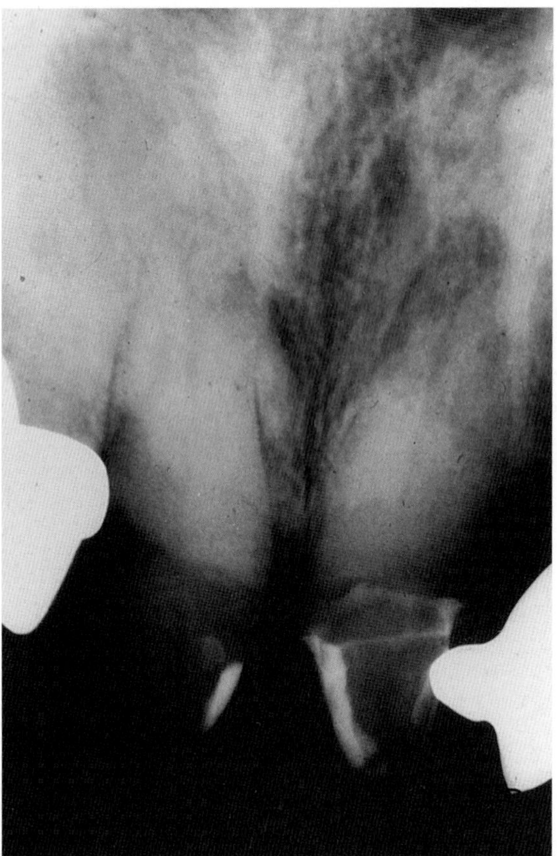

FIGURE 1-41 ■ Radiographic appearance of Paget disease, showing the traditional irregular radiopacities ("cotton-wool effect") in bone characteristic of this disease.

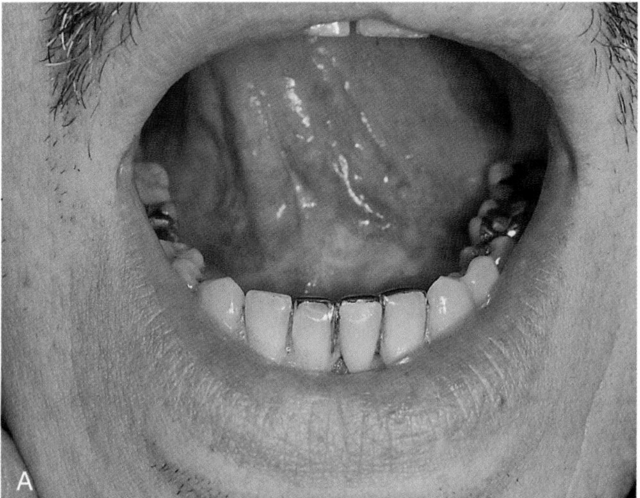

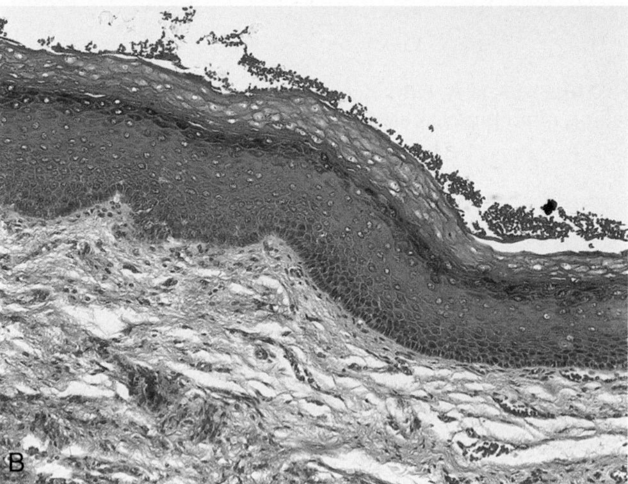

FIGURE 1-42 ■ **A,** A white lesion is seen on the anterior floor and ventral surface of the tongue. **B,** Microscopic examination of the white lesion showed a thickened keratin layer called *hyperkeratosis* and some atypical changes in the basal layer of the epithelium (mild epithelial dysplasia).

of this type of white lesion can vary from a thickening of the epithelium or surface keratin layer to epithelial dysplasia, which can be premalignant (Figure 1-42, *B*).

Surgical Diagnosis

The strength of a surgical diagnosis comes from surgical intervention. Diagnosis is made using the information gained during the surgical procedure for the traumatic bone cyst (Figure 1-43). A traumatic or simple bone cyst will appear as a radiolucency that scallops around the roots. Surgical intervention provides conclusive evidence when the lesion is opened and an empty void within the bone is found. The void usually fills with bone and heals after the surgical procedure. Lingual mandibular bone concavity, also referred to as a static bone cyst or Stafne bone cyst (Figure 1-44), is a developmental anomaly that is often bilateral. The radiolucent area is oval or eliptical in shape and is found anterior to the angle of the ramus and inferior to the mandibular canal. A CT scan would further confirm the diagnosis showing the invagination of the lingual aspect of the mandible. However, if the radiolucency is not in the classic location, surgical examination and biopsy would be necessary to confirm the diagnosis. There is no treatment necessary for lingual mandibular bone concavity.

Therapeutic Diagnosis

Nutritional deficiencies are common conditions to be diagnosed by therapeutic means. Although angular cheilitis (Figure 1-45) may be associated with a deficiency of the B-complex vitamins, it is most commonly a fungal condition and responds to topical application of an antifungal cream or ointment such as nystatin. A thorough patient history should be obtained to rule out a contributory nutritional deficiency.

Necrotizing ulcerative gingivitis (NUG) has distinct clinical features (Figure 1-46) and constitutional signs.

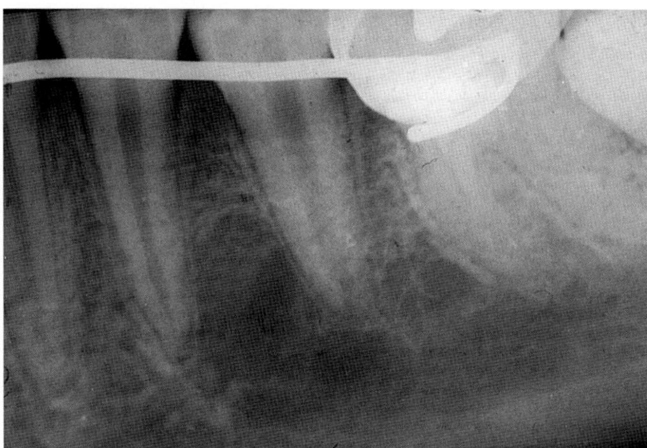

FIGURE 1-43 ■ Traumatic bone cyst. (Courtesy Dr. Edward V. Zegarelli.)

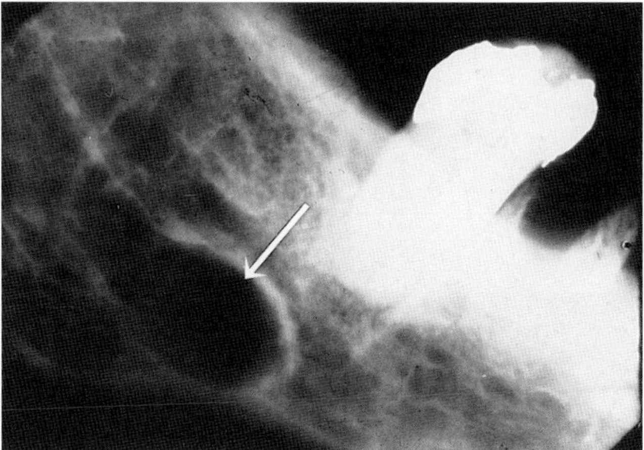

FIGURE 1-44 ■ *Arrow* points to a static (Stafne) bone cyst. (Courtesy Dr. Edward V. Zegarelli.)

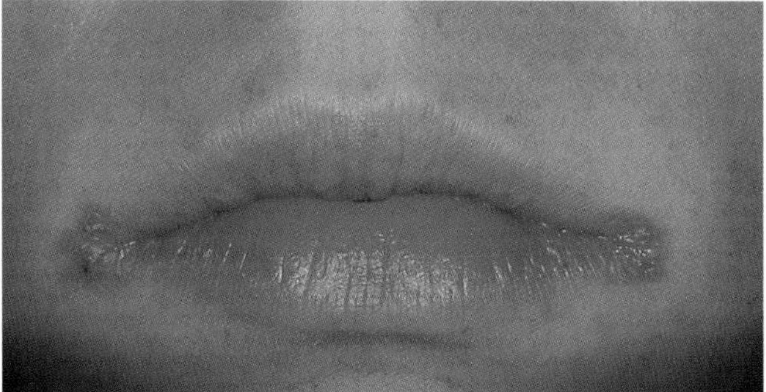

FIGURE 1-45 ■ Angular cheilitis.

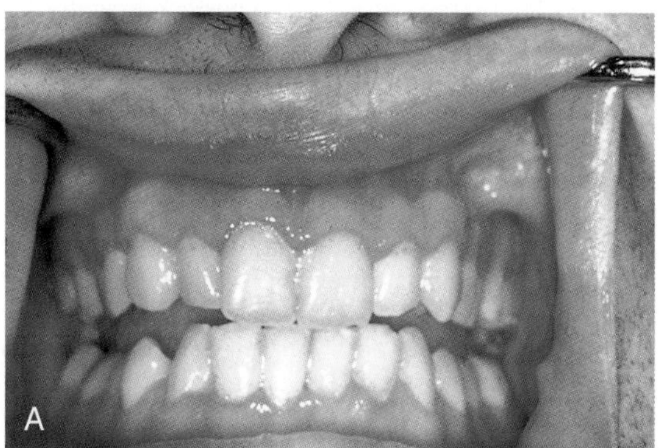

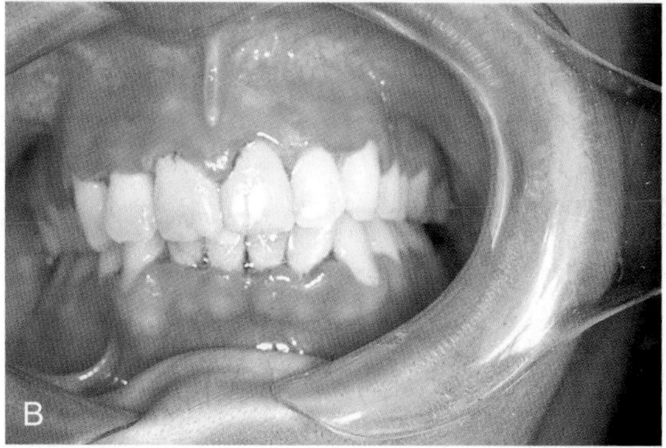

FIGURE 1-46 ■ **A,** Necrotizing ulcerative gingivitis (NUG). **B,** NUG. The clinician should note the gingival contours and punched-out, blunted papillae.

It responds to hydrogen peroxide rinses because the anaerobic bacteria that cause NUG cannot survive in an oxygenated environment. Prescribing hydrogen peroxide rinses and observing the results without culturing the bacteria applies the principle of therapeutic diagnosis because it is based solely on clinical and historical information with confirmation by the response of the condition to therapy. Antibiotic therapy can also be used in the treatment of NUG.

Differential Diagnosis

The differential diagnosis is that point in the diagnostic process when the practitioner decides which test or procedure is required to rule out the conditions originally suspected and establish the definitive or final diagnosis. All the previously discussed components are applied to the differential diagnosis. The final diagnosis emerges from a thorough evaluation of the suspected lesions (Box 1-1).

To arrive at a diagnosis, the data collection included the patient's medical and dental health histories, the history of the lesion in question, a clinical description and evaluation, and biopsy and microscopy reports. Box 1-1 illustrates the fact that arriving at a diagnosis involves a process. As stated previously, the diagnostic process can be thought of as a puzzle because the information from each diagnostic category becomes part of it. In the case presented in Box 1-1 the microscopic examination contributed most significantly

Box 1-1

Case Study

The following case study illustrates how the diagnostic processes work together and how the differential diagnosis is used.

An 11-year-old white girl came to the dental office with her mother. The mother was concerned about the interdental papilla on the child's labial aspect between the maxillary right central and lateral incisors (Figure 1-47). Nothing in the medical history explained the condition; the child had been wearing orthodontic appliances for about 1 year.

Clinically the interdental papilla was enlarged and had a papillary surface that bled easily when probed. The sessile lesion measured 5 mm cervicoincisally by 3 mm mesiodistally. No pain was felt in the area. Information pertinent to the history of the lesion was secured from the mother. The lesion had been there for about 1 year and was first noticed around the time the child began wearing braces. At times tags of the lesion or pieces of it "fell off" during brushing. The orthodontist "pulled most of it off" at one point, but it was never surgically removed or submitted for microscopic examination and seemed to grow back. Additional questioning revealed that the child had a wart on her foot within the last year. A biopsy was performed, and the tissue sample was placed in formalin and sent to an oral pathology laboratory with the following differential diagnosis:

- **Pyogenic granuloma:** The spongy inflammatory tissue was possibly caused by the mechanical irritation from the orthodontic bands, thereby causing pyogenic granuloma.
- **Papilloma:** On the basis of the papillary surface texture of the lesion, it was thought to be a papilloma.
- **Verruca vulgaris:** Because the child had a wart and could have spread the virus, verruca vulgaris was suggested. In addition, histologically a wart has lateral lipping, and it was thought that this could explain why pieces of the lesion fell off periodically during brushing. However, the surface of a verruca vulgaris is usually keratinized and therefore whiter than the lesion illustrated in Figure 1-47.

The microscopic examination revealed stratified squamous epithelium covering a core of loose and edematous fibrous connective tissue. The stroma contained numerous endothelium-lined, blood-filled capillaries and a dense infiltrate of lymphocytes, plasma cells, and neutrophils.

The definitive or final diagnosis was pyogenic granuloma.

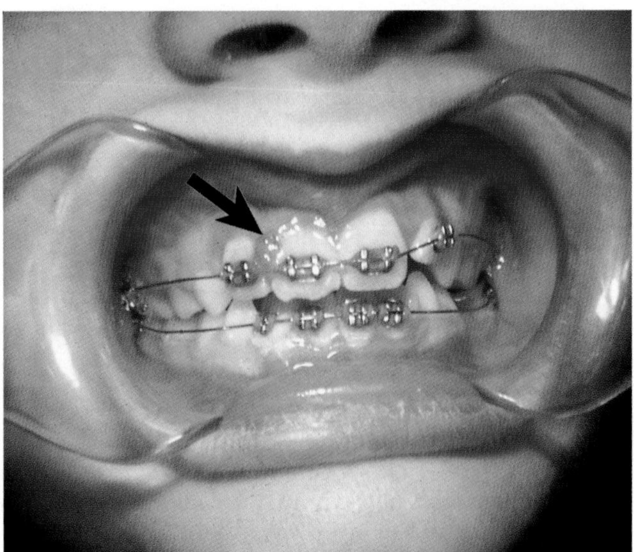

FIGURE 1-47 ■ *Arrow* points to a pyogenic granuloma between the patient's right maxillary central and lateral incisors. (Courtesy Dr. Victor M. Sternberg.)

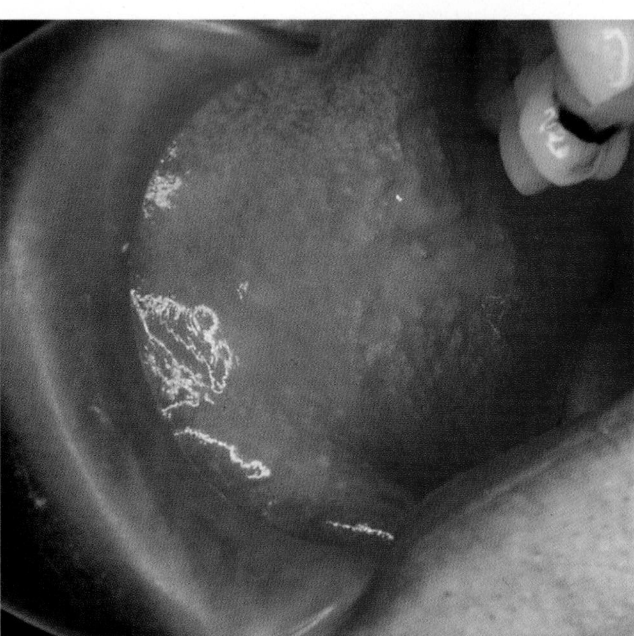

FIGURE 1-48 ■ Fordyce granules on the buccal mucosa.

to the definitive or final diagnosis. The differential diagnosis included three possible diagnoses; the biopsy and microscopic examinations provided conclusive information in the diagnostic process.

The hygienist can be effective in the preliminary evaluation of the lesion by calling it to the attention of the dentist and then gathering and preparing all the data for the clinician who will perform the biopsy. In addition, it is both challenging and stimulating to discuss diagnostic impressions with other professionals on the basis of the data available at the time.

VARIANTS OF NORMAL

FORDYCE GRANULES

Clusters of ectopic sebaceous glands are called **Fordyce granules.** They are most commonly observed on the lips and buccal mucosa. Clinically they appear as tiny yellow lobules in clusters and are usually distributed over the buccal mucosa or vermilion border of the involved lips. The surrounding tissue is normal. Because more than 80% of adults over 20 years of age have Fordyce granules, they are considered a variant of normal. Microscopically, Fordyce granules appear as normal sebaceous glands. They are asymptomatic and require no treatment (Figure 1-48).

TORUS PALATINUS

Torus palatinus or palatal torus is an exophytic growth of normal compact bone. Palatal tori are inherited and occur more frequently in women. They are asymptomatic, develop gradually, and are observed clinically in the midline of the hard palate. Palatal tori may take on various shapes and sizes, may be lobulated, and are covered by normal soft tissue. It is not unusual for the palatal torus to be traumatized, which can cause discomfort and possible ulceration on the surface of the torus. When the lesion is large, it may be seen as a radiopaque mass on the radiograph. No treatment is indicated unless the torus interferes with speech, swallowing, or a prosthetic appliance (Figure 1-49).

MANDIBULAR TORI

Outgrowths of normal dense bone found on the lingual aspect of the mandible in the area of the premolars above the mylohyoid ridge are **mandibular tori.** They are usually bilateral, often lobulated or nodular, can appear fused together, and have no predilection for either sex. Mandibular tori usually do not require treatment unless the patient needs a prosthodontic appliance (denture) and the tori interfere with proper fabrication and placement (Figure 1-50).

MELANIN PIGMENTATION

Melanin is the pigment that gives color to the skin, eyes, hair, mucosa, and gingiva. **Melanin pigmentation** of the oral mucosa or gingiva is most commonly observed in dark-skinned individuals (Figure 1-51; see Figure 1-18).

RETROCUSPID PAPILLA

A **retrocuspid papilla** is a sessile nodule on the gingival margin of the lingual aspect of the mandibular cuspids (see Figure 1-19).

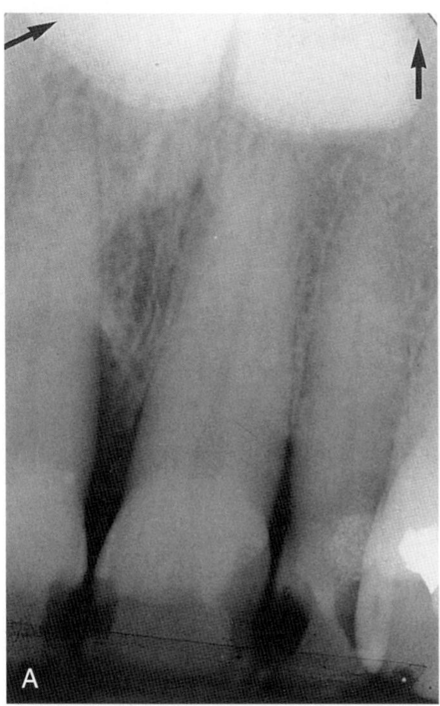

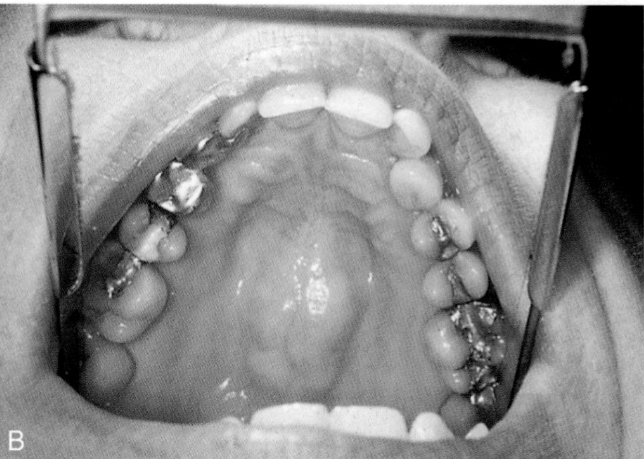

FIGURE 1-49 ■ **A,** Radiopaque appearance of torus palatinus. **B,** Clinical appearance of torus palatinus.

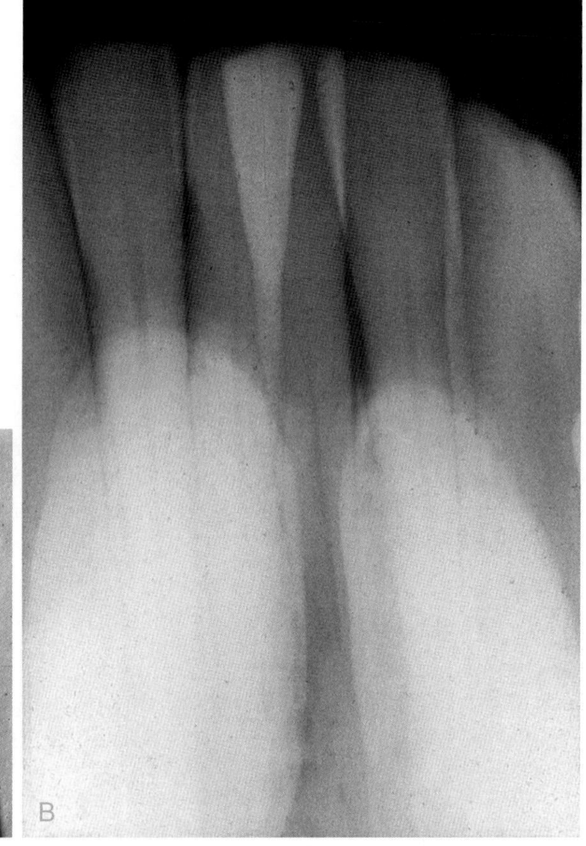

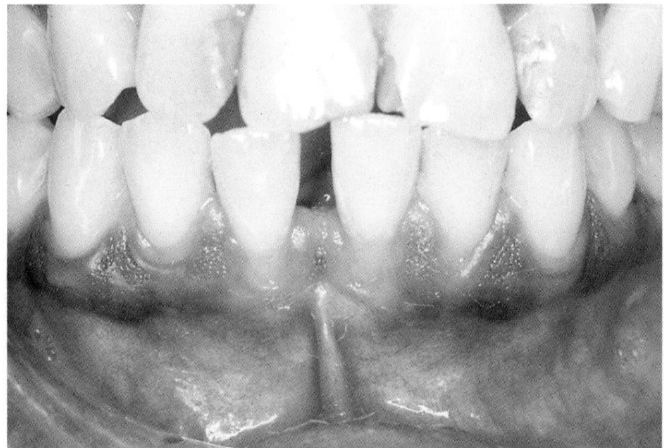

FIGURE 1-50 ■ **A,** Clinical appearance of lobulated mandibular tori. **B,** Radiopaque appearance of mandibular tori in same patient. (Courtesy Dr. Edward V. Zegarelli.)

FIGURE 1-51 ■ Melanin pigmentation of the mandibular gingiva.

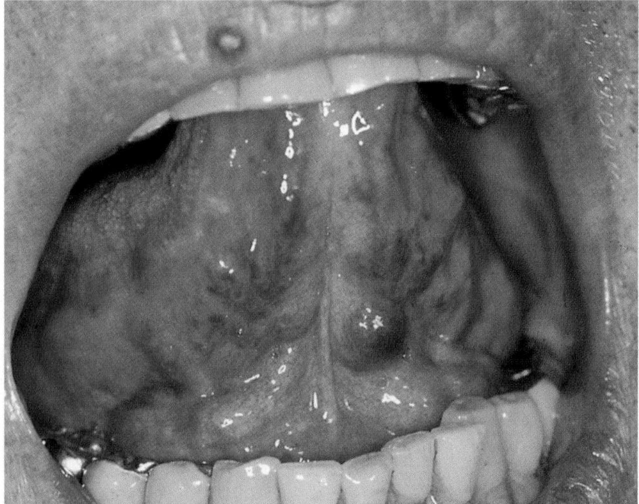

FIGURE 1-52 ■ Lingual varices. (Courtesy Dr. David Zegarelli.)

LINGUAL VARICOSITIES

Prominent lingual veins, called **lingual varicosities,** are usually observed on the ventral and lateral surfaces of the tongue. Clinically, red-to-purple enlarged vessels or clusters are seen. They are not associated with other systemic diseases; however, a relationship between varicosities in the legs and prominent lingual veins has been reported. Lingual varices are most commonly observed in individuals older than 60 years of age and therefore are thought to be related to the aging process (Figure 1-52).

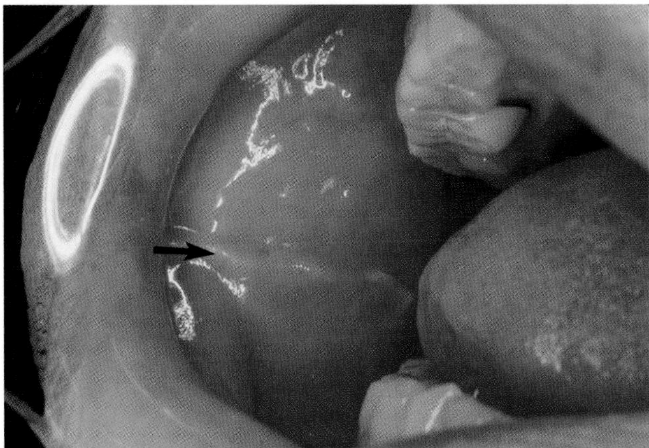

FIGURE 1-53 ■ *Arrow* points to linea alba on the buccal mucosa.

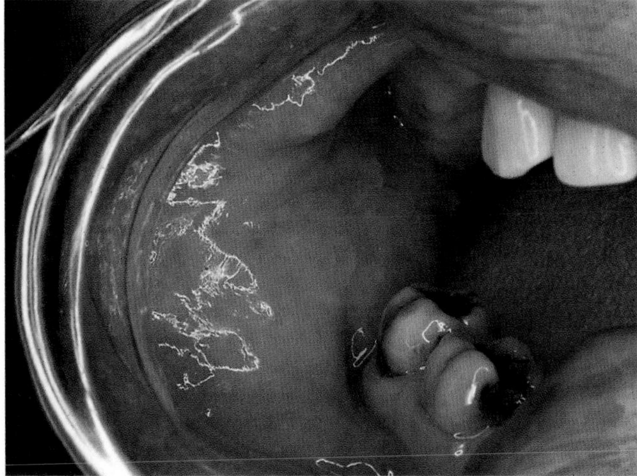

FIGURE 1-54 ■ Leukoedema of the buccal mucosa showing an opalescent, velvety texture.

LINEA ALBA

Linea alba is a "white line" that extends anteroposteriorly on the buccal mucosa along the occlusal plane. It may be bilateral and can be more prominent in patients who have a clenching or bruxing habit (Figure 1-53).

LEUKOEDEMA

A generalized opalescence is imparted to the buccal mucosa by **leukoedema.** It is most commonly observed in black adults (up to 85%), suggesting an ethnic predisposition. Leukoedema can also be seen in whites. Clinically a gray-white film is diffused throughout the buccal mucosa, giving the mucosa an opaque quality. If the mucosa is stretched, the opalescence becomes less prominent. The condition becomes more pronounced in smokers. The opalescence is an integral part of the buccal tissue and cannot be removed. Histologically significant intracellular edema in the spinous cells and acanthosis of the epithelium is seen. It is a benign anomaly that requires no treatment (Figure 1-54).

BENIGN CONDITIONS OF UNKNOWN CAUSE

LINGUAL THYROID NODULE

The thyroid gland begins to develop during the first month of fetal life and is located initially in the area of the foramen cecum on the posterior tongue. In normal development the thyroid gland descends to its normal location in the neck. When thyroid tissue either does not descend or remnants become entrapped in the tissue that makes up the tongue, a developmental anomaly called a **lingual thyroid nodule** results. Research has indicated a high predilection in females, and studies have linked the emergence of the lingual thyroid nodule with hormonal changes because it appears to be associated with puberty, pregnancy, and menopause. Clinically a lingual thyroid nodule is observed as a mass in the midline of the dorsal surface of the tongue posterior to the circumvallate papillae in the area of the foramen cecum. The lesion usually has a sessile base and is 2 to 3 cm in width. On histologic examination normal thyroid tissue is found. Treatment requires careful evaluation of the patient to determine whether the thyroid gland is present in its normal location. Surgical intervention is not always required.

MEDIAN RHOMBOID GLOSSITIS

The cause of **median rhomboid glossitis** is not clear. Research has suggested that it may be associated with a chronic fungal infection by *Candida albicans.* Clinically median rhomboid glossitis appears as a flat or slightly raised oval or rectangular erythematous area in the midline of the dorsal surface of the tongue, beginning at the junction of the anterior and middle thirds and extending posterior to the circumvallate papillae. It is devoid of filiform papillae; therefore its texture is smooth. If the remaining surface of the tongue is coated, the area appears more prominent. No specific treatment exists; however, sometimes an antifungal agent is applied, and the lesion resolves, but this is not always the case. Occasionally the condition resolves with no specific treatment at all (Figure 1-55).

GEOGRAPHIC TONGUE

The cause of **geographic tongue** (erythema migrans, benign migratory glossitis) is not clear. The familial occurrence of geographic tongue suggests that genetic factors play a role. Some investigators suggest that it is exacerbated by stress, and studies exist that associate the histologic findings with those found in psoriasis. The clinical appearance involves the dorsal and lateral borders of the tongue. Diffuse areas devoid of filiform papillae can be observed. These areas appear as erythematous patches that are surrounded by a white or yellow perimeter. The fungiform papillae appear distinct within the erythematous patch. The condition does not remain static; remission and changes in the depapillated areas appear to occur. Occasionally a patient complains of a burning discomfort associated with geographic tongue. Usually no treatment is indicated (Figure 1-56, *A*).

Ectopic geographic tongue is the term used to describe the condition when it is found on mucosal surfaces other than the tongue. In Figure 1-56, *B* it is seen in the mandibular anterior mucobuccal fold.

FISSURED TONGUE

The cause of **fissured tongue** is unknown. It is seen in about 5% of the population. Familial patterns of occurrence suggest that genetic factors are probably involved. Clinically the dorsal surface of the tongue appears to have deep fissures or grooves that may become irritated if food debris collects in them. No treatment is indicated for the condition. However, a patient with a fissured tongue may be advised to brush the tongue gently with a soft toothbrush to keep the fissures clean of debris and irritants (Figure 1-57; see Figure 1-20).

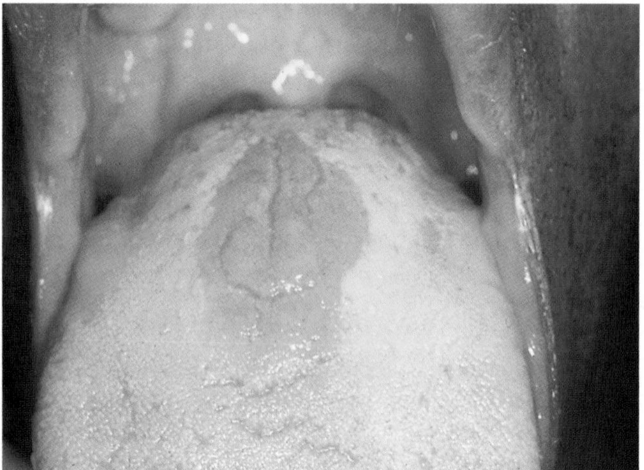

FIGURE 1-55 ■ Median rhomboid glossitis. (Courtesy Dr. Edward V. Zegarelli.)

HAIRY TONGUE

Hairy tongue is a condition in which the patient has an increased accumulation of keratin on the filiform papillae that results in a white, "hairy" appearance. This may be the result of either an increase in keratin production or a decrease in normal desquamation. Unless otherwise pigmented, the elongated filiform papillae are white (Figure 1-58). In the condition known as black hairy tongue, the papillae are a brown-to-black color because of chromogenic bacteria (Figure 1-59). Tobacco and certain foods may also discolor the papillae. Although the cause is unknown, hydrogen peroxide, alcohol, or chemical rinses have been suggested to stimulate the elongation of the filiform papillae that results in the appearance of hairy tongue.

Treatment involves directing the patient to brush the tongue gently with a toothbrush (wet with water only) to remove debris. The condition usually clears completely but may recur.

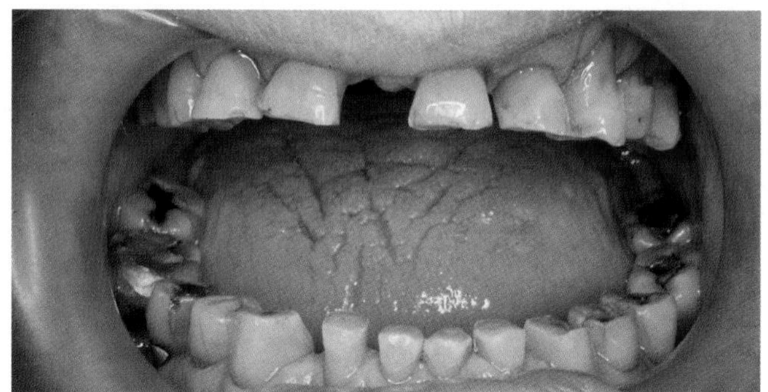

FIGURE 1-57 ■ Fissured tongue and attrition.

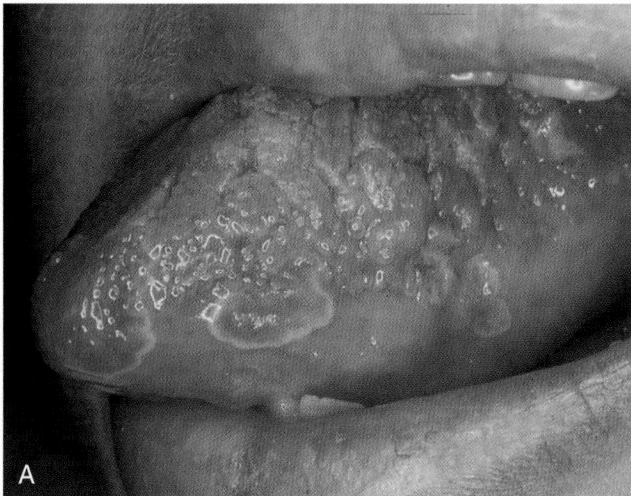

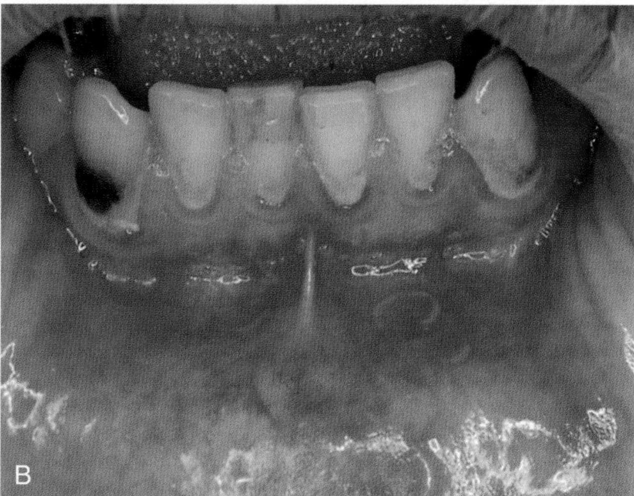

FIGURE 1-56 ■ **A,** Geographic tongue. **B,** Ectopic geographic tongue observed in the mandibular anterior mucosa.

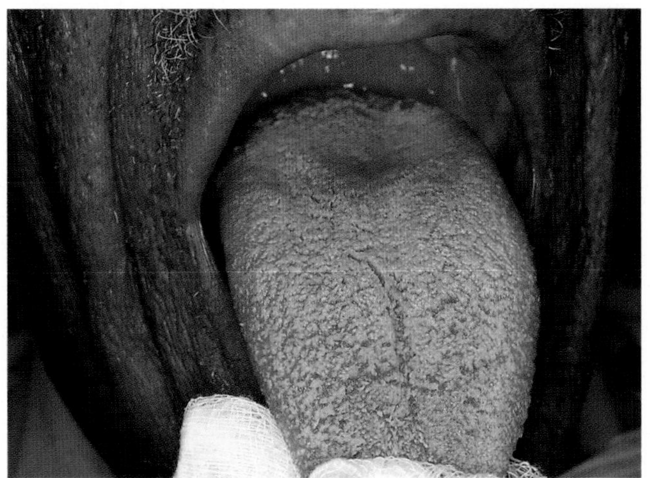

FIGURE 1-58 ■ White hairy tongue.

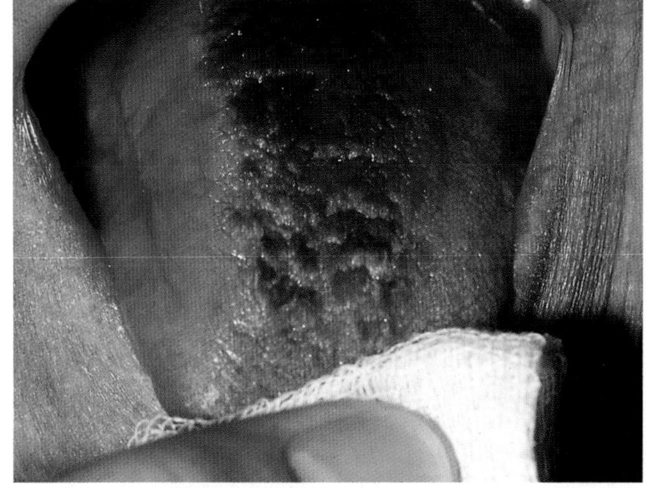

FIGURE 1-59 ■ Black hairy tongue.

Selected References

Books

Darby ML: *Mosby's comprehensive review of dental hygiene*, ed 6, St Louis, 2006, Mosby.

Neville BW et al: *Color atlas of clinical oral pathology*, Philadelphia, 1991, Lea & Febiger.

Neville BW et al: *Oral and maxillofacial pathology*, ed 3, Philadelphia, 2009, Saunders.

Regezi JA, Sciubba JJ: *Oral pathology: clinical pathologic correlations*, ed 5, St Louis, 2008, Saunders.

Stedman's Medical Dictionary for the Dental Professions, Illustrated, 1st Edition, 2007, Lippincott, Williams and Wilkins.

Journal Articles

Bouquot JE, Gundlach KKH: Odd tongues: the prevalence of common tongue lesions in 23,616 white Americans over 35 years of age, *Quintessence Int* 17:719, 1986.

Brannon RB, Pousson RR: The retrocuspid papillae: a clinical evaluation of 51 cases, *J Dent Hyg* 77:180, 2003.

Chapnick L: External root resorption: an experimental radiographic evaluation, *Oral Surg Oral Med Oral Pathol* 67:578, 1989.

Comfort M, Wu PC: The reliability of personal and family medical histories in the identification of hepatitis B carriers, *Oral Surg Oral Med Oral Pathol* 67:531, 1989.

Daley TD: Pathology of intraoral sebaceous glands, *J Oral Pathol Med* 22:241, 1993.

Ibsen OAC: Oral cancer: incidence, the diagnostic process, and screening techniques, *Dimensions Dent Hyg* 4(10):4, 2006.

Ibsen OAC: Diagnosing smoking-related lesions, *Dimensions Dent Hyg* 2(9):32-35, 2004.

Ibsen OAC: Putting the pieces together, *Dimensions Dent Hyg* 2(3):32-35, 2004.

Kalan A, Tarig M: Lingual thyroid gland: clinical evaluation and comprehensive management, *Ear Nose Throat J* 78:340, 1999.

Kaugars GE, Miller ME, Abbey LM: Odontomas, *Oral Surg Oral Med Oral Pathol* 67:2172, 1989.

Lydiatt DD, Hollins RR, Peterson GP: Multiple idiopathic root resorption: diagnostic considerations, *Oral Surg Oral Med Oral Pathol* 67:208, 1989.

McCann AL, Wesley RK: A method for describing soft tissue lesions of the oral cavity, *J Dent Hyg* 304, 1986.

Neupert EA, Wright JM: Regional odontodysplasia presenting as a soft tissue swelling, *Oral Surg Oral Med Oral Pathol* 67:193, 1989.

Pogrel MA, Cram D: Intraoral findings in patients with psoriasis with a special reference to ectopic geographic tongue (erythema circinata), *Oral Surg Oral Med Oral Pathol* 66:184, 1988.

Rosen DJ et al: Traumatic bone cyst resembling apical periodontitis, *J Periodontol* 68:1019, 1997.

Suzuki M, Sakae T: A familial study of torus palatinus and torus mandibularis, *Am J Phys Anthropol* 18:263, 1960.

REVIEW QUESTIONS

1. After arriving at a differential diagnosis, information from which one of the following categories will best establish a final or definitive diagnosis?
   A. Clinical
   B. Historical
   C. Microscopic
   D. Radiographic

2. The descriptive term that would best be used for a freckle is a:
   A. Bulla.
   B. Vesicle.
   C. Lobule.
   D. Macule.

3. Which one of the following terms describes the base of a lesion that is stalklike?
   A. Sessile
   B. Lobulated
   C. Pedunculated
   D. Macule

4. Clinical diagnosis can be used to determine the final or definitive diagnosis of all of the following *except*:
   A. Fordyce granules.
   B. Unerupted supernumerary teeth.
   C. Mandibular tori.
   D. Geographic tongue.

5. Radiographic diagnosis would contribute to the definitive diagnosis of all of the following *except:*
   A. Internal resorptions.
   B. Periapical cemento-osseous dysplasia.
   C. Odontomas.
   D. A retained deciduous tooth.

6. To determine the presence of blood dyscrasias, which one of the following would provide the most definitive information?
   A. Laboratory blood tests
   B. Bleeding during probing
   C. Pallor of the gingiva and mucosa
   D. Patient complaint of weakness

7. When an antifungal ointment or cream is used to treat suspected angular cheilitis, which one of the following diagnostic categories is being used?
   A. Clinical
   B. Therapeutic
   C. Laboratory
   D. Differential

8. Yellow clusters of ectopic sebaceous glands commonly observed on the buccal mucosa and evaluated through clinical diagnosis are most likely:
   A. Lipomas.
   B. Fibromas.
   C. Fordyce granules.
   D. Linea alba.

9. A slow-growing, bony hard exophytic growth on the midline of the hard palate is developmental and hereditary in origin. The diagnosis is determined through clinical evaluation. You suspect:
   A. Torus palatinus.
   B. Mixed tumor.
   C. Palatal cyst.
   D. Nasopalatine cyst.

10. The "white line" observed clinically on the buccal mucosa that extends from anterior to posterior along the occlusal plane is:
   A. Leukoedema.
   B. Leukoplakia.
   C. Linea alba.
   D. Lichen planus.

11. Which one of the following occurs as an erythematous area, is devoid of filiform papillae, is oval to rectangular in shape, and is on the midline of the dorsal surface of the tongue?
   A. Median rhomboid glossitis
   B. Geographic tongue
   C. Fissured tongue
   D. Lingual thyroid

12. Which one of the following diagnostic categories would the dental hygienist most easily apply to the preliminary evaluation of oral lesions?
   A. Microscopic
   B. Clinical
   C. Therapeutic
   D. Differential

13. These examples of exostoses are found on the lingual aspect of the mandible in the area of the premolars. They are benign, bony hard, and require no treatment. Radiographically they appear as radiopaque areas and are often bilateral. You suspect:
   A. Retrocuspid papilla.
   B. Lingual mandibular bone concavity.
   C. Genial tubercles.
   D. Mandibular tori.

14. Which one of the following terms is most often used when describing mandibular tori?
   A. Bullous
   B. Lobulated
   C. Sessile
   D. Pedunculated

15. Which of the following conditions is a benign anomaly, has a diffuse gray-to-white opaque appearance on the buccal mucosa, and is most commonly seen in adult black individuals?
   A. Leukoedema
   B. Linea alba
   C. Ectopic geographic tongue
   D. Lichen planus

16. A patient has the clinical signs of necrotizing ulcerative gingivitis. The hygienist has the patient begin hydrogen peroxide rinses without culturing the bacterial flora. This action applies to which one of the following diagnostic categories?
    A. Therapeutic
    B. Microscopic
    C. Clinical
    D. Final or definitive

17. A small circumscribed lesion usually less than 1 cm in diameter that is elevated and protrudes above the surface of normal surrounding tissue is called a:
    A. Bulla.
    B. Macule.
    C. Vesicle.
    D. Papule.

18. The base of a sessile lesion is:
    A. Broad and flat.
    B. Stemlike.
    C. Corrugated.
    D. Lobulated.

19. The identification of which one of the following is not determined by clinical diagnosis?
    A. Fordyce granules
    B. Tori
    C. Compound odontoma
    D. Retrocuspid papilla

20. Another term for geographic tongue is:
    A. Allergic tongue.
    B. Median rhomboid glossitis.
    C. Migratory glossitis.
    D. White hairy tongue.

21. The cause of supernumerary teeth is most likely:
    A. Genetic.
    B. Traumatic.
    C. Cystic.
    D. Systemic

22. Historical diagnosis can include the patient's:
    A. Age and sex.
    B. Family history.
    C. Medical history.
    D. All of the above.

23. Which condition is most often seen on the buccal mucosa?
    A. Melanin pigmentation
    B. Fordyce granules
    C. Nicotine stomatitis
    D. Angular cheilitis

24. Which one of the following is not considered a variant of normal?
    A. Migratory glossitis
    B. White hairy tongue
    C. Fissured tongue
    D. Hairy leukoplakia

25. Which cyst is often described as a radiolucency that scallops around the roots of the teeth involved?
    A. Stafne bone
    B. Traumatic bone
    C. Radicular
    D. Residual

CHAPTER 1 Synopsis

Condition/Disease	Cause	Age/Race/Sex	Location
Fordyce Granules	Variant of normal	Adults	Most common on the buccal mucosa and lips
Torus Palatinus	Genetic	More common in females Develops after age 13 Increased prevalence in Native Americans	Midline of palate
Mandibular Tori	Genetic	Develops after age 13	Lingual mandibular premolar area
Melanin Pigmentation	Variant of normal	Increased prevalence with increased skin pigmentation	Gingiva and oral mucosa Most prominent in dark-skinned individuals
Retrocuspid Papillae	Developmental	N/A	Lingual gingival margin of the mandibular cuspids
Lingual Varicosities	Aging process	Older adults	Most common on ventral and lateral surfaces of the tongue
Linea Alba	Clenching/bruxing habit	N/A	Buccal mucosa at occlusal plane
Leukoedema	Unknown	Black	Buccal mucosa
Lingual Thyroid Nodule	Developmental thyroid tissue entrapped in tongue	Affects women more than men	Midline of tongue posterior to circumvallate papillae in area
Median Rhomboid Glossitis	Unknown, associated with candida	Adults Rare in children	Midline of dorsal tongue
Geographic Tongue	Genetic Associated with stress Some cases associated with psoriasis	*	Dorsal and lateral borders of tongue
Hairy Tongue	Unknown Associated with smoking, peroxide rinses, alcohol	*	Dorsal midposterior tongue

N/A, Not applicable.
*Not included in text.

Clinical Features	Radiographic Features	Microscopic Features	Treatment	Diagnostic Process
Tiny, yellow lobules in clusters	N/A	Normal sebaceous gland lobules	None	Clinical
Bony hard exophytic structure	Radiopaque	Compact bone	None	Clinical
Bony hard exophytic structures	Radiopaque	Compact bone	None	Clinical
Most prominent in dark-skinned individuals Brown to gray-black pigmented mucosa	N/A	Melanin pigment in the basal cell layer of the epithelium and subjacent connective tissue	None	Clinical
Red, sessile nodule	N/A	Fibrous connective tissue with large stellate-shaped cells	None	Clinical
Red-to-purple enlarged blood vessels	N/A	Thick-walled blood vessels	None	Clinical
Anterior-posterior white line	N/A	Epithelial hyperplasia and hyperkeratosis	None	Clinical
Gray-white film that gives the mucosa an opalescent quality	N/A	Intracellular edema and acanthosis of the epithelium	None	Clinical
Exophytic mass	N/A	Normal thyroid tissue	None	Clinical
Flat or slightly raised erythematous, rectangular area anterior to the circumvallate papillae	N/A	Epithelial hyperplasia	None	Clinical
Erythematous, depapillated areas with white borders Occasional complaint of burning discomfort	N/A	Epithelial hyperplasia with tiny collections of neutrophils near the surface	None Avoid spicy foods	Clinical
Elongated filiform papillae (e.g., black, white, yellow)	N/A	N/A	Gently brush tongue without toothpaste	Clinical

chapter 2

Inflammation and Repair

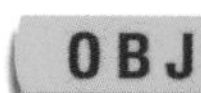

Margaret J. Fehrenbach, Joan A. Phelan

OBJECTIVES

After studying this chapter, the student will be able to:

1. Define each of the words in the vocabulary list for this chapter.
2. List the five classic signs of inflammation that occur locally at the site of inflammation.
3. List and describe three major systemic signs of inflammation.
4. List and describe the microscopic events of the inflammatory process.
5. Describe the microscopic events associated with each of the local signs of inflammation.
6. List the two types of white blood cells that are involved in acute inflammation and describe how each is involved.
7. Describe the differences between acute and chronic inflammation.
8. Define and contrast hyperplasia, hypertrophy, and atrophy.
9. Describe the microscopic events that occur during the repair of a mucosal wound.
10. Describe and contrast healing by primary intention, healing by secondary intention, and healing by tertiary intention.
11. List local and systemic factors that can impair healing.
12. Describe and contrast attrition, abrasion, and erosion.
13. Describe the pattern of erosion seen in bulimia.
14. Describe the relationship between bruxism and abrasion.
15. Describe the cause, clinical features, and treatment of each of the following: aspirin and phenol burns, electric burn, traumatic ulcer, frictional keratosis, linea alba, and nicotine stomatitis.
16. Describe the clinical features, cause (when known), treatment, and histologic appearance of each of the following: traumatic neuroma, post inflammatory melanosis, solar cheilitis, mucocele, ranula, necrotizing sialometaplasia, pyogenic granuloma, peripheral giant cell granuloma, chronic hyperplastic pulpitis, and irritation fibroma.
17. Describe the difference between a mucocele and a ranula.

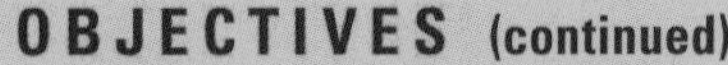

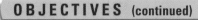

OBJECTIVES (continued)

18. Define sialolithiasis.
19. Describe the difference between acute and chronic sialadenitis.
20. Describe the clinical features, radiographic appearance, and histologic appearance of a periapical abscess, a periapical granuloma, and a periapical (radicular) cyst.
21. Describe and contrast internal and external tooth resorption.

VOCABULARY

Abscess A collection of pus that has accumulated in a cavity formed by the tissue.

Acute **(ah-kūt)** Of short duration or of short and relatively severe course.

Atrophy **(at'-ro-fe)** The decrease in size and function of a cell, tissue, organ, or whole body.

Central **(sen-'tral)** Within bone.

Chemotaxis **(ke″mo-tak'sis)** The directed movement of white blood cells to the area of injury by biochemical mediators.

Chronic **(kron'ik)** Persisting over a long time.

C-reactive protein A protein produced in the liver that becomes elevated during episodes of acute inflammation or infection.

Edema **(e-dē'mă)** Excess plasma or exudate in the interstitial space of the tissues that causes swelling.

Emigration **(em″əgra'shun)** The passage of white blood cells through the endothelium and wall of the microcirculation into the injured tissue.

Erythema **(er″ə-the'mah)** Redness of the skin or mucosa.

Exudate **(eks'u-dat)** Inflammatory fluid formed as a reaction to injury of tissues and blood vessels.

Fever **(fe'ver)** An elevation of body temperature to greater than the normal of 37° C (98.6° F).

Hyperemia **(hi″per-e'me-ah)** An excess of blood in a part of the body.

Hyperplasia **(hi″per-pla'ze-ah)** An enlargement of a tissue or organ resulting from an increase in the number of normal cells.

Hypertrophy **(hi-per'tro-fe)** An enlargement of a tissue or organ resulting from an increase in size but not in number of cells.

Inflammation **(in'flă-mā'shŭn)** A nonspecific response to injury that involves the microcirculation and its blood cells.

Local **(lo''kal)** Confined to a limited part; not general or systemic.

Lymphadenopathy **(lim-fad″ĕ-nop'ah-thē)** A condition associated with various disease processes that affect lymph nodes such that they become enlarged.

Macrophage **(mak'ro-fāj)** The second white blood cell to arrive at the site of injury; is involved in phagocytosis and also the immune response.

Margination **(mar'jĭ-nā-'shun)** A process during inflammation in which white blood cells tend to move to the periphery of the blood vessel wall.

Microcirculation **(mi″kro-sur-kūl-a'shin)** Small blood vessels, including arterioles, capillaries, and venules, all of which can be affected by local changes as the result of inflammation.

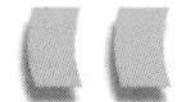

VOCABULARY (continued)

Necrosis (nĕ-kro′sis) The pathologic death of one or more cells or a portion of tissue or organ resulting from irreversible damage.

Neutrophil (nōō′tro-fil) The first white blood cell to arrive at the site of injury; the primary cell involved in acute inflammation; one of the white blood cells with a multilobed nucleus; also called a polymorphonuclear leukocyte.

Pavementing (pāv′ment-ing) Adherence of white blood cells to the walls of a blood vessel during inflammation.

Peripheral (pĕ-rif′er-al) Located away from the center; indicates that the location of a lesion is in the soft tissue surrounding a bone.

Phagocytosis (fag″o-si-tol′ĭ-sis) A process of ingestion and digestion by cells.

Leukocytosis (loo″ko-si-to′sis) A temporary increase in the number of white blood cells circulating in blood.

Purulent (pu′roo-lent) Containing or forming pus.

Regeneration (re-gen-er-a′-shun) The process by which injured tissue is replaced with tissue identical to that present before the injury.

Repair (re-pār′) The restoration of damaged or diseased tissues.

Serous (se′rus) Having a watery consistency relating to serum.

Systemic (sis-tem′ik) Pertaining to or affecting the body as a whole.

Wheal (hwēl) A localized swelling of tissue because of edema during inflammation, often accompanied by severe itching.

Inflammation, immunity, and **repair** are the body's responses to injury. Inflammation allows the human body to eliminate injurious agents, contain injuries, and begin the process of healing. This chapter begins with a description of the inflammatory response, tissue regeneration, and repair and continues with a description of oral lesions that occur in response to injury. Many of these lesions are quite common and are likely to be encountered when the dental hygienist examines the hard and soft tissues of the oral cavity. Lesions that occur as a result of destruction through activity of the immune responses are included in Chapter 3. Lesions that occur as a result of infection are included in Chapter 4.

INJURY

Injury is an alteration in the environment that causes tissue damage. Injury to oral tissues can be caused by many different factors. Physical injury can affect teeth, soft tissue, and bone. Chemical injury can occur from the application of caustic substances to oral tissues. Microorganisms can cause injury by invading oral tissues. Nutritional deficiencies can render oral tissues more susceptible to injury from other sources.

NATURAL (INNATE) DEFENSES AGAINST INJURY

The body has a number of natural or innate defenses to protect against injury. Intact skin or mucosa acts as a physical barrier to injury. Cilia and mucus in the respiratory system serve as a mechanical defense system. Stomach acid kills most of the microorganisms that are taken into the body through the mouth. Components of saliva and tears have antimicrobial activity. The flushing action of tears, saliva, urine, and diarrhea also removes foreign substances. The process of inflammation and the white blood cells that are brought to the area of injury initially through the process of inflammation are innate or inborn responses to injury.

INFLAMMATION

Inflammation is a nonspecific response to injury and occurs in the same manner, regardless of the nature of the injury. The extent and duration of the injury determine the extent and duration of the inflammatory response. The inflammatory response may be **local** and limited to the area of injury, or it may become **systemic** if the injury is extensive.

Inflammation of a specific tissue is denoted by the suffix *-itis* combined with the name of the tissue, such as in *tonsillitis, pulpitis,* and *gingivitis.*

The inflammatory response may be **acute** or **chronic**. If the injury is minimal and brief and its source is removed from the tissue, only **acute inflammation** occurs. The duration of acute inflammation is short, lasting only a few days. The tissue may return to its original state (regeneration), or repair of the tissue may begin immediately. If the inflammatory response is longer lasting, it is referred to as **chronic inflammation**. Chronic inflammation may last weeks, months, or even indefinitely. Chronic inflammation occurs if injury to the tissue continues. The inflammatory response is a dynamic process, changing continually.

Thus transitional stages exist during which the response is changing from one type of inflammation to the next and from an innate inflammatory response to an immune response (see Chapter 3). In addition, an acute inflammatory response may be superimposed over a chronic inflammatory response. Occasionally an overwhelming inflammatory response may lead to further injury. Repair of the tissue occurs only if the persistent source of injury is removed. Current research is demonstrating that chronic inflammation is a component of the pathogenesis of common disorders such as atherosclerosis, insulin resistance, colon cancer, and Alzheimer's disease. Research focused on proinflammatory markers such as C-reactive protein is attempting to determine the link between chronic inflammation and a number of seemingly unrelated degenerative disorders.

MICROSCOPIC EVENTS AND CLINICAL SIGNS OF INFLAMMATION

Microscopic events occur within the injured tissues during both acute and chronic inflammation. These events cause changes that can be observed clinically. The local clinical changes at the site of injury are called the five classic (cardinal) signs of inflammation: redness, heat, swelling, pain, and loss of normal tissue function (Table 2-1). Systemic signs of inflammation may be present when the response is more extensive; these signs are discussed later in this chapter.

The microscopic events of inflammation involve the small blood vessels or **microcirculation** (arterioles, capillaries, and venules) in the area of injury, red blood cells, white blood cells, and chemicals in the body called biochemical mediators (Figure 2-1). Normally, blood and the cells it contains flow through the microcirculation. Exchange of oxygen and nutrients needed for the health of the surrounding tissue occurs as plasma passes between the endothelium lining the vessel walls of the arterioles and capillaries. Plasma is the fluid component of blood in which the blood cells are suspended; it is composed mainly of water and proteins. Normally most of the plasma that leaves the microcirculation reenters the circulation through the venules. The lymphatic vessels carry away any excess plasma that does not reenter the blood vessels.

In inflammation the underlying microscopic events proceed faster than the visible clinical changes. The sequence of microscopic events that occur during the inflammatory response is as follows:

Table 2-1

Local and systemic clinical signs of inflammation and associated microscopic events

Clinical Feature	Associated Microscopic Events
Localized Signs of Inflammation	
Redness (erythema) and heat	Hyperemia resulting from dilation of microcirculation
Swelling	Permeability of microcirculation leads to exudate formation in the tissues
Pain	Pressure on nerves by exudate formation and release of biochemical mediators
Loss of normal tissue function	Events associated with swelling and pain
Systemic Signs of Inflammation	
Fever	Production of pyrogens affects the hypothalamus, which influences body temperature
Leukocytosis	An increase in the number of white blood cells circulating in blood
Elevated C-reactive protein	A protein produced in the liver and elevated in circulating blood when inflammation is present somewhere in the body
Lymphadenopathy	Hyperplasia and hypertrophy of lymphocytes

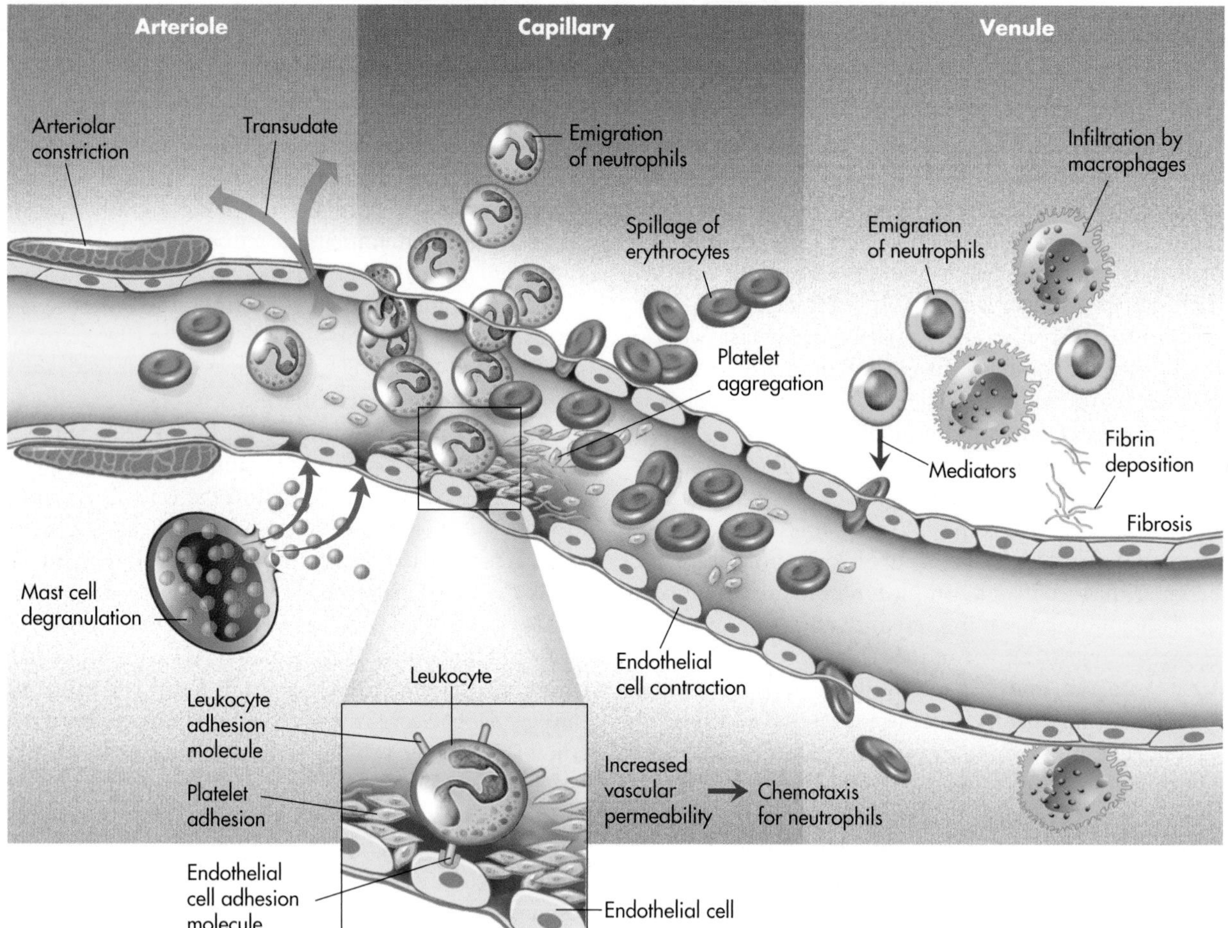

FIGURE 2-1 ■ Microscopic events during inflammation. (From McCance K, Huether S: *Pathophysiology,* ed 5, St Louis, 2005, Mosby Elsevier).

1. Injury to tissue
2. Constriction of the microcirculation
3. Dilation of the microcirculation
4. Increase in permeability of the microcirculation
5. Exudate leaving the microcirculation
6. Increase in blood viscosity in the microcirculation
7. Decrease in blood flow through the microcirculation
8. Margination and pavementing of white blood cells
9. Emigration of white blood cells from the microcirculation
10. Phagocytosis by white blood cells of foreign substances

The first microscopic event of the inflammatory response is a brief, immediate reflex constriction of the microcirculation in the area of the injury. This is followed, within seconds, by a dilation of the same small blood vessels. Dilation is an increase in the diameter of the vessels and is caused by biochemical mediators that are released at the time of the injury. Dilation of the microcirculation results in increased blood flow through the vessels. The increased blood flow that fills the capillary beds in the injured tissue is called **hyperemia.** Hyperemia is responsible for two clinical signs of inflammation: redness (**erythema**) and heat. Erythema is easily visible in most inflamed orofacial tissues. Local temperature changes may be more difficult to recognize.

While hyperemia is occurring, the permeability of the vessels of the microcirculation also increases. As a result, plasma flows into the injured tissues as a fluid that is called an **exudate.** Two main types of exudate are (1) serous and (2) purulent. **Serous** exudate is composed mainly of plasma with just a few white blood cells. **Purulent** exudate (suppuration) contains tissue debris and many white blood cells in addition to the plasma. The presence of exudate in the injured tissue helps to dilute injurious agents that may be present and carry injurious agents through the lymphatic vessels to the lymph nodes.

As the exudate escapes into the tissue, excess plasma collects in the interstitial space. This excess plasma in the interstitial space is called **edema** and results in localized enlargement or swelling of the tissue, another clinical sign of inflammation (Figure 2-2). If the swollen tissue area is injured further, the exudate flows out of the tissue as either a

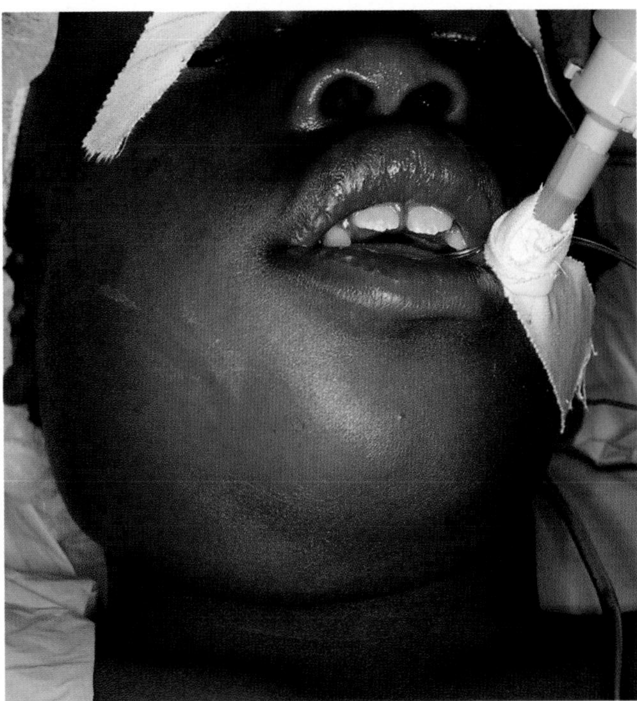

FIGURE 2-2 ■ Swelling caused by increased local edema associated with a dental infection. The patient was hospitalized for treatment of the swelling. (Courtesy Dr. Sidney Eisig.)

thin, clear fluid (serous exudate) or a thick, white-to-yellow pus (purulent exudate). An **abscess** is a collection of pus that has accumulated in a cavity formed by the tissue.

The formation of exudate may be so excessive that it interferes with repair of the tissue. The injured tissue may allow the excess exudate to drain by formation of a drainage passage that bores through the tissue, allowing drainage to the outside. This channel through the tissue is called a **fistula** (Figure 2-3); it is formed at the expense of healthy, functioning tissue in the area that is lost as the tissue becomes necrotic. Sometimes excessive exudate in damaged tissue has to be drained mechanically by making an incision in the surface of the swollen area and often placing a drainage tube in the site of the incision. This procedure is called incision and drainage and is usually accompanied by the administration of an antibiotic to treat infection and medication to reduce inflammation (Figure 2-4).

Exudate formation also results in another clinical sign of inflammation, pain, as the exudate presses on sensory nerves in the area. Some biochemical mediators present in inflamed tissue can also cause pain. The swelling and pain in tissue resulting from the inflammatory process may then cause a loss of normal tissue function, another clinical sign of inflammation.

In addition to exudate formation, blood vessel permeability leads to increased blood viscosity within the vessels because of the loss of plasma. The blood becomes thicker and cannot flow as easily. This eventually results in decreased flow through the microcirculation. As the blood flow slows down, the red blood cells begin to pile up in the center of the blood vessels, and the white blood cells are displaced to the periphery of the blood vessels. This movement of the white blood cells to the periphery is called **margination**. The white blood cells are now in position to adhere themselves to the inner walls of the injured blood vessels that have become "sticky" because of specific factors on the surfaces of the cells. This lining of the walls by white blood cells is called **pavementing** (Figure 2-5).

After pavementing the vessel walls, the white blood cells begin to escape from the blood vessels along with the plasma and enter the injured tissue. This process by which the white blood cells escape from the blood vessels is called **emigration**. Emigration occurs as a result of opening of the cellular junctions of the endothelium lining the blood vessels as its cells retract in size because of biochemical mediators.

This directed movement of white blood cells toward the site of the injury is called **chemotaxis**; biochemical mediators that enhance this directed movement are called chemotactic factors. Emigration and chemotaxis of the white blood cells to the area of injury allow these cells to be mobilized in the body's defense against the injury.

At first these cells try to wall off the site of the injury from the surrounding healthy tissue. Later in the injured tissue, the white blood cells also try to remove foreign substances from the site by ingesting and then digesting them. This is called **phagocytosis** (Figure 2-6). The foreign substances may include pathogenic microorganisms or tissue debris. The presence of these substances interferes with the repair process; therefore they must be removed for the inflammation to resolve and any necessary tissue repair to proceed.

WHITE BLOOD CELLS AND THEIR INVOLVEMENT IN THE INFLAMMATORY RESPONSE

Emigration of white blood cells (leukocytes) from the blood vessels into the site of injury and subsequent chemotaxis and phagocytosis are important components of the process of inflammation. Two types of white blood cells are involved initially in the inflammatory response: the **neutrophil** and the monocyte circulating in blood that becomes the **macrophage** in tissue. The neutrophil is sometimes called the **polymorphonuclear leukocyte** because it is the most prevalent of the white blood cells containing a multilobed nucleus. However, this term also includes other white blood cells; therefore neutrophil is a more specific name for this cell. Other cells within the blood and tissue such as the lymphocyte and plasma cell, eosinophil, and mast cell participate in both inflammatory and immune responses. The immune response and the involvement of these cells are included in Chapter 3.

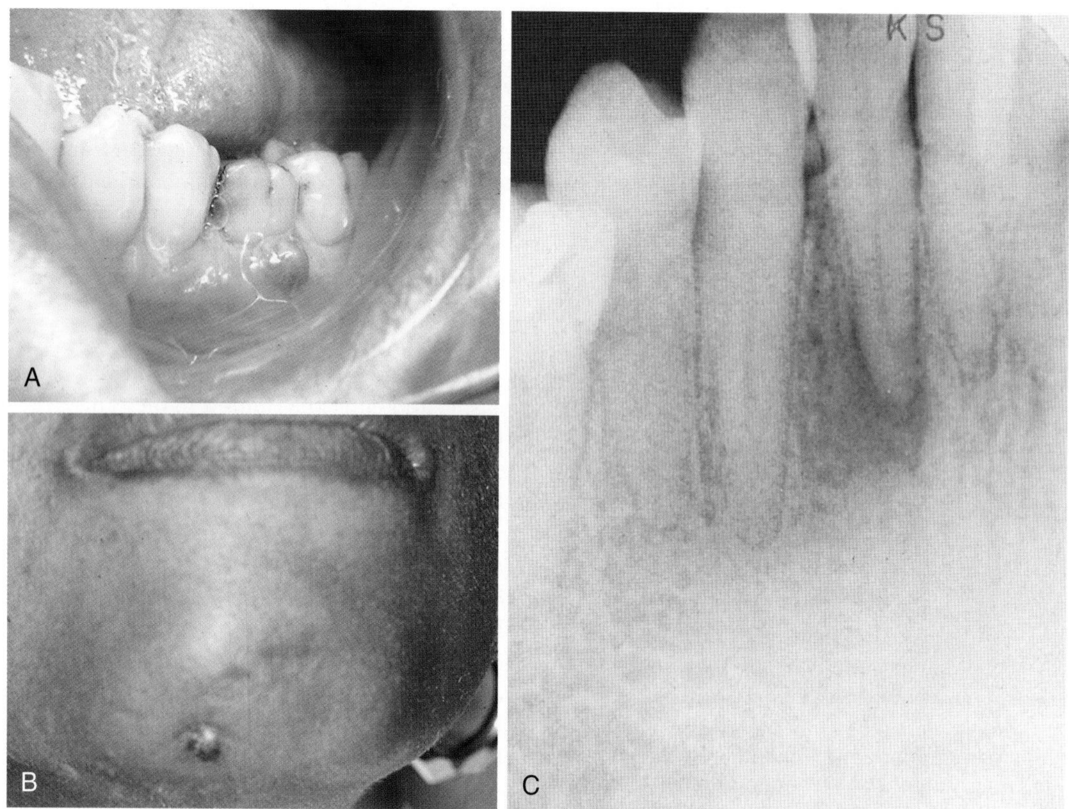

FIGURE 2-3 ■ Fistulas formed from periapical abscesses. **A,** A fistula formed from an abscess associated with a mandibular first molar. **B,** The opening of a fistulous tract from a mandibular incisor is noted on the skin of the chin. **C,** A periapical radiolucency at the area of abscess causing the fistula to the skin in **B.**

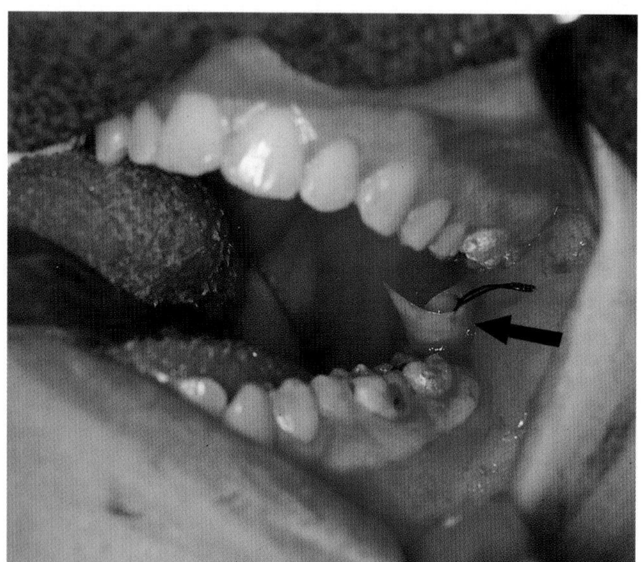

FIGURE 2-4 ■ An intraoral abscess has been incised, and a drain *(arrow)* placed to allow the escape of purulent exudate from the tissue. (Courtesy Dr. Sidney Eisig.)

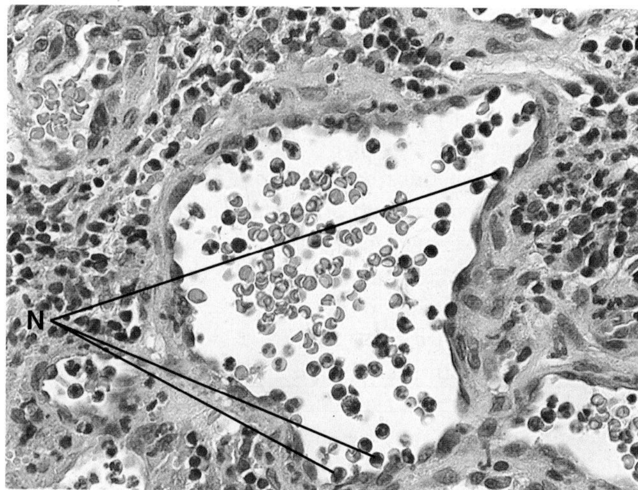

FIGURE 2-5 ■ Microscopic view of a blood vessel showing margination and pavementing are present during inflammation. Neutrophils *(N)* are seen at the periphery of a small blood vessel.

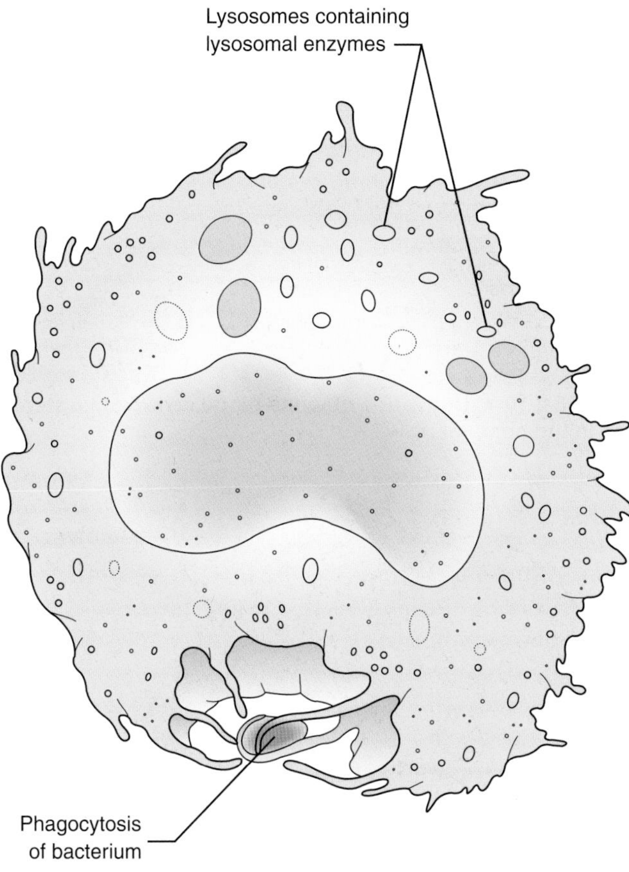

FIGURE 2-6 ■ Phagocytosis of a foreign substance (bacterium) by a white blood cell. The foreign substance will later be destroyed by digestion within the cell by lysosomal enzymes that are contained within lysosomes.

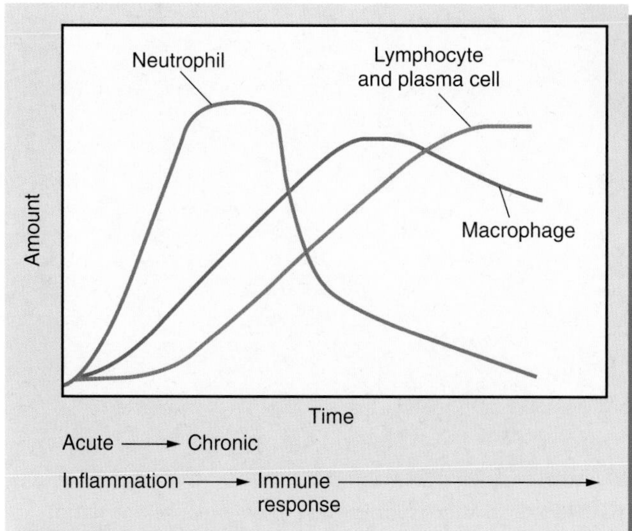

FIGURE 2-7 ■ Changes in the white blood cell population of the injured tissue over time, starting with acute inflammation, continuing to chronic inflammation, and the beginning of the immune response.

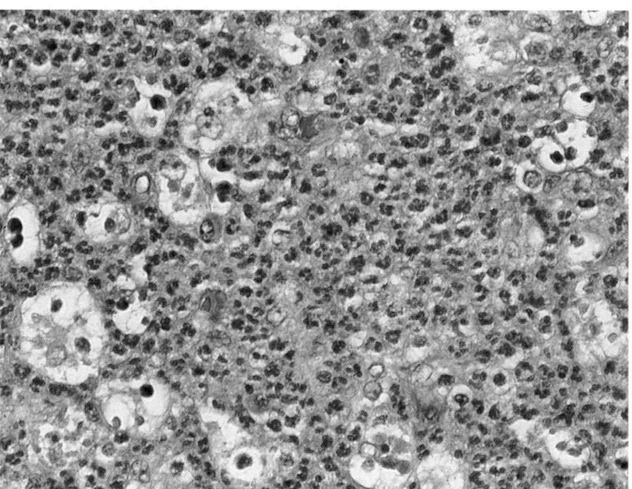

FIGURE 2-8 ■ Microscopic view of acute inflammation showing an increase in the number of neutrophils. Macrophages are also present.

As inflammation begins and continues over the 2-week time frame after an injury, changes take place in the types of white blood cells present in the tissue (Figure 2-7).

The neutrophil is the first cell to arrive at the site of injury and is the most common inflammatory cell present (Figure 2-8) during acute inflammation. The monocyte circulating in blood enters the tissue and becomes a macrophage. It is the second type of white blood cell to arrive at the site of injury. As inflammation continues, the number of neutrophils decreases. If the injury persists and chronic inflammation occurs, macrophages, lymphocytes, and plasma cells replace the neutrophils and become the predominant white blood cells in the tissue (Figure 2-9).

Neutrophils

Neutrophils are the first white blood cells recruited into the area of injury in response to chemotactic factors. The main function of the neutrophil is phagocytosis of substances such as pathogenic microorganisms and tissue debris. Lysosomal enzymes contained within vacuoles in the cytoplasm destroy substances after the cell has engulfed them. The removal of these substances from the site of injury is necessary to allow the process of healing to occur. The neutrophil dies shortly after phagocytosis; as a result, lysosomal enzymes and other damaging cellular substances that were meant only for intracellular destruction of foreign substances leak from the cells. This leakage can cause further tissue damage.

Neutrophils constitute 60% to 70% of the entire white blood cell population. Like all white blood cells, neutrophils are derived from stem cells in the bone marrow (Figure 2-10). Stem cells are undifferentiated cells in the spongy tissue that is found in the center shafts of certain long and flat bones of the body, such as the bones of the pelvis and sternum. When observed microscopically, neutrophils possess a multilobed nucleus, which is why they are sometimes called

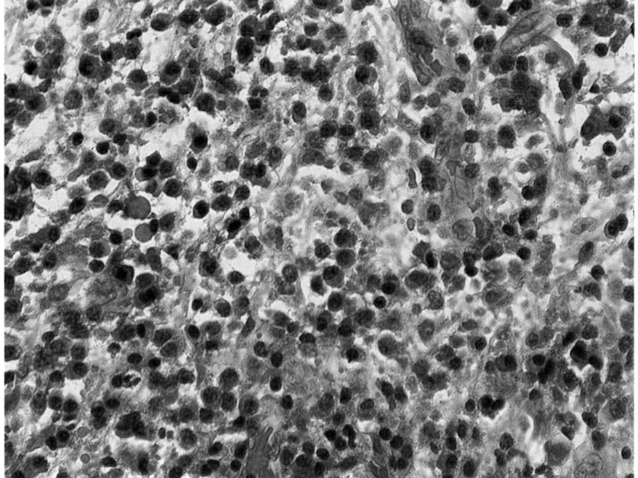

FIGURE 2-9 ■ Microscopic view of chronic inflammation and the beginning of the immune response, showing lymphocytes, and plasma cells.

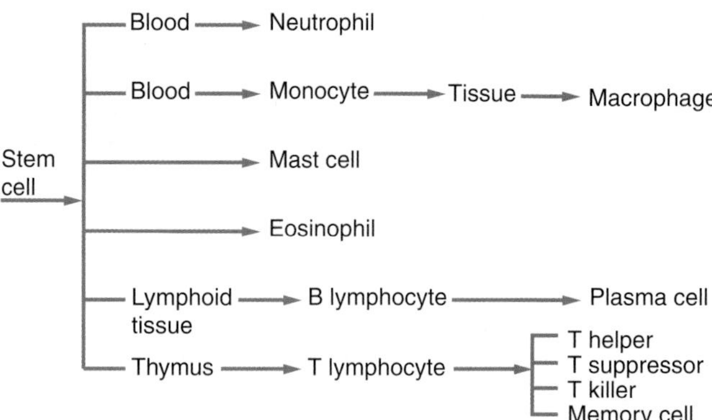

FIGURE 2-10 ■ Derivation of white blood cells from a stem cell in the bone marrow.

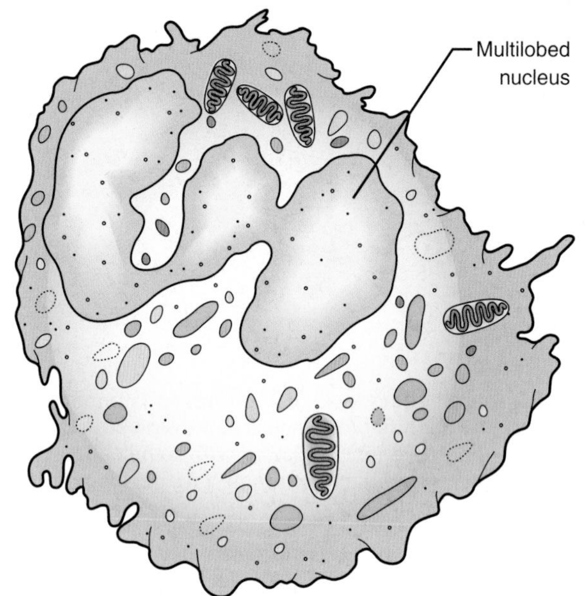

FIGURE 2-11 ■ A neutrophil has a multilobed nucleus and granular cytoplasm.

polymorphonuclear leukocytes, and a granular cytoplasm that contains enzymes called **lysosomal enzymes** (Figure 2-11). They are produced throughout life and are mobile cells.

Macrophages

The monocyte is the second white blood cell to emigrate from the blood vessels into the injured tissue, where it becomes a macrophage. Like neutrophils, monocytes are derived from stem cells in the bone marrow (see Figure 2-10). As a macrophage, it responds to chemotactic factors, is capable of phagocytosis, is mobile, and has lysosomal enzymes in its cytoplasm that assist in the destruction of foreign substances.

The macrophage is larger than its monocytic precursor. It has a single round nucleus and does not have granular cytoplasm (Figure 2-12). It constitutes 3% to 8% of the entire white blood cell population. The macrophage has a somewhat longer life span than the neutrophil. In addition to its role in phagocytosis, the macrophage is an important cell in the immune response (see Chapter 3).

BIOCHEMICAL MEDIATORS OF INFLAMMATION

Chemical agents in the body called biochemical or inflammatory mediators cause many of the events involved in the inflammatory response. Biochemical mediators are essential to the inflammatory response and can start or amplify the response. During the response, basic mediators of inflammation can recruit other mediators and immune mechanisms, thus escalating the overall process. Some biochemical mediators are circulating in blood, some come from endothelium, some from white blood cells, and some from platelets; others are produced by certain pathogenic microorganisms as they injure the tissue.

Three systems of plasma proteins circulating in the blood may be activated during inflammation: (1) the kinin system, (2) the clotting mechanism, and (3) the complement system. The activation of these plasma protein systems involves a sequential cascade of events. These systems are interrelated; interaction among the systems takes place during their activation, among their products, and within their various actions.

Kinin System

The kinin system mediates inflammation by causing increased dilation of the blood vessels at the site of injury and increasing the permeability of local blood vessels. This system is rapidly activated both by substances present in plasma and by those present in injured tissues. Its role is limited to the early phases of inflammation. Components of the kinin system also induce pain. The primary kinin is bradykinin.

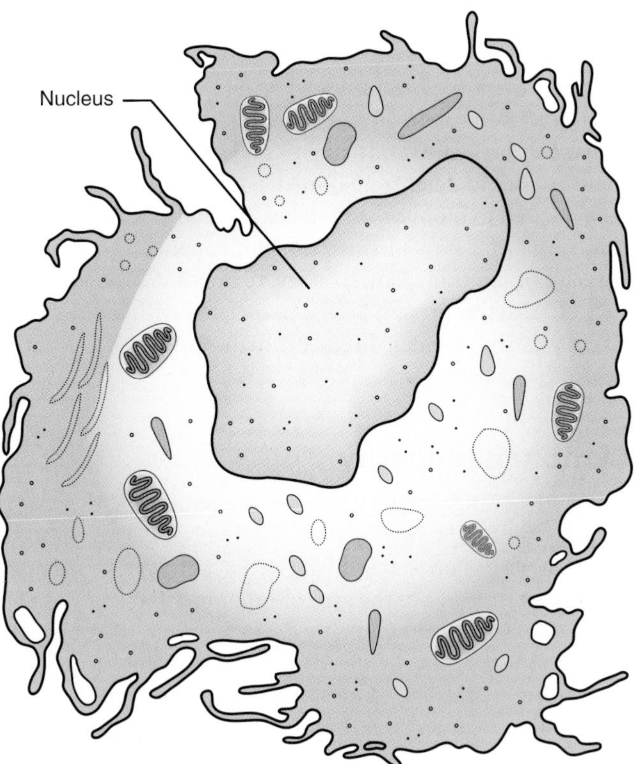

FIGURE 2-12 ■ A macrophage. This cell was a monocyte when circulating in blood.

Clotting Mechanism

The clotting mechanism functions primarily in the clotting of blood, which helps stop bleeding at the site of injury. It forms a fibrinous meshwork at the site of injury that protects adjacent tissues and keeps foreign substances corralled at the site. It also mediates inflammation because certain of its products that are activated when tissue is injured cause local vascular dilation and permeability by activating the kinin system. The clotting mechanism is also important in tissue repair since it forms a future framework for the repair process.

Complement System

The complement system is composed of a series of plasma proteins that are activated in a cascading fashion with one protein activating the next in the series. Components of the complement system function during both inflammation and immunity. Complement components can cause mast cells to release the granules in their cytoplasm that contain the biochemical mediator histamine and other mediators. Mast cells are a central cell in certain inflammatory reactions. They are located in large numbers in the loose connective tissue of skin and mucosa. When released, histamine causes an increase in vascular permeability and vasodilation. Other components of the complement system can cause cell death (cytolysis) by creating holes in the cell membrane. They also can form chemotactic factors for white blood cells and enhance phagocytosis. This enhancement of phagocytosis is called **opsonization.**

Other Biochemical Mediators of Inflammation

In addition to the biochemical mediators derived from circulating blood that have been described already, others are formed in the body during inflammation. Cell products from certain cells called cytokines effect the inflammatory response. These are described in Chapter 3 because they participate in the immune response. Prostaglandins are derived from cell membranes. They function in the inflammatory response by causing increased vascular dilation and permeability, tissue redness and pain, and changes in connective tissues. Lysosomal enzymes are released from the granules in white blood cells. They act as chemotactic factors and can cause damage to connective tissues and to the clot.

Endotoxin and lysosomal enzymes released by pathogenic microorganisms may also serve as biochemical mediators. Endotoxin, produced from the cell walls of gram-negative bacteria, can serve as a chemotactic factor, activate complement, and function as an antigen and damage bone tissue. During infection the lysosomal enzymes released from pathogenic microorganisms have a similar chemical composition and action to those released by white blood cells.

Antiinflammatory Drugs

Antiinflammatory drugs block or suppress the inflammatory response, preventing or reducing the clinical signs of inflammation and adverse reactions to the injury. Diseases and conditions such as asthma, arthritis, organ transplants, and surgical trauma are treated with nonsteroidal or steroidal antiinflammatory agents. Examples of nonsteroidal antiinflammatory agents (NSAIDs) include acetylsalicylic acid (aspirin) and ibuprofen. They exert their analgesic effects by inhibiting prostaglandin synthesis. Prednisone is a steroidal antiinflammatory drug. Another drug classification, antihistamines, reduces the effects of the mediator histamine.

Medications that are traditionally used to treat cancer such as methotrexate, sulfasalazine, leflunomide, cyclophosphamide, and mycophenolate are also being used to treat inflammatory diseases; the doses are significantly lower, and the risk of side effects tends to be considerably less than when prescribed in higher doses to treat cancer.

SYSTEMIC MANIFESTATIONS OF INFLAMMATION

In addition to the local features of inflammation, four major systemic signs may also occur: (1) fever, (2) an increase in the number of white blood cells (leukocytosis), (3) elevated C-reactive protein, and (4) enlargement of lymph nodes (lymphadenopathy) (see Table 2-1).

Fever

Body temperature is controlled by a regulatory center in the brain called the hypothalamic thermoregulatory center. **Fever** is a body temperature higher than 98.6° F (37° C) and is associated with a systemic inflammatory response. White blood cells and pathogenic microorganisms produce fever-producing substances known as pyrogens. Pyrogens exert their effects by action on the hypothalamus, the regulatory center in the brain that increases the temperature of the body by way of prostaglandins, producing fever.

The function of this increased body temperature is not clear. A moderately high fever may be helpful in combating some infections because increased temperature slows the growth of many pathogenic microorganisms. However, the body cannot tolerate excessively high fever for very long, and such fever could prove fatal. Drugs can be given to reduce high fever. Measuring body temperature with a thermometer is helpful in assessing whether a systemic inflammatory response is present.

Leukocytosis

Leukocytosis is an increase in the number of white blood cells circulating in blood. The normal value is 4,000 to 10,000/mm^3. The complete blood count is an initial blood test that can be used to evaluate a patient for infection. During a systemic inflammatory response, particularly a response to infection, there is an increase in the number of circulating white blood cells (leukocytosis). The number increases to 10,000 to 30,000/mm^3. This increase primarily involves neutrophils. The body increases the number of circulating white blood cells by increasing their formation and releasing immature forms from the bone marrow into the blood; this is called a "shift to the left." This increase is caused by biochemical mediators and is an attempt by the body to provide more cells for phagocytosis.

A complete blood count includes a "differential" white blood cell count. This measures the proportion of each white blood cell type and is useful in distinguishing a viral infection from a bacterial infection or an allergic reaction that involves eosinophils. These results provide a useful tool for evaluating patients but do not indicate the particular cause or site of inflammation in the body.

Elevated C-Reactive Protein

Another diagnostic laboratory test measures serum **C-reactive protein.** C-reactive protein is produced in the liver and plays the important role of interacting with the complement system. Normally low levels of C-reactive protein circulate in blood. Elevated C-reactive protein is present during episodes of acute inflammation or infection and may continue with chronic inflammation. Although a result above 10 mg/L is usually considered high for C-reactive protein, most infections and episodes of inflammation result in C-reactive protein levels at 100 mg/L. C-reactive protein levels drop as inflammation subsides.

C-reactive protein level can be used to help assess conditions such as rheumatoid arthritis and systemic lupus erythematosus and to determine if medication taken is effective. It may be used to monitor wound healing and as an early detection system for possible infections in patients who have had surgery, organ transplants, or severe burns. Chronically elevated C-reactive protein level is associated with an increased risk for cardiovascular disease. A high-sensitivity C-reactive protein (hs-CRP) assay is now available.

Lymphadenopathy

During the inflammatory process the lymph nodes enlarge or undergo **lymphadenopathy** (Figure 2-13). The enlarged lymph node or nodes, if located superficially, can be palpated as a mass or masses in the area of inflammation and possibly along the associated lymphatic drainage route (Figure 2-14). When palpated, the involved node feels firmer and larger than normal and may also be tender. Deeper lymph nodes may also be enlarged, but these cannot be palpated.

Lymphadenopathy results from changes in the lymphocytes that reside in the lymph node. Lymphocytes are white blood cells that mature in lymphoid tissue. They are the primary white blood cells of the immune response (see Chapter 3). They also travel from the lymph node to the tissues, where they are involved in the immune response. The changes in the lymphocytes cause the change in size of the lymph nodes. These changes include an increase in the number of cells **(hyperplasia)**, resulting from increased cell division, and an enlargement of individual cells **(hypertrophy)**, resulting from cellular maturation. The lymphoid tissue in Waldeyer's ring, which includes the pharyngeal and lingual tonsillar tissue, may also undergo these changes. These changes in the lymphocyte population occur during prolonged or chronic inflammation.

CHRONIC INFLAMMATION

Chronic inflammation results from injuries that persist, often for weeks or months, possibly indefinitely. In addition to neutrophils and monocytes, other white blood cells are involved, as is the proliferation of fibroblasts. The cells involved in chronic inflammation include macrophages, lymphocytes, and plasma cells. Repair takes place at the same time that chronic inflammation proceeds, but it cannot be completed until the source of the injury is removed.

A distinctive form of chronic inflammation is called **granulomatous inflammation**. It is characterized by the formation of **granulomas**, which are microscopic groupings of macrophages surrounded by lymphocytes and occasional plasma cells. Granulomas usually contain large macrophages that have multiple nuclei called multinucleated giant cells.

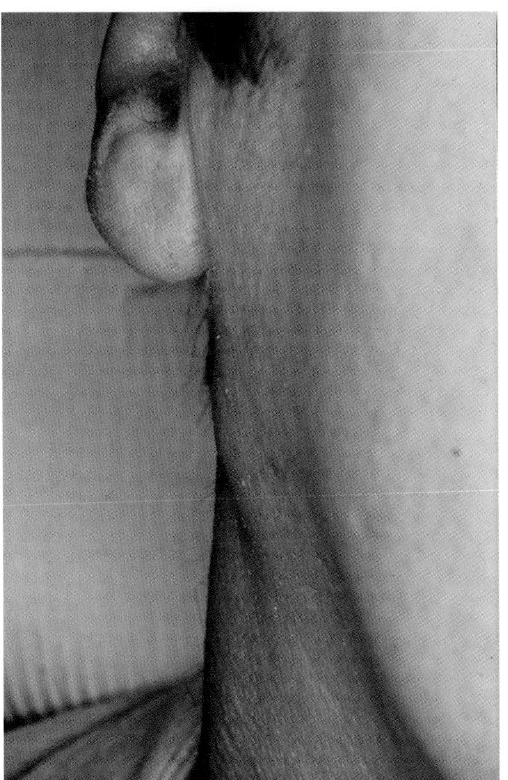

FIGURE 2-13 ■ Enlarged cervical lymph node.

Foreign substances in tissue and certain infections such as tuberculosis tend to stimulate the formation of granulomas. The body is unable to destroy the offending substances and tries to enclose them in a mass of inflammatory cells.

HYPERPLASIA, HYPERTROPHY, AND ATROPHY

A cell or its associated tissue or organ may respond to injury by undergoing an adaptive response such as hyperplasia, hypertrophy, or atrophy. Hyperplasia is defined as an increase in the number of cells in a tissue or organ whereby the size of the tissue or organ is increased in response to conditions that cause cellular stress. Pathologic hyperplasia frequently occurs in oral tissues. In the oral cavity an increase in the number of epithelial cells and the increased thickness of the epithelium commonly occur in response to chronic irritation (Figure 2-15). As surface epithelial cells are lost, division of deeper basal epithelial cells increases to replace the lost cells. The production of new cells is in excess of the original number of cells; thus the epithelium becomes thickened, and the tissue appears paler or whiter.

When the irritation subsides, the proliferation ceases; with time the epithelium usually returns to its normal size, and the color of the tissue returns to normal. However, sometimes the hyperplastic tissue persists even after the irritation

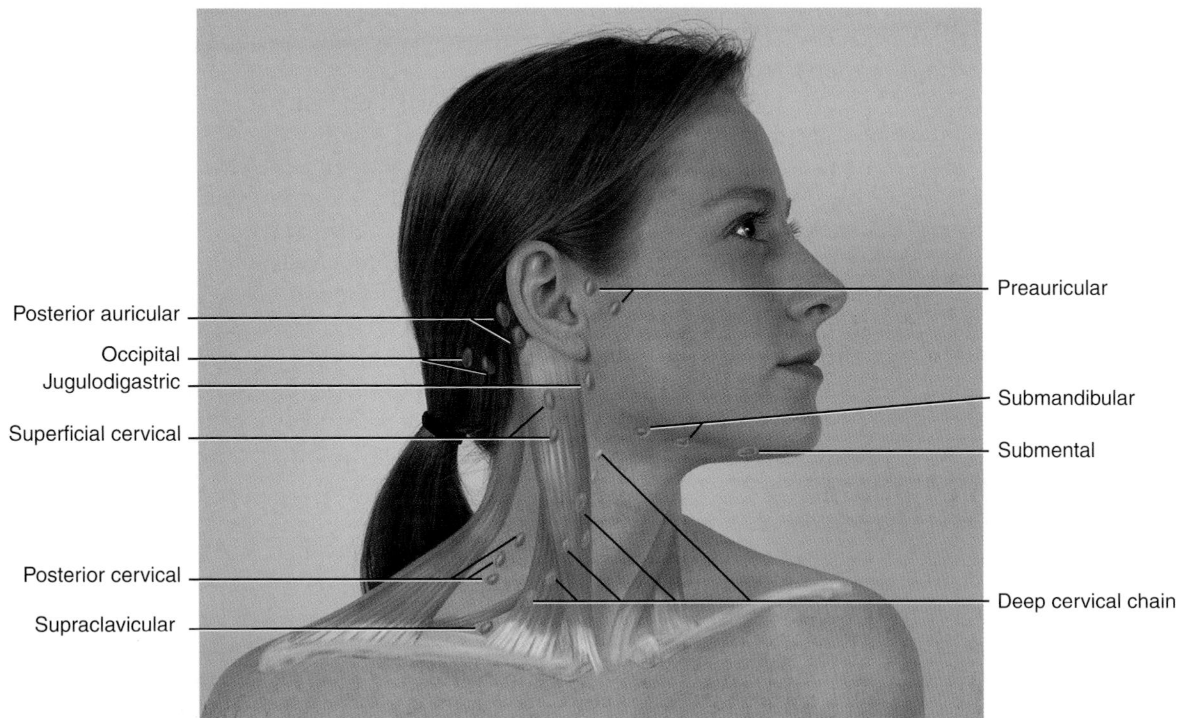

FIGURE 2-14 ■ Location of lymph nodes in the neck. (From Jarvis C: *Physical examination and health assessment,* ed 5, St Louis, 2008, Saunders Elsevier.)

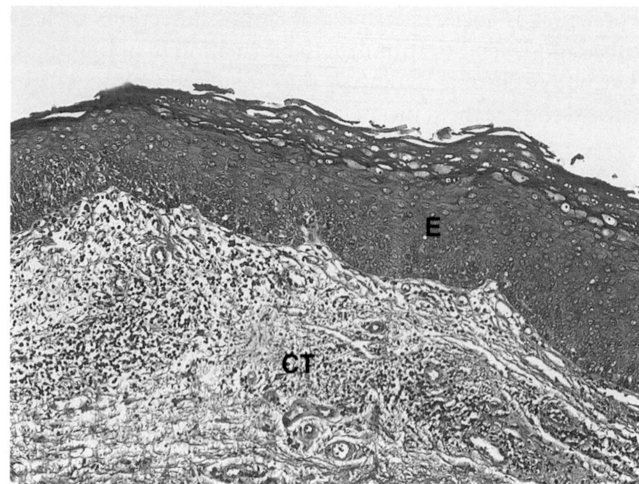

FIGURE 2-15 ■ Microscopic appearance of epithelial hyperplasia (low magnification). The epithelium *(E)* is thickened because of an increase in the number of cells. *CT,* underlying connective tissue.

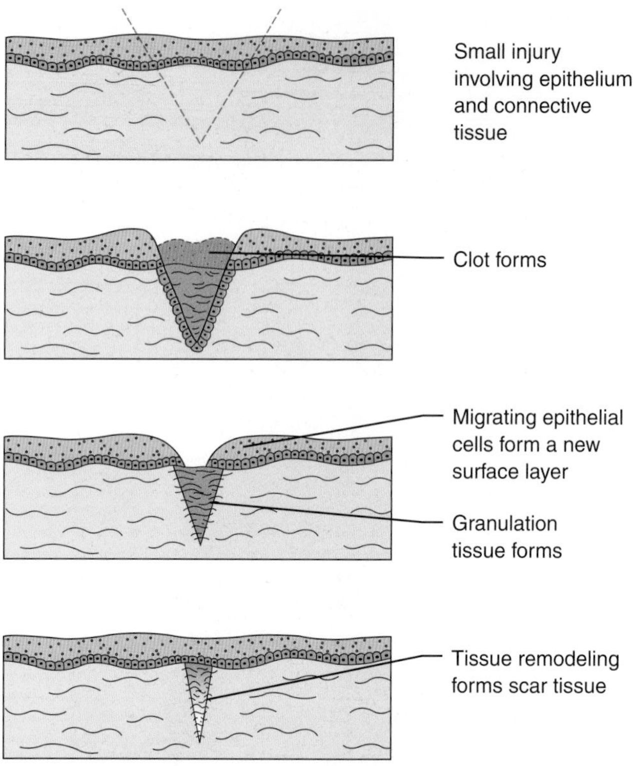

FIGURE 2-16 ■ Underlying microscopic events of the repair process from the day of injury to 2 weeks later.

is discontinued. Hyperplasia of fibrous connective tissue may also occur in response to chronic injury and is common in the oral cavity. Oral lesions caused by epithelial and fibrous hyperplasia are described later in this chapter.

In contrast, hypertrophy is a response to cellular stress that is defined as an increase in the size of a tissue or organ because of an increase in the size, not the number, of cells. For example, hypertrophy occurs in the smooth muscles of the uterus and the mammary glands in response to pregnancy, in cardiac muscle in response to long-standing high blood pressure, and in skeletal muscle in response to increased exercise. Hyperplasia and hypertrophy are often present together in one disease state.

Atrophy is the decrease in size and function of a cell, tissue, organ, or whole body in response to certain conditions of cellular stress. Atrophied cells are capable of increasing to their normal size after the stress is removed. Atrophy can be present in the muscular wasting that sometimes occurs in chronic disease states that do not allow mobility and thus function of the body ("use it or lose it"). It can also happen with changes in cellular growth, malnutrition, pressure, ischemia, or hormonal changes.

REGENERATION AND REPAIR

With resolution of the inflammatory response, the injured tissue undergoes wound healing as either regeneration or repair. When tissue damage has been slight, the inflamed area may return completely to its normal structure and function. This is called **regeneration.** Regeneration is the most favorable resolution of acute inflammation and involves complete removal of all cells, by-products, and inflammatory exudate that enter the tissue during inflammation and return of the microcirculation to its preinflammatory state.

In contrast, the process of repair takes place when complete return of the tissue to normal is not possible because the damage has been too great. Some tissues such as epithelium, fibrous connective tissue, and bone have the ability to undergo repair. Other tissues such as enamel do not.

Repair is the body's final defense mechanism in its attempt to restore injured tissue to its original state. During the repair process destroyed cells and tissue are replaced with live cells and new tissue components, but the repair process cannot be completed until the source of injury is removed or the injurious agents are destroyed. Repair is not always a perfect process. Functioning cells and tissue components are often replaced by nonfunctioning scar tissue. Many studies are currently investigating ways to enhance the repair process.

MICROSCOPIC EVENTS DURING REPAIR

After an injury microscopic events occur in both the epithelium and connective tissue (Figure 2-16). These events are different for each of these tissues but occur almost simultaneously and are dependent on each other for optimal healing. If the source of the injury is removed, the repair process for both tissues is usually completed in 2 weeks. The repair process is slightly different in mucosa than in skin because mucosal tissues are wet and a scab does not form. There are three phases to repair that occur during these 2 weeks: (1) inflammation, (2) proliferation, and (3) maturation.

Day of Injury

A clot forms as the blood flows into the injured tissue. The clot is produced in the area of injury as a result of activation of the clotting mechanism. The clot consists of a meshwork structure comprised of locally produced fibrin, aggregated (clumped) red blood cells, and platelets. Platelets (thrombocytes) are cellular fragments found in blood and are extremely important in the formation of a clot. There are 250,000 to 400,000 platelets per cubic milliliter within the blood. The number of platelets is measured within the panel of the complete blood count. Hereditary factors, drugs, extensive injury, or certain diseases may affect red blood cells, platelets, and other factors involved in the formation of the clot and thus prevent or delay tissue repair.

One Day after Injury

Acute inflammation is taking place in the area of future repair. The neutrophils emigrate from the microcirculation into the injured tissue, and phagocytosis of foreign substances and necrotic tissue occurs as part of the inflammatory response.

Two Days after Injury

The monocytes emigrate from the microcirculation into the injured area as macrophages. Macrophages continue phagocytosis in a manner similar to that of the neutrophils. Neutrophils are reduced in number as the chronic inflammatory process proceeds. Fibroblasts proliferate within the injured connective tissue as a result of biochemical mediators from macrophages. Fibroblasts become the most important cells during wound healing as they begin to produce and secrete new collagen fibers, using the fibrinous meshwork as a scaffold.

The initial tissue formed in the connective tissue portion of the injury is called **granulation tissue**. It is an immature tissue, with many more capillaries and fibroblasts than the usual connective tissue that clinically appears a vivid pink or red. Sometimes the growth of this tissue is excessive (exuberant). It may interfere with the repair process until it is removed surgically.

If the surface epithelium has been destroyed by the injury, the epithelial cells create a new surface tissue at the same time that granulation tissue forms in the injured connective tissue. The epithelial cells from the borders of the healing injured area lose their cellular junctions and become mobile. They then divide and migrate across the injured tissue, using the fibrinous meshwork as a guide to form a new surface layer.

In addition to serving as a guide for migrating epithelial cells and as a scaffold for forming connective tissue, the fibrinous meshwork of the clot serves to protect the two newly formed deeper tissues from further injury. Thus it is important for the clot to remain in place during this time to allow optimal repair in both tissues. Dressings placed over the clot may prove beneficial to the healing process in some injuries.

At the end of 2 days, lymphocytes and plasma cells begin to immigrate from the surrounding blood vessels into the injured area as chronic inflammation and an immune response begin. The macrophages already present in the area now assist the lymphocytes in the immune response occurring at the site of injury.

Seven Days after Injury

The fibrinous meshwork of the clot is digested by tissue enzymes and sloughs off, and the initial repair of the tissues is completed. Clinically the surface of the repaired injury remains redder than normal because of the thinness of the new surface epithelium and the increased vascularity of the new underlying connective tissue. If the source of the injury has been removed completely, the inflammatory and immune responses in the tissue have completed their cycles. The immature type of collagen fibers found in granulation tissue is still present and remains fragile and at risk of reinjury.

Two Weeks after Injury

The initial granulation tissue and its fibers have been remodeled, giving the tissue its full strength. The new tissue has undergone maturation and is now called scar tissue; it appears whiter or paler at the surface of the repaired injury because of the increased number of collagen fibers and decreased vascularity. The amount of scar tissue remaining after an injury depends on many factors such as heredity, the strength and flexibility needed in the tissue, the type of repair that has occurred, and the tissue involved; the oral mucosa is less prone to scar formation than the skin.

TYPES OF REPAIR

Healing by Primary Intention

This refers to the healing of an injury in which little loss of tissue takes place, such as in a surgical incision. In this type of healing the clean edges of the incision are joined with sutures to form only a small clot, and very little granulation tissue forms (Figure 2-17). Thus less scar tissue forms, and the patient retains more normal tissue. The use of sutures is an attempt to try to join the edges of the injury surgically so that healing by primary intention occurs and scarring is minimized.

Healing by Secondary Intention

This involves injury in which tissue is lost; thus the edges of the injury cannot be joined during healing. A large clot slowly forms, resulting in increased formation of granulation tissue (e.g., an extraction site) (Figure 2-18). After healing,

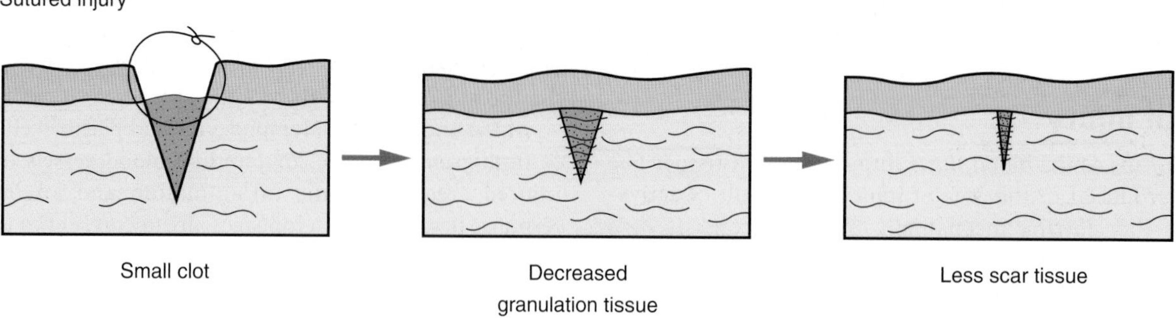

FIGURE 2-17 ■ Use of sutures in an unintentional injury to encourage healing by primary intention.

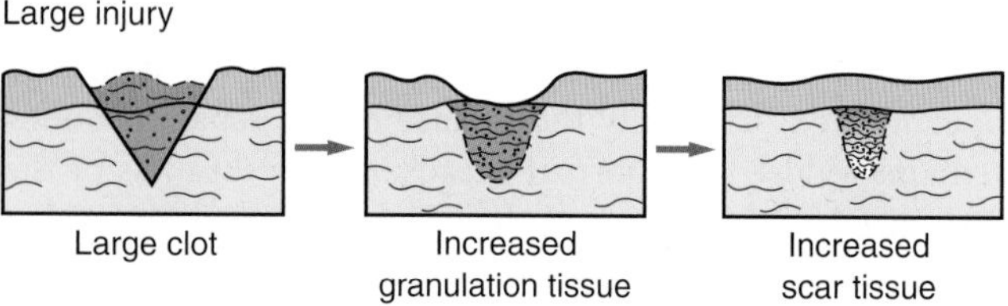

FIGURE 2-18 ■ Healing by secondary intention (without the use of sutures) in a large injury.

scar tissue increases, and normal tissue function is greatly reduced. This scar tissue formation can be so excessive that surgical correction is sometimes needed. Excessive scarring in skin that appears raised and extends beyond its original boundaries is called a **keloid** (Figure 2-19). A familial tendency to keloid formation has been noted.

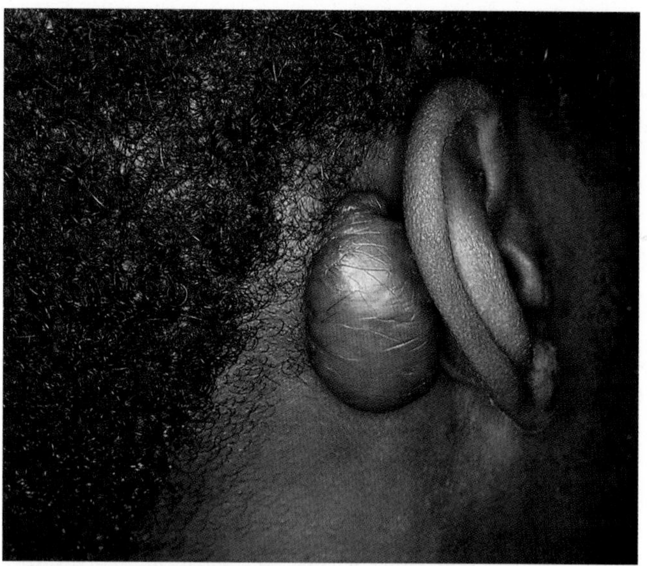

FIGURE 2-19 ■ Example of keloid formation (excessive scar tissue formation) after an injury. (Courtesy Dr. Harold Baurmash.)

Healing by Tertiary Intention

If infection occurs at the site of a surgical incision that is healing by primary intention, healing by tertiary intention may result. This transformation occurs because of an enlargement of the injured area and an increase in the magnitude and duration of the inflammatory and immune responses triggered by the presence of pathogenic microorganisms. In some cases an infected injury is left open, and the edges are not surgically joined until the infection is controlled. Waiting to perform surgical tissue repair until the infection is resolved is called healing by tertiary intention.

Factors That Impair Healing

Certain local factors impair healing; these include bacterial infection (primarily by *Streptococcus* species), tissue destruction and **necrosis**, hemorrhage into the tissue (hematoma), excessive movement of the injured tissue, and poor blood supply. Systemic factors such as those resulting from malnutrition (especially when protein, zinc, calcium, and vitamin C are severely reduced in the diet) can also impair healing. If the body is undergoing immunosuppression because of steroid use or chemotherapy, healing is also impaired. Certain genetic connective tissue disorders (osteogenesis imperfecta, Marfan syndrome) (see Chapter 6) and metabolic disorders resulting from age, renal failure, and diabetes mellitus (see Chapter 9) can reduce the effectiveness of the natural healing mechanism. Tobacco use has also been shown to impair healing.

BONE TISSUE REPAIR

Repair of a bone injury is similar to the process that takes place in fibrous connective tissue except that it involves the creation of bone tissue. Bone-forming cells called osteoblasts, which are found on the inner and outer surfaces of bone, produce this tissue. As with other tissues, nutrition, age, and tobacco use can influence the repair process of bone. At the site of the injury blood supply and growth factors can further modulate the process. Removal of osteoblast-producing tissues and excessive movement of the bone can interrupt healing. Inadequate movement of bone during the healing process can adversely affect repair. Injury, edema, or infection in the involved bone can delay repair.

INJURIES TO TEETH

ATTRITION

Attrition is the wearing away of tooth structure during mastication. It is a normal occurrence and happens as an individual ages. It involves the incisal, occlusal, and proximal surfaces of the teeth and is rarely seen on any other tooth surfaces unless teeth are abnormally placed in the arch (Figure 2-20). Attrition occurs in both deciduous and permanent dentitions; it is usually a slow process that starts as soon as the teeth are in contact and continues for the duration of the contact.

The first sign of attrition is the disappearance of the mamelons on incisal teeth and the flattening of the occlusal cusps (Figure 2-21). The rate of attrition is influenced by diet. A diet of more fibrous food causes greater attrition. Bruxism, the use of chewing tobacco, and certain occupations and environments in which abrasive dust particles enter the mouth accelerate attrition. Attrition increases as patients grow older, and the rate of attrition has been reported to be greater in men than in women.

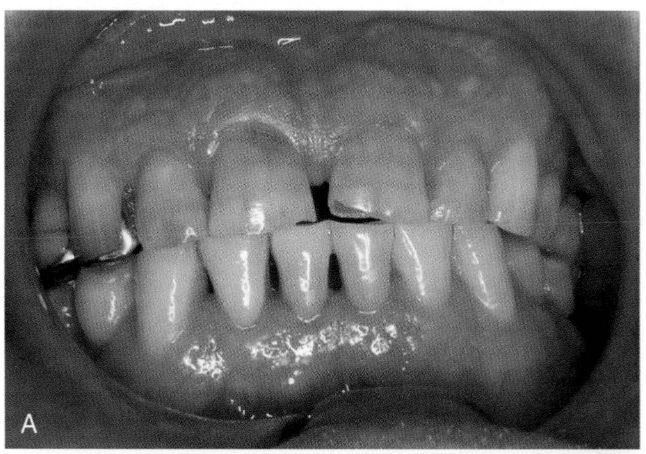

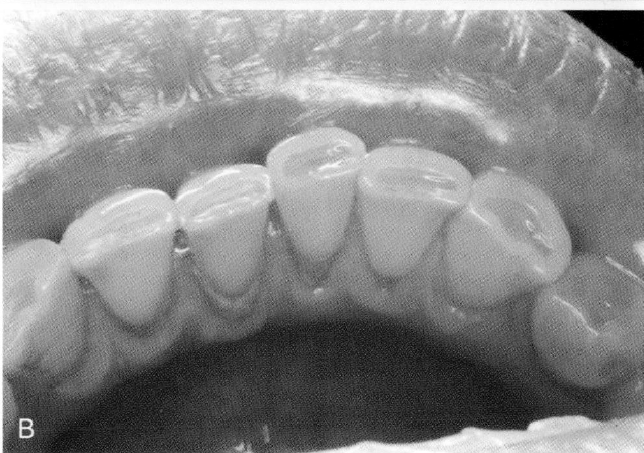

FIGURE 2-20 ■ **A,** Attrition of adult dentition. **B,** Attrition of adult dentition (incisal view).

Bruxism

Grinding and clenching the teeth together for nonfunctional purposes is called **bruxism.** The signs and symptoms resulting from bruxism and their extent are related to the intensity of the grinding and clenching. They are varied and include "wear facets" visible on enamel surfaces, an abnormal rate of attrition (Figure 2-22), hypertrophy of masticatory muscles (especially the masseter muscle), increased muscle tone, muscle tenderness, muscle fatigue, cheek biting, pain in the temporomandibular joint area (see Chapter 10), tooth mobility, and pulpal sensitivity to cold.

The incidence of bruxism varies greatly according to the population studied. In a university student population, 5% of individuals showed signs and symptoms of bruxism. In studies of patients with periodontal disease, 60% to 90% had evidence of bruxism. In children ages 2 to 5 years, the average prevalence reported was 20% to 30%, but the highest prevalence reported was 78%.

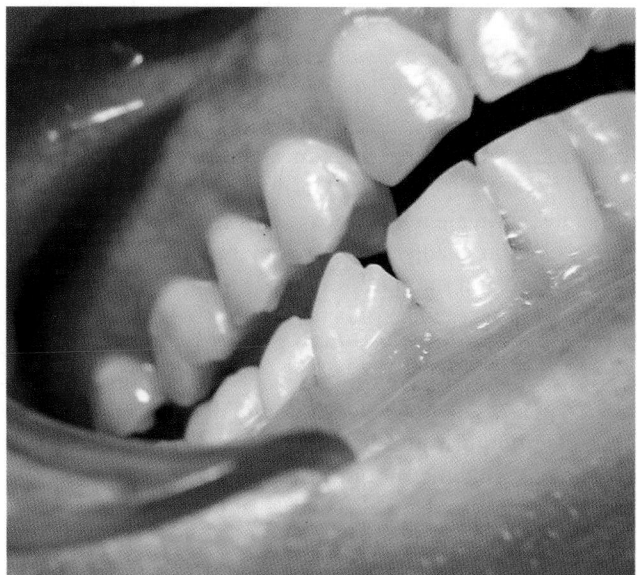

FIGURE 2-21 ■ Attrition has caused the flattening of the cusps (wear facets) of both the maxillary and mandibular cuspid teeth.

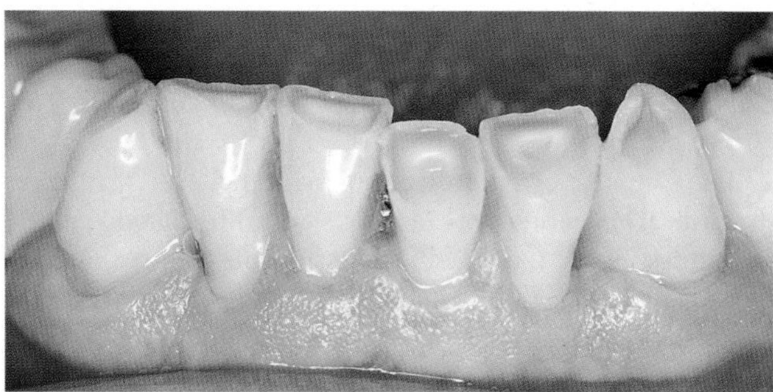

FIGURE 2-22 ■ Attrition of the mandibular anterior teeth resulting from bruxism.

The cause of bruxism is unclear. Local factors such as occlusal interferences in combination with stress and tension are considered to be triggering factors. A relationship has been reported between bruxism and anxiety, hostility, and hyperactivity. Other studies have characterized the individual who engages in bruxism as emotionally fragile with meticulous character traits, more headaches and muscle pains, and more success in school. Certain conditions such as seizure disorders have been related to bruxism. The higher prevalence of bruxism reported in certain occupations is possibly related to the amount of stress associated with those occupations.

Management of the individual with bruxism includes eliminating the occlusal interferences through occlusal adjustments and protecting the teeth and supporting tissues from further destruction by fabricating an acrylic splint that can be worn as a protective device.

The dental hygienist may identify signs of bruxism while taking the patient's history and during the oral examination. Active wear facets, muscle tenderness, and excessive attrition are clues to the presence of bruxism.

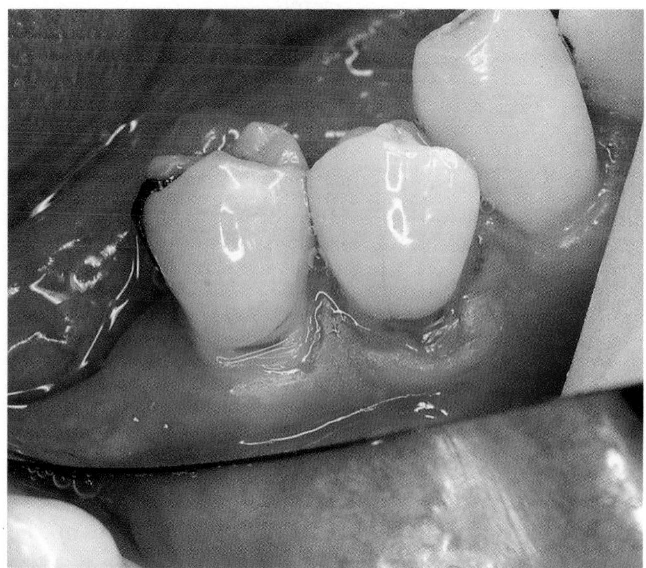

FIGURE 2-23 ■ Abrasion at the cervical area of mandibular bicuspids caused by toothbrushing.

ABRASION

Abrasion is the pathologic wearing away of tooth structure that results from a repetitive mechanical habit. It is most commonly seen in exposed root surfaces because the cementum and dentin are not as hard as enamel; however, abrasion also occurs on enamel surfaces. The process of abrasion is usually slow, and the dentin responds by laying down a protective layer of secondary dentin. Therefore pulpal exposure does not usually result.

Abrasion most frequently presents as a notching of the root surface in areas of gingival recession and may occur from an improper toothbrushing technique, most commonly a back-and-forth scrubbing motion using excessive pressure. The use of an abrasive dentifrice or a hard toothbrush may also cause abrasion (Figure 2-23). Today most dentifrices manufactured in the United States have a very low abrasive index, and toothbrushes with soft bristles are recommended. Other causes of abrasion include opening bobby pins with the teeth or holding needles or pins in the teeth. These practices result in a notching of the maxillary incisors. Musicians who play wind instruments may also exhibit forms of abrasion of the teeth in the area of the mouth where the instrument is placed, and pipe smokers may show evidence of abrasion in the area of pipe placement.

The diagnosis of abrasion can often be made by correlating the clinical appearance of the lesions with information gained from questioning the patient about possible factors that may be causing the lesions. The patient should be informed of the cause of the abrasion, and corrective measures should be taken to prevent further destruction of tooth structure. Restorative dental treatment to repair the defect may be appropriate.

ABFRACTION

Abfraction typically appears as wedge-shaped lesions at the cervical areas of teeth. These lesions occur in adults; the cause may be related to fatigue, flexure, fracture, and deformation of tooth structure as the result of biomechanical forces on the teeth. The weakened tooth structure is more susceptible to abrasion, particularly toothbrush abrasion. The lesions may be treated using composite or glass ionomer materials, but the forces on the teeth may result in dislodging of the restorations.

EROSION

Erosion is the loss of tooth structure resulting from chemical action. The loss may occur on the smooth facial or lingual surfaces of the teeth and on the proximal and occlusal surfaces (Figure 2-24). The area of erosion appears smooth and polished and is usually extensive, involving several teeth. If erosion occurs in an area where restorations exist, the tooth structure is lost around the restoration, making it appear as if the restoration is standing on its own. This phenomenon is not seen in abrasion or attrition because the restoration would be worn down along with the tooth surface.

Erosion may be seen in individuals who work in industries in which acid is used, such as battery manufacturing, plating companies, and soft-drink manufacturing. The erosion occurs because the workers breathe the acid in the air. Erosion of teeth associated with intraorally applied cocaine hydrochloride has been reported. Erosion of the facial surfaces of the teeth may also occur as a result of frequently sucking on lemons; erosion of the lingual surfaces of the teeth may occur as a result of chronic vomiting.

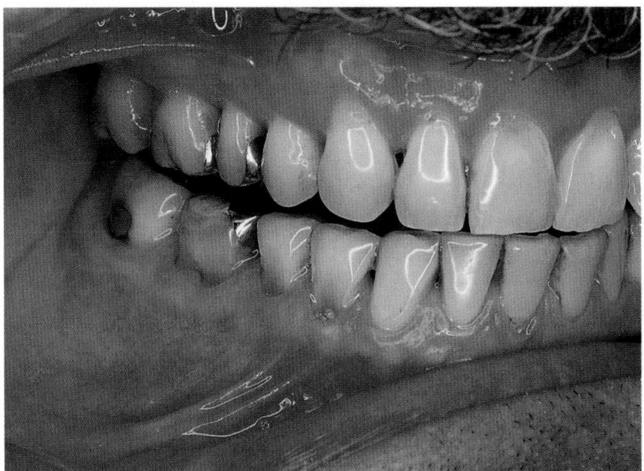

FIGURE 2-24 ■ Erosion of buccal and labial surfaces of teeth that occurred as a result of accidental exposure to sulfuric acid.

The location of erosion and abrasion cannot reliably identify the cause. The patient's history must be correlated with the location and cause.

Bulimia is an eating disorder characterized by food binges, usually of very high caloric intake, followed by self-induced vomiting. The frequent vomiting in an individual with bulimia results in generalized erosion of the lingual surfaces of teeth (Figure 2-25). Because of the pattern of erosion of the lingual surfaces of the teeth caused by frequent vomiting, the dental hygienist may be the first health care professional to identify a patient with bulimia and may assist in encouraging the patient to seek treatment. Bulimia differs from **anorexia nervosa**, another eating disorder, which is characterized by a distorted perception of body image, in addition to depression, intense fear of gaining weight, and self-imposed starvation. The patient with bulimia maintains a normal body weight but is secretive about eating habits. Vomiting after eating is a component of bulimia and not of anorexia nervosa. Electrolyte imbalance and signs of malnutrition may be present. Irritation of the oral mucosa and lips may occur, and there may be lesions on the back of the fingers caused by their continual use to induce vomiting.

Dental management of patients who vomit frequently includes an effort to minimize the effects of acid on tooth enamel by encouraging the daily use of fluoride rinse and toothpaste containing fluoride. Rinsing the mouth with water and thoroughly cleaning the teeth immediately after vomiting episodes also lessens the effects of acid.

METHAMPHETAMINE ABUSE

Recently the oral manifestations of **methamphetamine** abuse have been described. Acid content of methamphetamine, decreased salivary flow, and craving for high sugar–containing beverages combined with lack of oral hygiene care

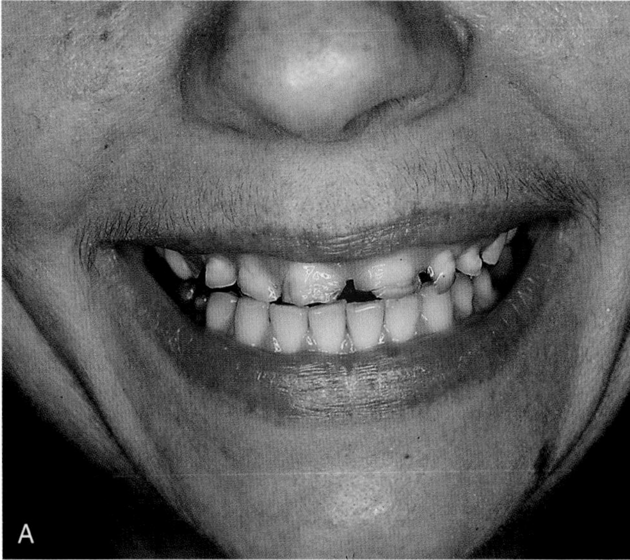

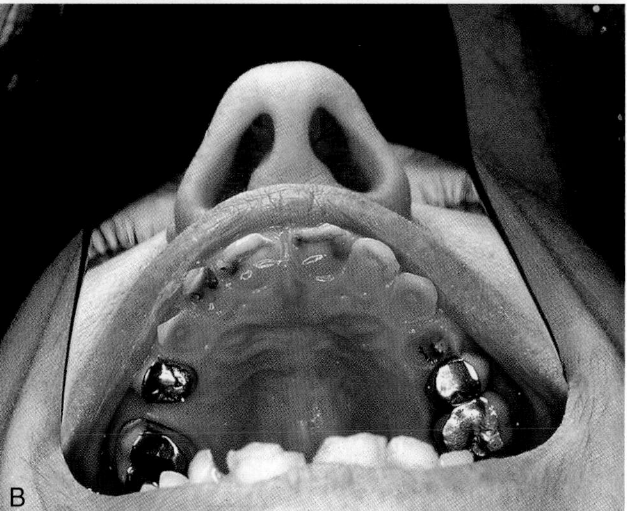

FIGURE 2-25 ■ Erosion caused by bulimia. **A,** Decreased tooth size. **B,** Erosion of maxillary lingual surfaces.

results in the extensive and rapid destruction of teeth that is called "**meth mouth**" (Figure 2-26).

INJURIES TO ORAL SOFT TISSUES

ASPIRIN BURN

An **aspirin burn** generally occurs when a patient with a toothache places an aspirin tablet directly on the painful tooth instead of swallowing it. Aspirin (acetylsalicylic acid) is an analgesic (pain reliever) and antiinflammatory agent that must be ingested to be effective. Topical application is a common misuse of aspirin. As a result of placing the aspirin on the soft tissue, the tissue becomes necrotic and appears white. The lesion is painful, and the necrotic tissue may separate from the underlying connective tissue and slough off, resulting in a large ulcer (Figure 2-27). Questioning the

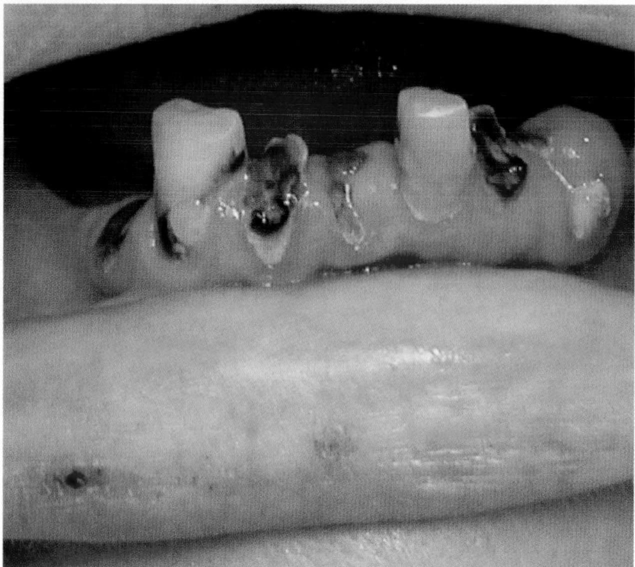

FIGURE 2-26 ■ Extensive dental destruction related to methamphetamine abuse. (Courtesy of Dr. Bobby Collins)

patient should reveal the cause of the lesion, and the diagnosis is generally made without the need for biopsy of the tissue. An aspirin burn is painful and heals slowly because of the extent of destruction. However, the ulcer usually heals spontaneously in 7 to 21 days. The patient requires appropriate treatment of the painful tooth and medication for symptomatic relief of pain until the ulcer heals.

PHENOL BURN

Phenol is used in dentistry as a cavity-sterilizing and cauterizing agent. When phenol comes into contact with the soft tissues, a whitening of the exposed area occurs as a result of tissue destruction. The surface tissue may slough off, exposing the underlying connective tissue. The resulting ulcer is painful, and the duration of healing depends on the extent of the destruction. The phenol should be removed immediately to minimize the destruction. If phenol is ingested, the patient should drink large amounts of water and be referred for medical evaluation. Other agents used in dental treatment may also cause mucosal burns (Figure 2-28, *A*).

Phenol is also a component of some over-the-counter products that are advertised for relief of oral pain. Patients frequently misuse these preparations for oral ulcers, and the resulting destruction, in addition to being quite painful, may mask the clinical and microscopic diagnostic characteristics of the original ulcer.

ELECTRIC BURN

Electric burns in the oral area are usually seen in infants and young children who have bitten or chewed a live electric cord or have inserted something into an electric socket. The electric current can cause a great deal of destruction of the

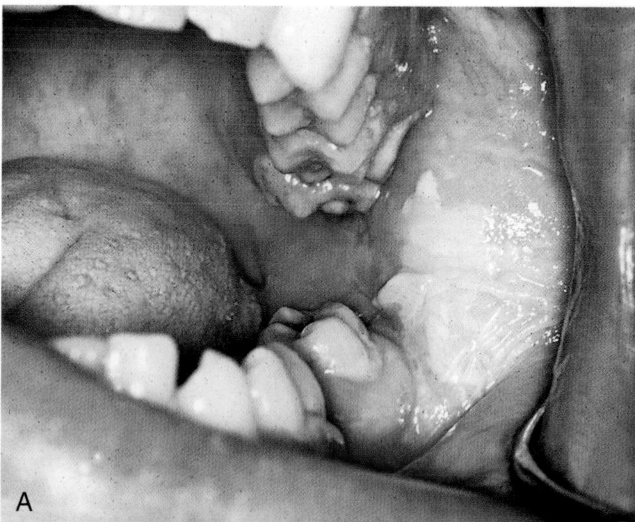

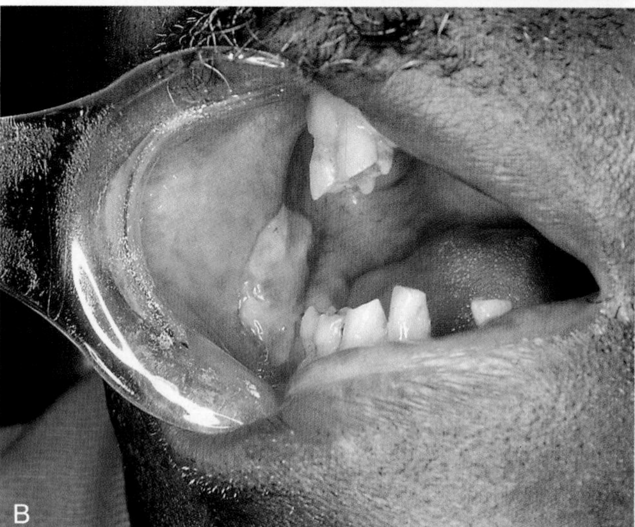

FIGURE 2-27 ■ **A** and **B,** Aspirin burns.

oral tissues. Any tissue in the area may be damaged, including the permanent tooth buds. Permanent disfigurement and scarring may result from this type of injury. Treatment may require a multidisciplinary approach that includes plastic surgery, oral surgery, and orthodontics.

OTHER BURNS

Mucosal burns from hot food are common. They occur most often on the palate and tongue (Figure 2-28, *B*). Over-the-counter products containing hydrogen peroxide or eugenol can also cause mucosal necrosis.

LESIONS ASSOCIATED WITH COCAINE USE

Lesions located at the midline of the hard palate that vary from ulcers to keratotic lesions to exophytic reactive lesions have been reported to result from the smoking of crack

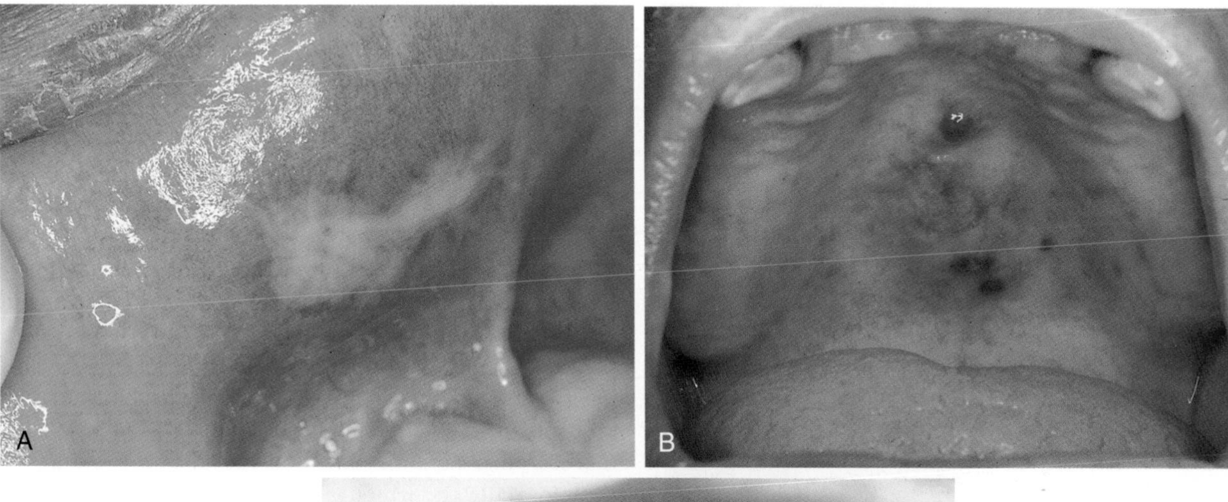

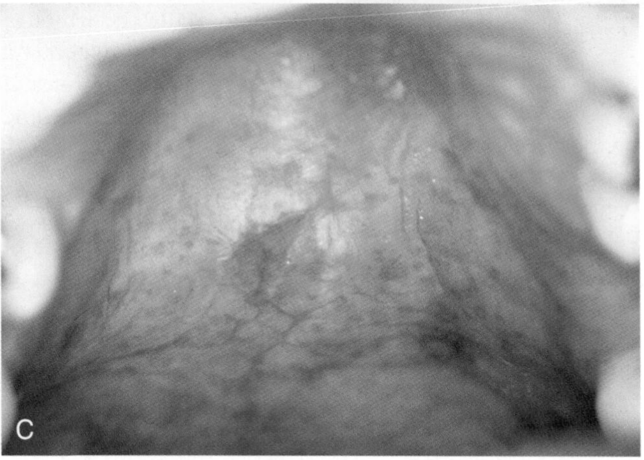

FIGURE 2-28 ■ Mucosal burns. **A,** Chemical burn caused by contact with caustic material during endodontic treatment. **B,** Thermal burn of palate caused by contact with hot soup. **C,** Ulcer of midline of palate caused by heat generated during the use of crack cocaine. (**C** reprinted by permission of ADA Publishing Co., Inc. from Mitchell-Lewis DA et al: Identifying oral lesions associated with crack-cocaine use, *J Am Dent Assoc* 125:1104, 1994. Copyright 1994, American Dental Association.)

cocaine (Figure 2-28, *C*). When crack cocaine is smoked, the crack pipe directs extremely hot smoke to this part of the hard palate. Identification of these lesions is based on their location and the history of recent smoking of crack cocaine. Necrotic ulcers of the tongue and epiglottis related to smoking free-base cocaine have also been reported.

LESIONS FROM SELF-INDUCED INJURIES

Habits of which the patient may or may not be aware can cause injury. Chronic lip, cheek, or tongue biting (see Figure 2-31, B) and trauma to the gingiva by a fingernail (see Figure 2-30, A) are examples of habits that may cause oral lesions. These lesions range from ulceration to epithelial hyperplasia and hyperkeratosis. Ulcers caused by continual self-induced injuries may be of long duration and require biopsy and histologic examination to confirm the diagnosis. Treatment of self-induced lesions depends on the amount and type of destruction and may involve psychotherapy.

HEMATOMA

A **hematoma** is a lesion that results from the accumulation of blood within tissue as a result of trauma. In the oral cavity a hematoma appears as a red-to-purple-to–bluish-gray mass, most frequently seen on the labial or buccal mucosa (Figure 2-29). The size may vary from small to large, depending on the extent of the trauma. No treatment is required because the lesion will spontaneously resolve.

TRAUMATIC ULCER

A **traumatic ulcer** occurs as a result of some form of trauma (Figure 2-30). Sources of trauma vary. Biting the cheek, lip, or tongue may result in a traumatic ulcer, as can irritation from a complete or partial denture or mucosal injury from sharp edges of food. The removal of a dry cotton roll from the oral tissue after a dental procedure can cause a traumatic ulcer, and it is not uncommon to see a patient present for a dental hygiene appointment with a traumatic injury to the gingival

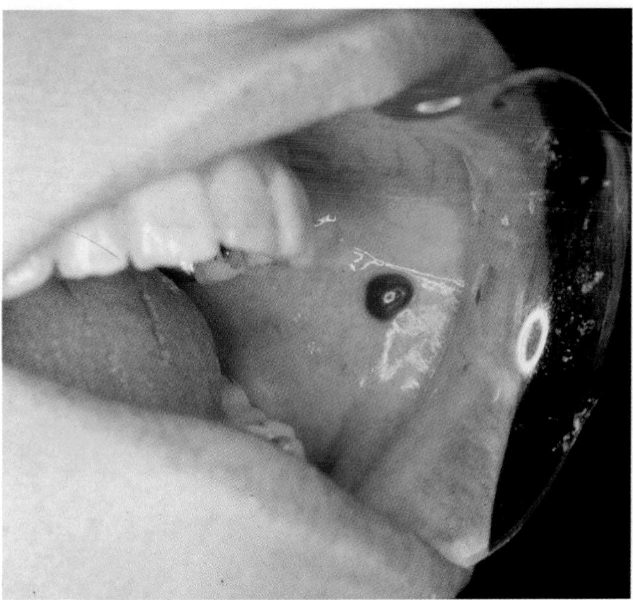

FIGURE 2-29 ■ Hematoma on the buccal mucosa.

tissues or vestibular mucosa that results from overzealous brushing before the appointment. Persistent trauma may result in a hard (indurated), raised lesion called a **traumatic granuloma** (see Figure 2-30, *D*).

Traumatic ulcers are usually diagnosed on the basis of the relationship of the history to the lesion. Healing is usually uneventful and occurs in 7 to 14 days unless the trauma persists. If trauma persists, ulcers may last for weeks to months. The patient is followed until healing is ensured. If an ulcer does not heal in 7 to 14 days, a biopsy is usually indicated. Microscopically the inflammatory infiltrate associated with a traumatic ulcer includes many eosinophils in addition to neutrophils, lymphocytes, and plasma cells. Persistent traumatic granulomas often heal rapidly following biopsy.

FRICTIONAL KERATOSIS

Chronic rubbing or friction against an oral mucosal surface may result in hyperkeratosis, a thickening of the keratin on the surface. This results in an opaque, white appearance of the tissue and represents a protective response. It is analogous to a callus on the skin. An example of frictional keratosis is an increase in surface keratin that results from chronic cheek and tongue chewing and chewing on edentulous alveolar ridges (Figure 2-31). Frictional keratosis is not associated with malignancy.

The diagnosis of frictional keratosis is made by identification of the trauma causing the lesion, elimination of the cause, and observing the resolution of the lesion. The keratosis may take a while to disappear on keratinized surfaces such as the gingiva.

Frictional keratosis must be distinguished from other white lesions. White lesions that are not caused by trauma and arise spontaneously are called **leukoplakia.** Leukoplakia may be a premalignant lesion (see Chapter 7). Biopsy is indicated for any questionable lesion.

LINEA ALBA

Linea alba is a white raised line that forms most commonly on the buccal mucosa at the occlusal plane and is usually considered a variant of normal (Figure 2-32). In some patients the line becomes prominent as a result of a teeth-clenching habit. The line follows the pattern of the teeth at the occlusal plane. Although it is most commonly seen on the buccal mucosa, linea alba may form on the labial mucosa as well. Histologically the white raised line is caused by epithelial hyperplasia and hyperkeratosis. No treatment is indicated. The prominence of linea alba may be helpful in evaluating the severity of the clenching habit.

NICOTINE STOMATITIS

Nicotine stomatitis is a benign lesion on the hard palate most typically associated with pipe and cigar smoking; however, it also occurs with cigarette smoking. The development of the lesion indicates that the patient is smoking heavily. The intensity of smoking required to produce this lesion increases the patient's risk for development of malignancy elsewhere in the oral cavity and respiratory tract.

The initial response of the palatal mucosa to the heat from these substances is an erythematous appearance. Over time keratinization occurs and results in increasing opacification. After the increase in keratinization, raised red dots are seen at the openings of the ducts of the minor salivary glands on the palatal surface (Figure 2-33). The minor salivary glands become inflamed as a result of obstruction by keratin at the mucosal opening of the ducts. The palate may develop a very similar clinical appearance as a result of the chronic intake of very hot liquids.

TOBACCO POUCH KERATOSIS

Individuals who chew tobacco may develop a white lesion in the area where the tobacco is habitually placed. The mucobuccal fold is the most common location. The epithelium usually has a granular or wrinkled appearance in early lesions. Long-standing lesions may be more opaquely white and have a corrugated surface (Figure 2-34). The lesion often disappears when the tobacco is no longer placed in the area.

Long-term exposure to smokeless tobacco has been associated with an increased risk of squamous cell carcinoma. Lesions that do not resolve require biopsy and may show atypical dysplastic epithelium. In addition, the patient with this habit has an increased risk of caries, periodontal disease, attrition, and staining.

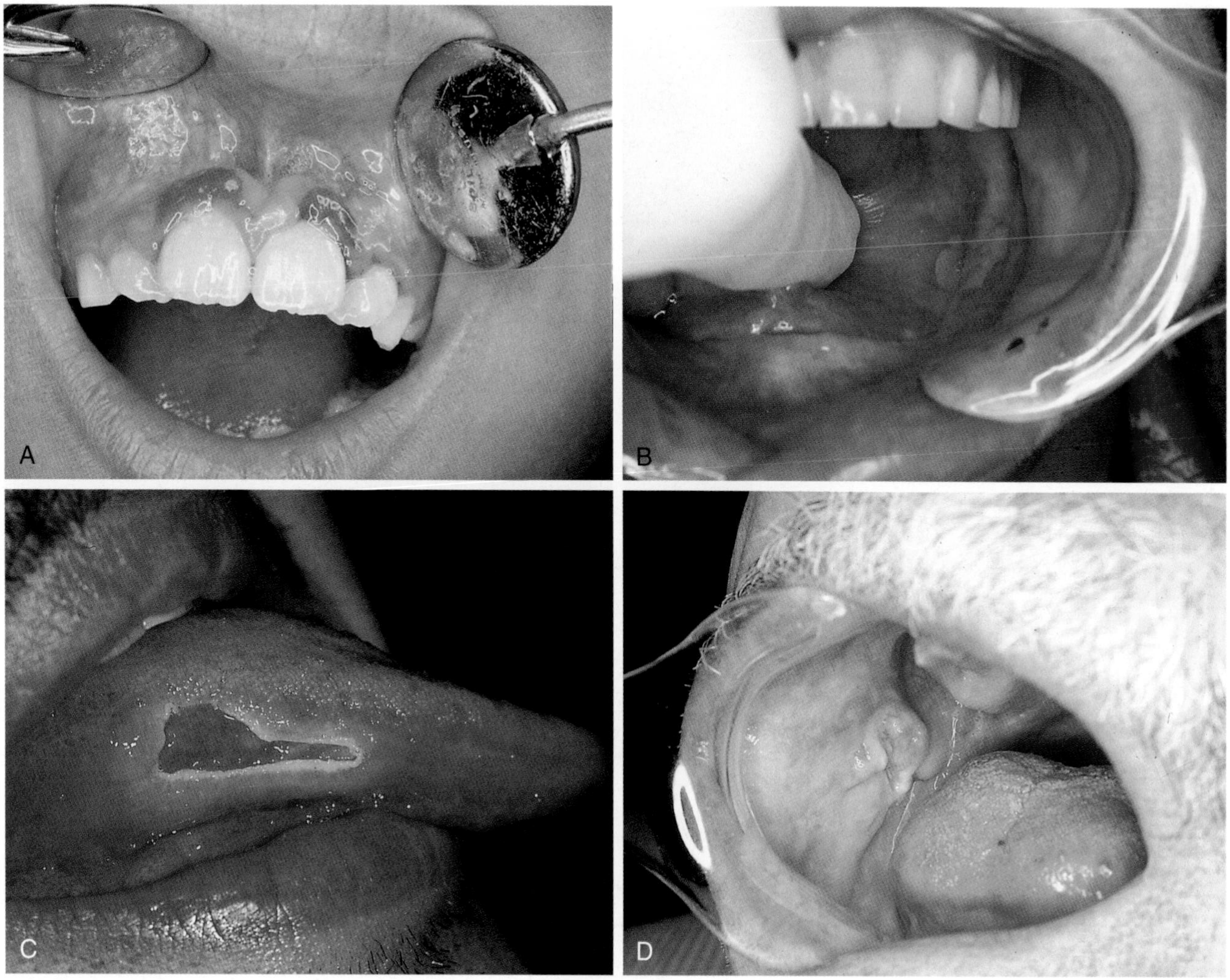

FIGURE 2-30 ■ **A,** Traumatic ulceration caused by irritation of gingiva by fingernails. **B,** Traumatic ulcer caused by denture. **C,** Traumatic ulcer on lateral tongue caused by chronic trauma to tongue by teeth. **D,** Traumatic ulcer (traumatic granuloma) of buccal mucosa.

TRAUMATIC NEUROMA

A **traumatic neuroma** is a lesion caused by injury to a peripheral nerve. Nerve tissue is encased in a sheath composed of Schwann cells and their fibers. When this sheath is disrupted, the nerve loses its framework. When a nerve and its sheath are damaged, the proximal end of the damaged nerve proliferates into a mass of nerve and Schwann cells mixed with dense fibrous scar tissue. In the oral cavity injury to a nerve may occur from injection of local anesthesia, surgery, or other sources of trauma.

Traumatic neuromas are often painful. The pain may range from pain on palpation to severe and constant pain. Most traumatic neuromas occur in adults, and the mental foramen is the most common location. However, a traumatic neuroma may occur in other locations as well. Although the clinical features, particularly the pain that is characteristic, may suggest that a lesion is a traumatic neuroma, the diagnosis is made on the basis of a biopsy and microscopic examination. Traumatic neuromas are treated by surgical excision, and recurrence is rare.

AMALGAM TATTOO

An **amalgam tattoo** is a flat, bluish-gray lesion of the oral mucosa that results from the introduction of amalgam particles into the tissues (Figure 2-35, *A*). This may occur at the time of placement or removal of an amalgam restoration or at the time of tooth extraction if a piece of amalgam fractures off a restoration and remains in the tissue. The metallic particles disperse in the connective tissue and result in a permanent area of pigmentation. Over time the mercury-silver-tin amalgam changes, and it is mainly silver that remains in the tissue.

Amalgam tattoos may be seen in any location in the oral cavity but are most commonly found on the gingiva or edentulous alveolar ridge. The posterior region of the mandible is the most common location.

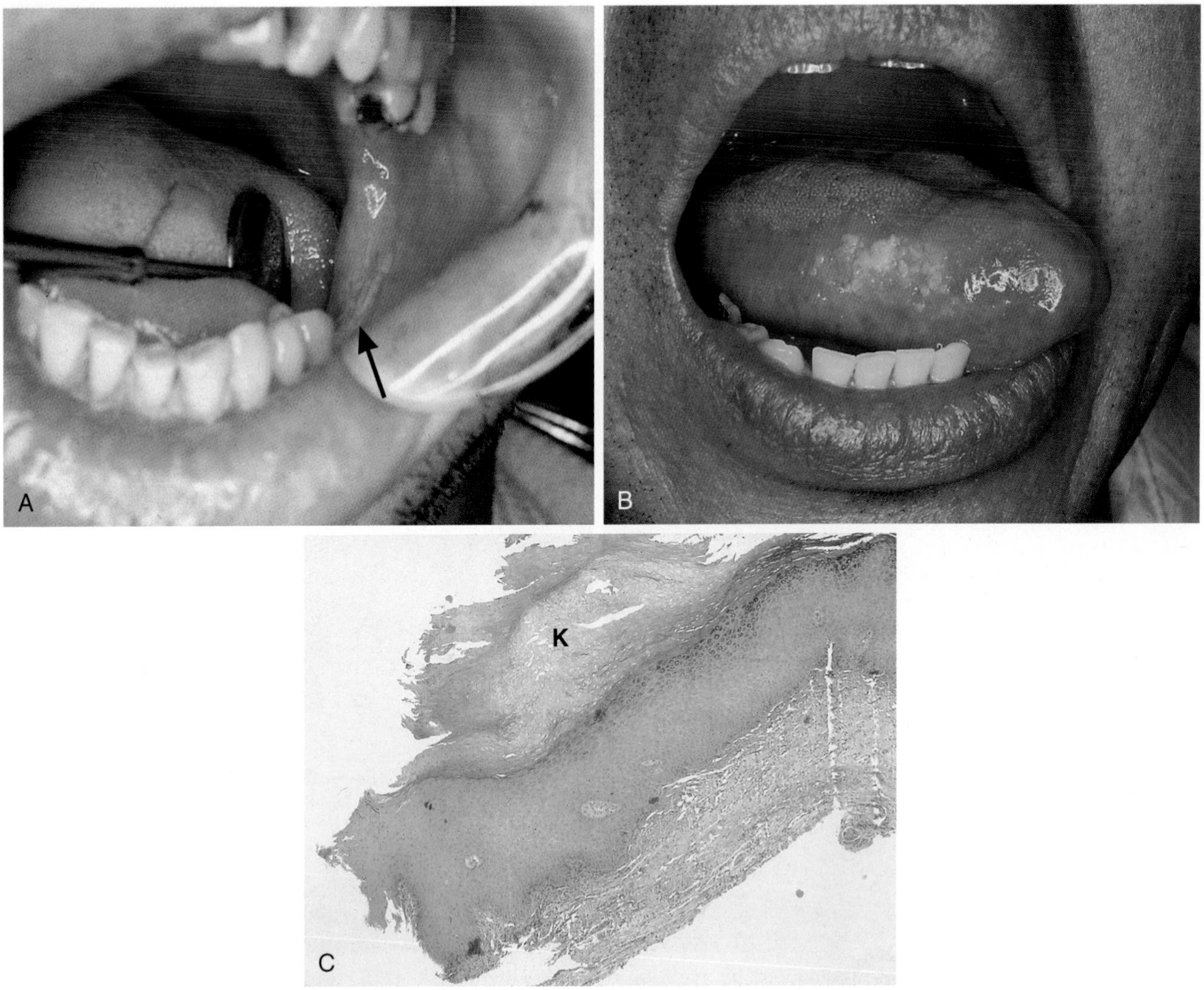

FIGURE 2-31 ■ Frictional keratosis caused by an opposing third molar (indicated by *arrow*) **(A)**, and chronic tongue chewing **(B)**. **C,** Microscopic appearance of hyperkeratosis (low magnification) showing an increase in surface keratin *(K)*.

An amalgam tattoo is usually diagnosed on the basis of clinical appearance of the pigmented area. Often the particles of amalgam can be seen on a periapical radiograph (Figure 2-35, *B*). As amalgam particles diffuse in the tissue over time, the size of the amalgam tattoo may increase. Biopsy may be necessary to distinguish an amalgam tattoo from a melanocytic lesion, particularly if it is located in an area other than the gingiva or alveolar ridge. Once the diagnosis of amalgam tattoo has been established, treatment is generally not indicated.

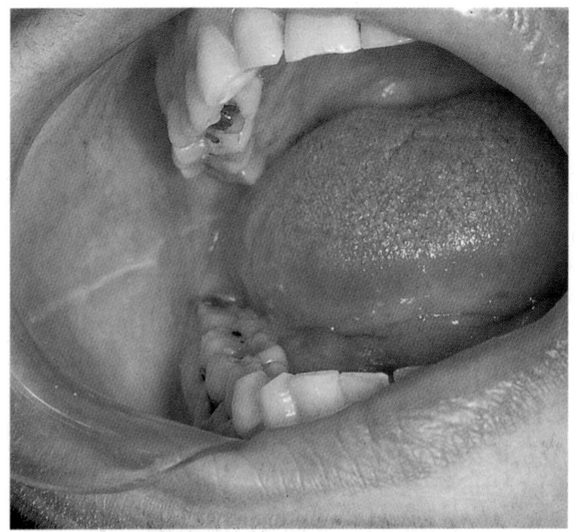

FIGURE 2-32 ■ Linea alba.

MELANOSIS

Normal physiologic pigmentation of the oral mucosa is common, particularly in dark-skinned individuals (see Figures 1-18 and 1-51). Melanin pigmentation may also occur after inflammation (Figure 2-36). The **oral melanotic macule** is

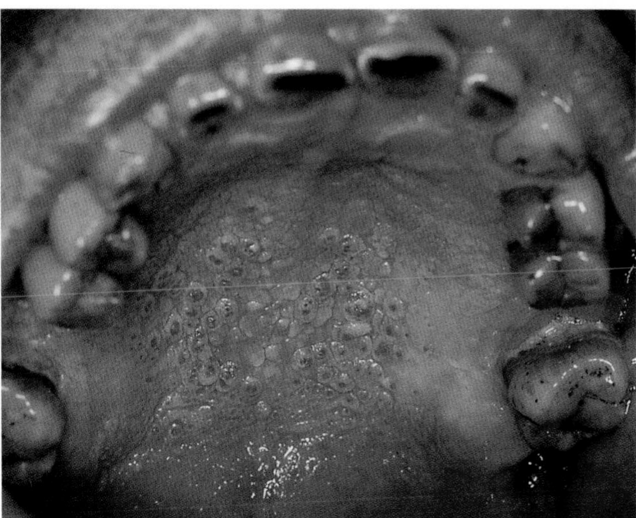

FIGURE 2-33 ■ Nicotine stomatitis.

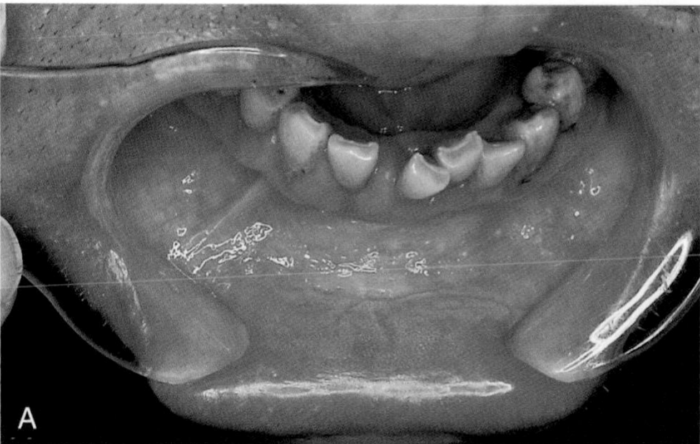

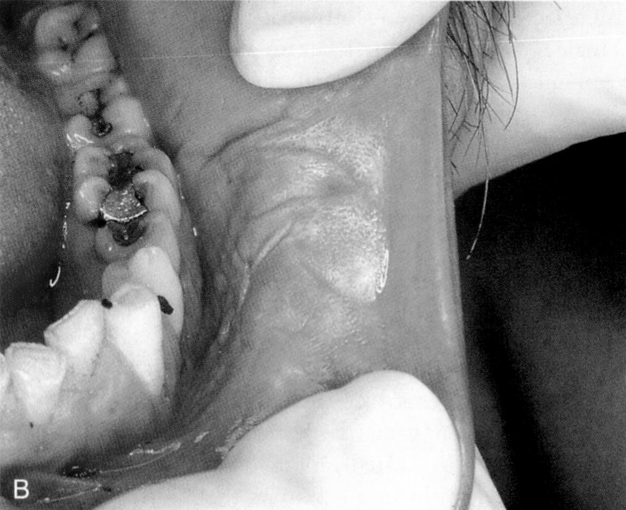

FIGURE 2-34 ■ Tobacco pouch keratosis. Note the rough texture of the surface. **A,** Labial mucosa. **B,** Anterior buccal mucosa.

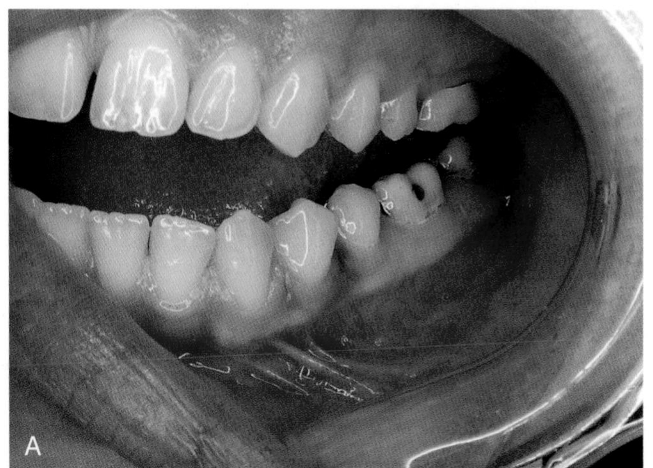

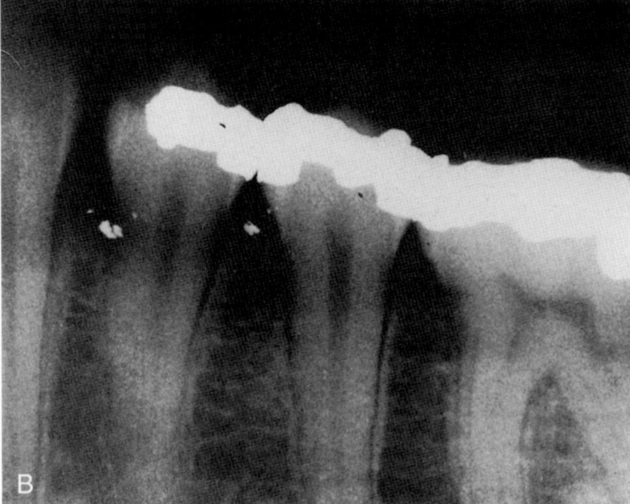

FIGURE 2-35 ■ **A,** This bluish-gray pigmentation of the gingiva is an amalgam tattoo. **B,** Periapical radiograph showing amalgam particles in the gingival tissue.

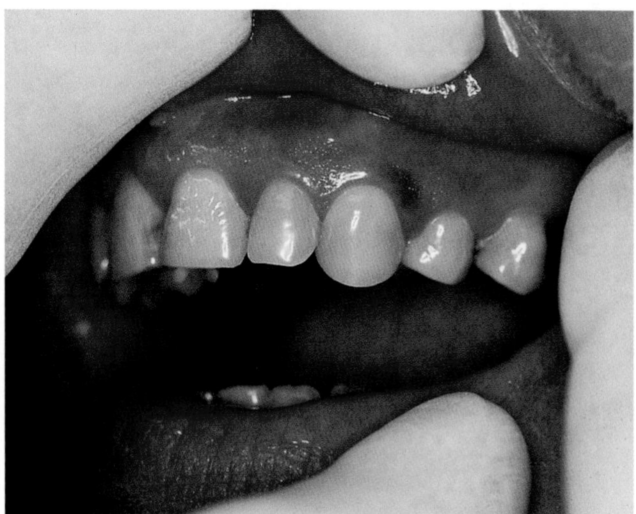

FIGURE 2-36 ■ Posttraumatic melanin pigmentation. Area of melanin pigmentation on the gingiva after healing of a traumatic injury.

a flat, well-circumscribed brown lesion of unknown cause. These are usually small (<1 cm in diameter) and may require biopsy and histologic examination for diagnosis. A similar lesion may occur on the vermilion of the lips. When occurring on the lips, the lesion may darken with exposure to sunlight.

Another type of melanosis is called **smoker's melanosis** or **smoking-associated melanosis.** In this type of melanosis the melanin pigmentation is associated with smoking, and the intensity is related to the amount and duration of smoking. The pigmentation fades when smoking is discontinued. However, this may take months to years. The anterior labial gingiva is the most commonly affected site. Women are affected more frequently than men. A relationship to female hormones and birth control pills has been suggested. Oral mucosal melanin pigmentation may also be associated with genetic, bone, and systemic diseases (see Chapters 6, 8, and 9).

SOLAR CHEILITIS

Sun exposure, particularly in fair-skinned individuals, can result in degeneration of the tissue of the lips, called **solar cheilitis** (Figure 2-37). Solar cheilitis is also called **actinic cheilitis.** The development of this condition is related to the total cumulative exposure to sunlight and the amount of skin pigmentation; it may be seen in individuals of various ages. The lower lip is usually more severely involved than the upper lip. The epithelium is thinner than normal and often exhibits abnormal maturational changes (epithelial dysplasia). Degenerative changes are seen microscopically in the connective tissue.

The vermilion of the lips is affected. The color appears pale pinkish and mottled. The interface between the lips and the skin is indistinct, with fissures appearing at right angles to the skin and vermilion junction. The lips are dry and cracked.

No specific treatment is indicated. However, a strong relationship exists between these epithelial and connective tissue changes and the development of basal cell carcinoma and squamous cell carcinoma of the skin and squamous cell carcinoma of the vermilion of the lip. The risk is greater for the lower lip than the upper lip. Smoking may increase this risk. Biopsy is indicated for persistent scaling or ulceration. Identification of patients at high risk and with early indications of sun damage can be helpful in preventing future lesions. Patients at risk should be advised to avoid sun exposure and use sun-blocking agents for protection.

MUCOCELE

A **mucocele** is a lesion that forms when a salivary gland duct is severed and the mucous salivary gland secretion spills into the adjacent connective tissue. An inflammatory response occurs, granulation tissue forms, and the mucus is walled off to form a cystlike structure lined by compressed granulation tissue. This is not a true cyst because the cystic space is not lined by epithelium.

A mucocele presents as a swelling in the tissue that often increases and decreases in size over time. The lower lip is the most common site of occurrence (Figure 2-38). However, mucoceles may form in any area of the oral mucosa in which minor salivary glands are found. On the lower lip they are usually lateral to the midline. If a mucocele is near the surface, it may appear bluish. The color of the mucosa is normal if the mucocele is deeper in the tissue. A mucoepidermoid carcinoma may clinically resemble a mucocele and should be considered in the differential diagnosis. Most mucoceles occur in children and adolescents. However, they may occur in adults as well. If they are chronic or persistent, treatment is by surgical excision and removal of the adjacent minor salivary glands.

Occasionally an epithelium-lined cystic structure occurs in association with a salivary gland duct. This is also called a **mucocele, mucous cyst,** or **mucous retention cyst** (Figure 2-39) and occurs much less frequently than the type described previously. Most of these are not true cysts but rather dilated salivary gland ducts that are believed to develop as a result of salivary duct obstruction. A ballooning of the duct occurs, which appears microscopically as an epithelium-lined cyst. Mucous cysts usually occur in adults older than 50 years of age. They may occur anywhere in the oral cavity where minor salivary glands are found and are treated by removal of the affected minor salivary glands.

Ranula is a term used for a mucocele-like lesion that forms unilaterally on the floor of the mouth (Figure 2-40). It is associated with the ducts of the sublingual and submandibular glands. The name *ranula* is derived from *rana,* the

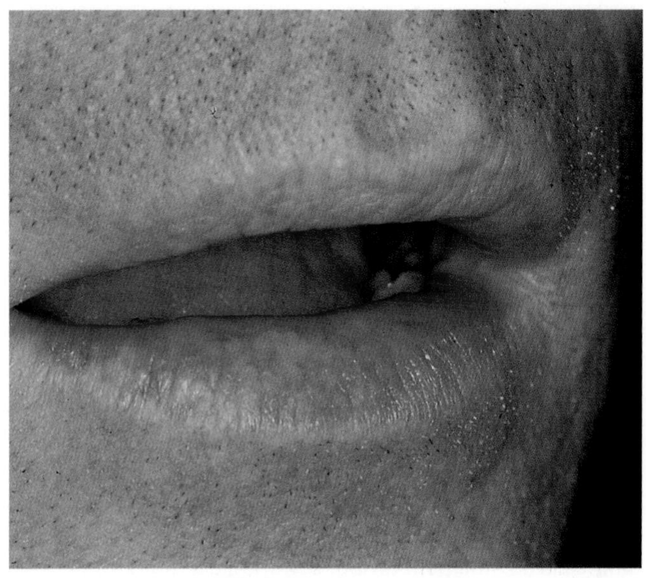

FIGURE 2-37 ■ Solar cheilitis.

Latin word for frog. The clinical appearance of the ranula resembles the outpouching that occurs under the jaw of the frog when croaking. Although obstruction of the duct is considered to be the most likely cause for its development, histologically a ranula may resemble either a mucocele or a mucous cyst. Ranulas are treated by surgery; and the cause of obstruction, often a salivary gland stone, must be removed.

NECROTIZING SIALOMETAPLASIA

Necrotizing sialometaplasia is a benign condition of the salivary glands characterized by moderately painful swelling and ulceration in the affected area (Figure 2-41). Histologically necrosis of the salivary glands is seen. The salivary gland duct epithelium is replaced by squamous epithelium (metaplasia) and appears microscopically as islands of squamous epithelium deep in the connective tissue. If the duration of the ulcer is prolonged, a biopsy is needed to establish the diagnosis. However, the ulcer heals spontaneously by secondary intention, usually within a few weeks. The junction of the hard and soft palates is most often affected. Necrotizing sialometaplasia is thought to result from blockage of the blood supply to the area of the lesion.

SIALOLITH

A **sialolith** is a salivary gland stone. Sialoliths occur in both major and minor salivary glands and form by precipitation of calcium salts around a central core. They may cause

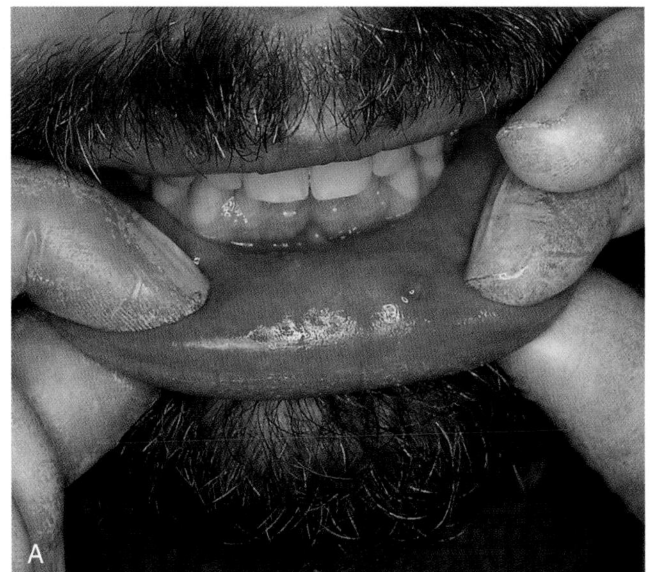

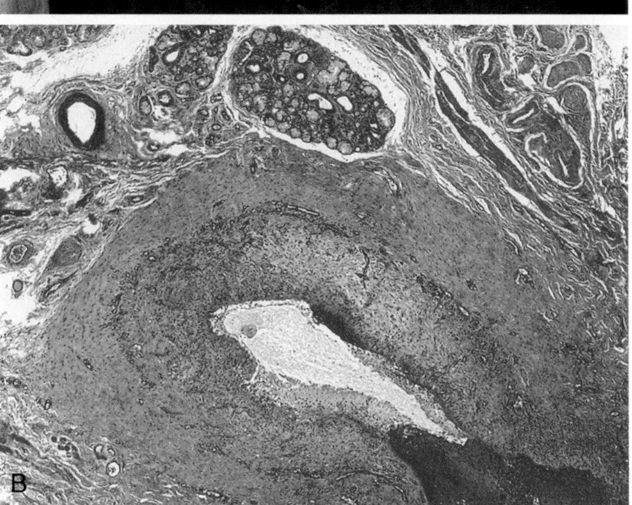

FIGURE 2-38 ■ Mucocele of the lower lip. **A,** Fluid-filled lesion is seen on the lower lip. **B,** Microscopic appearance of a mucocele showing a cystlike space lined by granulation tissue (low magnification).

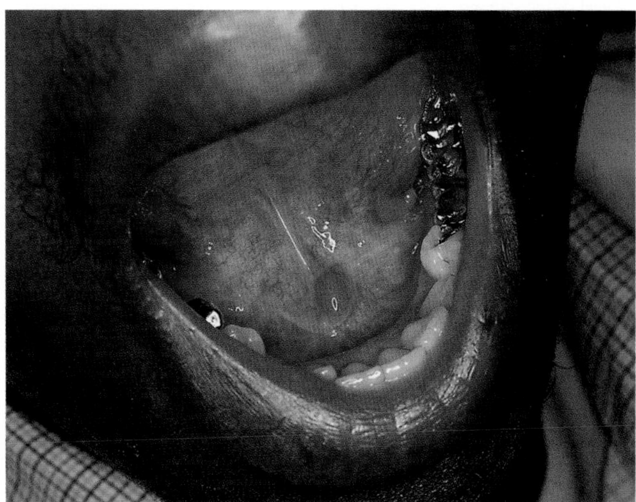

FIGURE 2-39 ■ Mucocele (mucous cyst) of the floor of the mouth.

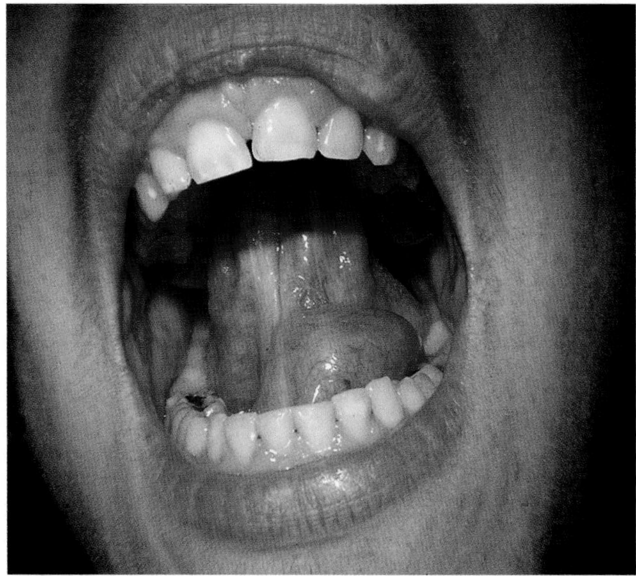

FIGURE 2-40 ■ Ranula.

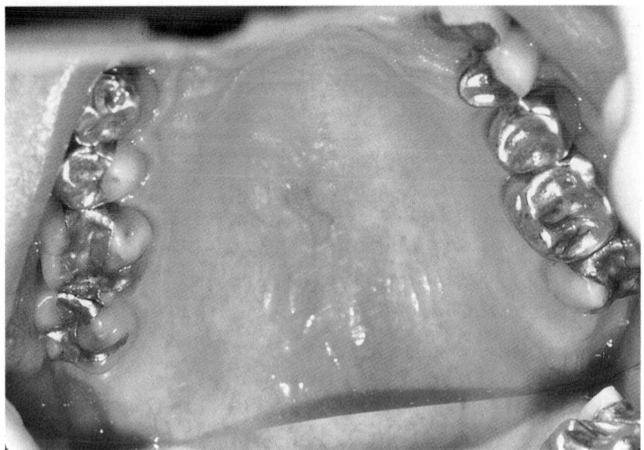

FIGURE 2-41 ■ Necrotizing sialometaplasia.

obstruction of the involved salivary gland; when they occur in the floor of the mouth, they can often be seen as a radiopaque structure on an occlusal radiograph (Figure 2-42).

ACUTE AND CHRONIC SIALADENITIS

Both **acute** and **chronic sialadenitis** may occur as a result of obstruction of a salivary gland duct. They may also occur as a result of infection. In some cases the cause cannot be identified. Sialadenitis presents as a painful swelling of the involved salivary gland, usually one of the major glands. Diagnosis may require injection of a radiopaque dye into the gland, followed by taking a radiograph of the gland (sialography). Antibiotics may be necessary in cases of infection.

REACTIVE CONNECTIVE TISSUE HYPERPLASIA

Reactive connective tissue hyperplasia consists of proliferating, exuberant granulation tissue and dense fibrous connective tissue. These lesions result from overzealous repair. They may occur as a response to a single event or as a chronic low-grade injury. The reason for the exuberant overgrowth of reparative tissue is not known.

Periapical inflammation, radicular cyst, and **internal** and **external tooth resorption** are included in this classification because they are also examples of lesions associated with proliferating inflamed tissue.

PYOGENIC GRANULOMA

A **pyogenic granuloma** is a commonly occurring intraoral lesion that is characterized by a proliferation of connective tissue containing numerous blood vessels and inflammatory cells. It occurs as a response to injury. The term *pyogenic granuloma* is a misnomer. The lesion does not produce pus (pyogenic) and is not a true granuloma.

The pyogenic granuloma (Figure 2-43) is usually ulcerated and soft to palpation and bleeds easily. It is deep red to purple because of the vascularity of the proliferating tissue. It is generally elevated and may be either sessile or pedunculated. When ulcerated, the fibrin membrane on the surface appears yellowish white. The gingiva is the most common location of occurrence, but the lesion also occurs in other areas such as the lips, tongue, and buccal mucosa. Pyogenic granulomas may vary considerably in size, from a few millimeters to several centimeters. They usually develop rapidly and then remain static. Although they are most common in teenagers and young adults, they may occur at any age. Some studies show predominance in females.

Pyogenic granulomas often occur in pregnant women and have been called **pregnancy tumors** (Figure 2-44). The lesions are identical to those seen in men and nonpregnant women and may be caused by changing hormonal levels and increased response to plaque. However, they often regress after delivery. Similar gingival lesions also occur during puberty.

The pyogenic granuloma is treated by surgical excision if it does not resolve spontaneously. Occasionally the lesion may recur if the injurious agent (e.g., calculus) remains.

PERIPHERAL GIANT CELL GRANULOMA

A **giant cell granuloma** is a lesion that contains many multinucleated giant cells and well-vascularized connective tissue. Red blood cells and chronic inflammatory cells are also seen in this lesion. The cause of the giant cell granuloma is not clear. It occurs only in the jaws, seems to originate from the periodontal ligament or the periosteum, and is thought to be a response to injury. The giant cell granuloma occurs both on the gingiva (peripheral giant cell granuloma) and within bone (central giant cell granuloma). The term **peripheral** pertains to lesions occurring outside the bone, generally on the gingiva or alveolar mucosa, and the term **central** refers to a lesion occurring within the maxilla and mandible. The description of the central giant cell granuloma is included in Chapter 8.

The **peripheral giant cell granuloma** always occurs on the gingiva or alveolar process, usually anterior to the molars. It is considered a reactive lesion, usually occurring as a result of local irritating factors. Peripheral giant cell granulomas associated with dental implants have been reported. The peripheral giant cell granuloma may resemble the pyogenic granuloma in clinical appearance (Figure 2-45). Peripheral giant cell granulomas may vary in size from 0.5 to 1.5 cm in diameter and are usually dark red because of the numerous blood vessels present. The lesion may occur at any age but has been reported to be more frequent in people between 40 and 60 years of age and more common in women than men. Peripheral giant cell granulomas may cause superficial destruction of the alveolar bone; they are treated by surgical excision of the lesion and generally do not recur.

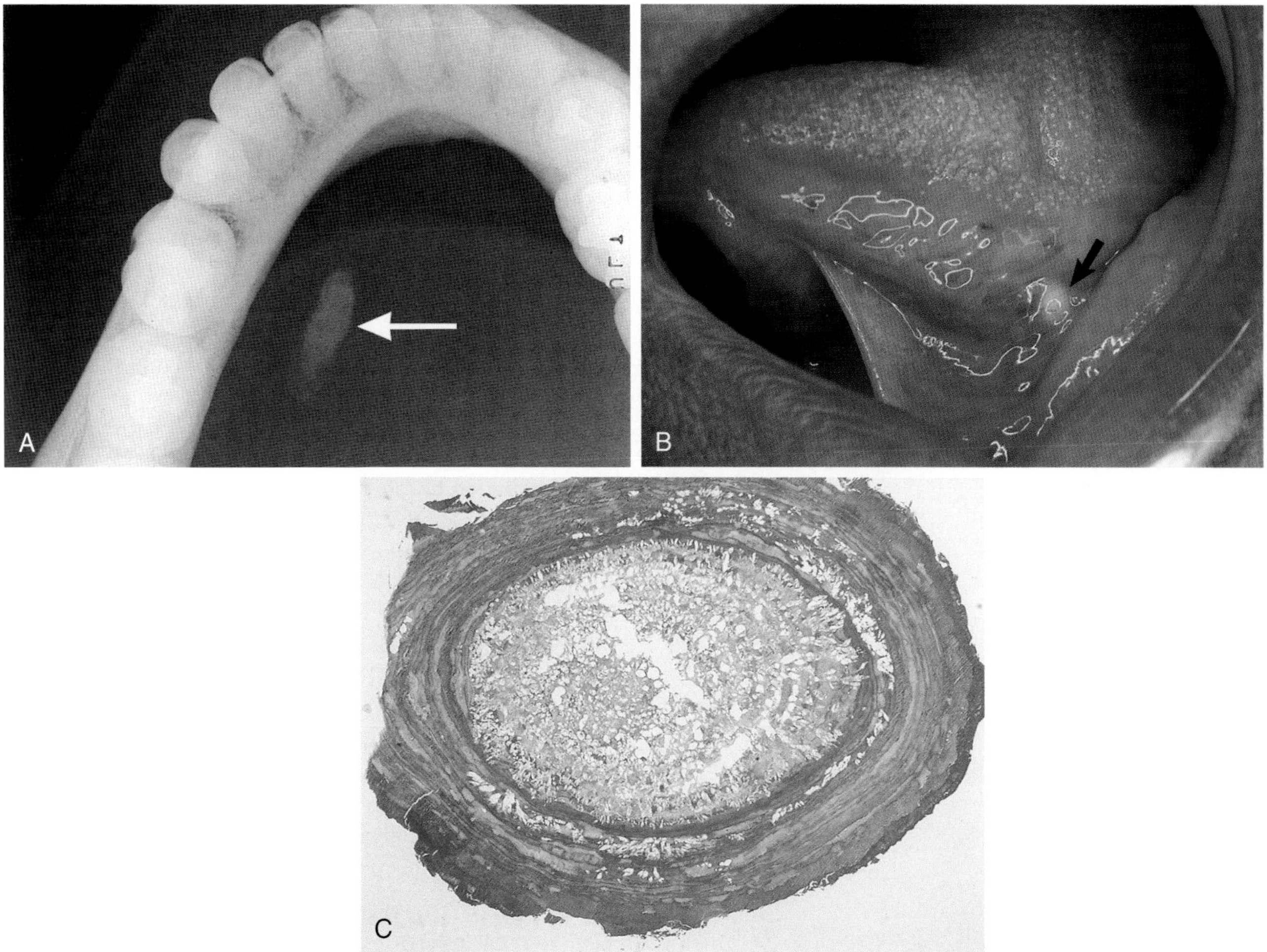

FIGURE 2-42 ■ Sialoliths. **A,** Occlusal radiograph showing a sialolith *(arrow)* in Wharton's duct. **B**, Sialolith *(arrow)* in a minor salivary gland on the floor of the mouth. **C,** Microscopic appearance of a sialolith showing concentric rings. (**A** courtesy Dr. Barry Wolinsky.)

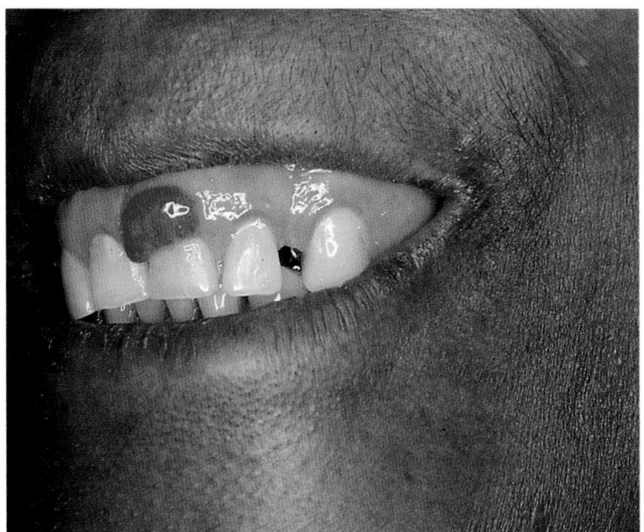

FIGURE 2-43 ■ Pyogenic granuloma.

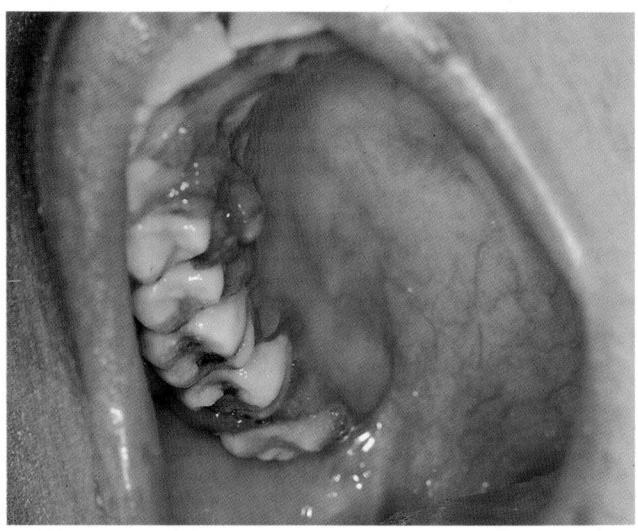

FIGURE 2-44 ■ Pyogenic granuloma of pregnancy (pregnancy tumor).

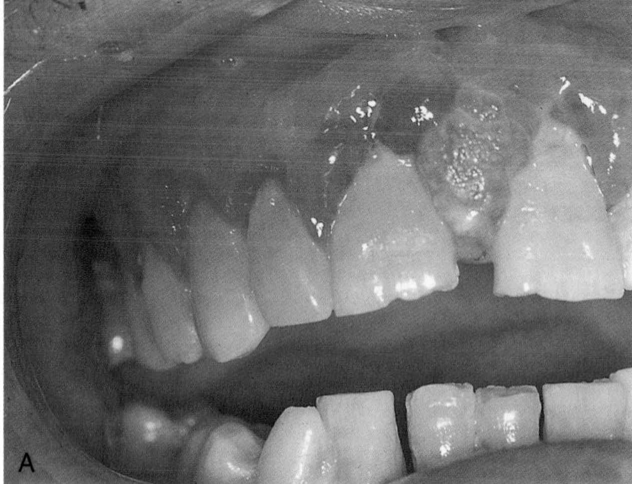

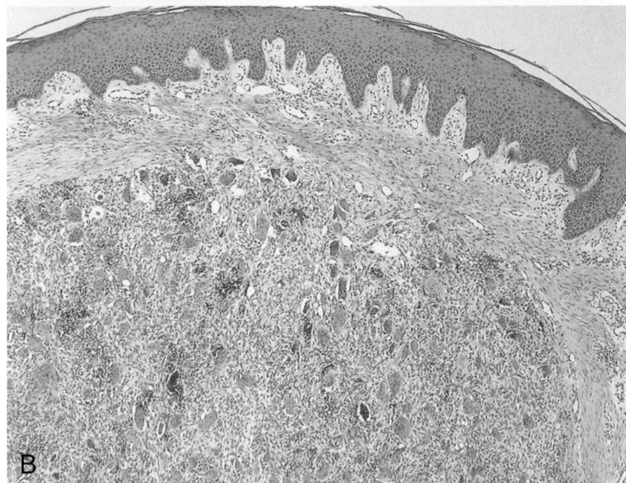

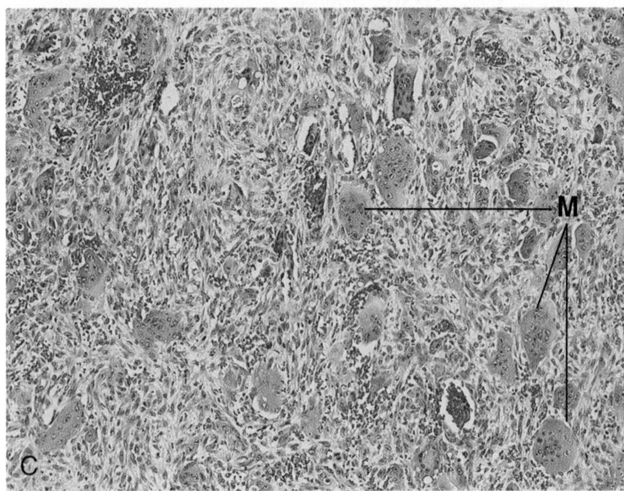

FIGURE 2-45 ■ **A,** Peripheral giant cell granuloma. **B** and **C,** Microscopic appearance of a peripheral giant cell granuloma. Low magnification **(A)** shows the surface epithelium. Higher magnification **(C)** shows multinucleated giant cells *(M),* capillaries, and fibroblasts.

IRRITATION FIBROMA

The irritation fibroma (also known as **fibroma** or **traumatic fibroma**) is a broad-based, persistent exophytic lesion that is composed of dense, scarlike connective tissue containing few blood vessels (Figure 2-46). It occurs as a result of chronic trauma or an episode of trauma. The irritation fibroma is usually a small lesion. Most are less than 1 cm in diameter; fibromas greater than 2 cm in diameter are rare. The fibroma occurs most frequently on the buccal mucosa. It also occurs on the gingival, tongue, lips, and palate. The color of the irritation fibroma is usually lighter than that of the surrounding mucosa. The surface is covered by stratified squamous epithelium and may appear opaque and white if it has a thick keratin surface, or it may be ulcerated because of local secondary trauma.

An irritation fibroma is removed surgically. Many benign soft tissue tumors resemble the irritation fibroma in clinical appearance. Excision and microscopic examination of the tissue are important for diagnosis if the clinician is unsure about the nature of the lesion. Irritation fibromas usually do not recur at the same site, but additional lesions may occur as a response to additional trauma.

The **peripheral ossifying fibroma** is a common gingival lesion. The cause is not known. It is thought to originate from the cells forming the periodontal ligament. However, it is not clear whether this lesion is a reactive or neoplastic lesion. The peripheral ossifying fibroma is included in Chapter 7.

DENTURE-INDUCED FIBROUS HYPERPLASIA

Denture-induced fibrous hyperplasia is commonly called **epulis fissuratum** or **inflammatory hyperplasia.** This lesion is caused by an ill-fitting denture and is located in the vestibule along the denture border. It is composed of dense, fibrous connective tissue surfaced by stratified squamous epithelium, the same type of tissue seen in the irritation fibroma. The lesion is usually somewhat larger than the irritation fibroma. It is arranged in elongated folds of tissue into which the denture flange fits (Figure 2-47). The surface of the lesion is often ulcerated. Because this lesion does not resolve even with prolonged removal of the denture, treatment involves surgical removal of the excess tissue and construction of a new denture.

PAPILLARY HYPERPLASIA OF THE PALATE

Papillary hyperplasia of the palate, or **palatal papillomatosis,** is a form of denture stomatitis. It is almost always associated with a removable full or partial denture or an orthodontic appliance. The palatal mucosa, most commonly the vault area, is covered by multiple erythematous papillary projections that give the area a granular or "cobblestone" appearance (Figure 2-48).

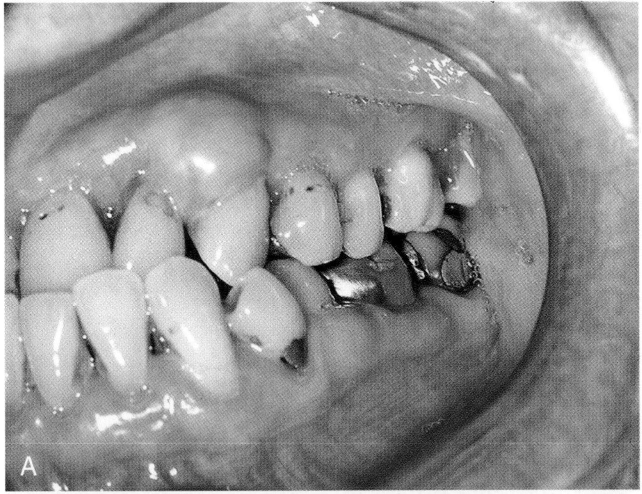

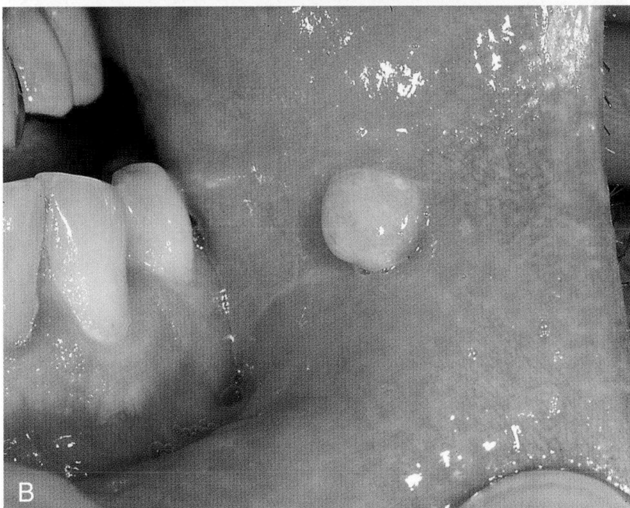

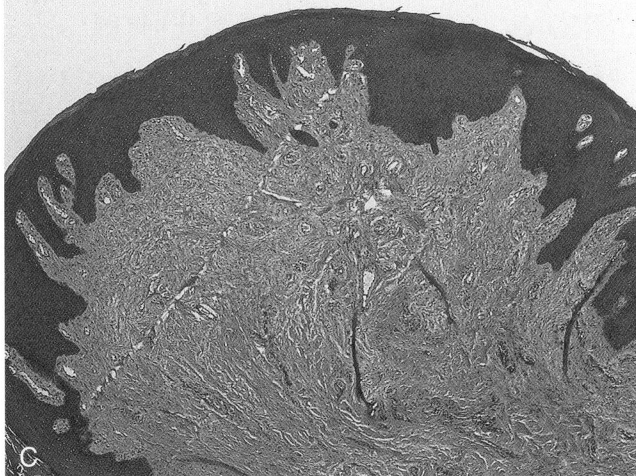

FIGURE 2-46 ■ Irritation fibroma. **A,** Development of fibroma followed by the healing of a periodontal abscess. **B,** Irritation fibroma of the buccal mucosa. **C,** Microscopic appearance of a fibroma. (**A** courtesy Dr. Murray Schwartz.)

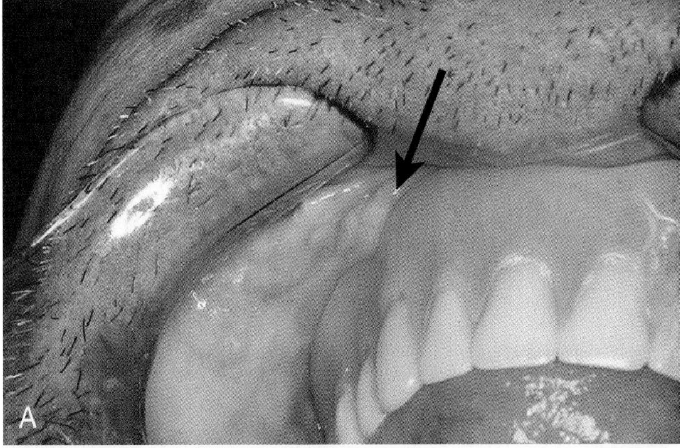

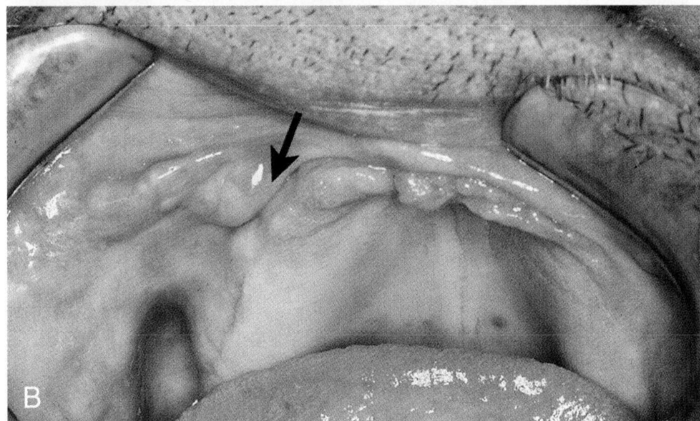

FIGURE 2-47 ■ Denture-induced fibrous hyperplasia (epulis fissuratum). **A,** With denture; **B,** without denture.

Each of the papillary projections consists of fibrous connective tissue, usually chronically inflamed and surfaced by stratified squamous epithelium. The precise cause of this type of hyperplasia is not known. It is usually related to an ill-fitting upper denture or other removable prosthetic device that is worn continuously, 24 hours a day. Surgical removal of the hyperplastic papillary tissue before construction of a new denture generally is necessary.

GINGIVAL ENLARGEMENT

Gingival enlargement is characterized by an increase in the bulk of the free and attached gingiva, especially that involving the interdental papillae (Figure 2-49). No stippling is seen, and the gingival margins are rounded. The tissue consistency may vary from soft to firm, and the appearance may vary from erythematous to a normal pink color, depending on the degree of inflammation. Gingival enlargement may be generalized or localized and may vary from mild focal enlargement of interdental papillae to severe generalized gingival enlargement that may cover the crowns of the teeth. The enlarged tissue may appear red, a normal mucosal color, or paler, depending on the amount of inflammation and degree of vascularity. Although generally called **gingival hyperplasia,** enlargement of the gingiva may also be the result of hypertrophy.

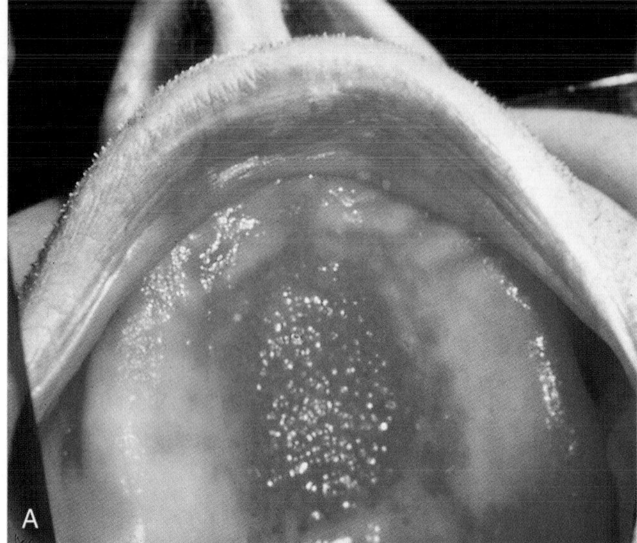

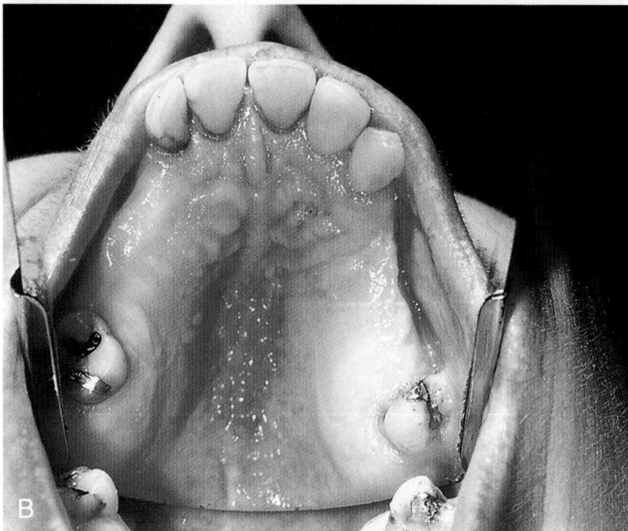

FIGURE 2-48 ■ Papillary hyperplasia of the palate. **A,** Full denture. **B,** Partial denture. (Courtesy Dr. Edward V. Zegarelli.)

Most cases are the result of an unusual tissue response to chronic inflammation associated with local irritants such as plaque or calculus. Hormonal changes such as those occurring in pregnancy and puberty and certain drugs such as phenytoin, calcium channel blockers, and cyclosporine can increase the tissue response to local factors (see Chapter 9). Hereditary forms of gingival fibromatosis occur, beginning in early childhood (see Chapter 6). In some cases the cause of gingival hyperplasia cannot be identified.

If the tissue is inflamed and bleeds easily, biopsy and histologic examination may be necessary to rule out the gingival enlargement that may occur in individuals with leukemia (see Chapter 7).

Gingivoplasty (reshaping the gingiva) or gingivectomy (removing gingival tissue) may be necessary to recontour the gingival tissue. Meticulous oral hygiene is helpful in reducing additional hyperplasia.

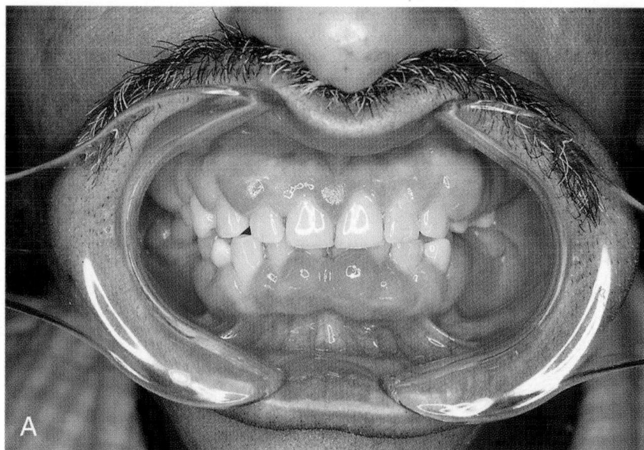

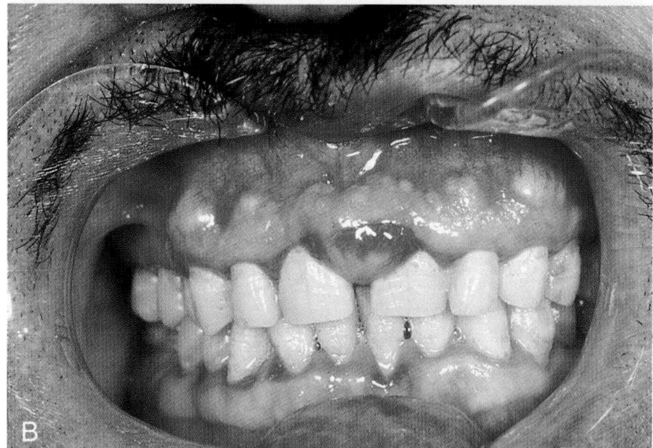

FIGURE 2-49 ■ Gingival enlargement. **A,** Fibrous; **B,** inflamed.

CHRONIC HYPERPLASTIC PULPITIS

Chronic hyperplastic pulpitis, or **pulp polyp,** is an excessive proliferation of chronically inflamed dental pulp tissue. In children and young adults it occurs in teeth with large, open carious lesions; primary and permanent molars are often affected. Chronic hyperplastic pulpitis appears as a red or pink nodule of tissue that often fills the entire cavity in the tooth, with tissue protruding from the pulp chamber (Figure 2-50). It is usually asymptomatic; because the hyperplastic tissue contains so few nerves, it is usually insensitive to manipulation. The proliferation of pulp tissue rather than pulpal necrosis, which can also result from dental caries, may be related to the large root opening and blood supply of the tooth involved.

The hyperplastic tissue is granulation tissue. Inflammatory cells, primarily lymphocytes and plasma cells and sometimes neutrophils, are commonly present. The tissue is generally surfaced by stratified squamous epithelium. Because no epithelium exists in normal pulp tissue, this epithelium is thought to result from desquamation of the surface oral mucosa. Chronic hyperplastic pulpitis is treated by either extraction or endodontic treatment of the involved tooth.

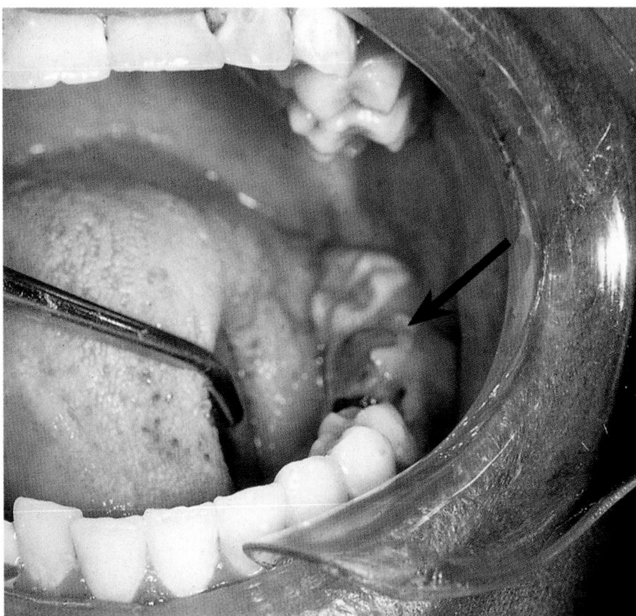

FIGURE 2-50 ■ Chronic hyperplastic pulpitis (pulp polyp) *(arrow).*

INFLAMMATORY PERIAPICAL LESIONS

Dental caries or trauma to a tooth may result in a variety of responses: inflammation, infection, chronic hyperplastic pulpitis, and necrosis of the dental pulp. The inflammatory process begins in the dental pulp and then extends into the periapical area (the area surrounding the apical portion of the tooth root at the site of the apical foramen). This condition occurs because, once the inflammatory process has been established in the dental pulp, the only route it can follow is through the root canal into the periapical area. The presence of accessory canals may lead to areas of inflammation located on the lateral portion of the tooth root.

PERIAPICAL ABSCESS

An acute **periapical abscess** is composed of a purulent exudate, or pus, surrounded by connective tissue containing neutrophils and lymphocytes. The patient complains of severe pain, which is the result of inflammation. The inflammatory exudate puts pressure on nerves, and chemical mediators can also cause pain. The periapical abscess may develop directly from the inflammation in the pulp, but it more commonly develops in an area of previously existing chronic inflammation. The pus that forms seeks a path of least resistance and finds either a channel or a fistula out of the tissue, or it spreads to contiguous areas through oral and facial tissue spaces (see Figure 2-3). The tooth associated with the abscess is usually quite painful and may be slightly extruded from its socket. If the acute abscess develops directly from pulpal inflammation, there may be no radiographic changes except for a slight thickening of the apical periodontal ligament space. If the abscess develops in a preexisting area of periapical chronic inflammation, a distinct radiolucent area is seen at the apex.

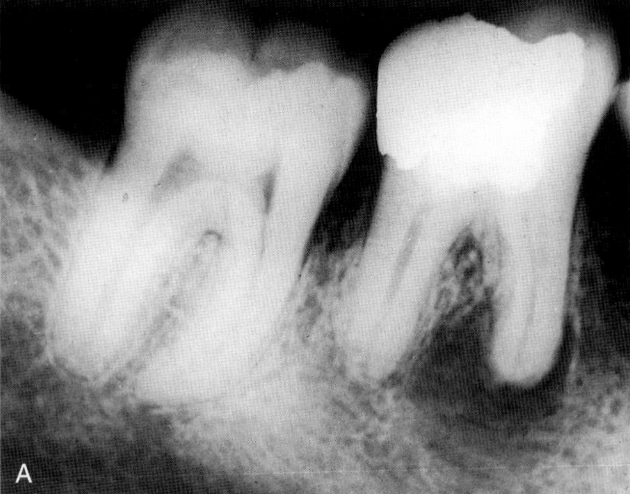

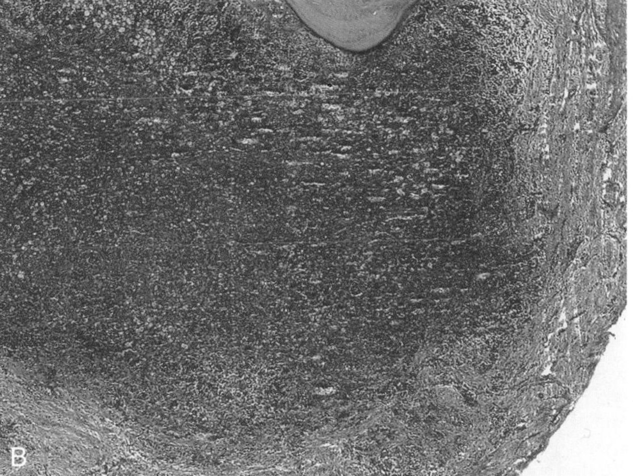

FIGURE 2-51 ■ **A,** Radiograph of a periapical granuloma. **B,** Microscopic appearance of a periapical granuloma showing a collection of inflammatory cells at the apex of a tooth (low magnification). (**A** courtesy Dr. Herbert Frommer.)

The clinician treats a periapical abscess by establishing drainage, by either opening the pulp chamber or extracting the tooth. If the abscess has extended into adjacent tissue, an incision may be necessary to establish drainage. The patient may also be given antibiotic therapy.

DENTAL OR PERIAPICAL GRANULOMA

A **periapical granuloma** is a localized mass of chronically inflamed granulation tissue that forms at the opening of the pulp canal, generally at the apex of a nonvital tooth root (Figure 2-51). This is a chronic process from the outset. Most cases are completely asymptomatic. Sometimes the tooth is sensitive to pressure and percussion because of the inflammation in the apical area. The tooth may also appear slightly

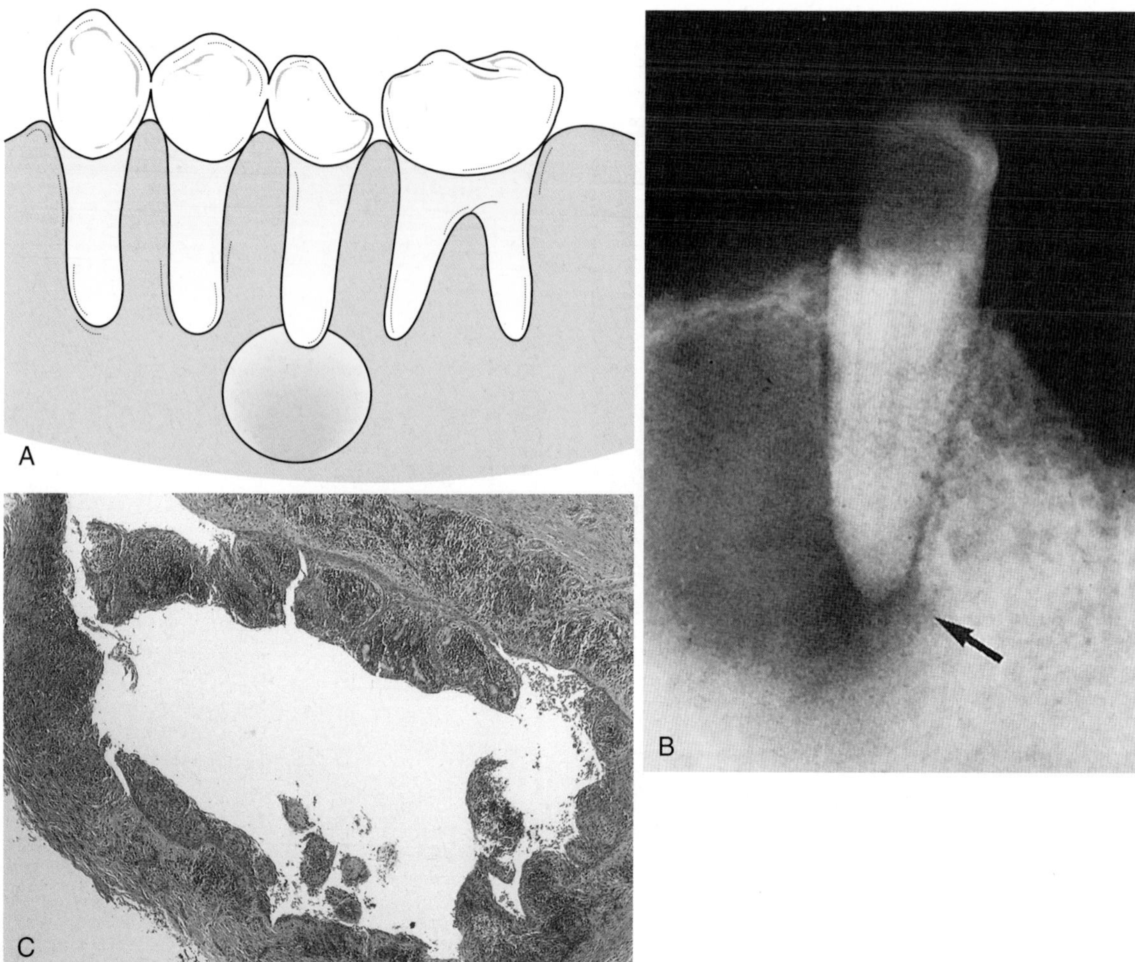

FIGURE 2-52 ■ Radicular cyst. **A,** A radicular cyst located around the root of an erupted tooth. **B,** Radiograph showing a well-circumscribed radiolucency around the root of a tooth. **C,** Microscopic features of a radicular cyst.

extruded from its socket. The radiographic change may vary from a slight thickening of the periodontal ligament space in the area of inflammation to a diffuse radiolucency to a distinct, well-circumscribed radiolucency surrounding the root apex.

The periapical granuloma is composed of granulation tissue containing lymphocytes, plasma cells, and macrophages. Neutrophils may also be present, and areas of dense fibrous connective tissue are often seen. The periapical granuloma is different from the granuloma or granulomatous inflammation, which is a distinctive type of inflammation characteristic of certain diseases (e.g., tuberculosis). Epithelial rests of Malassez, which are remnants of tooth-forming tissue, are often present in the periapical granuloma. The periapical granuloma is treated by root canal therapy or extraction of the tooth.

RADICULAR CYST (PERIAPICAL CYST)

A **radicular cyst,** or **periapical cyst,** is a true cyst consisting of a pathologic cavity lined by epithelium. It occurs in association with the root of a nonvital tooth (Figure 2-52). It is the most commonly occurring cyst in the oral region. The epithelial lining of the cyst develops in a periapical granuloma as a result of proliferation of the epithelial rests of Malassez.

A periapical cyst develops when the epithelium within the inflamed connective tissue of the periapical granuloma proliferates, forming an epithelial mass that increases in size through division of the peripheral cells. The peripheral cells are the equivalent of the basal cell layer of the epithelium. As the cells in the central portion of the mass become increasingly separated from the source of nutrition in the connective tissue, they degenerate centrally, forming a cavity (lumen) that is lined by epithelium and filled with fluid. Histologically the tissue surrounding this epithelial-lined cystic cavity is similar to that seen in the periapical granuloma.

Most periapical cysts are asymptomatic and discovered on radiographic examination. The radiographic appearance of the radicular cyst is the same as that of the periapical granuloma. It appears as a radiolucency, usually well circumscribed, that is attached to a tooth root. It is not possible to differentiate reliably a periapical granuloma from a radicular

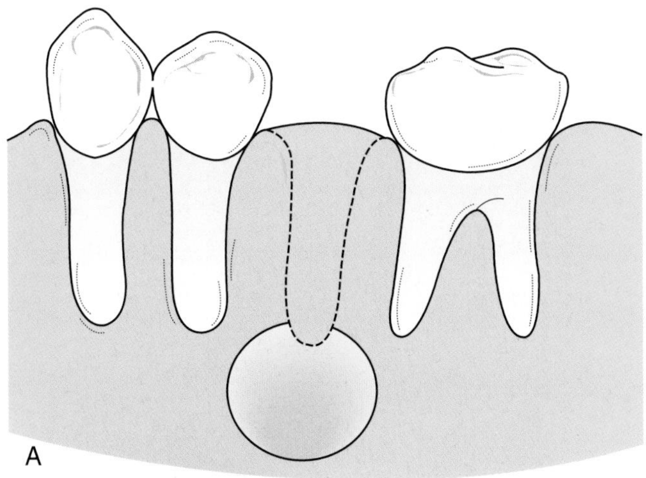

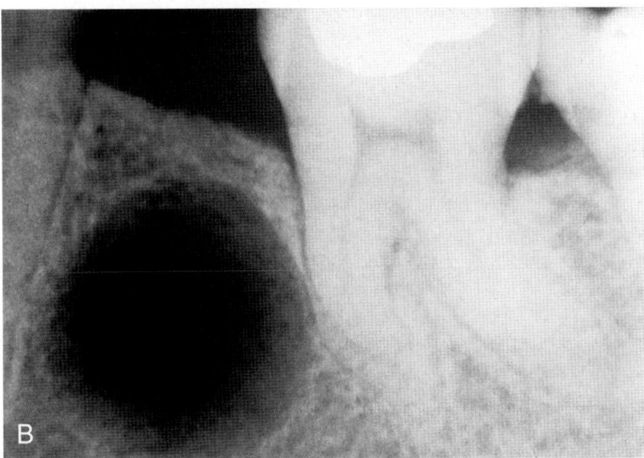

FIGURE 2-53 ■ **A,** A residual cyst. **B,** Radiograph of a residual cyst showing radiolucency at the site of a previously extracted tooth. (Courtesy Drs. Paul Freedman and Stanley Kerpel.)

cyst on the basis of the radiographic appearance alone. A periapical cyst may form in association with any tooth. The cyst may occur lateral to the tooth root rather than at the apex if it is associated with a lateral pulp canal. Other types of cysts can resemble a periapical cyst radiographically; therefore removal of the cyst and microscopic examination of the tissue are necessary.

The radicular cyst is treated by root canal therapy, apicoectomy, or extraction and curettage of the periapical tissues. A **residual cyst** forms when the tooth is removed and all or part of a periapical cyst is left behind (Figure 2-53). Radiographically a residual cyst is a well-circumscribed radiolucency located at the site of tooth extraction. It is treated by surgical removal of the cyst.

RESORPTION OF TEETH

Tooth structure can be resorbed in the same manner as bone. This occurs normally in the process of exfoliation of deciduous teeth and may also occur in other situations. Resorption of the tooth structure beginning at the outside of the tooth is called external resorption. This usually involves the root of a tooth but can occasionally involve the crown of an impacted tooth.

Like bone resorption, tooth resorption can occur when inflammatory tissue is present. Resorption of the root of a tooth sometimes occurs when a periapical granuloma is present. Bone resorption as a response to pressure allows orthodontic tooth movement to occur. Pressure can also cause resorption of tooth structure. This can occur from excessive occlusal or orthodontic forces and with benign and malignant tumors. When a tooth that has been avulsed is reimplanted, the root is resorbed and replaced by bone. Occasionally resorption may involve the crown of an impacted tooth or the roots of teeth, and the cause cannot be identified. This is called **idiopathic tooth resorption.**

External root resorption first appears as a slight raggedness or blunting of the root apex and can proceed to severe loss of tooth substance (Figure 2-54). The condition is not reversible, but progression of the process can be avoided if the cause can be identified and removed. Resorption of impacted teeth can also occur. Generalized root resorption may also occur after orthodontic tooth movement.

Internal tooth resorption can occur in any tooth. Usually only a single tooth is involved. In some cases no cause can be identified. However, it is usually associated with an inflammatory response in the pulp. If the process occurs in the coronal part of the tooth, it may be seen clinically as a pinkish area in the crown. The dental hard tissue has resorbed and is thinner than normal, and the pink color results from the vascular, inflamed connective tissue that can be seen through the remaining enamel and dentin. When the process involves the root, it can be seen only radiographically. A round-to-ovoid radiolucent area associated with the pulp is seen in the central portion of the tooth.

Root canal treatment can be performed successfully if internal resorption is discovered early. If not treated, the process can extend through the dental hard tissue and cause a perforation. After this perforation occurs, the tooth must be extracted.

FOCAL SCLEROSING OSTEOMYELITIS

Focal sclerosing osteomyelitis, also called **condensing osteitis,** is a change in bone near the apexes of teeth that is thought to be a reaction to low-grade infection. Radiographically a radiopaque area is seen extending below the roots of the involved tooth (Figure 2-55). The tooth most commonly associated with focal sclerosing osteomyelitis is the mandibular first molar. Occasionally the mandibular second molar and the mandibular premolars may also be involved.

Radiographically focal sclerosing osteomyelitis appears as a radiopaque area extending below the roots of the tooth. The borders may be diffuse or well defined. Occasionally the periphery of the area is radiolucent; in other cases a

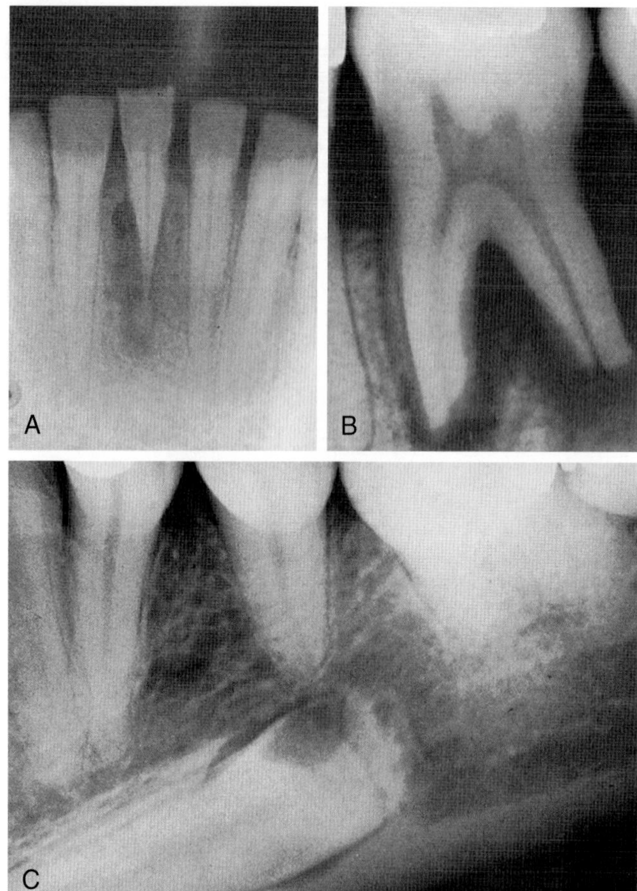

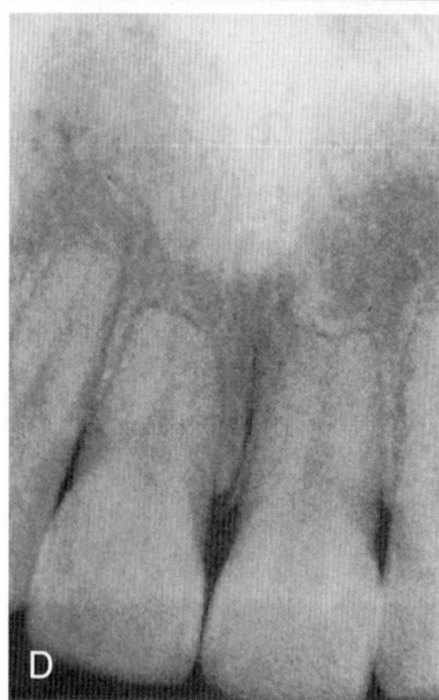

FIGURE 2-54 ■ Tooth resorption. **A,** Root resorption of a mandibular anterior tooth associated with chronic inflammation. **B,** Resorption of tooth structure and bone because of chronic inflammation. **C,** Idiopathic resorption of an impacted tooth. **D,** Generalized root resorption associated with orthodontic tooth movement. (**A** courtesy Dr. Gerald P. Curatola.)

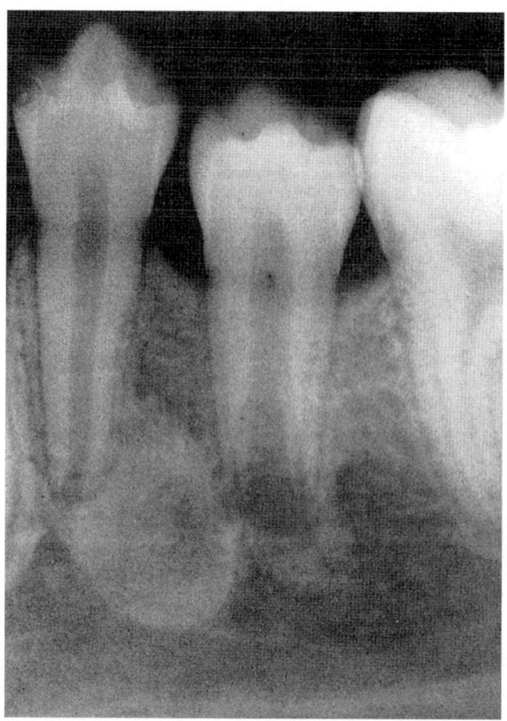

FIGURE 2-55 ■ Focal sclerosing osteomyelitis (condensing osteitis).

central radiolucency surrounded by radiopacity is seen. Microscopically it is dense bone with little marrow or connective tissue. Generally very little inflammation is present. Focal sclerosing osteomyelitis is often associated with a carious or restored tooth. It is generally asymptomatic. However, pain may be associated if pulpal inflammatory disease is present. Focal sclerosing osteomyelitis may be present at any age, but it is typically first seen in young adults.

Diagnosis of focal sclerosing osteomyelitis usually can be made on the basis of the characteristic radiographic appearance. Occasionally biopsy may be necessary to rule out other radiopaque lesions such as osteoma, complex odontoma, or ossifying fibroma. Treatment is not necessary. The sclerotic bone remains even after treatment of the involved tooth.

ALVEOLAR OSTEITIS ("DRY SOCKET")

Alveolar osteitis or **"dry socket"** is a postoperative complication of tooth extraction. The most frequently affected area is the socket of an extracted mandibular third molar. After the extraction of the tooth, the blood clot breaks down and is lost before healing has taken place. Pain develops several days after the extraction. On examination the tooth socket appears empty, and the bone surfaces exposed. The patient complains of pain, bad odor, and bad taste. Because no infection exists, fever, swelling, and erythema are not present. Treatment of alveolar osteitis is directed at relief of pain and includes gentle irrigation and insertion of a medicated dressing.

Selected References

Books

Bath-Balogh M, Fehrenbach MJ: *Illustrated dental embryology, histology, anatomy*, ed 2, St Louis, 2006, Saunders.

Fehrenbach MJ, Herring SW: *Illustrated anatomy of the head and neck*, ed 3, St. Louis, 2007, Saunders.

McCance K, Huether S: *Pathophysiology*, ed 5, St Louis, 2005, Mosby.

Kumar V, Cotran RS, Robbins SL: *Robbins basic pathology*, ed 8, Philadelphia, 2007, Saunders.

Neville BW et al: *Oral and maxillofacial pathology*, ed 3, St Louis, 2009, Saunders.

Regezi JA, Sciubba JJ: *Oral pathology: clinical-pathologic correlations*, ed 5, St Louis, 2008, Saunders.

Journal Articles

Inflammation and Repair

Broughton II G, Janis JE, Attinger CE: Wound healing: an overview, *Plast Reconstr Surg* 117(7 Suppl):S1e, 2006.

Eming SA, Krieg T, Davidson JM: Inflammation in wound repair: molecular and cellular mechanisms, *J Invest Dermatol* 127:(3), 514, 2007.

Kobayashi SD et al: Neutrophils in the innate immune response, *Arch Immunol Ther Exp (Warsz)* 53(6):505, 2005.

Krishnamoorthy S, Honn KV: Inflammation and disease progression, *Cancer Metastasis Rev* 25(3):481, 2006.

Krishnaswamy G, Ajitawi O, Chi DS: The human mast cell: an overview, *Methods Mol Biol* 315:13, 2006.

Moore K: An anatomy of an infection: overview of the infectious process, *Crit Care Nurs Clin North Am* 19(1):9, 2007.

Rankin JA: Biological mediators of acute inflammation, *AACN Clin Issue* 15(1):3, 2004.

Zamai L et al: NK cells and cancer, *J Immunol* 178(7):4011, 2007.

Lesions From Physical and Chemical Injuries to the Oral Tissues

Axell T, Hedin C: Epidemiologic study of excessive oral melanin pigmentation with special reference to the influence of tobacco habits, *Scand J Dent Res* 90:432, 1982.

Bouquot JE, Seime RJ: Bulimia nervosa: dental perspectives, *Pract Periodontics Aesthet Dent* 9:655, 1997.

Buchner A, Hansen LS: Amalgam pigmentation (amalgam tattoo) of the oral mucosa, *Oral Surg Oral Med Oral Pathol* 49:39, 1980.

Ferguson MM et al: Enamel erosion related to wine making, *Occup Med* 46:159, 1996.

Gandara BK, Truelove EL: Diagnosis and management of dental erosion, *J Contemp Dent Pract* 1:16, 1999.

Geurtsen W: Rapid general dental erosion by gas-chlorinated swimming pool water: review of the literature and case report, *Am J Dent* 13:291, 2000.

Gormley MB et al: Thermal trauma: a review of 22 electrical burns of the lip, *J Oral Surg* 30:531, 1972.

Greer RO, Paulsion TC: Oral tissue alterations associated with the use of smokeless tobacco by teenagers, *Oral Surg Oral Med Oral Pathol* 56:275, 1983.

Hanemura H et al: Periodontal status and bruxism: a comparative study of patients with periodontal disease and occlusal parafunctions, *J Periodontol* 58:173, 1987.

Imbery TA, Edwards P: Necrotizing sialometaplasia: literature review and case reports, *J Am Dent Assoc* 127:1087, 1996.

Järvinen V et al: Dental erosion and upper gastrointestinal disorders, *Oral Surg Oral Med Oral Pathol* 64:298, 1988.

Kapila YL, Kashani H: Cocaine-associated rapid gingival recession and dental erosion: a case report, *J Periodontol* 68:485, 1997.

Lineberry TW et al: Methamphetamine abuse: a perfect storm of complications, *Mayo Clin Proc* 81:77, 2006.

Little JW: Eating disorders: dental implications, *Oral Surg Oral Med Oral Pathol Oral Radiol Endod* 93:138, 2002.

Maron FS: Enamel erosion resulting from hydrochloric acid tablets, *J Am Dent Assoc* 127:781, 1996.

Mitchell-Lewis DA et al: Identifying oral lesions associated with crack cocaine use, *J Am Dent Assoc* 125:1104, 1994.

Needleman HL, Berkowitz RJ: Electric trauma to the oral tissues of children, *J Dent Child* 41:19, 1974.

Nemcovsky CE, Artizi Z: Erosion-abrasion lesions revisited, *Compend Contin Educ Dent* 17:416, 1996.

Owens BM, Gallien GS: Noncarious dental "abfraction" lesions in an aging population, *Compend Contin Educ Dent* 16:552, 1995.

Owens BM, Johnson WW, Schuman NJ: Oral amalgam pigmentation (tattoos): a retrospective study, *Quintessence Int* 23:805, 1992.

Owens BM, Schuman NJ, Johnson WW: Oral amalgam tattoos: a diagnostic study, *Compendium* 14:210, 1993.

Piotrowski BT, Gillette WB, Handcock EB: Examining the prevalence and characteristics of abfraction-like cervical lesions in a population of US veterans, *J Am Dent Assoc* 132:1694, 2001.

Pollman L, Berger F, Pollman S: Age and dental abrasion, *Gerodontics* 3:94, 1987.

Pullinger AG, Seligman DA: The degree to which attrition characterizes differentiated patient groups of temporomandibular disorders, *J Orofac Pain* 7:196, 1990.

Rawlinson A: Case report: labial cervical abrasion caused by misuse of dental floss, *Dent Health (London)* 26:3, 1987.

Richmond NL: Update on dental erosion: office and home treatment for hypersensitive teeth, *J Indiana Dent Assoc* 66:29, 1987.

Roberts MW, Li SH: Oral findings in anorexia nervosa and bulimia nervosa: a study of 47 cases, *J Am Dent Assoc* 115:497, 1987.

Robertson PB, Walsh MM, Greene JC: Oral effects of smokeless tobacco use by professional baseball players, *Adv Dent Res* 11:307, 1997.

Rossie KM, Guggenheimer J: Thermally induced 'nicotine' stomatitis: a case report, *Oral Surg Oral Med Oral Pathol* 70:597, 1990.

Rugh JD, Harlan J: Nocturnal bruxism and temporomandibular disorders, *Adv Neurol* 49:329, 1988.

Rytomaa I et al: Bulimia and tooth erosion, *Acta Odontol Scand* 56:36, 1998.

Simmons MS, Thompson DC: Dental erosion secondary to ethanol-induced emesis, *Oral Surg Oral Med Oral Pathol* 64:731, 1987.

Sist T, Green G: Traumatic neuroma of the oral cavity, *Oral Surg Oral Med Oral Pathol* 51:394, 1981.

Welsh RA, Donely C: The association between occlusion and attrition, *Aust Orthod J* 12:138, 1992.

Wray A, McGuirt F: Smokeless tobacco usage associated with oral carcinoma, *Arch Otolaryngol Head Neck Surg* 119:929, 1993.

Zimmers PL, Gobetti JP: Head and neck lesions commonly found in musicians, *J Am Dent Assoc* 125:1487, 1994.

Reactive Connective Tissue Hyperplasia

Bodner L et al: Growth potential of peripheral giant cell granuloma, *Oral Surg Oral Med Oral Pathol Oral Radiol Endod* 83:548, 1997.

Bonetti F et al: Peripheral giant cell granuloma: evidence for osteoclastic differentiation, *Oral Surg Oral Med Oral Pathol* 70:471, 1990.

Brown RS et al: Nitrendipine-induced gingival hyperplasia: first case report, *Oral Surg Oral Med Oral Pathol* 70:593, 1990.

Brunet L et al: Prevalence and risk of gingival enlargement in patients treated with anticonvulsant drugs, *Eur J Clin Invest* 31:781, 2001.

Cloutier M et al: An analysis of peripheral giant cell granuloma associated with dental implant treatment, *Oral Surg Oral Med Oral Pathol Oral Radiol Endod* 103:618, 2007.

Daley TD, Nartey NO, Wysocki GP: Pregnancy tumor: an analysis, *Oral Surg Oral Med Oral Pathol* 72:196, 1991.

Daley T, Wysocki G, Day C: Clinical and pharmacologic correlations in cyclosporine-induced gingival hyperplasia, *Oral Surg Oral Med Oral Pathol* 62:417, 1986.

Fay AA et al: Felodipine-influenced gingival enlargement in an uncontrolled type 2 diabetic patient, *J Periodontol* 76:1217, 2005.

Gould A, Escobar V: Symmetrical gingival fibromatosis, *Oral Surg Oral Med Oral Pathol* 51:62, 1981.

Lederman D et al: Gingival hyperplasia associated with nifedipine therapy: report of a case, *Oral Surg Oral Med Oral Pathol* 57:620, 1984.

Miranda J et al: Prevalence and risk of gingival enlargement in patients treated with nifedipine, *J Periodontol* 72:605, 2001.

Proia NK et al: Smoking and smokeless tobacco-associated human buccal cell mutations and their association with oral cancer—a review, *Cancer Epidemiol Biomarkers Prev* 15:1061, 2006.

Roberson JB, Crocker DJ, Schiller T: The diagnosis and treatment of central giant cell granuloma, *J Am Dent Assoc* 128:81, 1997.

Silverstein LH et al: The late development of oral pyogenic granuloma as a complication of pregnancy: a case report, *Compendium* 17:192, 1996.

Zain RB, Fei YJ: Fibrous lesions of the gingiva: a histopathologic analysis of 204 cases, *Oral Surg Oral Med Oral Pathol* 70:466, 1990.

Inflammatory Periapical Lesions

Gunraj MN: Dental root resorption, *Oral Surg Oral Med Oral Pathol Oral Radiol Endod* 88:647, 1999.

Harris EF, Butler MI: Patterns of incisor root resorption before and after orthodontic correction in cases with anterior open bites, *Am J Orthod Dentofacial Orthop* 101:112, 1992.

Harris EF, Robinson QC, Woods MA: An analysis of causes of apical root resorption in patients not treated orthodontically, *Quintessence Int* 24:417, 1993.

REVIEW QUESTIONS

1. Which of the following is the body's initial response to injury?
   A. The immune response
   B. The inflammatory response
   C. Repair
   D. Hyperplasia

2. What type of inflammation occurs if the injury is minimal and brief and the source is removed from the tissue?
   A. Fatal
   B. Acute
   C. Chronic
   D. Life-threatening

3. In the inflammatory response, the first microscopic event is:
   A. Dilation of the microcirculation.
   B. Increased permeability of the microcirculation.
   C. Formation of exudate.
   D. Constriction of the microcirculation.

4. Which one of the following conditions is a chronic inflammatory lesion?
   A. Necrotizing sialometaplasia
   B. Periapical granuloma
   C. Aphthous ulcer
   D. Aspirin burn

5. The directed movement of white blood cells to the area of injury is called:
   A. Pavementing.
   B. Margination.
   C. Chemotaxis.
   D. Hyperemia.

6. Which cells are most common in chronic inflammation?
   A. Neutrophils
   B. Macrophages and lymphocytes
   C. Lymphocytes and plasma cells
   D. Neutrophils and lymphocytes

7. The macrophage has many functions. Which of the following is not a function of the macrophage?
   A. Phagocytosis
   B. Removal of large foreign matter
   C. Removal of inhaled particles
   D. Formation of antibodies

8. Which of the following is the term used to describe blood plasma and proteins that leave the blood vessels and enter the surrounding tissues during inflammation?
   A. Hyperemia
   B. Hypertrophy
   C. Margination
   D. Exudate

9. The process of phagocytosis directly involves the:
   A. Ingestion of foreign substances by white blood cells.
   B. Escape of plasma fluids and proteins from the microcirculation into the surrounding tissues.
   C. Displacement of white blood cells to the blood vessel walls.
   D. Attachment of white blood cells to the blood vessel walls.

10. Which of the following statements is INCORRECT concerning the neutrophil? The neutrophil:
   A. Makes up 30% of white blood cells.
   B. Contains lysosomal enzymes.
   C. Is a cell whose main function is phagocytosis.
   D. Has a multilobed nucleus.

11. During the process of inflammation, the second type of white blood cell to emigrate from the blood vessel into the injured tissue is the:
   A. Neutrophil.
   B. Red blood cell.
   C. Lymphocyte.
   D. Monocyte.

12. Components of the complement system mediate the inflammatory process by:
   A. Decreasing vascular permeability.
   B. Releasing histamine granules from neutrophils.
   C. Causing cytolysis of cells.
   D. Decreasing phagocytosis.

13. Two days after injury, granulation tissue can be described as:
   A. Immature vascular connective tissue.
   B. Exudate.
   C. Keloids.
   D. Ulceration.

14. The enlargement of superficial lymph nodes that occurs as a systemic sign of inflammation is:
   A. Called leukocytosis.
   B. Regulated by the hypothalamus.
   C. Caused by changes in their lymphocytes.
   D. A process that involves only the lymph nodes in the submental area.

15. Which statement concerning repair in the body is true?
   A. Repair can be completed with the injurious agents present.
   B. Functioning cells and tissue components are always replaced by functioning scar tissue.
   C. Repair always results in regeneration.
   D. The process of repair is initiated by the inflammatory response.

16. The clot that forms during repair:
   A. Consists of fibrous connective tissue.
   B. Serves as a guide for migrating epithelial cells.
   C. Forms after skin injury, but not after mucosal injury.
   D. Only occurs with healing by secondary intention.

17. Healing by secondary intention refers to healing of an injury when:
   A. The incision has clean edges joined by sutures.
   B. Only a small clot forms.
   C. An infection forms in the injured area.
   D. The patient has increased formation of granulation tissue.

18. An increase in the size of an organ or tissue resulting from an increase in the number of its cells is termed:
   A. Hyperemia.
   B. Hyperplasia.
   C. Inflammation.
   D. Hypertrophy.

19. Normal bone tissue repair can be delayed by:
   A. Maintenance of osteoblast-producing tissues.
   B. Inadequate movement of bone tissue.
   C. Removal of an area of edema.
   D. Reduction in amount of tissue infection.

20. Which one of the following would appear as a pigmented lesion?
   A. Amalgam tattoo
   B. Traumatic ulcer
   C. Frictional keratosis
   D. Aspirin burn

21. Which of the following statements is false?
   A. Attrition is the wearing away of tooth structure during mastication.
   B. Bruxism is the same as mastication.
   C. Erosion is the loss of tooth structure resulting from chemical action.
   D. Abrasion is caused by mechanical, repetitive habits.

22. Loss of tooth structure associated with bulimia is caused by:
    A. Attrition.
    B. Erosion.
    C. Bruxism.
    D. Abrasion.

23. An aspirin burn:
    A. Occurs as a result of an overdose of aspirin.
    B. Is usually painless.
    C. Results from a misuse of aspirin.
    D. Usually takes several weeks to heal.

24. A patient has a generalized white appearance of the palate. Tiny erythematous dots can be seen, surrounded by a thickened raised white-to-gray area. Overall the palate appears wrinkled. This condition is most likely:
    A. Papillary hyperplasia of the palate.
    B. Nicotine stomatitis.
    C. An aspirin burn.
    D. Necrotizing sialometaplasia.

25. The primary and most common cause of a mucocele is:
    A. Inflammation.
    B. Tumor formation.
    C. Severing of or trauma to a minor salivary gland duct.
    D. A sialolith.

26. A ranula is located on the:
    A. Lower lip.
    B. Buccal mucosa.
    C. Retromolar area.
    D. Floor of the mouth.

27. Which one of the following would not occur on the gingiva?
    A. Irritation fibroma
    B. Pyogenic granuloma
    C. Giant cell granuloma
    D. Epulis fissuratum

28. Generalized loss of tooth structure primarily on the lingual surfaces of maxillary anterior teeth is associated with:
    A. Erosion.
    B. Attrition.
    C. Abrasion.
    D. Abfraction.

29. External tooth resorption occurs as a result of:
    A. Caries.
    B. Salivary gland dysfunction.
    C. Chronic inflammation.
    D. Medication.

30. Which one of the following is considered to be the most likely cause of necrotizing sialometaplasia?
    A. Loss of blood supply
    B. Radiation therapy
    C. Smoking
    D. A sialolith

31. The most common site for a mucocele to occur is the:
    A. Floor of the mouth.
    B. Tongue.
    C. Buccal mucosa.
    D. Lower lip.

32. The peripheral giant cell granuloma only occurs on the:
    A. Gingiva or alveolar mucosa.
    B. Hard palate.
    C. Buccal mucosa.
    D. Floor of the mouth.

33. A sialolith is:
    A. Chronic inflammation of a salivary gland.
    B. Acute inflammation of a salivary gland.
    C. A pooling of saliva in the connective tissue.
    D. A salivary gland stone.

34. Which of the following statements is false?
    A. A periapical cyst develops from a periapical granuloma.
    B. A periapical abscess always causes radiographic periapical changes.
    C. A periapical granuloma is a circumscribed area of chronically inflamed tissue.
    D. A periapical cyst is also called a radicular cyst.

35. Epulis fissuratum results from irritation caused by:
    A. A denture flange.
    B. Denture adhesive.
    C. Poor suction from the denture in the palatal vault.
    D. An allergic reaction to the acrylic in the denture.

36. Which of the following statements is true?
    A. A traumatic neuroma is never painful.
    B. Necrotizing sialometaplasia is considered a denture-related lesion.
    C. Chronic hyperplastic pulpitis is the same as gingival hyperplasia.
    D. Gingival enlargement may be caused by medication.

37. Loss of tooth structure caused by chemical action describes:
    A. Abrasion.
    B. Drug allergy.
    C. Erosion.
    D. Attrition.

38. Which of the following cysts is characteristically associated with a tooth that is nonvital on pulp testing?
    A. Residual cyst
    B. Radicular cyst
    C. Dentigerous cyst
    D. Dermoid cyst

39. Which cyst results when a tooth is extracted without removing the periapical cystic sac?
    A. Radicular
    B. Primordial
    C. Residual
    D. Periodontal

40. The most common cause of the radicular cyst is:
    A. Deep restorations without a base.
    B. Caries.
    C. Occlusal trauma.
    D. Toothbrush abrasion at the cemento-enamel junction.

41. The wearing away of tooth structure through an abnormal mechanical action defines:
    A. Attrition.
    B. Abrasion.
    C. Erosion.
    D. Germination.

42. Which one of the following is not associated with attrition?
    A. Toothpaste
    B. Bruxism
    C. Mastication
    D. Age

43. Heavy plaque and calculus, mouth breathing, orthodontic appliances, and overhanging restorations best describe some of the causative factors for:
    A. Phenytoin (Dilantin) hyperplasia.
    B. A reaction from nifedipine (Procardia).
    C. Irritation fibromatosis.
    D. Chemical fibromatosis.

44. The central giant cell granuloma:
    A. May occur on the tongue.
    B. May present as a multilocular radiolucency.
    C. Is histologically the same as a pyogenic granuloma.
    D. Occurs primarily in men older than 60 years of age.

45. During examination of the dentition, the dental hygienist notes the presence of active wear facets. This indicates that the patient is:
    A. Chewing too vigorously.
    B. A bruxer.
    C. A vegetarian.
    D. Lip biting.

46. A patient has a loss of tooth structure on the labial surfaces of the anterior teeth and reports a high intake of citrus fruit juices. The hygienist would most likely suspect:
    A. Abrasion.
    B. Bulimia.
    C. Bruxism.
    D. Erosion.

47. The amalgam tattoo represents amalgam particles in the tissue and is most commonly observed in the oral cavity on the:
    A. Lateral borders of the tongue.
    B. Anterior palate near the rugae.
    C. Floor of the mouth.
    D. Posterior gingiva and edentulous ridge.

48. A pink protruding mass in the occlusal surface of a mandibular first or second molar is most likely:
    A. A pulpal granuloma.
    B. Caused by caries.
    C. A pulp polyp.
    D. All of the above.

49. Which of the following drugs does NOT cause gingival enlargement?
    A. Dilantin
    B. Cyclosporine
    C. Procardia
    D. Tetracycline

50. Traumatic ulcers are usually diagnosed on the basis of:
    A. The patient's medical history.
    B. The clinical appearance and history of the ulcers.
    C. The results of a biopsy and histologic examination.
    D. A therapeutic diagnosis.

CHAPTER 2 Synopsis

Condition/Disease	Cause	Age/Race/Sex	Location
Injuries to Teeth			
Attrition	Mastication	Men are affected more than women	Occlusal/incisal surfaces Proximal
Abrasion	Repetitive mechanical habit	*	Dependent on cause
Abfraction	Biomechanical forces on teeth	Adults	Cervical regions of teeth
Erosion	Chemical action	*	Dependent on cause
"Meth Mouth"	Methamphetamine abuse	*	Generalized
Injuries to Soft Tissues			
Chemical Burn (e.g., aspirin, phenol)	Caustic chemical in contact with mucosa	*	Site of contact
Electric Burn	Live electric cord in contact with mucosa	Infants and young children	Site of contact
Thermal Burn	Hot food or liquid	*	Site of contact
Cocaine Use	Crack cocaine Cocaine hydrochloride	*	Midpalate Site of contact
Hematoma	Trauma	*	Site of trauma Most common sites are the buccal/labial mucosa
Traumatic Ulcer	Trauma to mucosa	*	Site of trauma
Frictional Keratosis	Chronic friction against mucosal surface	*	Site of friction
Linea Alba	Teeth clenching/habit	*	Buccal mucosa at occlusal plane
Nicotine Stomatitis	Smoking pipe smoking	*	Hard palate

N/A, Not applicable.
*No significant information.
†Not covered in this text.

Clinical Features	Radiographic Features	Microscopic Features	Treatment	Diagnostic Process
Flattening of tooth surfaces	N/A	N/A	Prevention Restoration	Clinical
Loss of tooth structure at site of wear	N/A	N/A	Prevention Restoration	Clinical
Wedge-shaped notching at cervical areas of involved teeth	N/A	N/A	Restoration May not require treatment	Clinical
Loss of tooth structure Smooth polished surface	N/A	N/A	Prevention Restoration	Clinical
Generalized extensive destruction of tooth structure	Generalized destruction of teeth	N/A	Restoration Extraction of teeth	Clinical Historical
Painful ulcer with necrotic surface	N/A	†	Palliative	Clinical
Tissue destruction	N/A	†	Tissue repair	Clinical
Painful erythema and superficial ulceration	N/A	†	None/palliative	Clinical
Painful ulceration and erythema Necrotic ulcers	N/A	†	Elimination of cause	Clinical
Red-to-purple-to–bluish-black mass lesion Size depends on extent of trauma	N/A	†	None	Clinical
Painful, mucosal ulceration	N/A	Ulcer with eosinophils present in inflammatory infiltrate	Elimination of cause	Clinical
White mucosal surface	N/A	Hyperkeratosis	Elimination of cause	Clinical
Anterior-to-posterior white line	N/A	Epithelial hyperplasia and hyperkeratosis	None	Clinical
White, opacification of the palatal mucosa with raised red dots	N/A	Hyperkeratosis with inflamed minor salivary glands	Elimination of cause	Clinical

Continued

CHAPTER 2 Synopsis (continued)

Condition/Disease	Cause	Age/Race/Sex	Location
Tobacco Pouch Keratosis	Chewing tobacco	*	Site where tobacco is habitually placed
Traumatic Neuroma	Injury to a peripheral nerve	*	Site of injured nerve
Amalgam Tattoo	Particles of amalgam in connective tissue	*	Most common on gingiva and edentulous alveolar ridge
Smoker's Melanosis	Smoking	†	Anterior labial gingiva
Solar (Actinic) Cheilitis	Sun exposure	Adults	Vermilion of lips
Mucocele	Severed salivary gland duct	Any age	Most common: lower lip
Ranula	Obstruction/severing of salivary gland duct	*	Floor of mouth
Necrotizing Sialometaplasia	Compromised blood supply to area	*	Most common: junction of the hard and soft palate
Sialolith	Precipitation of calcified material around a central core	*	Major and minor salivary glands
Sialadenitis	Infection Obstruction of salivary gland duct	*	Symptomatic when involving major salivary glands
Reactive Connective Tissue Hyperplasia			
Pyogenic Granuloma	Response to injury Puberty Pregnancy	*	Most common: gingiva Also other areas

N/A, Not applicable.
*No significant information.
†Not covered in this text.

Clinical Features	Radiographic Features	Microscopic Features	Treatment	Diagnostic Process
Granular-to-white, wrinkled appearance	N/A	Hyperkeratosis and epithelial hyperplasia Sometimes *epithelial atypia*	Elimination of cause	Clinical Microscopic
Painful, submucosal nodule	N/A	Mass of nerve	Surgical excision	Microscopic
Bluish-gray macule	Tiny radiopacity	Black granular material in connective tissue	No treatment after identification	Clinical Microscopic Radiographic
Diffuse grayish-brown color of gingiva	N/A	Melanin pigment in basal layer of epithelium and in underlying connective tissue	None Fades with decreased smoking	Clinical
Indistinct, fissured skin-mucosal interface	N/A	Degenerative changes in connective tissue	Protect lips and skin from sun exposure	Clinical
Localized tissue swelling that increases/decreases in size	N/A	Extravasated mucus in tissue surrounded by granulation tissue	Excision May spontaneously resolve	Clinical Microscopic
Fluid-filled swelling that increases/ decreases in size	N/A	Resembles mucocele or mucous cyst	Surgery	Clinical
Moderately painful swelling and ulceration Acute onset	N/A	Necrosis of the salivary glands Replacement of salivary duct epithelium with squamous epithelium	Spontaneous resolution	Microscopic
Obstruction of the gland Hard nodule in soft tissue	Floor of the mouth: radiopaque structure	Calcified structure arranged in concentric rings	Surgical removal of stone	Clinical Radiographic Microscopic
Painful swelling of gland	N/A	Acute or chronic inflammatory infiltrate in salivary gland	Antibiotic if infection	Clinical Laboratory Microscopic
Deep red-purple exophytic lesion, usually ulcerated	N/A	Ulcerated granulation tissue	Surgical excision	Microscopic

Continued

CHAPTER 2 Synopsis (continued)

Condition/Disease	Cause	Age/Race/Sex	Location
Giant Cell Granuloma Peripheral	Unknown	Any age More frequent between 40 and 60 years of age More common in women than men	Gingiva
Irritation Fibroma	Trauma	*	Common on the gingiva Many other oral locations
Denture-Induced Fibrous Hyperplasia (Epulis Fissuratum) *not precancerous	Ill-fitting denture Continuous wearing of denture	*	Vestibule along a denture border
Papillary Hyperplasia of the Palate	Removable prosthesis	*	Hard palate
Gingival Enlargement (Hyperplasia)	Response to chronic inflammation Idiopathic Drug reaction Hormonal changes Genetic	* *puffy gingiva; lots of bleeding; odor of blood fr. iron!	Gingiva: generalized or localized
Chronic Hyperplastic Pulpitis	Dental caries	Children and young adults	Primary or permanent molars
Inflammatory Periapical Lesions			
Periapcial Abscess	Inflammation of the dental pulp Preexisting periapical chronic inflammation	*	Roots of primary or permanent teeth

N/A, Not applicable.
*No significant information.
†Not covered in this text.

Clinical Features	Radiographic Features	Microscopic Features	Treatment	Diagnostic Process
Deep-red exophytic lesion	N/A	Many multinucleated giant cells in well-vascularized connective tissue	Surgical excision	Microscopic
Broad-based, pink, exophytic lesion	N/A	Dense fibrous connective tissue usually surfaced by normal epithelium	Surgical excision	Microscopic
Elongated folds of exophytic tissue surrounding denture phalange	N/A	Dense fibrous connective tissue surfaced by epithelium that may be hyperplastic and ulcerated	Surgical excision Fabrication of new denture	Clinical Microscopic
Mucosa surfaced by multiple, erythematous papillary projections	N/A	Papillary projections composed of fibrous connective tissue (usually inflamed) surfaced by squamous epithelium	Surgical removal of papillary tissue Fabrication of new denture	Clinical
Increase in the bulk of the free and attached gingival No stippling Erythematous to normal color	N/A	Connective tissue (usually inflamed) surfaced by squamous epithelium	Gingivectomy Meticulous oral hygiene	Clinical Microscopic
Red or pink nodule protruding from the pulp chamber of a tooth with a large, open carious lesion	N/A	Granulation tissue surfaced by squamous epithelium	Extraction of tooth or endodontic treatment	Clinical
Pain, swelling, fistula, slight extrusion of tooth	None Thickening of periodontal ligament space Periapical radiolucency	Acute inflammatory infiltrate	Establish drainage	Clinical

Continued

CHAPTER 2 Synopsis (continued)

Condition/Disease	Cause	Age/Race/Sex	Location
Periapical Granuloma	Pulpal inflammation and necrosis	*	Roots of primary or permanent teeth
Radicular Cyst (Periapical Cyst)	Nonvital tooth	*	Roots of primary or permanent teeth
Resorption of Teeth **External Resorption** **Internal Resorption**	 Chronic inflammation Chronic pulpal inflammation		 Roots of primary or permanent teeth Dental hard tissue within root or crowns
Focal Sclerosing Osteomyelitis	Low-grade chronic infection	*	Bone adjacent to any tooth Mandibular first molar most common
Alveolar Osteitis ("Dry Socket")	Postoperative complication of tooth extraction	*	Extraction site

N/A, Not applicable.
*No significant information.
†Not covered in this text.

Clinical Features	Radiographic Features	Microscopic Features	Treatment	Diagnostic Process
Asymptomatic Tooth sensitive to percussion Slight extrusion of tooth	Slight thickening of periodontal ligament space Periodontal radiolucency	Chronic inflammatory infiltrate	Root canal therapy Extraction	Radiographic Microscopic
Most are asymptomatic	Radiolucency associated with the root of a nonvital tooth	Space lined by epithelium surrounded by an infiltrate of chronic inflammatory cells	Root canal therapy Apicoectomy Extraction and curettage of the extraction site	Radiographic Microscopic
Asymptomatic Asymptomatic May see pinkish color if crown involved	Blunting of root apex to severe loss of root substance Round to avoid radiolucency in the central part of the tooth	N/A N/A	Identify and remove cause Root canal therapy Extraction	Radiographic Radiographic
Asymptomatic	Radiopaque area below roots of the tooth	Dense bone	None	Radiographic
Pain develops several days after extraction	N/A	N/A	Gentle irrigation Insertion of medicated dressing	Clinical

chapter 3

Immunity

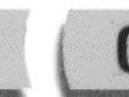

Margaret J. Fehrenbach, Joan A. Phelan

OBJECTIVES

After studying this chapter, the student will be able to:

1. Define each of the words in the vocabulary list for this chapter.
2. Describe the primary difference between an immune response and an inflammatory response.
3. List and describe the two main types of lymphocytes, their origins, and their activities.
4. List the activities of macrophages.
5. Using the cells involved, describe the difference between antibody-mediated (humoral) immunity and cell-mediated immunity.
6. Describe the difference between passive and active immunity.
7. Give one example of passive immunity and one example of active immunity.
8. List and describe four types of hypersensitivity reactions and give an example of each.
9. Define autoimmunity and describe how it results in disease.
10. Define immunodeficiency and describe how it results in disease.
11. Describe and contrast the clinical features of each of the three types of aphthous ulcers.
12. List three systemic diseases associated with aphthous ulcers.
13. Describe and compare the clinical features of urticaria, angioedema, contact mucositis, fixed drug eruption, and erythema multiforme.
14. Describe the clinical and histologic features of lichen planus.
15. List the triad of systemic signs that comprise Reactive Arthritis (Reiter syndrome) and describe the oral lesions that occur in this condition.
16. Name the two cells that characterize Langerhans cell disease histologically. Describe the acute disseminated form, chronic disseminated form, and chronic localized form and state the names that traditionally have been used for each of these conditions.

OBJECTIVES (continued)

17. Describe the oral manifestations of each of the following autoimmune diseases: Lupus erythematosus, pemphigus vulgaris, mucous membrane pemphigoid, and Behçet syndrome.
18. Define desquamative gingivitis, describe the clinical features, and list three diseases in which desquamative gingivitis may occur.
19. Describe the components of Behçet syndrome.

VOCABULARY

Acantholysis (āk″an-thol′ĭ-sis) Dissolution of the intercellular bridges of the prickle cell layer of the epithelium.

Acquired immune response A response of the body to injury that has memory of past exposure to a foreign substance and responds more quickly to a foreign substance when encountered a second time.

Allergy (al′er-je) A hypersensitive state acquired through exposure to a particular allergen; reexposure to the same allergen elicits an exaggerated reaction.

Anaphylaxis (an″ah-fĭ-lak′sis) A severe type of hypersensitivity or allergic reaction in which the exaggerated immunologic reaction results from the release of vasoactive substances such as histamine; the reaction occurs on reexposure to a foreign protein or other substance after sensitization.

Antibody (an″tĭ-bod″e) A protein molecule, also called an immunoglobulin, which is produced by plasma cells and reacts with a specific antigen.

Antigen (an′′tĭ-jen) Any substance able to induce a specific immune response.

Autoantibody (aw″to-an′tĭ-bod″e) An antibody that reacts against an antigenic constituent of the person's own tissues.

Autoimmune disease (aw″to-ĭ-mun′dĭ-zēz′) A disease characterized by tissue injury caused by a humoral or cell-mediated immune response against constituents of the body's own tissues.

B lymphocyte (B cell) (B lim′fo-sīt) A lymphocyte, that matures without passing through the thymus; the B cell can later develop into a plasma cell that produces antibodies.

Cell-mediated immunity (sel me′de-a″ted ĭ-mu′nĭ-te) Immunity in which the predominant role is played by T lymphocytes.

Cytokine (sī′tō-kīn) Cell product produced by the cells involved in the immune response.

Humoral immunity (hu′mor-l ĭ-mu′nĭ-te) Immunity in which B lymphocytes and antibodies play the predominant role.

Hypersensitivity (hi″per-sen″sĭ-tiv′ĭ-te) A state of altered reactivity in which the body reacts to a foreign agent with an exaggerated immune response.

Immune complex (ĭ-m ū′n kom′pleks) A combination of antibody and antigen.

Immunodeficiency (ĭ-m″u-no-dĕ-fish′en-se) A deficiency of the immune response resulting from hypoactivity or decreased numbers of lymphoid cells.

Immunoglobulin (Ig) (ĭ-m″u-no-glob′u-lin) A protein, also called an antibody, synthesized by plasma cells in response to a specific antigen.

LE cell A cell that is a characteristic of lupus erythematosus (LE) and other autoimmune diseases; it is a mature neutrophil that has phagocytized a spherical inclusion derived from another neutrophil.

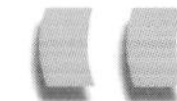

VOCABULARY (continued)

Lymphoid tissue **(lim'foid tish'u)** Tissue composed of lymphocytes supported by a meshwork of connective tissue.

Macrophage **(mak'ro-fāj)** A large tissue-bound mononuclear phagocyte derived from monocytes circulating in blood; macrophages become mobile when stimulated by inflammation and interact with lymphocytes in an immune response.

Mucositis **(mu″ko-sĭ'tis)** Mucosal inflammation.

Natural killer cell **(NK cell)** A lymphocyte that is part of the body's initial innate immunity, which by unknown mechanisms is able to directly destroy cells recognized as foreign.

Nikolsky's sign **(nĭ-kol'skē sīn)** In some bullous diseases such as pemphigus vulgaris and bullous pemphigus the superficial epithelium separates easily from the basal layer on exertion of firm, sliding manual pressure.

Rheumatoid factor **(roo'mah-toid fak'tor)** A protein, immunoglobulin M (IgM), found in serum and detectable on laboratory tests; it is associated with rheumatoid arthritis and other autoimmune diseases.

T lymphocyte (T cell) **(T lim'fo-sīt)** A lymphocyte that matures in the thymus before migrating to tissues; the T lymphocyte is responsible for cell-mediated immunity and may modulate the humoral immune response.

Thymus **(thī'mus)** A lymphoid organ located high in the chest, which is large in an infant and gradually shrinks in size.

Xerophthalmia **(ze″rof-thal'me-ah)** Abnormal dryness of the eyes.

Xerostomia **(ze″ro-sto'me-ah)** Patient complaint of dryness of the mouth usually caused by decreased salivary flow.

The acute inflammatory response, which is described in Chapter 2, is a rapid first line of defense against tissue injury and disease-producing microorganisms. The acquired immune response, described in this chapter, occurs after the inflammatory response and generally is necessary for complete recovery. This chapter begins with a description of the acquired immune response and includes the oral diseases that result from harmful effects of the immune response. Surveillance against neoplastic cells also involves the immune response. The neoplastic process is described in Chapter 7.

THE ACQUIRED IMMUNE RESPONSE

Like the inflammatory response, the **acquired immune response** defends the body against injury, particularly from foreign substances such as microorganisms. The immune response differs from the inflammatory response in that it has the capacity to remember past instances of injury and responds more quickly to a foreign substance that is encountered again. It works amid the background of an already activated inflammatory and innate immune response and a working repair process. The innate immune response does not involve memory. It is described along with inflammation in Chapter 2. The acquired immune response involves a complex network of white blood cells. As with inflammation, the immune response may also result in an increased level of injury and disease.

ANTIGENS

Antigens are the foreign substances against which the immune system defends the body. These substances are mainly proteins and are often microorganisms and their toxins. The immune system tolerates the normal components of the body (self) and their normal diversity. Antigens are substances that the immune system recognizes as foreign (nonself). Transformed human cells such as tumor cells or cells infected by viruses can be antigens. Human tissue, as in the case of an organ transplant, tissue graft, or incompatible blood transfusion, can also be an antigen. In diseases called **autoimmune diseases,** parts of an individual's own body become antigens. Disease occurs when the immune response identifies components of self as antigen or doesn't recognize foreign material as antigen.

CELLULAR INVOLVEMENT IN THE IMMUNE RESPONSE

Many cells are involved in the immune response. These cells can produce cell products or **cytokines** that are active during the immune response. The primary white blood cells involved in the immune response are lymphocytes. These cells are able to recognize and respond to an antigen when it is in contact with receptor sites on the surface of the cell. Lymphocytes, like other white blood cells, are derived from stem cells in the bone marrow. Lymphocytes constitute 20% to 25% of the white blood cell population. They are mobile antigen-sensitive cells with a long life. They have a round nucleus and only a small amount of cytoplasm. Different types of lymphocytes have different functions. The two main types of lymphocyte are called **B lymphocytes (B cells)** and **T lymphocytes (T cells)** (Figure 3-1).

A third type of lymphocyte is called the **natural killer cell (NK cell).** This is a large lymphocyte that is part of the body's innate immunity and not directly involved in acquired immunity. NK cells and their activities are described in Chapter 2. NK cells have the ability to destroy foreign cells early in their appearance since they recognize them as foreign without first having to recognize them as specific antigens. They are usually located within the microcirculation and not in the outlying tissue. This cell seems to be active against viruses and cancer cells. However, in several immunodeficiency diseases, including acquired immunodeficiency syndrome, NK cell function is abnormal.

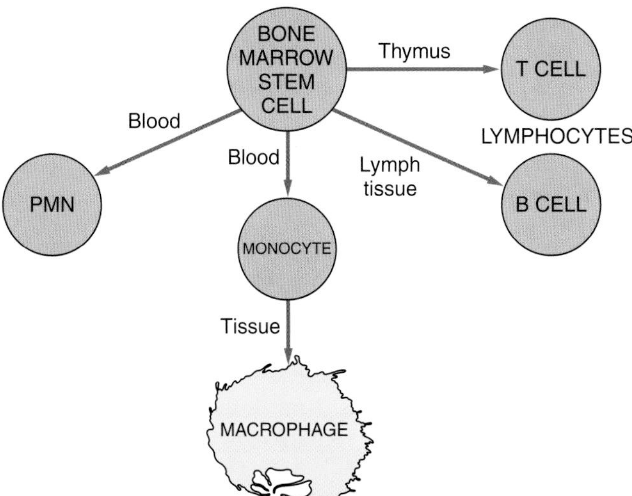

FIGURE 3-1 ■ Differentiation between B and T lymphocytes. The primary cell of the immune response is the lymphocyte. The two main types of lymphocytes are (1) the B lymphocyte and (2) the T lymphocyte. Lymphocytes, like other white blood cells, are derived from stem cells in the bone marrow. *PMN*, Polymorphonuclear neutrophil.

B LYMPHOCYTES

B lymphocytes develop from the stem cells in the bone marrow and then reside and mature in **lymphoid tissue.** Lymphoid tissue is found in lymph nodes and many other body locations, including pharyngeal and lingual tonsillar tissues. When antigen stimulates B lymphocytes, they travel to the site of injury. Two main types of B cells develop when a B cell is stimulated by an antigen: the **plasma cell** and the B memory cell. The B memory cell retains the memory of the antigen. In the presence of an antigen recognized by the memory B, this cell duplicates in a process called clonal selection; all of these newly formed B cells retain the capacity to recognize the previously encountered antigen.

Plasma cells have a round, pin-wheel–shaped nucleus and visible cytoplasm. Plasma cells produce proteins called **antibodies.** Antibodies, also called **immunoglobulins (Igs),** are secreted into the blood serum. Five different types of immunoglobulins exist: IgA, IgD, IgE, IgG, and IgM (Table 3-1). They all have variations of the same basic structure (Figures 3-2 and 3-3).

Specific antibodies are produced in response to specific antigens by a specific plasma cell. This specificity is a characteristic function of the immune response. The level of a specific antibody in the blood is called the **antibody titer** and can be measured by diagnostic laboratory tests. This is helpful in the diagnosis of some infectious diseases.

Antibodies can combine with antigen, forming an **immune complex.** The portion of the antibody that recognizes and binds to the antigen is called its **antigenic determinate.** The formation of an immune complex usually renders the antigen inactive. Immune complexes may also be involved in certain disease states.

T LYMPHOCYTES

After they develop from the bone marrow stem cell, the T lymphocytes travel to the **thymus** and then are processed into mature cells. The thymus is a primary lymphoid organ located high in the chest. It is quite large in infants and shrinks as an individual matures.

T cells depend on unique cell surface molecules called the **major histocompatibility complex** to help them recognize antigen fragments. Different types of T cells have different functions in the immune response. Some are memory cells similar to those within the B cell population; others are T-helper cells that increase the functioning of the B lymphocytes (enhancing the antibody response) and are easily identifiable by the T4 cell marker (Figure 3-4). T-suppressor cells, which usually carry the T8 marker, suppress or "turn off" the functioning of the B lymphocytes. T-cytotoxic cells, which also carry the T8 marker, are active in surveillance against virally infected cells or tumor cells by directly attacking these cells. T cells within cell-mediated immunity also orchestrate, regulate, and coordinate the overall immune response.

Table 3-1

Known immunoglobulins (antibodies)

Immunoglobulin	Description
IgA	Has two subgroups: serous in the blood and secretory in the saliva and other secretions; aids in defense against proliferation of microorganisms in body fluids
IgD	Functions in the activation of B lymphocytes
IgE	Involved in hypersensitivity reactions since it can bind to mast cells and basophils and bring about the release of biochemical mediators such as histamine
IgG	Major antibody in blood serum; can pass the placental barrier and forms the first passive immunity for the newborn
IgM	Involved in early immune responses because of its involvement with IgD in the activation of B cell lymphocytes

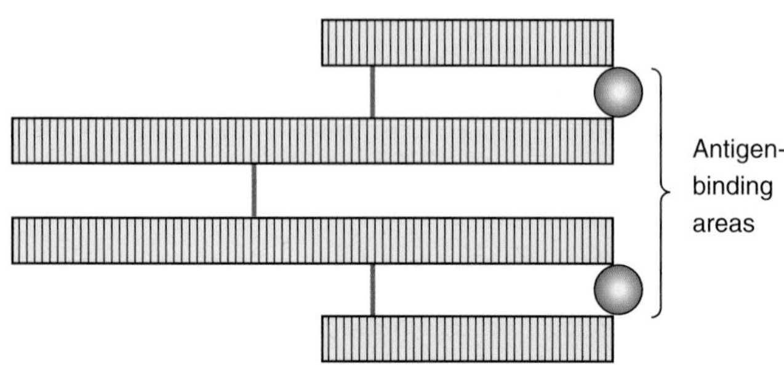

FIGURE 3-2 ■ The basic structure of an antibody or immunoglobulin (Ig) includes four protein chains consisting of two identical heavy polypeptide chains and two identical light chains, shaped to form a Y. The sections that make up the tips of the arms of the Y vary greatly, creating a pocket uniquely shaped to enfold a specific antigen. This is called the variable region. The stem of the Y serves to link the antibody to other participants in the immune response. This area is identical in all antibodies of the same class and is called the constant region.

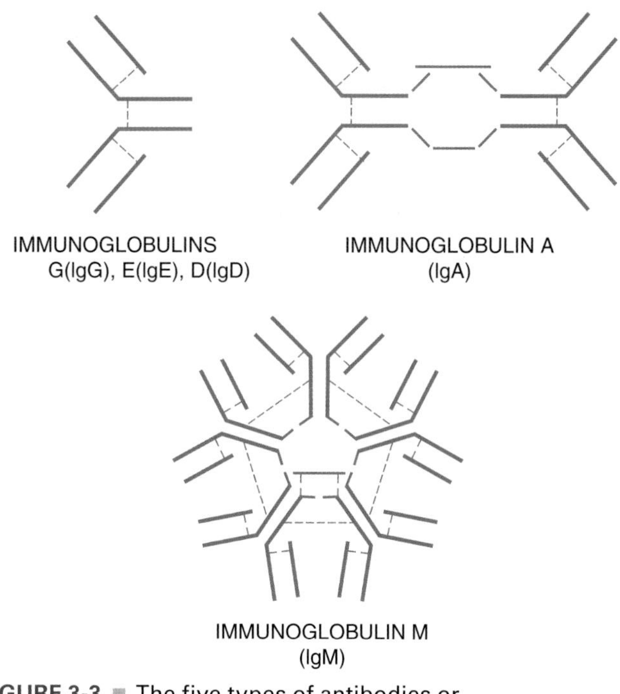

FIGURE 3-3 ■ The five types of antibodies or immunoglobulins include the same basic structure arranged differently. This variation in structure allows them to function differently.

MACROPHAGES

Not only are **macrophages** present in the connective tissue during inflammation (see Chapter 2 for their role and a description of the cell), but they are also involved in the immune response to an antigen. Macrophages are active in phagocytosis of foreign substances and help both the B cells and T cells during the immune response. After phagocytosis of an antigen at the injury site, the macrophages then act as antigen-processing cells for the lymphocytes. This stimulates the lymphocytes to travel from the lymphoid tissue to the injury site.

Thus macrophages serve as a link between the inflammatory and immune responses since, in addition to phagocytosis, macrophages can also act as antigen-presenting cells. When activated, macrophages can function in many different ways, always amplifying the immune response. Unlike lymphocytes, macrophages do not remember the encountered antigen and need to be reactivated during each encounter.

CYTOKINES

Cytokines are proteins that are made by cells and are able to affect the behavior of other cells. They are produced by the cells of the immune system and play a prominent role in the activation of the immune response. Cytokines are one way that lymphocytes communicate with each other and with other immune system cells. B or T lymphocytes produce cytokines that are called lymphokines. Different cytokines have different functions (Table 3-2). They can activate macrophages and enhance the ability of macrophages to destroy foreign cells. These types of cytokines may also be involved in various other functions concerning leukocytes, fibroblasts, and endothelial cells. Macrophages produce cytokines called monokines. One of the first cytokines to be discovered was interferon. Produced by T cells and macrophages (as well as

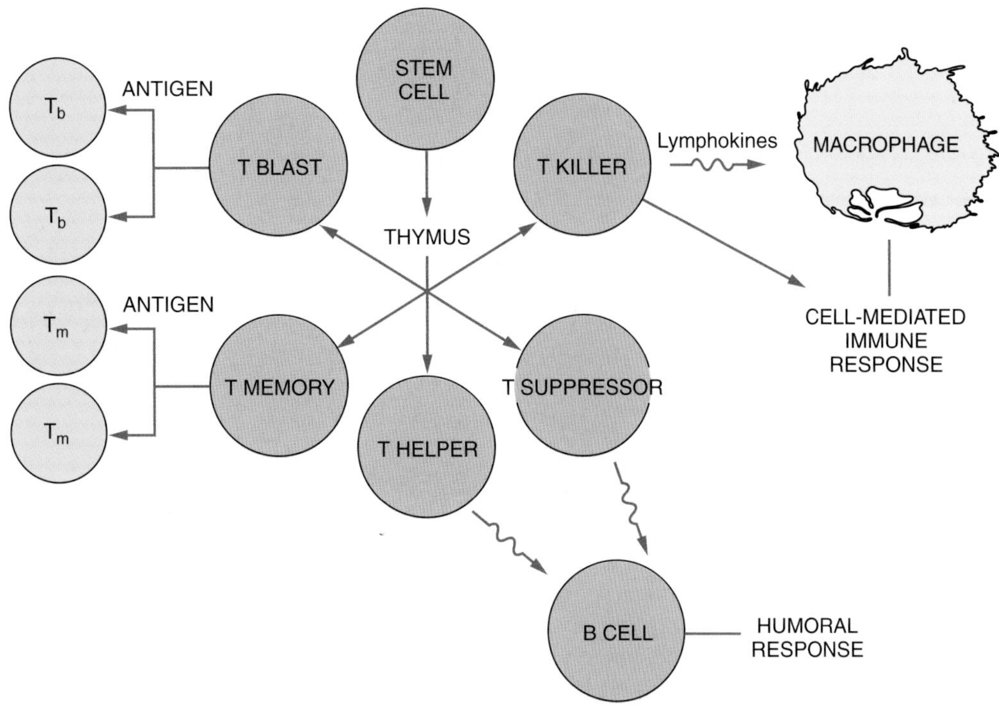

FIGURE 3-4 ■ Various types of T lymphocytes and their involvement in the immune response.

Table 3-2

Cytokines and their functions during the immune response

Cytokine	Function
Interleukins	Stimulates leukocyte proliferation and other functions
Macrophage chemotactic factor	Stimulates macrophage emigration
Migration inhibitory factor	Inhibits macrophage activity
Macrophage-activating factor	Activates macrophages to produce and secrete lysosomal enzymes
Lymphotoxin	Destroys fibroblasts
Interferons	Various functions involving leukocytes, fibroblasts, and endothelial cells
Tumor necrosis factor	Various functions involving leukocytes and fibroblasts

by cells outside the immune system), interferons are a family of proteins with antiviral properties. Chemokines are a family of small cytokines; their name is derived from their ability to induce directed chemotaxis in nearby responsive cells. They may be involved in controlling infection as part of the immune response such as in an infection with the human immunodeficiency virus.

MAJOR DIVISIONS OF THE IMMUNE RESPONSE

Historically the immune system has been described as two major divisions that differ in their response to an antigen. However, these divisions are interrelated, and present understanding of immune responses recognizes that these divisions are not distinctly separate mechanisms. The immune response to an antigen can take one of two forms (Figure 3-5): **humoral immunity** and **cell-mediated immunity.** Humoral (antibody-mediated) immunity involves the production of antibodies with the B lymphocytes as the primary cells. Humoral immunity is responsible for protection against many bacteria and viruses. The other division of the immune system, cell-mediated immunity or cellular immunity, involves lymphocytes, usually T cells, working alone or assisted by macrophages. The cell-mediated division regulates both major responses.

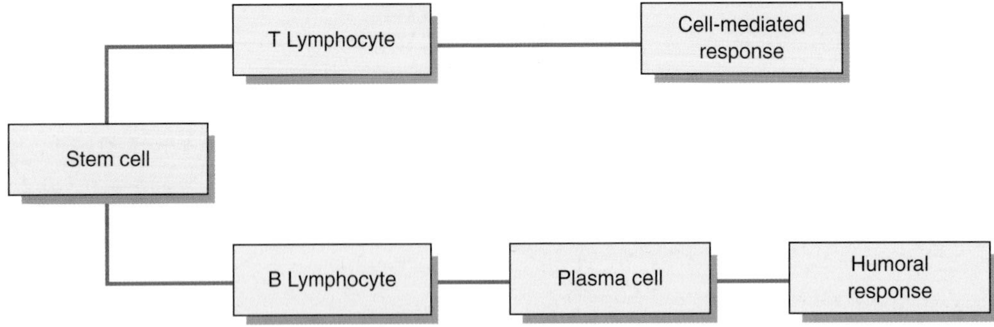

FIGURE 3-5 ■ Major divisions of the immune response.

MEMORY AND IMMUNITY

Memory is a characteristic function of the acquired immune response. This contrasts with the inflammatory response, which is not capable of memory. Certain lymphocytes retain the memory of an antigen after an initial encounter. For this reason, the immune response to that antigen is much more rapid and is stronger the next time it is encountered. Immunity is this increased responsiveness that results from the retained memory of an already encountered antigen.

TYPES OF IMMUNITY

PASSIVE IMMUNITY

Two types of immunity occur: passive and active. Using antibodies produced by another person to protect an individual against infectious disease is called **passive immunity.** This type of immunity can occur naturally or it can be acquired. **Natural passive immunity** occurs when antibodies from a mother pass through the placenta to the developing fetus. These antibodies protect a newborn infant from disease while the infant's own immune system matures.

Passive immunity can also be acquired through an injection of antibodies against a microorganism to which the person has not previously developed antibodies. This is used to confer immediate protection against the disease caused by that microorganism. These antibodies are collected from individuals who have already had the disease and have naturally produced antibodies to the disease-causing microorganism. This type of passive immunity is short-lived but can act immediately. It is used because the unprepared immune system of an individual takes longer to produce antibodies, and in the meantime the disease may develop. Acquired passive immunity, using hepatitis B immunoglobulin, may be provided to dental personnel who do not have immunity to hepatitis B after needlestick or other occupational exposure incidents.

ACTIVE IMMUNITY

Active immunity can occur naturally or be acquired. It occurs naturally when a microorganism causes the disease. Protection against further attack by that microorganism is conferred to the individual if the body recovers from the disease. A less risky way of achieving active immunity is by an acquired or artificial means. A person is injected with or ingests either altered pathogenic microorganisms or products of those microorganisms. The altered microorganism or product cannot produce infection but is able to act as an antigen. This is called a vaccine, and the process is called vaccination. When the pathogenic microorganism is encountered after vaccination, the immune system produces a stronger, faster response and prevents development of the disease. This production of acquired immunity is called **immunization.**

Immunization lowers the risk of a microorganism causing disease because it safely prepares the immune system to fight future attacks by the disease-causing microorganism. In some cases more than one exposure to the antigen is needed to ensure adequate immunity. A repeated exposure by way of a vaccination is called a booster. Immunization by vaccination is used to protect children and adults against many diseases. Dental personnel should be vaccinated against the hepatitis B virus because of their high risk of occupational exposure to that virus.

IMMUNOPATHOLOGY

Immunopathology is the study of immune reactions involved in disease. The immune response helps defend the body against disease-producing antigens, but it can also malfunction and cause tissue damage. Immunopathology includes diseases caused by malfunctioning of the immune system. Hypersensitivity reactions and autoimmune diseases are examples of conditions in which damage is caused by the immune response.

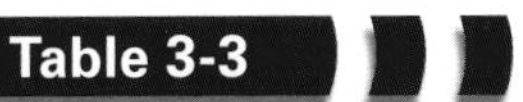

Examples of hypersensitivity reactions

Type of Reaction	Examples
Type I (anaphylactic type)	Hay fever, asthma, anaphylaxis
Type II (cytotoxic type)	Autoimmune hemolytic anemia
Type III (immune complex type)	Autoimmune diseases
Type IV (cell-mediated type)	Granulomatous disease (e.g., tuberculosis)

HYPERSENSITIVITY

Hypersensitivity reactions are also called allergic reactions (**allergy**) and comprise the same types of reactions that occur when the immune response is fighting microorganisms and protecting the body against disease. However, hypersensitivity reactions are exaggerated immunopathologic responses; tissue destruction occurs as a result of the immune response. Four main types of hypersensitivity reactions occur; they are classified by the nature of the immune response that causes the disease (Table 3-3).

Type I Hypersensitivity

Type I hypersensitivity is a reaction that occurs immediately (within minutes) after exposure to a previously encountered antigen (allergen) such as pollen, latex, or penicillin. In type 1 hypersensitivity plasma cells produce IgE as a response to the antigen. IgE causes mast cells to release their granules containing histamine. This results in edema caused by increased dilation and permeability of blood vessels and in constriction of smooth muscle in the bronchioles of the lungs. This type of hypersensitivity includes hay fever and more serious conditions, including asthma and **anaphylaxis.** Anaphylaxis can be life threatening because the individual may not be able to breathe as a result of the oropharyngeal tissue swelling and constriction of the bronchioles.

Type II Hypersensitivity

In type II hypersensitivity antibody combines with an antigen that is bound to the surface of tissue cells, usually a circulating red blood cell. Activated complement components, IgG and IgM antibodies in blood, participate in this type of hypersensitivity reaction. The result is the destruction of the tissue that has the antigen on the surface of its cells. This type of reaction occurs in incompatible blood transfusions and in rhesus (Rh) incompatibility. In Rh incompatibility the mother's antibodies cross the placenta and destroy the newborn's red blood cells, resulting in hemolytic anemia.

Type III Hypersensitivity

In type III hypersensitivity immune complexes are formed between microorganisms and antibody in the circulating blood. The complexes leave the blood and are deposited in various body tissues or in a localized area. In either case the deposition results in the initiation of an acute inflammatory response. Neutrophils are attracted to the tissues in which the complexes have been deposited. As a result of phagocytosis and death of the neutrophils, lysosomal enzymes are released, causing tissue destruction. This type of hypersensitivity occurs in autoimmune diseases such as systemic lupus erythematosus. Systemic lupus erythematosus is discussed later in this chapter.

Type IV Hypersensitivity

Type IV hypersensitivity involves a cell-mediated immune response rather than a humoral (antibody) response. T lymphocytes that have been introduced to an antigen previously either cause damage to the tissue cells or recruit other cells that cause the damage. This type of hypersensitivity reaction is also called **delayed hypersensitivity** and is put to use when diagnosing tuberculosis. A visible skin reaction occurs if the individual tested has previously been exposed to the organism that causes tuberculosis. This type of hypersensitivity is also responsible for the rejection of tissue grafts and transplanted organs. New strategies for prevention of rejection, such as therapeutic antibodies against specific T-cell receptors, may produce fewer long-term side effects than the chemotherapies now routinely used.

Hypersensitivity to Drugs

Drugs can act as antigens and cause an immunologically induced inflammatory response. Many factors influence the risk of an allergic (hypersensitivity) reaction to a drug. The route of administration influences how the reaction will be manifested and its severity. Although topical administration of drugs may cause a greater number of reactions than oral (swallowed) or parenteral (administered by injection) routes of administration, the reaction that occurs after parenteral administration may be more widespread and severe because the allergen (the antigen eliciting the response) can be carried quickly to many parts of the body by the circulating blood. The presence of infection may increase the risk of an allergic reaction. Patients with multiple allergies are more likely to have allergic reactions to drugs, and patients with autoimmune diseases such as systemic lupus erythematosus commonly have adverse reactions to medication. Children are less likely than adults to have an allergic reaction to a drug.

Drugs can cause any of the previously described hypersensitivity reactions. Type I allergy to a drug can include anaphylaxis, urticaria (hives), and angioedema (localized swelling). A systemic anaphylactic reaction is more likely to occur with an injected drug but can also occur with a drug administered orally and can be fatal. For example, penicillin may cause a systemic anaphylactic reaction in approximately one in 10,000 patients. It causes about 300 deaths per year in the United States.

The classic example of a type III allergy is called *serum sickness*. This name was given to a reaction that occurred frequently when patients were given large amounts of horse antitoxin serum to provide passive immunity in the treatment of diphtheria and tetanus. This is no longer the method by which passive immunity to these diseases is provided. This reaction can occur in response to other foreign agents. Penicillin is the single most common cause of serum sickness. However, other drugs such as barbiturates can also cause this reaction. The symptoms of serum sickness include fever, painful swelling of the joints (arthritis), renal disturbance or failure, edema around the eyes, cardiac inflammation, and skin lesions.

Drugs can also cause a type IV hypersensitivity reaction. This T cell–mediated allergic reaction can occur in response to topically applied substances and can produce contact dermatitis and **mucositis.**

AUTOIMMUNE DISEASES

The immune system learns to differentiate between the body's own cells and tissues and foreign substances early in embryologic development. This recognition and the nonresponsiveness of the immune system to the body's own cells and tissues are called **immunologic tolerance**. In autoimmune diseases, also called **connective tissue diseases,** the recognition mechanism breaks down, and certain body cells are no longer tolerated. The immune system treats body cells as antigens. An autoimmune disease may involve a single cell type or a single organ or may be even more extensive, involving multiple organs. Tissues and even entire organs may be damaged. An example is the T cells that attack pancreatic cells contributing to diabetes mellitus. Genetic factors may play a role in the predisposition of an individual to autoimmune disease, and viral infection may also be involved. Several autoimmune diseases have oral manifestations. These are described later in this chapter.

IMMUNODEFICIENCY

Immunodeficiency is a type of immunopathologic condition that involves a deficiency in number, function, or interrelationships of the involved white blood cells and their products. This condition may be congenital (present at birth) or acquired (developed after birth). Immunodeficiency may be inherited genetically, or it can be caused by numerous other factors. When a person's immune system is not functioning adequately, infections and tumors may develop. Studies have shown that stress and depression may be associated with decreased levels of immune function. Acquired immunodeficiency syndrome, which is discussed in Chapter 4, is an example of an immunodeficiency that has numerous oral manifestations.

ORAL DISEASES WITH IMMUNOLOGIC PATHOGENESIS

APHTHOUS ULCERS

Aphthous ulcers, also known as **canker sores** or **aphthous stomatitis,** are painful oral ulcers for which the cause remains unclear. They frequently recur in episodes. Three forms of recurrent aphthous ulceration exist: (1) minor, (2) major, and (3) herpetiform. The three forms differ in the size and duration of the ulcers. Aphthous ulcers are common ulcers in the oral cavity, occurring in about 20% of the general population. However, a dramatic variation in occurrence takes place, from as high as 57% of a professional school population to 5% of patients studied in a large inner city hospital. The first episode of these ulcers usually occurs in adolescence, and they are somewhat more common in females than in males. The clinical appearance and location are important in establishing the diagnosis.

Trauma is the most commonly reported precipitating factor in the development of aphthous ulcers. They are often reported to occur after trauma to the oral mucosa during dental procedures (e.g., in the area of film placement or at the site of injection of local anesthetics). Some patients may experience aphthous ulcers as a result of manipulation of oral tissues during dental hygiene treatment. Emotional stress has also been suggested as a contributing factor. Some patients associate the initiation of aphthous ulcers with eating certain foods such as citrus fruits. However, it is possible that patients perceive these foods as causative because of the sensitivity of the ulcers to foods with a high acid content. The recurrence of aphthous ulcers has been associated with menstruation, whereas pregnancy has been found to produce a decrease in the episodes. These ulcers occur in association with certain systemic diseases such as:

- Behçet syndrome
- Crohn disease
- Ulcerative colitis
- Cyclic neutropenia
- Sprue (gluten intolerance)
- Intestinal lymphoma
- PFAPA syndrome (Periodic Fever, Aphthous stomatitis, Pharyngitis, Adenitis)

Substantial evidence indicates that aphthous ulcers have an immunologic pathogenesis. Patients in whom aphthous ulcers develop have slightly elevated levels of a ies to oral mucous membranes. Histologically an ir of lymphocytes is present in the lesion, suggestin cell-mediated immunity may be important in develo of the ulcers. The infiltrate contains primarily T-helpe in the prodromal stage, T-cytotoxic cells in the ulcer phase, and T-helper cells again in the healing stage. T-cytotoxic cells are probably responsible for the ulcerat However, the specific antigen to which they are respond has not yet been identified.

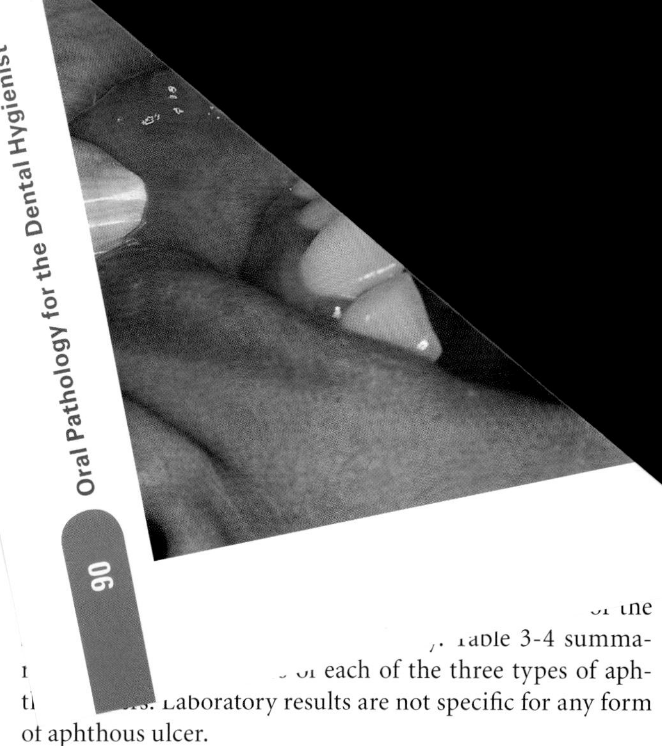

Minor Aphthous Ulcers

Minor aphthous ulcers are the most commonly occurring type. They appear as discrete, round-to-oval ulcers that can be as large as 1 cm in diameter and exhibit a yellowish-white fibrin surface surrounded by a halo of erythema (Figure 3-6). The ulcers occur on the movable mucosa of the oral cavity (the mucosa not covering bone) and occasionally extend onto the gingiva. They occur on the labial and buccal mucosa, the maxillary and mandibular vestibular mucosa, the ventral and lateral borders of the tongue, and the soft palate and oropharynx. Minor aphthous ulcers are more common in the anterior than the posterior part of the mouth. The ulcers often have a prodromal period of 1 to 2 days, which is characterized by a burning sensation or soreness in the area in which the ulcer will form. Aphthous ulcers are exquisitely painful, and single or multiple lesions may be present. The ulcers heal spontaneously in 7 to 10 days.

Major Aphthous Ulcers

Major aphthous ulcers (Sutton disease, periadenitis mucosa necrotica recurrens) are larger than 1 cm in diameter and are deeper and last longer than minor

... of the ... Table 3-4 summa- ... of each of the three types of aph- ... Laboratory results are not specific for any form of aphthous ulcer.

The location of the ulcers is important in differentiating between recurrent aphthous ulcers and recurrent intraoral ulceration caused by the herpes simplex virus (see Table 4-2). When they occur intraorally, ulcers resulting from the herpes simplex virus appear on keratinized mucosa. This is the mucosa of the palate and gingiva (i.e., the mucosa fixed to bone).

Frequently a biopsy is necessary for diagnosing major aphthous ulcers because they may clinically resemble squamous cell carcinoma or deep fungal infections.

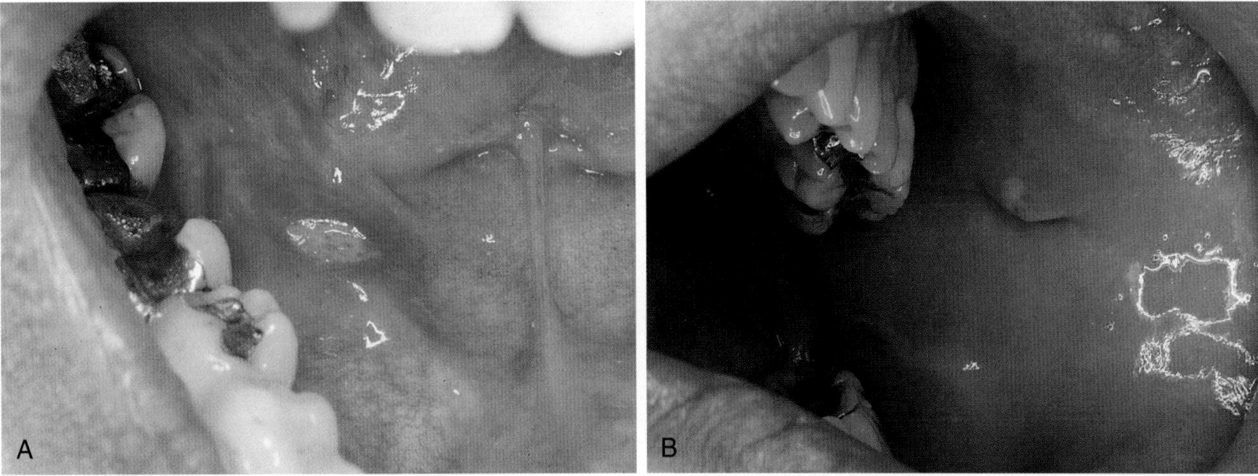

FIGURE 3-6 ■ **A,** Example of a minor aphthous ulcer. **B,** Minor aphthous ulcer on the buccal mucosa on the papilla of Stenson's duct.

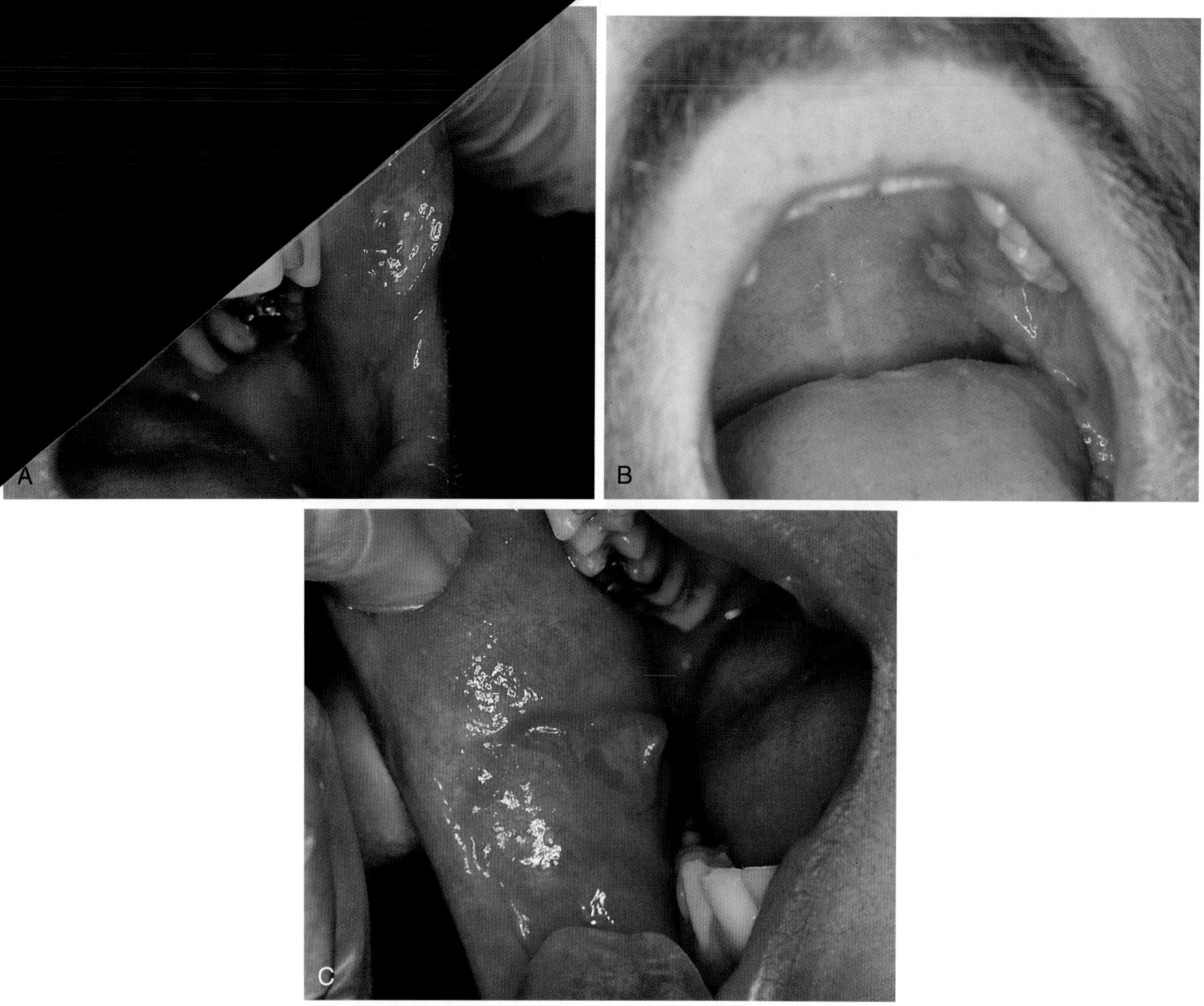

FIGURE 3-7 ■ Examples of major aphthous ulcers. **A,** Labial mucosa. **B,** Soft palate. **C,** Buccal mucosa.

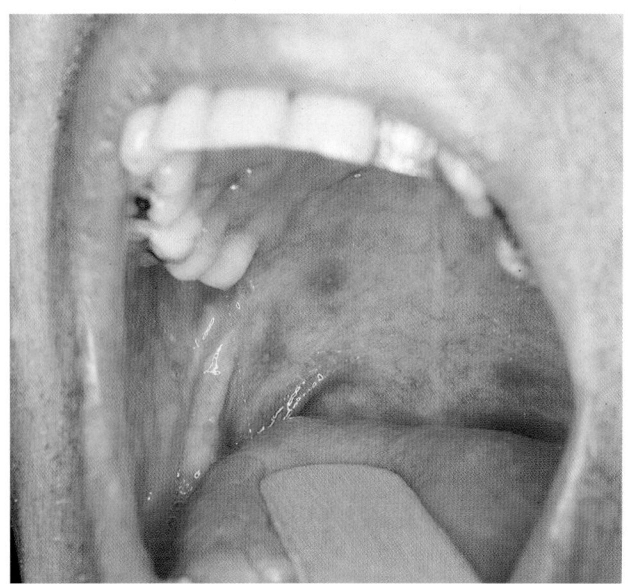

FIGURE 3-8 ■ Herpetiform aphthous ulcers.

Herpetiform aphthous ulcers may be difficult to distinguish clinically from primary herpetic gingivostomatitis. However, no systemic signs or symptoms exist as in primary herpes simplex infection. Herpetiform aphthous ulcers have been reported to respond to topical application of liquid tetracycline. This response may be helpful in confirming the diagnosis of herpetiform aphthous ulcers because true herpes simplex ulceration does not respond to this treatment.

When a patient develops multiple aphthous ulcers, it is important to consider that they might be associated with a systemic disease. Identification of signs and symptoms that may suggest systemic disease should be considered when reviewing the patient's medical history. These include the presence of chronic gastrointestinal symptoms such as diarrhea and discomfort (Crohn disease, ulcerative colitis, sprue, intestinal lymphoma), arthritis and skin lesions (Behçet syndrome), and periodic fevers in a child (cyclic neutropenia and PFAFA syndrome).

Table 3-4

Clinical features of the three types of recurrent aphthous ulcers

Feature	Minor	Major	Herpetiform
Size	Small, 3-5 mm	Large, 5-10 mm	Very small, 1-2 mm
Location	Unattached mucosa	Unattached mucosa	Unattached mucosa
Most common area	Anterior	Posterior	Anywhere
Number	1-5	1-10	1-100
Scarring	No	Yes	No
Pain	Yes	Yes	Yes
Appearance	Shallow	Deep	Ulcers coalesce

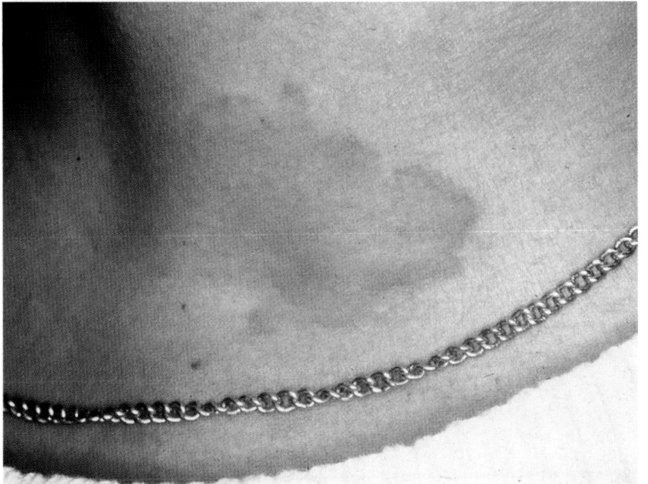

FIGURE 3-9 ■ Urticaria.

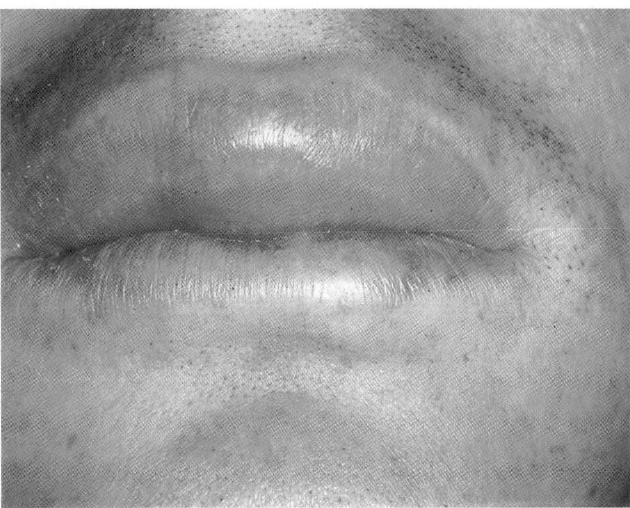

FIGURE 3-10 ■ Angioedema. (Courtesy Dr. Edward V. Zegarelli.)

Treatment

The local application of topical steroids and topical nonsteroidal antiinflammatory agents is helpful in the management of aphthous ulcers. These drugs are most effective when applied very early in the development of the ulcer. Occasionally systemic steroids may be necessary for managing patients with major aphthous ulcers. Topical application of liquid tetracycline is also helpful, particularly in the diagnosis of herpetiform ulcerations when the diagnosis is not clear and the differential diagnosis includes viral infection. The use of topical steroids is contraindicated for viral ulcers; therefore accurate diagnosis is important. Topical anesthetics can help to decrease the pain of aphthous ulcers.

URTICARIA AND ANGIOEDEMA

Urticaria and angioedema are similar lesions. **Urticaria,** also called **hives** (Figure 3-9), appears as multiple areas of well-demarcated swelling of the skin, usually accompanied by itching (pruritus). The lesions are caused by localized areas of vascular permeability in the superficial connective tissue beneath the epithelium. **Angioedema** (Figure 3-10) is a similar lesion that appears as a diffuse swelling of tissue caused by permeability of deeper blood vessels. The skin covering the swelling appears normal, and angioedema is usually not accompanied by itching. Urticaria and angioedema both may occur in acute self-limited episodes. Occasionally chronic or recurrent forms may occur.

In many cases of urticaria and angioedema the cause cannot be identified. Infection, trauma, emotional stress, and certain systemic diseases have been reported to cause these lesions. Ingested allergens are frequent causes of urticaria.

Several mechanisms are capable of causing the increased vascular permeability that results in urticaria and angioedema, including the release of the chemical mediator histamine from mast cells stimulated by IgE antibodies (type I hypersensitivity) and the activation of IgG or IgM antibodies along with trauma, causing vascular permeability.

Acetylsalicylic acid (aspirin) and nonsteroidal antiinflammatory drugs such as ibuprofen can produce a nonspecific effect that can cause vascular permeability. A rare hereditary form of angioedema exists in which uncontrolled activation of the complement cascade occurs, resulting in prolonged vascular permeability.

The diagnoses of urticaria and angioedema are based on the clinical appearance of the lesions and the patient's history. Avoidance of the causative agent, if identified, is important in managing patients with recurring urticaria and angioedema. Immediate treatment is essential. Antihistaminic drugs are the principal method of treatment. Angioedema involving the larynx and pharynx can cause asphyxiation and therefore may be fatal.

CONTACT MUCOSITIS AND DERMATITIS

Contact mucositis and **contact dermatitis** are lesions that result from the direct contact of an allergen with the skin or mucosa. The development of these conditions involves a T cell–mediated immune response and is an example of type IV hypersensitivity. The exact underlying immunologic basis is not always clear.

In contact mucositis the mucosa becomes erythematous and edematous, often accompanied by burning and pruritus (Figure 3-11, *A*). The mucositis occurs at the point at which the offending agent has contacted the mucosa, giving it a smooth, shiny appearance that is firm to palpation. Small vesicles and ulcers may appear in the affected areas. In contact dermatitis the initial lesion may be erythematous, with swelling and vesicles. Later the area becomes encrusted with a scaly, white epidermis.

Topical antibiotics, antihistamines, preservatives in local anesthetics, and components of topical medication are common causes of allergic reactions. Acrylics, metal-based alloys, epoxy resins, and the flavoring agents in chewing gum and dentifrices all have been reported to cause contact mucositis.

Contact dermatitis, particularly that affecting the hands, may occur in response to the materials used in dentistry. The routine use of gloves in dental care has decreased the incidence of this type of dermatitis, but latex gloves and glove powder have also been responsible for contact dermatitis in some individuals (Figure 3-11, *B*).

Skin testing for sensitivity to a particular substance can help confirm the agent that caused the lesion. However, first the substance has to be identified. Topical and systemic corticosteroids may be used in the management of these lesions in some patients.

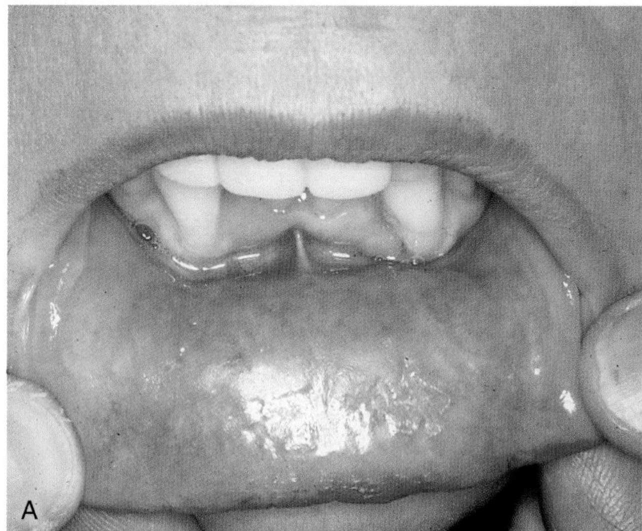

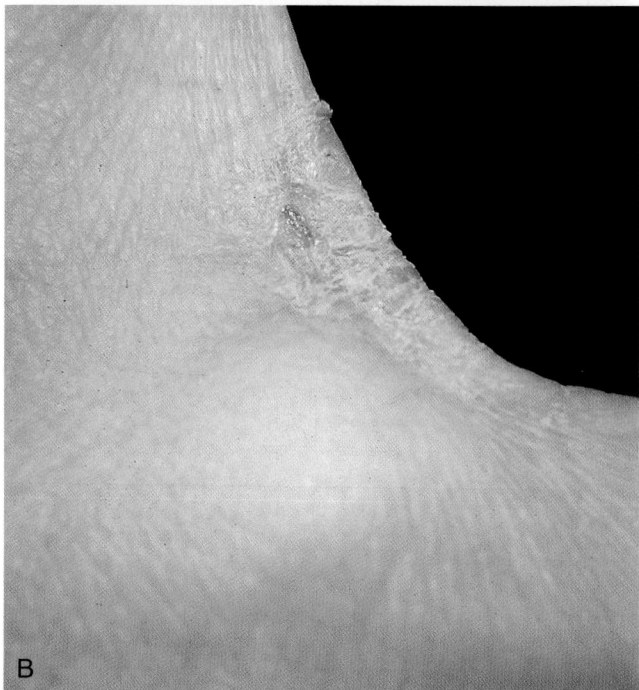

FIGURE 3-11 ■ **A,** Contact mucositis from acrylic. **B,** Contact dermatitis from latex gloves (seen here on the skin between the thumb and index finger). (**A** courtesy Dr. Edward V. Zegarelli.)

FIXED DRUG ERUPTIONS

Fixed drug eruptions are lesions that appear in the same site each time a drug is introduced. The lesions generally appear suddenly after a latent period of several days and subside when the drug is discontinued. They appear again when the drug is reintroduced, usually with greater intensity. Clinically there may be single or multiple slightly raised, reddish patches or clusters of macules on the skin or rarely the mucous membranes. Pain and pruritus may be associated with these lesions.

The fixed drug eruption is a type of allergic reaction (type III hypersensitivity) in which immune complexes are deposited along the endothelial wall of blood vessels. The ensuing inflammatory reaction causes vasculitis and subsequent damage to the vessel wall, giving rise to erythema and edema of the superficial layers of the skin or mucosa. If possible, the

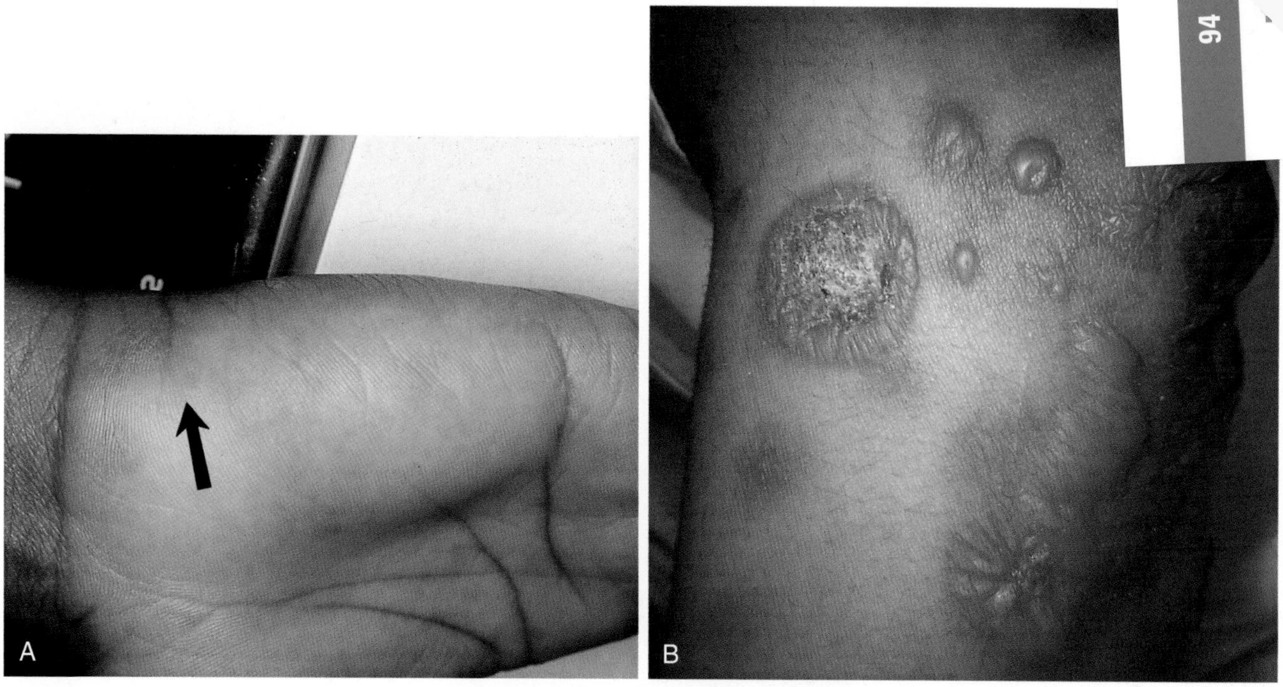

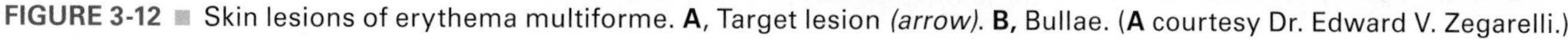

FIGURE 3-12 ■ Skin lesions of erythema multiforme. **A**, Target lesion *(arrow)*. **B**, Bullae. (**A** courtesy Dr. Edward V. Zegarelli.)

drug causing the reaction should be identified, and its use discontinued.

ERYTHEMA MULTIFORME

Erythema multiforme is an acute, self-limited disease that affects the skin and mucous membranes. The cause is not clear, but some evidence exists that it is a hypersensitivity reaction.

Erythema multiforme most commonly occurs in young adults and affects men more commonly than women. The characteristic skin lesion is called a target, iris, or bull's eye lesion and consists of concentric rings of erythema alternating with normal skin color. The color is darkest at the center of the lesion (Figure 3-12). The term *erythema multiforme* refers to the variety of skin lesions that can occur, which range from macules to plaques to bullae. Erythema multiforme can affect the oral mucosa either alone or in association with skin lesions. Skin lesions can occur without oral lesions. The oral lesions are usually ulcers (Figure 3-13, A&B). However, erythematous areas may also occur. The ulcers frequently form on the lateral borders of the tongue. Crusted and bleeding lips are frequently seen in erythema multiforme, and gingival involvement is rare. The disease usually has an explosive onset, and systemic symptoms are mild or lacking. It may be chronic on occasion, or there may be recurrent acute episodes. The most severe form of erythema multiforme is called **Stevens-Johnson syndrome** (Figure 3-13, *C*). Mucosal lesions are more extensive and painful, genital mucosa and the mucosa of the eyes may be involved, and lips are generally encrusted and bloody.

Although the cause of erythema multiforme is not clear, in some cases triggering factors can be identified. Infections such as herpes simplex, tuberculosis, and histoplasmosis have been associated with episodes of erythema multiforme, as have malignant tumors and drugs such as barbiturates and sulfonamides.

Diagnosis

The diagnosis of erythema multiforme is made on the basis of the clinical features and the exclusion of other diseases. The microscopic appearance is nonspecific. Biopsy and histologic examinations are sometimes helpful in excluding other diseases with similar clinical features but more distinctive histologic features.

Treatment and Prognosis

Topical corticosteroids may be helpful in mild cases of erythema multiforme, but systemic corticosteroid treatment is usually needed. Eye lesions in Stevens-Johnson syndrome may lead to scarring and blindness. Systemic antiviral medication is sometimes used to attempt to decrease recurrent episodes thought to be stimulated by herpes simplex virus infection.

LICHEN PLANUS

Lichen planus is a benign, chronic disease affecting the skin and oral mucosa. In some patients this disease may affect both the skin and the oral mucosa. In others either oral

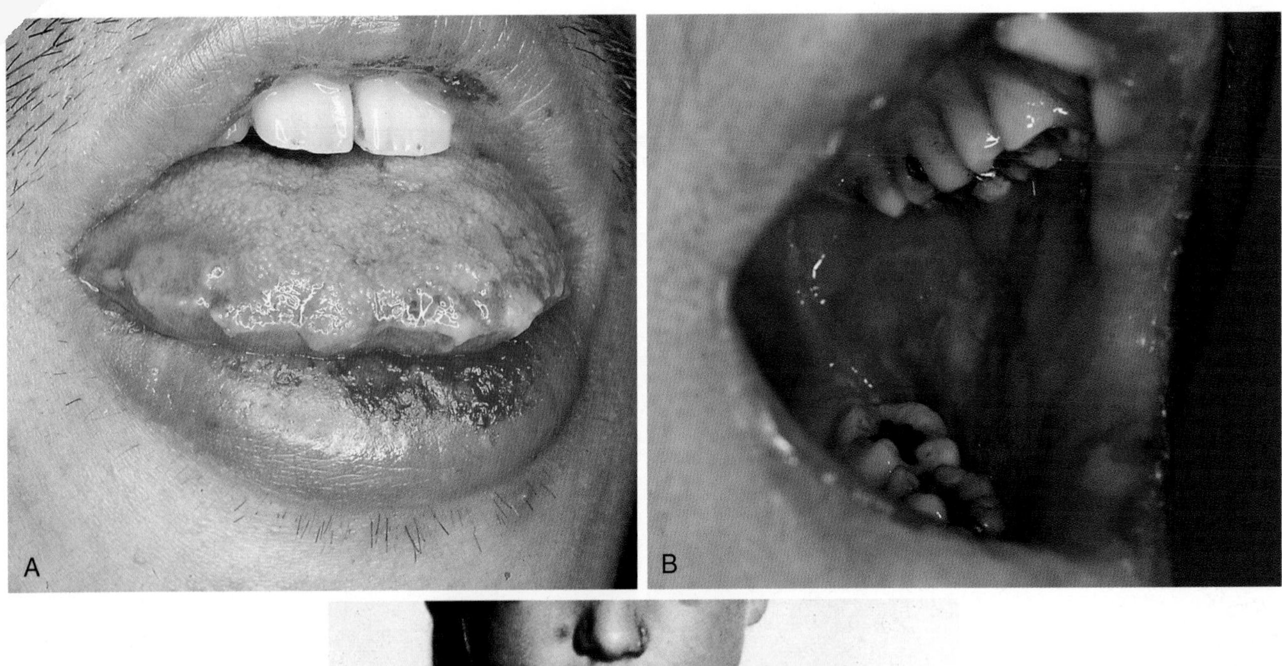

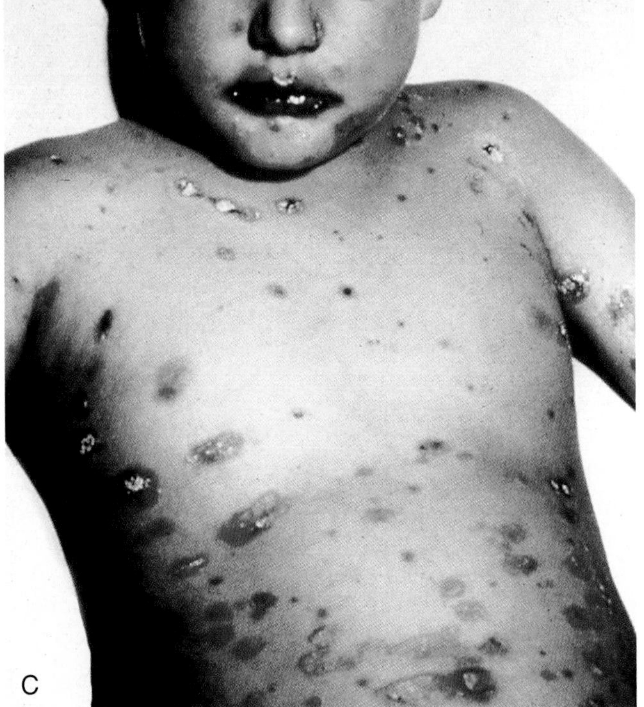

FIGURE 3-13 ■ Oral lesions of erythema multiforme. **A,** Crusted lip lesions with edema, ulceration, and erythema. **B,** Erythematous and ulcerated lesions of the lips and buccal mucosa. **C,** Stevens-Johnson syndrome. (**C** courtesy Dr. Sidney Eisig.)

mucosa or skin alone may be affected. The lesions have a characteristic pattern of interconnecting lines called **striae**, resembling the pattern of the plant lichen as it grows on rocks and trees.

The classic appearance of lichen planus affecting the oral mucosa is an arrangement of interconnecting white lines and circles (Figure 3-14). The slender white lines are called Wickham's striae. The fundamental lesion is a small, papular, pinhead-sized, domed or hemispheric, glistening white nodule on the mucosa. The clinical appearance depends on the arrangement of these minute papules and striae. The most common location is the buccal mucosa. However, lichen planus also occurs on the tongue, lips, floor of the mouth, and gingiva. Lesions of lichen planus are frequently distributed symmetrically in the oral cavity.

The prevalence of lichen planus in the general population of the United States has been reported to be about 1%. In one study of 100 cases, the age of individuals affected ranged

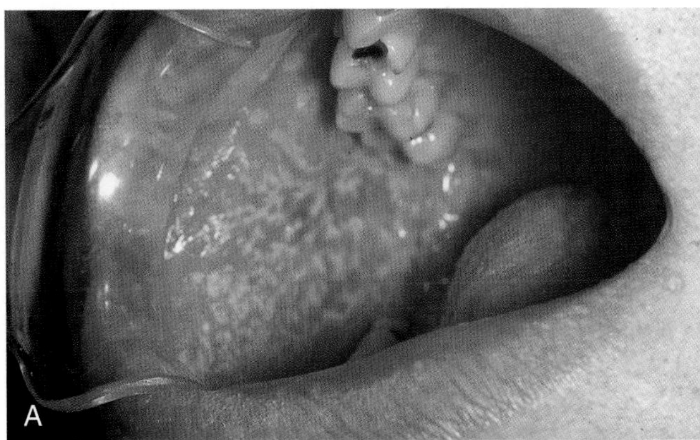

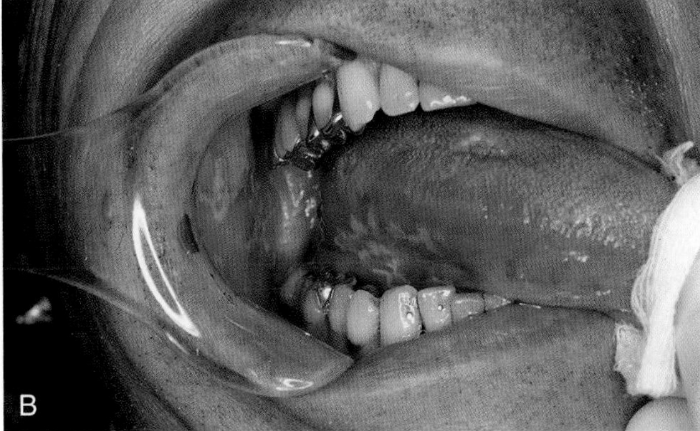

FIGURE 3-14 ■ **A** and **B,** Two examples of the oral lesions of lichen planus. (**A** courtesy Dr. Edward V. Zegarelli.)

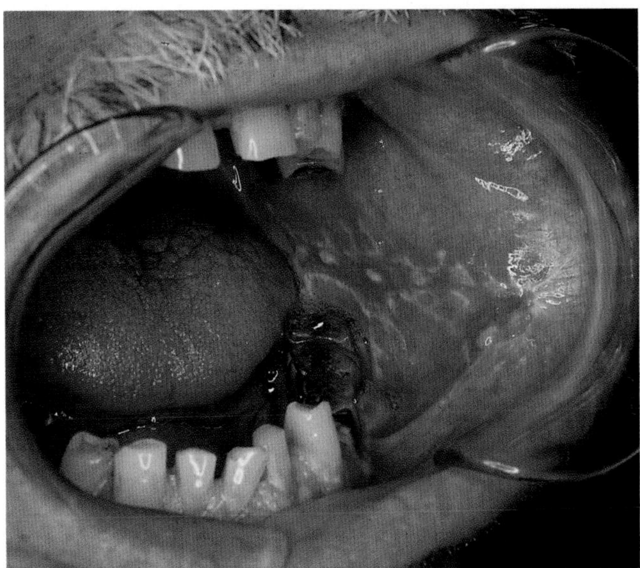

FIGURE 3-15 ■ Lichen planus. Erosion of the mucosa appears as erythema adjacent to white striae.

from 13 to 78 years. However, the disease is most common in middle age. A slight female predominance has been suggested. In another reported study of 200 cases, most were found to be asymptomatic and were discovered on routine oral examination.

Many factors have been implicated in lichen planus; however, the cause remains unknown. Erosive lesions do tend to worsen with emotional stress. Many drugs and chemicals have been shown to produce lichenoid lesions, but these have a different histologic appearance from true lichen planus.

Types of Lichen Planus

Several forms of lichen planus have been described. The most common is **reticular lichen planus.** In this form the lesions are composed of Wickham's striae along with slightly raised white plaquelike areas. Those in which the epithelium separates from the connective tissue and erosions, bullae, or ulcers form are called **erosive** and **bullous lichen planus** (Figure 3-15).

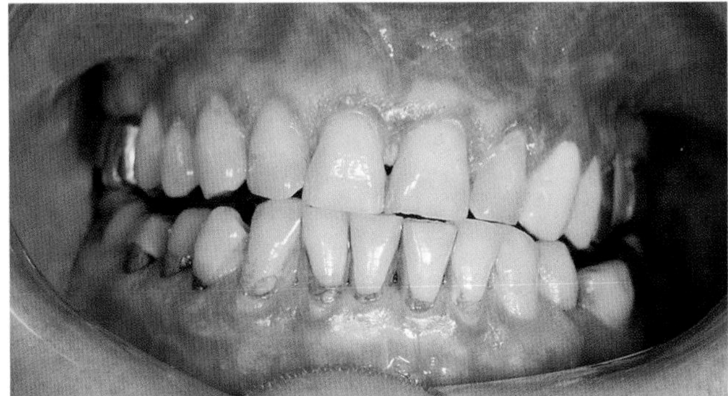

FIGURE 3-16 ■ Lichen planus. The gingival lesions of lichen planus are described clinically as desquamative gingivitis. (Courtesy Dr. Edward V. Zegarelli.)

Gingival lesions clinically described as **desquamative gingivitis** can also be caused by lichen planus (Figure 3-16). In addition to the gingival lesions, striated lesions generally occur elsewhere.

The skin lesions of lichen planus are 2- to 4-mm papules (Figure 3-17). Wickham's striae may also be present, as may pruritus. Lesions can occur anywhere on the skin, but the most common sites are the lumbar region, the flexor surfaces of the wrist, and the anterior surface of the ankles. Some patients have only skin lesions, some have only oral lesions, and others have both skin and oral lesions.

Diagnosis

The diagnosis of lichen planus is made on the basis of the distinctive clinical and histologic appearance of biopsy tissue (Figure 3-18). The epithelium is generally parakeratotic and may be either hyperplastic or atrophic. The characteristic microscopic features include degeneration of the basal

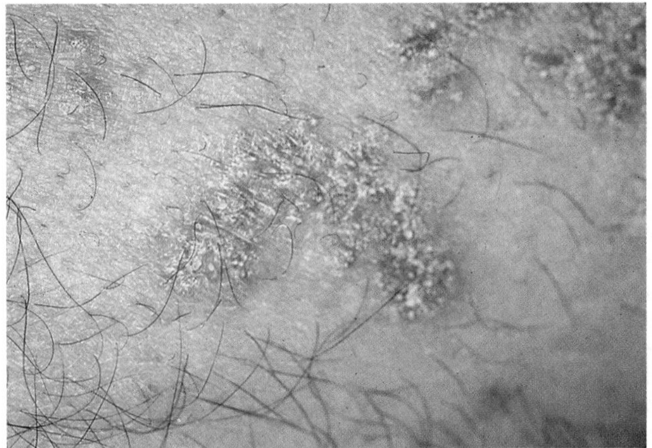

FIGURE 3-17 ■ Skin lesions of lichen planus.

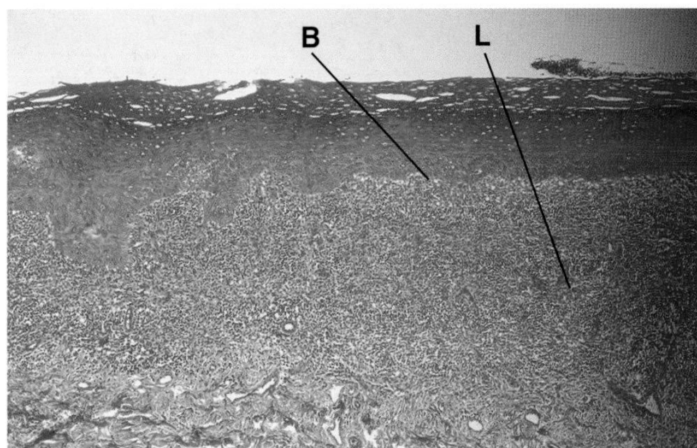

FIGURE 3-18 ■ Lichen planus seen by low-power microscopy. The reader should note the degeneration of the basal cell layer of the epithelium *(B)* and the bandlike infiltrate of lymphocytes *(L)*.

cell layer of the epithelium in small-to-extensive areas, sawtooth-shaped rete ridges, and a broad band of lymphocytes in the connective tissue immediately subjacent to the epithelium. In erosive areas the separation of the epithelium from the connective tissue occurs at the interface of the epithelium and connective tissue. Epithelial atypia and dysplasia may also occur in lesions that appear clinically as lichen planus, and it has been suggested that these lesions may be premalignant.

Treatment and Prognosis

Lichen planus is a chronic disease. Treatment is indicated only when lesions are symptomatic. Erosive lesions usually respond quickly when topical corticosteroid medication is applied. Improvement of gingival lesions with meticulous oral hygiene has been reported. If a drug can be identified as the causative agent of lichenoid-appearing lesions, discontinuation of the drug should cause the lesions to disappear. However, at times it is not possible to discontinue the drug.

Studies have been reported that suggest that patients with lichen planus may be at increased risk for the development of squamous cell carcinoma. Therefore regular oral soft tissue examination and biopsy of any lesions not consistent with lichen planus are recommended.

REACTIVE ARTHRITIS (REITER SYNDROME)

Reactive arthritis (Reiter syndrome) classically comprises the triad of arthritis, urethritis, and conjunctivitis. However, all the components of the syndrome may not be present. Polyarteritis is generally the most prominent component of this syndrome. (A **syndrome** is a group of signs and symptoms that occur together. Other syndromes are described elsewhere in this text.) The cause of this syndrome is not clear. An antigenic marker called HLA-B27 is present in most patients with reactive arthritis suggesting a genetic influence. An abnormal immune response to a microbial antigen is considered the most likely mechanism of occurrence. Reactive arthritis is far more prevalent in men (10:1) than in women (15:1). Reactive arthritis characteristically develops 1 to 4 weeks after venereal or gastrointestinal infection and is usually benign and self-limited.

The arthritis of this condition usually involves the joints of the lower extremities (knees and ankles). It may be asymmetric and migratory, chronic and recurrent.

Radiographically a periosteal proliferation can be detected on the heels, ankles, metatarsals, phalanges, knees, and elbows. Fever, malaise, and weight loss may be associated with the arthritis. The urethritis usually precedes the other lesions. No infectious organisms can be identified. The conjunctivitis is usually mild, but some individuals experience iritis (inflammation of the iris).

Skin and mucous membrane lesions are seen in many patients with reactive arthritis. Oral lesions occur almost anywhere in the oral cavity (Figure 3-19). Aphthouslike ulcers, erythematous lesions, and areas of depapillation of the tongue that mimic geographic tongue have been described in patients with reactive arthritis.

Diagnosis

The diagnosis of reactive arthritis is made on the basis of the clinical signs and symptoms along with identification of the HLA-B27 antigenic marker.

Treatment and Prognosis

The disease lasts from weeks to months. The patient may experience spontaneous remission, but recurrent attacks are common. Aspirin or other nonsteroidal antiinflammatory drugs are generally used for treatment.

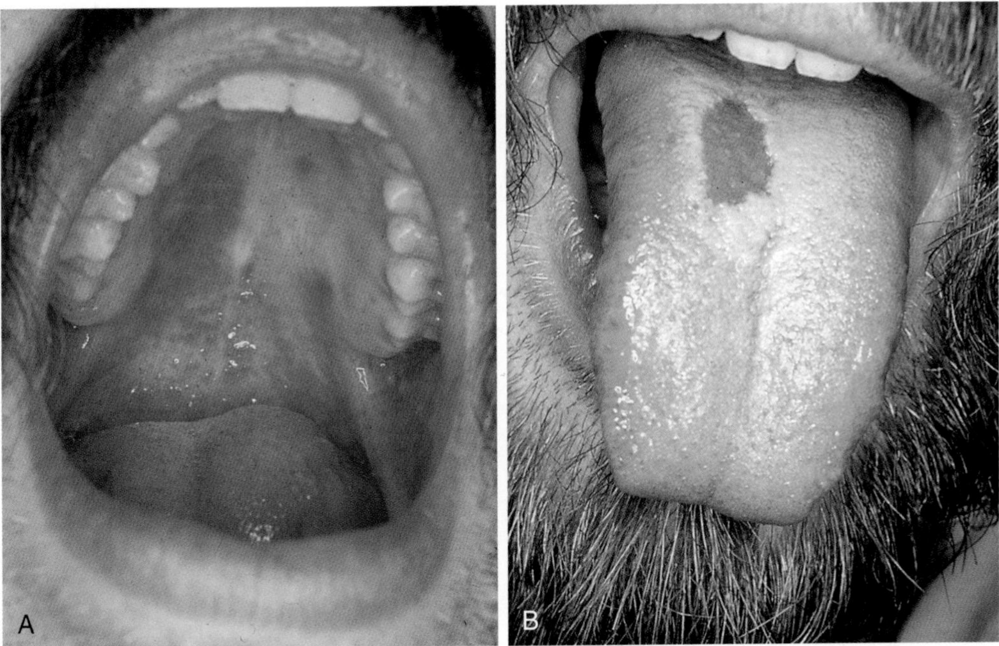

FIGURE 3-19 ■ **A** and **B,** Lesions are present on the palate and tongue in this patient with reactive arthritis.

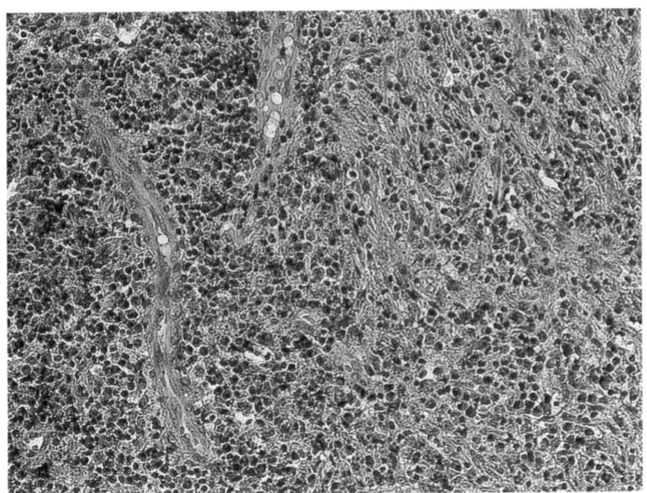

FIGURE 3-20 ■ Langerhans cell disease seen by high-power microscopy.

LANGERHANS CELL DISEASE

Langerhans cell disease was formerly called histiocytosis X. Traditionally three entities were grouped under the category of histiocytosis X: (1) Letterer-Siwe disease, (2) Hand-Schüller-Christian disease, and (3) solitary eosinophilic granuloma. Histologically all are characterized by a combination of Langerhans cells and eosinophils (Figure 3-20). Langerhans cells were originally called histiocytes and were responsible for the name histiocytosis X. In all three diseases the proliferating cell is the Langerhans cell. The presence of eosinophils is thought to result from the production of an eosinophilic chemotactic factor produced by the macrophage.

The Langerhans cell (a type of macrophage) is an immunologically competent cell of the mononuclear phagocyte series and participates in cell-mediated immunity. The cause and pathogenesis of Langerhans cell disease remains unclear. A reactive process, a primary immunodeficiency disease, and a neoplastic process have all been suggested.

Letterer-Siwe disease (acute disseminated form) is an acute fulminating disorder that usually affects children younger than 3 years of age. The course of the disease is usually so rapid that significant oral involvement does not often occur. The disease resembles a lymphoma in that it generally has a rapidly fatal course that sometimes responds to chemotherapy.

The chronic disseminated or multifocal form of Langerhans cell disease has been called **Hand-Schüller-Christian disease.** This form occurs in children, usually younger than 5 years of age. A classic triad is seen in about 25% of patients. All changes are caused by localized collections of Langerhans cells. The triad includes single-to-multiple, well-defined or "punched-out" radiolucent areas in the skull (may also occur in the jawbones); unilateral or bilateral exophthalmos; and diabetes insipidus that is caused by collections of macrophages in the sella turcica area, affecting the pituitary gland.

Oral manifestations of the chronic disseminated form of the disease include sore mouth with or without ulcerative lesions, halitosis, gingivitis, unpleasant taste, loose and sore teeth, early exfoliation of teeth, and nonhealing extraction sites. A characteristic loss of supporting alveolar bone occurs, mimicking advanced periodontal disease (Figure 3-21).

A solitary or chronic localized form has been called **eosinophilic granuloma of bone.** This form primarily affects older

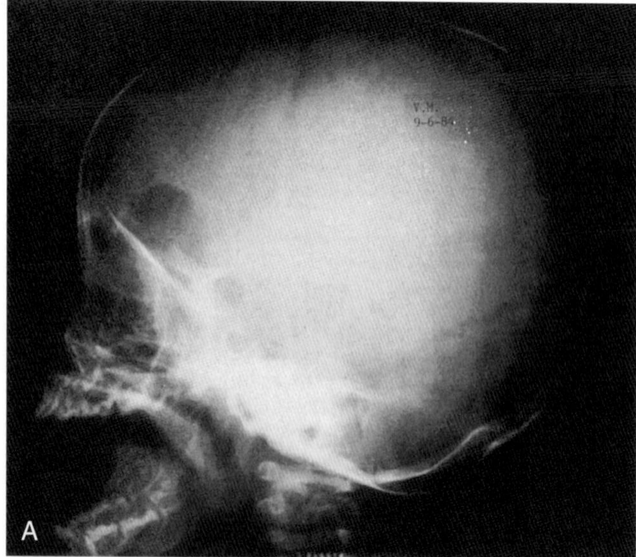

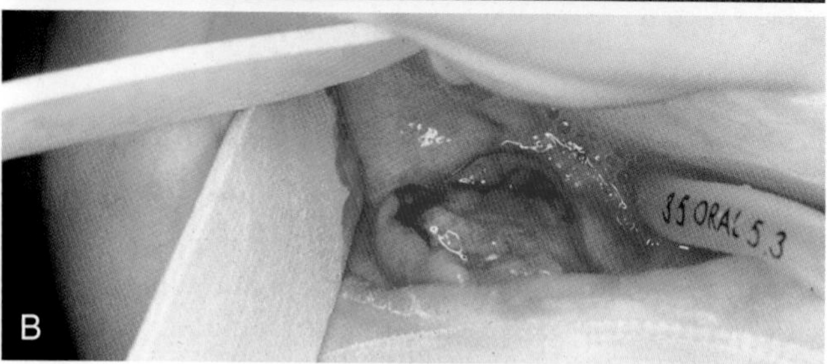

FIGURE 3-21 ■ Langerhans cell disease. Chronic disseminated form also known as Hand-Schüller-Christian disease. **A,** Skull radiograph. **B,** Ulcerated lesion of the mandible. (Courtesy Dr. Sidney Eisig.)

children and young adults. Males are affected twice as commonly as females. The skull and mandible are commonly involved with eosinophilic granuloma. The radiographic appearance varies, and the lesion may resemble periodontal disease or periapical inflammatory disease; or it may appear as a well-circumscribed radiolucency with or without a sclerotic border (Figure 3-22). Cases of multifocal eosinophilic granuloma have also been reported.

Treatment

Eosinophilic granuloma is treated by conservative surgical excision; recurrence is rare. Low-dose radiation therapy may also be used for treatment.

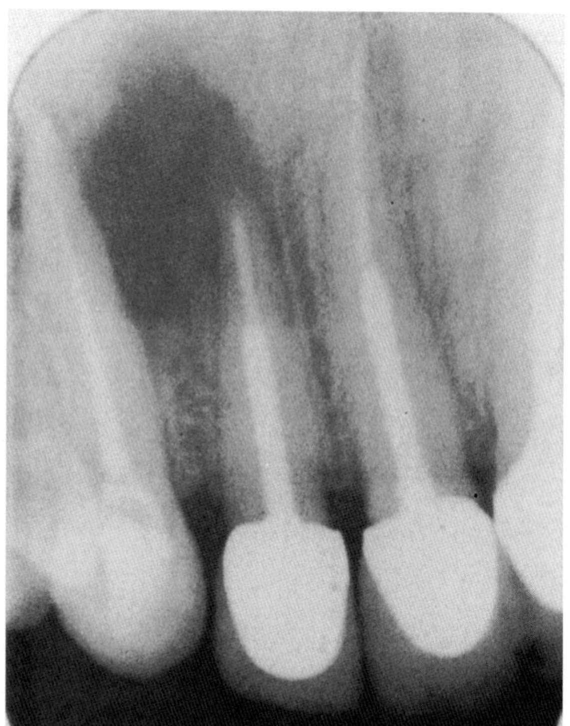

FIGURE 3-22 ■ Radiograph of eosinophilic granuloma. (Courtesy Drs. Paul Freedman and Stanley Kerpel.)

Table 3-5

Autoimmune diseases that affect the oral region

Disease	Oral Manifestation
Sjögren syndrome	Xerostomia
Lupus erythematosus	White, erosive lesions of the oral mucosa
Pemphigus vulgaris	Mucosal ulceration, bullae
Benign mucous membrane pemphigoid	Mucosal ulceration, desquamative gingivitis
Behçet syndrome	Aphthous ulcers
Pernicious anemia*	Mucosal atrophy, mucosal ulceration, loss of filiform and fungiform papillae

*Described in Chapter 9.

AUTOIMMUNE DISEASES THAT AFFECT THE ORAL CAVITY

Several autoimmune diseases affect the oral cavity (Table 3-5). In this type of disease tissue damage occurs because the immune system treats the person's own cells and tissues as antigens. An individual with one autoimmune disease has an increased risk of developing another. Although these are systemic diseases, they are included in this chapter because of their relationship to immunity.

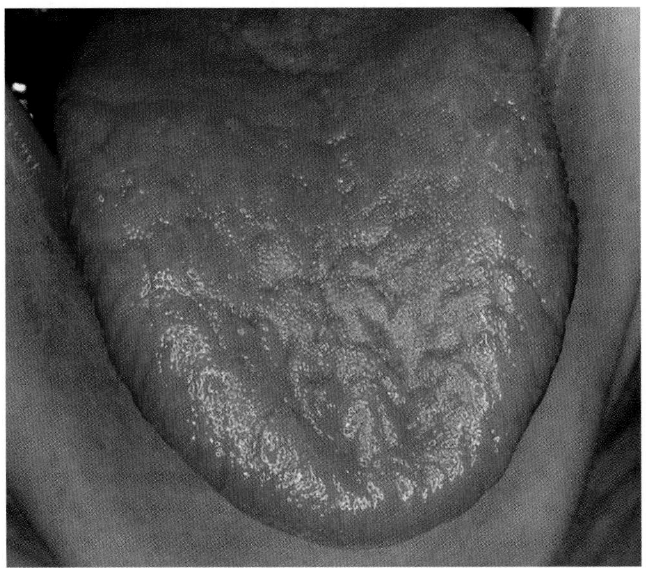

FIGURE 3-23 ■ Sjögren syndrome. This patient had severe xerostomia. The filiform papillae are lacking.

SJÖGREN SYNDROME

Sjögren syndrome is an autoimmune disease that affects the salivary and lacrimal glands, resulting in a decrease in saliva and tears. This combination of dry mouth and dry eyes is sometimes called **sicca** (dry) **syndrome.** Decreased salivary flow (**hyposalivation**) results in dry mouth (**xerostomia**); decreased lacrimal flow results in dry eyes (**xerophthalmia**). The eye damage that occurs in Sjögren syndrome is called **keratoconjunctivitis sicca.** Other secretory glands such as sweat glands and glands that lubricate the vagina can also be affected. The specific cause of Sjögren syndrome is not known. Both cellular and humoral immunity are involved.

In some patients only the mouth and eyes are involved. In others the autoimmune process can be more extensive. Many patients (about 50%) with Sjögren syndrome have another autoimmune disease such as rheumatoid arthritis or systemic lupus erythematosus. Lacrimal and salivary gland involvement without the presence of another autoimmune disease is called **primary Sjögren syndrome.** When another autoimmune disease accompanies salivary and lacrimal gland involvement, the combination is called **secondary Sjögren syndrome.**

The oral manifestation of Sjögren syndrome is xerostomia (dry mouth), which occurs as a result of decreased salivary flow and causes the mucosa to become erythematous. Patients complain of oral discomfort. Lack of saliva causes the mouth to feel sticky. Lips are cracked and dry, and a generalized loss of filiform and fungiform papillae occurs on the dorsum of the tongue (Figure 3-23). Patients with xerostomia are at high risk for the development of caries, periodontal disease, and oral candidiasis.

Both major and minor salivary glands are affected. Parotid gland enlargement, usually bilateral and symmetric,

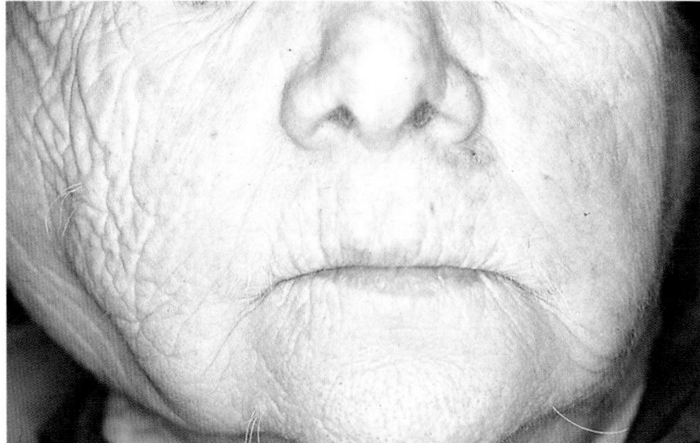

FIGURE 3-24 ■ Bilateral parotid gland swelling seen in Sjögren syndrome. (Courtesy Dr. Louis Mandel.)

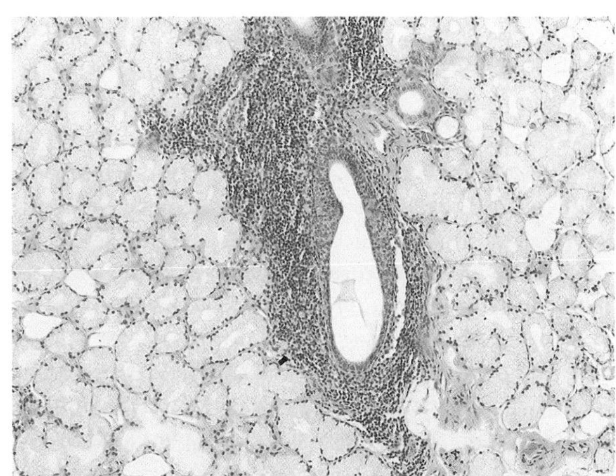

FIGURE 3-25 ■ Microscopy of a minor salivary gland from a patient with Sjögren syndrome. (Courtesy Dr. Harry Lumerman.)

occurs in about 50% of patients (Figure 3-24). The characteristic histologic appearance of these enlarged glands consists of replacement of the glands by lymphocytes and the presence of islands of epithelium called epimyoepithelial islands. Biopsy of the minor salivary glands is often performed to confirm a diagnosis of Sjögren syndrome. The minor glands show aggregates of lymphocytes surrounding the salivary gland ducts (Figure 3-25).

In addition to the oral findings, patients with decreased lacrimal flow that results in **xerophthalmia** complain of burning and itching of the eyes and photophobia (abnormal visual intolerance to light). Severe eye involvement may lead to ulceration and opacification of the cornea. Twenty percent of patients with Sjögren syndrome also have **Raynaud phenomenon,** which is a disorder affecting the fingers and toes. Cold and emotional stress trigger the reaction, which is characterized by an initial pallor of the skin that results from vasoconstriction and reduced blood flow. The initial pallor is followed by cyanosis, which occurs because of the decreased blood flow. When the skin is rewarmed, the blood vessels dilate, and the hyperemia results in a reddening of the skin. Finally, in minutes to hours the color returns to normal. Raynaud phenomenon can occur alone or in association with other autoimmune diseases, as well as in Sjögren syndrome. Patients with Sjögren syndrome might also complain of myalgia, arthralgia, and chronic fatigue.

Laboratory abnormalities are commonly found in patients with this syndrome. Ninety percent of patients with Sjögren syndrome have a positive reaction to **rheumatoid factor**, which is an antibody to IgG that is present in serum. It is an antibody to an antibody. Patients with other autoimmune diseases such as rheumatoid arthritis also react positively to rheumatoid factor. Other **autoantibodies,** called *anti-Sjögren syndrome A* and *anti-Sjögren syndrome B*, are also found in patients with Sjögren syndrome. Other laboratory abnormalities include mild anemia, a decreased white blood cell count, an elevated erythrocyte sedimentation rate, and a diffuse elevation of serum immunoglobulins.

Diagnosis and Management

The diagnosis of Sjögren syndrome is made when at least two of its three components are present: (1) xerostomia, (2) keratoconjunctivitis sicca, and (3) rheumatoid arthritis or another autoimmune disease. Xerostomia can result from conditions other than autoimmune disease. Measurement of stimulated and unstimulated salivary flow and biopsy of minor salivary glands (see Figure 3-25) can be helpful in the diagnosis of Sjögren syndrome. A characteristic pattern is seen in a parotid sialogram (Figure 3-26). The pattern reflects the lack of functioning glandular elements.

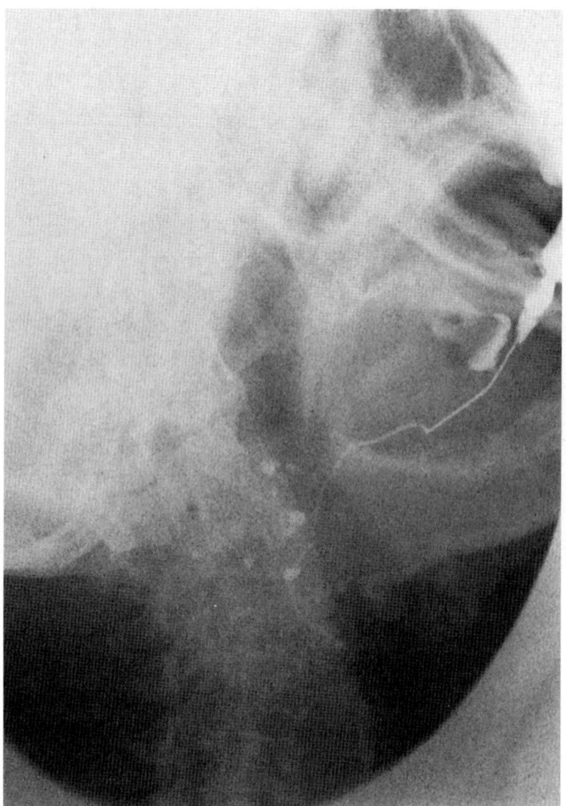

FIGURE 3-26 ■ Sialogram of Sjögren syndrome. (Courtesy Dr. Louis Mandel.)

Keratoconjunctivitis is confirmed by eye examination. Lacrimal flow is measured using filter paper. Special examination techniques are necessary to demonstrate the corneal erosions.

For most patients the course of the disease is chronic and benign. However, patients with Sjögren syndrome are at risk for the development of other more serious autoimmune diseases, lymphoma, and Waldenström macroglobulinemia (a disorder characterized by a high concentration of IgM in serum) and therefore should be monitored by a physician.

Treatment

Sjögren syndrome is usually treated symptomatically. Nonsteroidal antiinflammatory agents are used for the arthritis. In severe cases corticosteroids and other immunosuppressive drugs may be necessary. Saliva substitutes are helpful, and for some patients the use of a humidifier at night makes the xerostomia more tolerable. Sugarless gum or lozenges may be used to stimulate saliva production. However, the greater the destruction of salivary gland tissue, the less saliva will be stimulated. An "artificial tears" formula containing methylcellulose helps to protect the eye from the drying effects of the disease. Glasses provide shielding and are helpful to minimize the drying effects of wind. Pilocarpine may also be used in some patients to increase salivary flow.

Maintaining good oral hygiene and using fluoride toothpaste and daily fluoride rinses can minimize the effects of xerostomia. The interval between recall appointments should be sufficiently short to ensure early detection and treatment of root caries. The toothbrush and other oral hygiene aids may need modification if arthritis affects the movement of hands and arms.

SYSTEMIC LUPUS ERYTHEMATOSUS

Systemic lupus erythematosus (SLE) is an acute and chronic inflammatory autoimmune disease of unknown cause. The disorder affects women eight times more frequently than men, predominantly during the childbearing years. It occurs three times more frequently in black women than in white women. SLE is a syndrome rather than a specific disease entity and includes a wide spectrum of disease activity and signs and symptoms that range from lesions confined to the skin such as discoid lupus erythematosus to a widespread, debilitating, life-threatening disease with multiple-organ

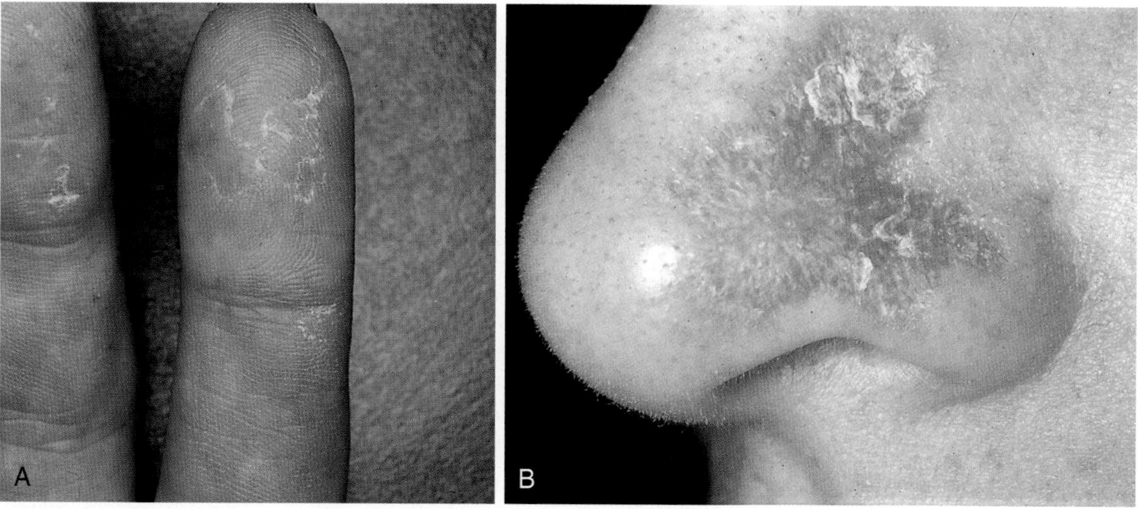

FIGURE 3-27 ■ **A** and **B,** Two examples of skin lesions in lupus erythematosus. (**B** courtesy Dr. Edward V. Zegarelli.)

involvement. SLE is usually chronic and progressive, with periods of remission and exacerbation.

Both cellular and humoral immunity are impaired in SLE. It has been suggested that cellular immunity is primarily affected, resulting in deregulation of the humoral response. Antigen and antibody complexes are deposited in various organs and stimulate an inflammatory response, which may be responsible for the tissue damage that occurs in SLE. Autoantibodies to the patient's deoxyribonucleic acid (DNA) (antinuclear antibodies) are present in serum. These circulating antibodies are responsible for the positive antinuclear antibody and lupus erythematosus laboratory test results. Production of these antibodies is enhanced by estrogen. Antibodies to lymphocytes are present in some patients. Evidence exists for a genetic component in the pathogenesis of SLE.

Clinical Features

Skin lesions are among the most common signs of the disease, occurring in 85% of individuals (Figure 3-27). The most common skin lesion is an erythematous rash involving areas of the body exposed to sunlight. The classic "butterfly" rash occurs over the bridge of the nose, and there may be erythematous lesions on the fingertips. The lesions can heal with scarring in the center as they continue to spread at the periphery. They tend to worsen when exposed to sunlight. Atrophy and hypopigmentation or hyperpigmentation can follow these lesions. Other skin lesions such as bullae, purpura, a discoid rash, vitiligo, or subcutaneous nodules can also occur.

Arthritis and arthralgia are common manifestations of SLE. Any joint can be involved, and symptoms resemble rheumatoid arthritis but without severe deformities. Raynaud phenomenon occurs in 15% of patients. Myalgia and myositis also occur. A retinal vasculitis causes degeneration of the nerve fiber layer of the retina and can cause loss of vision. Psychoses and depression are signs of central nervous system involvement, and seizures can be present. Involvement of the pleura may cause shortness of breath and chest pain. Pericarditis, cardiac arrhythmias, and endocarditis may be seen late in the disease. Kidney involvement is common. Thrombocytopenia may also occur in patients with SLE.

Oral lesions accompany skin lesions in about 25% of patients with discoid lupus erythematosus, which is the mildest form of this autoimmune disease. Oral lesions appear as erythematous plaques or erosions. White striae radiating from the center of the lesion are usually present. The lesions may resemble lichen planus but are less symmetric in their distribution. The involvement of the oral mucosa in this disease is usually mild (Figure 3-28). Petechiae and gingival bleeding may be present in patients with severe thrombocytopenia. Sjögren syndrome may be present in some patients with SLE.

Diagnosis

The diagnosis of systemic lupus erythematosus is usually based on the classic multiorgan involvement and the presence of antinuclear antibodies in serum. **LE cells,** mature neutrophils that have phagocytized a spherical inclusion derived from another neutrophil, may be identified in circulating blood. The diagnosis of SLE is difficult if the onset is slow and insidious. The histologic appearance of oral lesions resembles that of lichen planus. Microscopically destruction

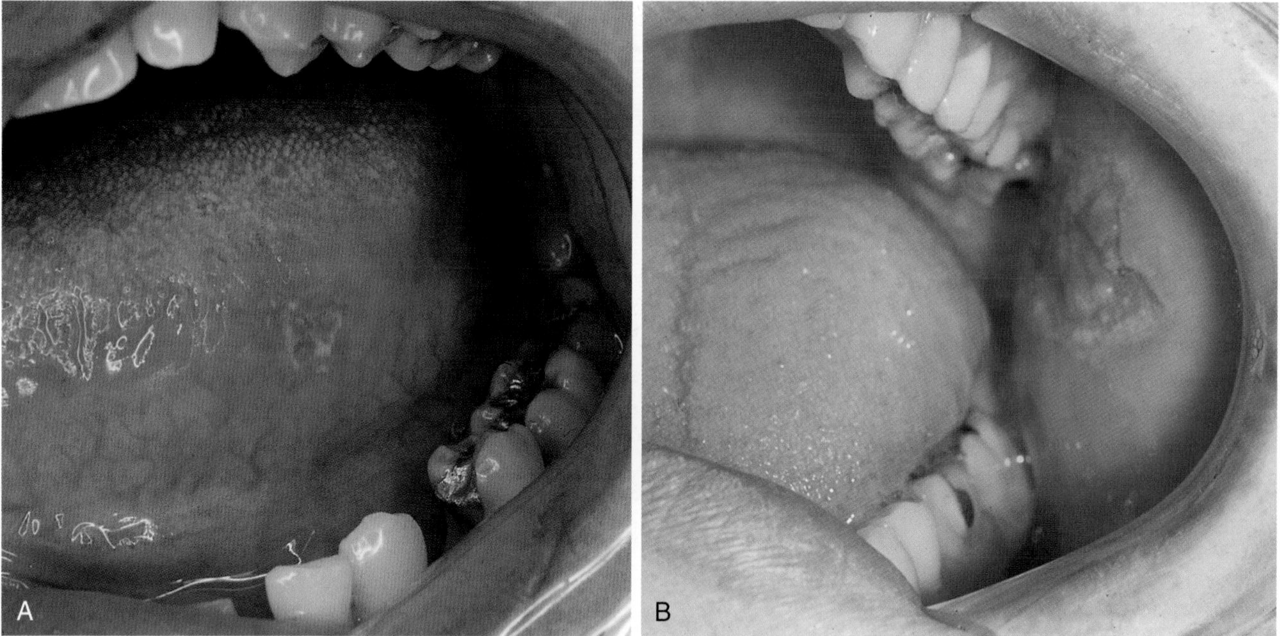

FIGURE 3-28 ■ **A** and **B,** Oral lesions in lupus erythematosus.

of the basal cells is seen, as in lichen planus. However, the inflammatory infiltrate is distributed around blood vessels in the connective tissue rather than in a subepithelial band. Direct immunofluorescence and immunohistochemical testing of skin and mucosal lesions shows granular and linear deposits of immunoglobulins along the basement membrane area.

Treatment and Prognosis

Once the diagnosis of SLE is made, the decision as to whether treatment is indicated depends on the degree of disease activity. This once-fatal disease is now managed with several drugs. Aspirin and nonsteroidal antiinflammatory agents are used for mild signs and symptoms. Hydroxychloroquine, an antimalarial agent, and corticosteroids combined with other immunosuppressive agents such as azathioprine and cyclophosphamide are also used. If the course of the disease is mild and only a few organs are involved, the prognosis is excellent. The disease can also be fatal. Kidney involvement can be associated with severe hypertension and rapid onset of renal failure, which is a cause of death in patients with SLE. Other common causes of death include hemorrhage secondary to thrombocytopenia, nervous system involvement, and infection.

SLE is an extremely complex disease. A consultation with the patient's physician should take place before initiating dental treatment. Antibiotic prophylaxis to prevent bacterial endocarditis may be necessary. The extent of systemic involvement and the drugs being used for treatment should be clarified.

PEMPHIGUS VULGARIS

Pemphigus vulgaris is a severe, progressive autoimmune disease that affects the skin and mucous membranes. It is characterized by intraepithelial blister formation that results from breakdown of the cellular adhesion between epithelial cells. This type of epithelial cell separation is called **acantholysis.** The patient with pemphigus vulgaris has circulating autoantibodies that are reactive against components of the epithelial cell attachment mechanism. The higher the titer of circulating antibodies, the greater the epithelial destruction. These autoantibodies are also found in surrounding epithelial cells. Pemphigus vulgaris is the type of pemphigus seen most frequently. Three other forms of pemphigus are (1) pemphigus vegetans, (2) pemphigus foliaceus, and (3) pemphigus erythematosus. These are much rarer conditions, but all are characterized by epithelial acantholysis. No sex predilection exists. A broad age range has been reported, including both children and elderly individuals. Most cases occur in the fourth and fifth decades of life. Genetic and ethnic factors have been reported. Although it is a relatively rare condition, pemphigus vulgaris is often seen in Ashkenazi Jews.

In more than 50% of cases of pemphigus vulgaris the first signs of disease occur in the oral cavity. Oral lesions can precede cutaneous lesions by many months. The appearance of oral lesions ranges from shallow ulcers to fragile vesicles or bullae.

Because the bullae are so fragile, they rupture soon after they form; the detached epithelium remains as a gray membrane (Figure 3-29). Ulcers are painful and range in size from small to very large. Gentle finger pressure with movement on

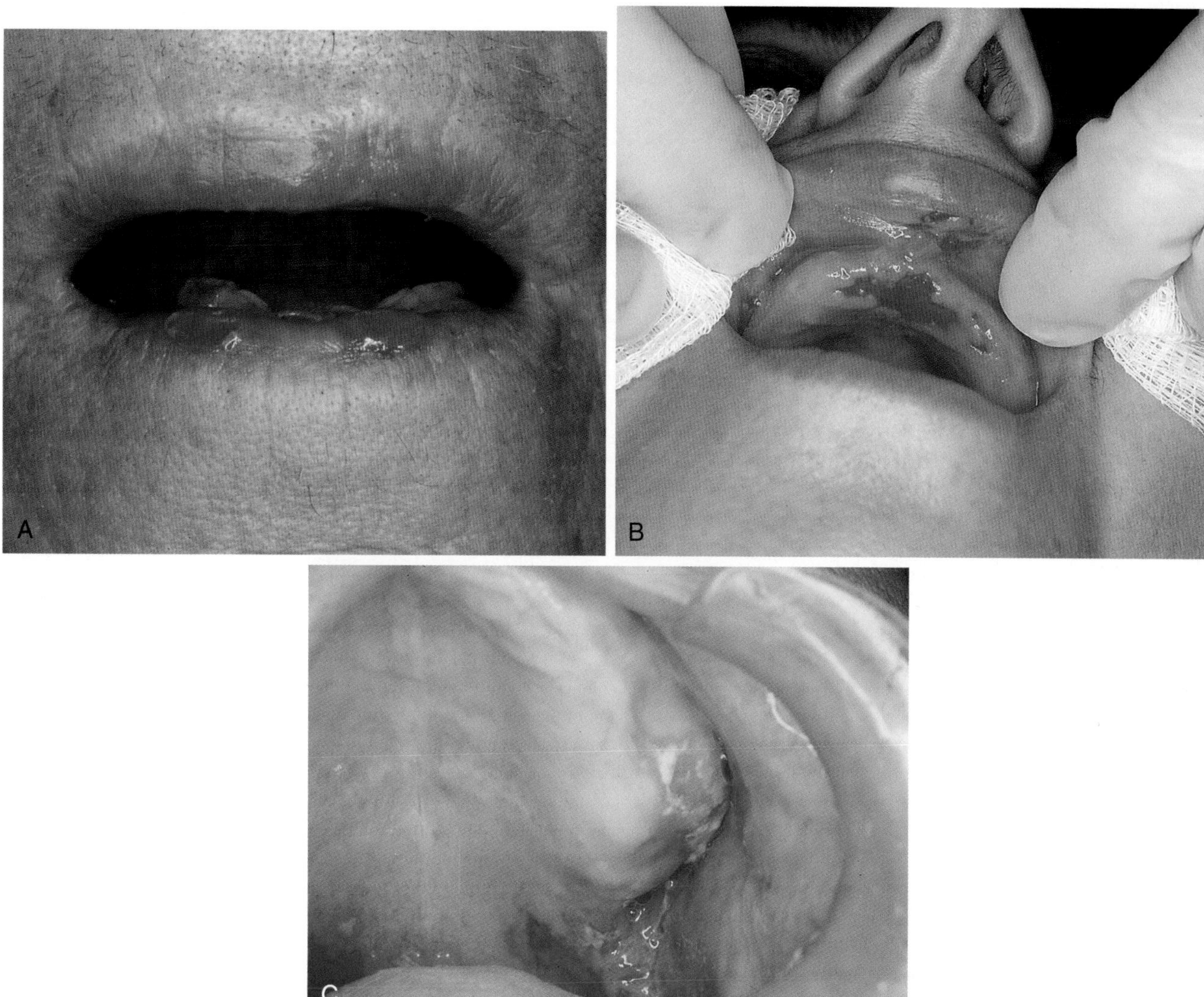

FIGURE 3-29 ■ **A** to **C,** Examples of oral lesions in pemphigus vulgaris. (**B** courtesy Dr. Fariba Younai; **C** courtesy Dr. Sidney Eisig.)

clinically normal mucosa can produce a cleavage in the epithelium and result in the formation of a bulla. This is called **Nikolsky's sign.**

Skin lesions in pemphigus vulgaris include erythema, vesicles, bullae, erosions, and ulcers. Microscopic examination of tissue shows an intact basal layer of epithelium attached to the underlying connective tissue (Figure 3-30). The loss of attachment between the epithelial cells results in detached cells that appear rounded. These rounded cells are called **acantholytic cells** or **Tzanck cells** and are present in the area of separation. Tzanck cells may also be seen on cytologic smear, but the diagnosis must be confirmed by biopsy.

Diagnosis

The diagnosis of pemphigus vulgaris is made by biopsy, microscopic examinations, and direct or indirect immunofluorescence. Direct immunofluorescence is performed on biopsy tissue and identifies autoantibodies present in the tissue. The tissue is viewed through a special microscope (in pemphigus vulgaris fluorescence is seen surrounding the cells in the prickle cell layer). In indirect immunofluorescence the patient's serum is used to detect the presence of circulating autoantibodies. Eighty percent of patients with pemphigus vulgaris have the identifiable circulating autoantibodies.

Treatment and Prognosis

Treatment generally involves high doses of corticosteroids. Other immunosuppressive drugs such as azathioprine and methotrexate are often used in addition to systemic corticosteroids. The amount of autoantibodies present in the patient's serum correlates with the severity of lesions; therefore this concentration of autoantibodies is used to monitor the success of drug treatment. Pemphigus vulgaris was at one time a life-threatening disease. Today the mortality rate is

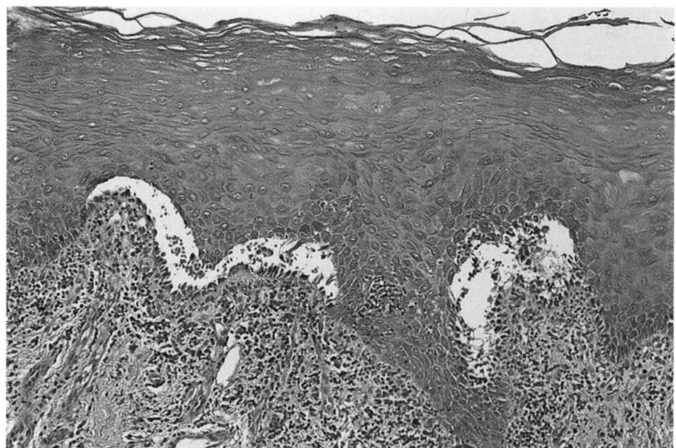

FIGURE 3-30 ■ Pemphigus vulgaris seen by microscopy. The reader should note the acantholysis of the epithelium and the intact basal layer attached to the connective tissue.

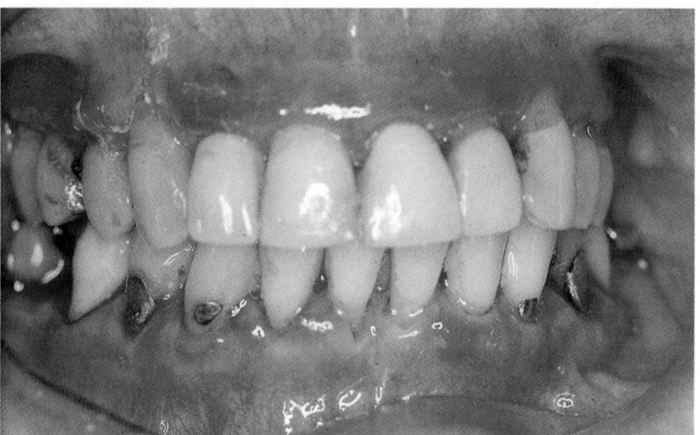

FIGURE 3-31 ■ Cicatricial pemphigoid (desquamative gingivitis). (Courtesy Dr. Victor M. Sternberg.)

about 8% to 10% in 5 years and is related to the complications of corticosteroid treatment rather than to the disease itself. The titer of circulating autoantibodies is used to determine disease activity and response to treatment.

Other autoimmune diseases may occur in association with pemphigus vulgaris. Among them are lupus erythematosus, rheumatoid arthritis, and Sjögren syndrome.

MUCOUS MEMBRANE PEMPHIGOID

Mucous membrane pemphigoid is also known as **cicatricial pemphigoid** and **benign mucous membrane pemphigoid.** It is a chronic autoimmune disease that affects the oral mucosa, conjunctiva, genital mucosa, and skin. It is not as severe as pemphigus vulgaris. Lesions may heal with scarring. The name cicatricial pemphigoid refers to this healing with scarring. Autoantibodies and complement components have been identified at the basement membrane of the epithelium. Lesions occur as a result of cleavage of the epithelium from the underlying connective tissue in this area.

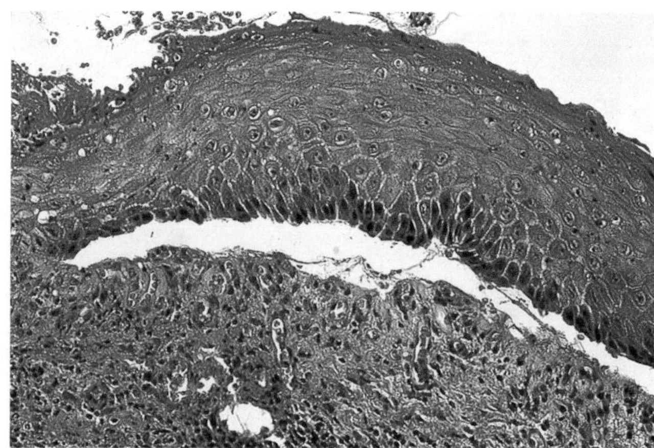

FIGURE 3-32 ■ Cicatricial pemphigoid seen by microscopy. Note the separation of the epithelium from the connective tissue at the basement membrane area.

The most common site for mucous membrane pemphigoid lesions is the gingiva. The gingival lesions have been called **desquamative gingivitis** (Figure 3-31). The appearance ranges from erythema to ulceration and involves both the free and the attached gingiva. However, desquamative gingivitis is a clinical and descriptive term, and similar lesions can be seen in lichen planus and pemphigus vulgaris. In this disease as in pemphigus vulgaris, a Nikolsky's sign can be produced on normal-appearing tissue by gentle friction. Bullae, erosions, and ulcers can also occur in other locations in the oral cavity. Bullae are thick walled and much less fragile than those of pemphigus vulgaris, and they may persist for 24 to 48 hours.

Diagnosis

The diagnosis of mucous membrane pemphigoid is made by biopsy and histologic examination. On microscopic examination the epithelium appears to detach from the connective tissue at the basement membrane (Figure 3-32). No degeneration of the epithelium occurs. An inflammatory infiltrate, usually with prominent plasma cells and eosinophils, is seen in the connective tissue. Direct immunofluorescence shows a linear pattern of fluorescence at the basement membrane. Indirect immunofluorescence (identifying autoantibodies in serum) is usually not helpful in the diagnosis of cicatricial pemphigoid.

Treatment and Prognosis

Mucous membrane pemphigoid is a chronic disease that follows a benign course. Gingival involvement can occur alone, or more extensive lesions can be present. Topical corticosteroid application is helpful in the management of mild cases. In more severe cases high doses of systemic corticosteroids may be necessary. The disease may be difficult to control and slow to respond to therapy.

Patients may experience episodes of exacerbation followed by periods of remission. An ophthalmologic consultation to rule out the presence of eye lesions should be considered. If eye lesions are present, severe damage to the cornea, conjunctiva, and eyelid can occur.

BULLOUS PEMPHIGOID

Some investigators have suggested that bullous and mucous membrane pemphigoid are variants of a single disease. However, differences exist between the two diseases that make this questionable. Eighty percent of patients with bullous pemphigoid are older than 60 years of age, and no sex predilection exists. Unlike mucous membrane pemphigoid, in bullous pemphigoid circulating autoantibodies are usually detectable; and unlike pemphigus vulgaris, the circulating autoantibodies do not correlate with disease activity. Oral lesions are less common in bullous pemphigoid than in mucous membrane pemphigoid, occurring in only about one third of patients. When they occur, the gingival lesions are very similar to those of mucous membrane pemphigoid, and other mucosal lesions are more extensive and painful. As in mucous membrane pemphigoid, the microscopic appearance of bullous pemphigoid shows a cleavage of the epithelium from the connective tissue at the basement membrane.

High doses of systemic corticosteroids and nonsteroidal antiinflammatory drugs are used in the management of bullous pemphigoid. The disease is chronic with periods of remission and is usually not life threatening.

BEHÇET SYNDROME

Behçet syndrome is a chronic, recurrent autoimmune disease consisting primarily of oral ulcers, genital ulcers, and ocular inflammation. No sex predilection exists, and the mean age of onset is 30 years. There is an increased prevalence of this syndrome in individuals from the Mediterranean region and Asia. Evidence for an immunologic pathogenesis includes the identification of antibodies to human mucosa in patients with Behçet syndrome and the association between Behçet syndrome HLA B5 and HLA B51.

The oral ulcers that occur in Behçet syndrome are very similar in appearance to aphthous ulcers (Figure 3-33). They are painful and recurrent. The lesions range in size from a few millimeters to several centimeters. The genital ulcers are usually small and located on the scrotum or base of the penis and the labia majora. The ocular lesions usually begin with photophobia and can develop into conjunctivitis and uveitis. The skin lesions show a papular pattern of pustules and are most common on the trunk and limbs.

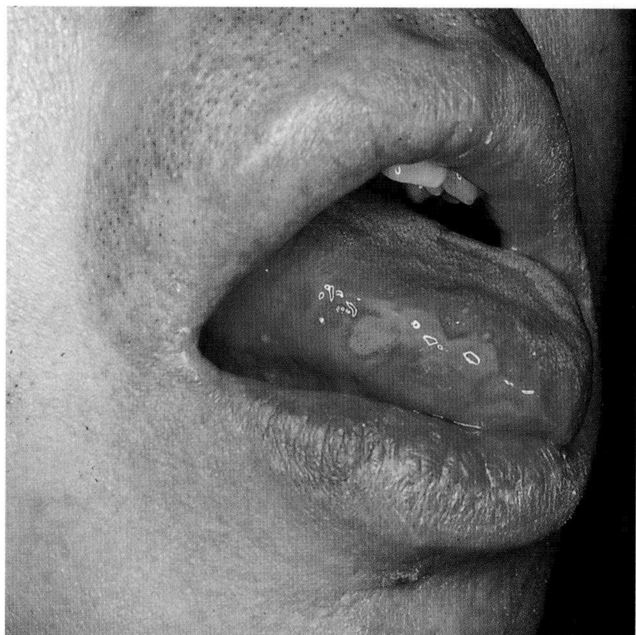

FIGURE 3-33 ■ Oral lesion seen in Behçet syndrome. Aphthouslike oral mucosal ulcer.

Diagnosis

The diagnosis of Behçet syndrome requires that two of the three principal manifestations (oral, genital, and ocular) be present. A pustular lesion that develops after a needle puncture is highly suggestive of Behçet syndrome.

Treatment and Prognosis

Systemic and topical corticosteroids are used in the management of Behçet syndrome. Chlorambucil is used for the ocular lesions. Occasionally other immunosuppressive drugs are needed.

Selected References

Books

Bath-Balogh M, Fehrenbach MJ: *Illustrated dental embryology, histology, anatomy,* ed 2, St Louis, 2006, Saunders.

Fehrenbach MJ, Herring SW: *Illustrated anatomy of the head and neck,* ed 3, St Louis, 2007, Saunders.

Kumar V, Cotran RS, Robbins SL: *Robbins basic pathology,* ed 8, Philadelphia, 2007, Saunders.

McCance K, Huether S: *Pathophysiology,* ed 5, St Louis, 2005, Mosby.

Neville BW, et al: *Oral and maxillofacial pathology,* ed 3, St Louis, 2009, Saunders.

Parham P: *The immune system,* New York, 2000, Garland Publishing.

Journal Articles

Al-Johani KA, Fedele S, Porter SR. Erythema multiforme and related disorders, *Oral Surg Oral Med Oral Pathol Oral Endod* 103:642, 2007.

Anderson KE et al: Contact dermatitis: a review, *Contact Dermatitis* 16:55, 1987.

Antoon JW, Miller RL: Aphthous ulcers: a review of the literature of etiology, pathogenesis, diagnosis and treatment, *J Am Dent Assoc* 101:803, 1980.

Ardekian L et al: Clinical and radiographic features of eosinophilic granuloma in the jaws: review of 41 lesions treated by surgery and low-dose radiotherapy, *Oral Surg Oral Med Oral Pathol Oral Radiol Endod* 87:238, 1999.

Atkinson JC, Fox PC: Sjögren's syndrome: oral and dental considerations, *J Am Dent Assoc* 124:74, 1993.

Barnard NA et al: Oral cancer development in patients with oral lichen planus, *J Oral Pathol Med* 22:241, 1993.

Barrett AW, Scully CM, Eveson JW: Erythema multiforme involving gingiva, *J Periodontol* 64:910, 1993.

Baudet-Pommel M et al: Early dental loss in Sjögren's syndrome, *Oral Surg Oral Med Oral Pathol* 78:181, 1994.

Chaplin DD: Part 1. Overview of the human immune response, *J Allergy Clin Immunol* 117(2 Suppl Mini-Primer) S430, 2006.

Eisenberg E: Lichen planus and oral cancer: is there a connection between the two? *J Am Dent Assoc* 123:104, 1992.

Epstein JB et al: Oral lichen planus: progress in understanding its malignant potential and the implications for clinical management, *Oral Surg Oral Med Oral Radiol Endod* 96:32, 2003.

Escudier M, Baraw J, Scully C: Number VII Behçet's disease (Adamantiades syndrome), *Oral Dis* 12:78, 2005.

Eversole LR: Immunopathology of oral mucosal ulcerative, desquamative, and bullous diseases, *Oral Surg Oral Med Oral Pathol* 77:555, 1994.

Feder HM: Periodic fever, aphthous stomatitis, pharyngitis, adenitis: a clinical review of a new syndrome, *Curr Opin Pediatr* 12:253, 2000.

Gawkrodger DJ, Stephenson TJ, Thomas SE: Squamous cell carcinoma complicating lichen planus: a clinico-pathological study of three cases, *Dermatology* 188:36, 1994.

Holmstrup P, Schiotz AW, Westergaard J: Effect of dental plaque control on gingival lichen planus, *Oral Surg Oral Med Oral Pathol* 69:585, 1990.

Jorizzo JL et al: Oral lesions in systemic lupus erythematosus: do ulcerative lesions represent a necrotizing vasculitis? *J Am Acad Dermatol* 27:389, 1992.

Katz RW, Brahim JS, Travis WD: Oral squamous cell carcinoma arising in a patient with long-standing lichen planus: a case report, *Oral Surg Oral Med Oral Pathol* 70:282, 1990.

Krippaehne JA, Montgomery MT: Erythema multiforme: a literature review and case report, *Spec Care Dentist* 12:125, 1992.

Loh HS, Quah TC: Histiocytosis X (Langerhans cell histiocytosis) of the palate: case report, *Aust Dent J* 35:117, 1990.

Lozada-Nur F, Gorsky M, Silverman S Jr: Oral erythema multiforme: clinical observations and treatment of 95 patients, *Oral Surg Oral Med Oral Pathol* 67:36, 1989.

MacPhail LA et al: Recurrent aphthous ulcers in association with HIV infection: description of ulcer types and analysis of T-lymphocyte subsets, *Oral Surg Oral Med Oral Pathol* 71:678, 1991.

Manton SL, Scully C: Mucous membrane pemphigoid: an elusive diagnosis? *Oral Surg Oral Med Oral Pathol* 66:37, 1988.

Miller MF, Ship II, Ram C: A retrospective study of the prevalence and incidence of recurrent aphthous ulcers in a professional population, 1958-1971, *Oral Surg Oral Med Oral Pathol* 43:532, 1977.

Miller RL, Gould AR, Bernstein ML: Cinnamon-induced stomatitis venenata, *Oral Surg Oral Med Oral Pathol* 73:708, 1992.

Panush RS et al: Retraction of the suggestion to use the term "Reiter's syndrome": sixty five years later, *Arthritis Rheum* 56:693, 2007.

Porter SR, Scully C, Standen GR: Autoimmune neutropenia manifesting as recurrent oral ulceration, *Oral Surg Oral Med Oral Pathol* 78:178, 1994.

Raghoebar GM, Brouwer TJ, Schoots CJ: Pemphigus vulgaris of the oral mucosa: report of two cases, *Quintessence Int* 22:199, 1991.

Reiche EM, Morimoto HK, Nunes SM. Stress and depression-induced immune dysfunction: implications for the development and progression of cancer, *Int Rev Psychiatry* 17:515, 2005.

Rodu B, Mattingly G: Oral mucosal ulcers: diagnosis and management, *J Am Dent Assoc* 123:83, 1992.

Schofield JK, Tatnall FM, Leigh IM: Recurrent erythema multiforme: clinical features and treatment in a large series of patients, *Br J Dermatol* 34:63, 1993.

Sciubba JJ: Sjögren's syndrome: pathology, oral presentation and dental management, *Compend Contin Educ Dent* 15:1084, 1994.

Spina AM, Levine HJ: Latex allergy: a review for the dental professional, *Oral Surg Oral Med Oral Pathol Oral Radiol Endod* 87:5, 1999.

Tasher D, Somekh E, Dalal: PFAPA syndrome: new clinical aspects disclosed, *Arch Dis Child* 91:981, 2006.

Vincent SD, Lilly GE, Baker KA: Clinical, historical and therapeutic features of cicatricial pemphigoid: a literature review and open therapeutic trial with corticosteroids, *Oral Surg Oral Med Oral Pathol* 76:453, 1993.

Vincent SD, et al. Oral lichen planus: the clinical, historical and therapeutic features of 100 cases, *Oral Surg Oral Med Oral Pathol* 70:165, 1990.

Walker DM. Oral mucosal immunology: an overview, *Ann Acad Med Singapore* 33(4 Suppl):27, 2004.

Woo S-B, Sonis ST: Recurrent aphthous ulcers: a review of diagnosis and treatment, *J Am Dent Assoc* 127:1202, 1996.

Yazici H, Barnes CG: Practical treatment recommendations for pharmacotherapy of Behçet's syndrome, *Drugs* 42:796, 1991.

Zegarelli DJ: The treatment of oral lichen planus, *Ann Dent* 52:3, 1993.

REVIEW QUESTIONS

1. The immune system usually defends the body against foreign substances that are called:
   A. Plasma cells.
   B. Antibodies.
   C. Antigens.
   D. Lymphocytes.

2. Memory is an important function of the immune system because:
   A. It retains the memory of the antibody.
   B. It allows faster future immune responses.
   C. It allows faster inflammatory responses.
   D. It weakens future immune responses.

3. Immunization with a vaccine works by:
   A. Increasing the risk of an antigen-causing disease.
   B. Using antibodies produced by another person.
   C. Passing antibodies from the mother to the fetus.
   D. Producing active acquired immunity.

4. A B lymphocyte is a cell in the immune system that:
   A. Is derived from a precursor stem cell.
   B. Matures and resides in the thymus.
   C. Is produced from plasma cells.
   D. Is active in foreign substance surveillance.

5. A macrophage is a cell in the immune system that:
   A. Retains the memory of the encountered antigen.
   B. Produces antibodies.
   C. Undergoes B cell phagocytosis initially during inflammation.
   D. Can be activated by lymphokines.

6. Which statement is true of NK cells?
   A. NK cells do not circulate.
   B. NK cells secrete antibodies.
   C. NK cells are part of the body's innate immunity.
   D. NK cells are T lymphocytes.

7. In which type of immunopathologic disease are the cells of the body no longer tolerated and treated by the immune system as antigens?
   A. Hypersensitivity
   B. Immunodeficiency
   C. Hyperplasia
   D. Autoimmune disease

8. During the anaphylactic type of hypersensitivity reaction, the plasma cells:
   A. Produce antibody called IgE.
   B. React with lymphocytes.
   C. Combine with antigen.
   D. Form immune complexes with antigen.

9. Which type of hypersensitivity reaction involves activated complement?
   A. Type I
   B. Type II
   C. Type III
   D. Anaphylaxis

10. What type of lymphocyte matures in the thymus, produces lymphokines, and can increase or suppress the humoral immune response?
    A. T lymphocyte
    B. Plasma cell
    C. NK cell
    D. Macrophage

11. In the immune system antibodies are proteins that are:
    A. Also called immunoglobulins.
    B. Also called cytokines.
    C. Directly produced by lymphocytes.
    D. Directly produced from mast cells.

12. Which of the following type(s) of immunologic disease involve a decreased number or activity of lymphoid cells?
    A. Autoimmunity
    B. Hypersensitivity
    C. Immunodeficiency
    D. Immunization

13. The humoral immune response involves the production of:
    A. Antigens.
    B. Antibodies.
    C. Autoimmune cells.
    D. Toxins.

14. The measurement of a specific antibody level in the blood is called:
    A. Phagocytosis.
    B. Immunization.
    C. Titer.
    D. Pavementing.

15. Which type of immunity may be provided immediately to dental personnel after needlestick accidents?
    A. Natural passive immunity
    B. Acquired passive immunity
    C. Natural active immunity
    D. Acquired active immunity

16. Which of the following situations would result in the least risk of drug allergy?
    A. Application of topical medication
    B. Presence of infection
    C. Presence of multiple allergies
    D. Use with children

17. Which of the following is involved in the regulation of both humoral and cell-mediated immunity?
    A. Humoral immunity
    B. Cell-mediated immunity
    C. Innate immunity
    D. The bone marrow

18. Which of the following is involved in the communication between lymphocytes within the immune system?
    A. Histamine
    B. Complement
    C. Bradykinin
    D. Cytokines

19. All of the following are examples of hypersensitivity reactions except:
    A. Systemic lupus erythematosus.
    B. Urticaria.
    C. Angioedema.
    D. Contact mucositis.

20. Reiter syndrome is:
    A. An infectious disease.
    B. An immunodeficiency disease.
    C. An immunologic disorder.
    D. More common in women than in men.

21. Which one of the following types of hypersensitivity reactions is referred to as delayed hypersensitivity?
    A. Type I
    B. Type II
    C. Type III
    D. Type IV

22. The "target lesion" on the skin is associated with which of the following diseases?
    A. Behçet syndrome
    B. Systemic lupus erythematosus
    C. Lichen planus
    D. Erythema multiforme

23. Tzanck cells are seen in which of the following conditions?
    A. Pemphigus vulgaris
    B. Erythema multiforme
    C. Systemic lupus erythematosus
    D. Behçet syndrome

24. The oral lesions in Reiter syndrome may resemble:
    A. Nicotine stomatitis.
    B. Lichen planus.
    C. Angioedema.
    D. Geographic tongue.

25. Apththous ulcers are seen in each all of the following systemic diseases EXCEPT:
    A. Behçet syndrome.
    B. Langerhans cell disease.
    C. Ulcerative colitis.
    D. Cyclic neutropenia.

26. The two cell types that histologically characterize Langerhans cell disease are:
    A. Lymphocytes and plasma cells.
    B. Fibroblasts and lymphocytes.
    C. Eosinophils and mononuclear cells.
    D. Neutrophils and lymphocytes.

27. Which one of the following is the form of Langerhans cell disease that is characterized by a triad of symptoms?
    A. Letterer-Siwe disease
    B. Hand-Schüller-Christian disease
    C. Eosinophilic granuloma
    D. Behçet syndrome

28. The most benign type of Langerhans cell disease is:
    A. Hand-Schüller-Christian disease.
    B. Eosinophilic granuloma.
    C. Letterer-Siwe disease.
    D. Chronic disseminated reticulosis.

29. The most characteristic oral manifestation of Sjögren syndrome is:
    A. Xerostomia.
    B. Geographic tongue.
    C. Erythema multiforme.
    D. Acute disseminated reticulosis.

30. Which of the following statements is false?
    A. The bullae in pemphigus vulgaris are more fragile than those in bullous pemphigoid.
    B. Acantholysis of the epithelium is seen in pemphigus vulgaris.
    C. In pemphigoid the separation of the epithelium from the connective tissue occurs at the basement membrane.
    D. Skin lesions are common in mucous membrane pemphigoid.

31. Which is the most distinct and definitive characteristic that distinguishes pemphigus from pemphigoid?
    A. Size of the ulcerations
    B. Age and sex of the patient
    C. The histologic findings
    D. Nikolsky's sign

32. Desquamative gingivitis may be seen in:
    A. Cicatricial pemphigoid.
    B. Pemphigus vulgaris.
    C. Lichen planus.
    D. All of the above.

33. In angioedema involvement of which of the following tissues could create a life-threatening situation for the patient?
    A. Lips
    B. Mucosa
    C. Eyelids
    D. Epiglottis

34. Which of the following is a pathologic condition that produces a characteristic butterfly-shaped lesion on the face and oral ulcers, occurs more frequently in females than males, and for which the result of a blood test is important to diagnosis?
    A. Pemphigus
    B. Erosive lichen planus
    C. Desquamative gingivitis
    D. Lupus erythematosus

CHAPTER 3 Synopsis

Condition/Disease	Cause	Age/Race/Sex	Location
Oral Diseases With Immunologic Pathogenesis			
Minor Aphthous Ulcer	Unclear immunologic pathogenesis involving cell-mediated immunity Trauma is most common participating factor	More common in younger than older individuals Affects women more than men	Oral mucosa not covering bone Anterior more than posterior
Major Aphthous	Unclear immunologic pathogenesis involving cell-mediated immunity	*	Oral mucosa not covering bone Often occur in the posterior oral cavity
Herpetiform Aphthous Ulcers	Unclear immunologic pathogenesis involving cell-mediated immunity	*	Anywhere in the oral cavity
Urticaria (Hives)	Type 1 hypersensitivity Release of 1gG, 1gM—often to ingested allergen Infection, trauma, emotional stress also associated with urticaria Localized vascular permeability in superficial connective tissue	*	Skin
Angioedema	Type I hypersensitivity Trauma, release of 1gG or 1gM Permeability of deeper blood vessels	*	Skin or mucosa
Contact Mucositis	Direct contact of allergen with mucosa	*	Mucosa in contact with allergen

N/A, Not applicable.
*No significant information.
†Not covered in this text.

Clinical Features	Radiographic Features	Microscopic Features	Treatment	Diagnostic Process
Painful, discrete, round-to-oval, yellowish white ulcers Halo of erythema Up to 1 cm in diameter Spontaneous healing in 7-10 days	N/A	Ulcer with lymphocytic infiltrate	Topical corticosteroids	Clinical
Painful Greater than 1 cm in diameter Often deeper than minor aphthous ulcers May last several weeks Often heal with scarring	N/A	May require biopsy for diagnosis to rule out other causes of ulceration	Topical or systematic corticosteroids Biopsy to rule out ulceration from other cause	Clinical Microscopic
Painful, very tiny 1- to 2-mm ulcers Often occurs in groups Resolve spontaneously	N/A	Unclear	Topical corticosteroids Topical tetracycline	Clinical
Multiple areas of well- demarcated swelling accompanied by itching (pruritus) Self-limiting episodes	N/A	†	Identification and avoidance of causative agent Antihistaminic drugs	Clinical
Diffuse swelling of tissue Usually no itching Self-limiting episodes	N/A	†	Identification of causative agent Antihistaminic drugs	Clinical
Smooth, shiny, firm mucosa with erythema and edema May form vesicles Often itching or burning sensation	N/A	†	Identification of causative agent Topical and systematic corticosteroids	Clinical

Continued

CHAPTER 3 Synopsis (continued)

Condition/Disease	Cause	Age/Race/Sex	Location
Contact Dermatitis	Direct contact of allergen with skin	*	Skin in contact with allergen
Fixed Drug Eruptions	Type III hypersensitivity	*	Same site each episode Usually skin Occasionally oral mucosa
Erythema Multiforme	Unclear Evidence for hypersensitivity reaction that in some cases may be associated with infection agents	Most frequent in young adults Affects men more than women	Skin and mucous membranes
Lichen Planus	Unknown	Broad age range Increased prevalence in middle age Affects women more than men	Skin and oral mucosal lesions Oral mucosa: buccal mucosa, tongue, labial mucosa, floor of mouth, gingival
Reactive Arthritis (Reiter Syndrome)	Abnormal immunologic response to infectious agent Genetic influence presence of HLA-B27	Affects men much more than women (10 to 15:1)	Conjunctiva Urethra Oral mucosa Skin Knee and ankle joints

N/A, Not applicable.
*No significant information.
†Not covered in this text.

Clinical Features	Radiographic Features	Microscopic Features	Treatment	Diagnostic Process
Erythema; swelling vesicles to encrusted, scaly, white appearance	N/A	†	Identification of causative agent Topical and systematic corticosteroids	Clinical
Lesions appear when drug is introduced and subside when drug is discontinued with increasing intensity Single-to-multiple raised, reddish patches or clusters of macules Pain/ pruritus may be present	N/A	†	Identification and discontinuation of causative drug	Clinical
Skin: characteristic target lesion, also macules, plaques, bullae Mucosa: erythema, ulcers, crusted, bleeding lips Severe form: Stevens-Johnson syndrome Explosive onset	N/A	Nonspecific	Identification of causative agent if possible Topical/systematic corticosteroids	Clinical
Oral lesions Wickham's striae Erosive and plaquelike lesions may occur Gingival lesions: desquamative gingivitis	N/A	Degeneration of the basal layer of the epithelium Broad band of lymphocytes in the connective tissue subjacent to the epithelium	None if asymptomatic Topical corticosteroids if symptomatic Follow-up evaluation	Clinical Microscopic
Syndrome triad Arthritis Urethritis Conjunctivitis Skin lesions Oral lesions Aphthouslike ulcers Lesions resembling geographic tongue	N/A	†	ASA and nonsteroidal antiinflammatory drugs	Clinical

Continued

CHAPTER 3 Synopsis (continued)

Condition/Disease	Cause	Age/Race/Sex	Location
Langerhans Cell Disease	Unclear: suggestive reactive process, immunologic disease, neoplastic process		
Acute disseminated form (Letterer-Siwi disease)		Affects children under 3 years of age	Disseminated disease
Chronic disseminated multifocal form (Hand-Schüller Christian disease)		Affects children under 5 years of age	Multiple locations
Solitary disseminated (multifocal form)			
Solitary (chronic) localized form (Eosinophilic granuloma)	Unclear—suggested reactive process, immunologic disease, neoplastic process	Affects older children and young adults Affects males more than females (2:1)	Bone: skull and mandible are commonly involved
Sjögren Syndrome	Autoimmune disease Decreased lacrimal flow Decreased salivary flow	*	Eyes: oral cavity

N/A, Not applicable.
*No significant information.
†Not covered in this text.

Clinical Features	Radiographic Features	Microscopic Features	Treatment	Diagnostic Process
Erythematous lesions				
†	N/A	†	Chemotherapy Poor Prognosis	Clinical Microscopic
Classic triad skull radiolucencies Exophthalmos Diabetes insipidus	Radiolucencies ("punched out") of skull Maxilla/mandible radiolucencies, including alveolar bone	Infiltrate of Langerhans cells (macrophages) and eosinophils	†	Clinical Microscopic
Oral: sore mouth with or without ulceration halitosis; gingivitis; unpleasant taste; loose, sore teeth; early exfoliation of teeth				
N/A	Radiolucency May resemble periodontal disease or may be well circumscribed radiolucency May be multifocal	Infiltrate of Langerhans cell (macrophages) and eosinophils	Conservative surgical excision Low-dose radiation treatment	Microscopic
Primary Sjögren syndrome: Dry eyes (xerophthalmia) Dry mouth (xerostomia) Secondary Sjögren's syndrome: Dry eyes (xerophthalmia) Dry mouth (xerostomia) Another autoimmune disease	Sialogram shows characteristic features (see text)	Salivary gland changes: lymphocytic infiltration and epimyoepithelial islands	Xerostomia Saliva substitutes Saliva stimulation Pilocarpine	Clinical Radiographic Microscopic Laboratory

Continued

CHAPTER 3 Synopsis (continued)

Condition/Disease	Cause	Age/Race/Sex	Location
Systemic Lupus Erythematosus	Autoimmune disease	Affects women more than men (8:1), blacks more than whites (3:1)	Multiple sites Skin Mucous membranes Joints Eyes Central nervous system Kidneys Heart and others
Pemphigus Vulgaris	Autoimmune disease	Affects children and adults Most common in fourth to fifth decade More common in Ashkenazic Jews	Mucous membranes Skin
Cicatricial Pemphigoid (mucosal pemphigoid, benign mucous membrane pemphigoid)	Autoimmune disease	Adults	Mucous membranes Most common: gingiva May affect eyes
Bullous Pemphigoid	Autoimmune disease	80% affected are over 60 years old	Mucous membranes Skin
Behçet Syndrome	Autoimmune disease	Mean age of onset 30 years	Mucous membranes Oral Genital Ocular

N/A, Not applicable.
*No significant information.
†Not covered in this text.

Clinical Features	Radiographic Features	Microscopic Features	Treatment	Diagnostic Process
Oral lesions Erythematous plaques or erosions White striations radiating from center of lesion	N/A	Destruction of the basal layer of the epithelium with inflammatory infiltrate around blood vessels Immunohistochemical testing Granular and linear deposits of immunoglobulins along basement membrane zone	Antiinflammatory and immunsuppresive agents	Laboratory Microscopic Clinical
Progressive involvement of mucous membranes and skin Oral lesions Painful, erythema, vesicles, bullae, erosions Positive Nikolsky's sign	N/A	Intact basal layer attached to the underlying connective tissue Acantholysis of the prickle cell layer Tzanck cells	Corticosteroids and other immuno-suppressive agents	Laboratory Microscopic
Oral lesion Desquamative gingivitis Bullae, erosions, ulcers Lesions heal with scarring	N/A	Epithelium detaches from the connective tissue at the basement membrane	Topical/systemic corticosteroids	Microscopic
Oral lesions as in cicatricial pemphigoid but less common	N/A	Epithelium detaches from the connective tissue at the basement membrane	Systemic corticosteroids and other antiinflammatory agents	Microscopic
Oral lesions Aphthouslike ulcers	N/A	†	Corticosteroids and other immuno-suppressive agents	Clinical

chapter 4

Infectious Diseases

Joan A. Phelan

OBJECTIVES

After studying this chapter, the student will be able to:

1. State the difference between an inflammatory and an immune response to infection.
2. Describe the factors that allow opportunistic infection to develop.
3. List two examples of opportunistic infections that can occur in the oral cavity.
4. For each of the following infectious diseases, name the organism causing it, list the route or routes of transmission of the organism and the oral manifestations of the disease, and describe how the diagnosis is made: impetigo, tuberculosis, actinomycosis, syphilis (primary, secondary, tertiary), verruca vulgaris, condyloma acuminatum, and primary herpetic gingivostomatitis.
5. Describe the relationship between streptococcal tonsillitis and pharyngitis and scarlet fever and rheumatic fever.
6. List and describe four forms of oral candidiasis.
7. Describe the clinical features of herpes labialis.
8. Describe the clinical features of recurrent intraoral herpes simplex infection and compare them with the clinical features of minor aphthous ulcers.
9. Describe the clinical characteristics of herpes zoster when it affects the skin of the face and oral mucosa.
10. List two oral infectious diseases for which a cytologic smear may assist in confirming the diagnosis.
11. List four diseases associated with the Epstein-Barr virus.
12. List two diseases caused by coxsackieviruses that have oral manifestations.
13. Describe the spectrum of human immunodeficiency virus (HIV) disease, including initial infection and the development of acquired immunodeficiency syndrome (AIDS).
14. List and describe the clinical appearance of five oral manifestations of HIV infection.

VOCABULARY

Granuloma (gran″u-lo′mah) A tumorlike mass of inflammatory tissue consisting of a central collection of macrophages, often including multinucleated giant cells, surrounded by lymphocytes.

Granulomatous disease (gran″u-lom′ah-tus dĭ-zēz′) A disease characterized by the formation of granulomas.

Incubation period (in″ku-ba′shĕn pir-ē-ĕd) The period between the infection of an individual by a pathogen and the manifestation of the disease it causes.

Malaise (mah-lāz′) A vague, indefinite feeling of discomfort, debilitation, or lack of health.

Opportunistic infection (op″or-tu-nis′tik in-fek′shun) A disease caused by a microorganism that does not ordinarily cause disease but becomes pathogenic under certain circumstances.

Paresthesia (par″ĕs-the′zhĕ) An abnormal sensation such as prickling or tingling.

Pathogenic microorganism (path-o-jen′ik mi″kro-or′gan-izm) A microorganism that causes disease.

Pruritus (proo-ri′tĕs) Itching.

Subclinical infection (sĕb-klinĭ-kel) An infectious disease not detectable by the usual clinical signs.

Whitlow (hwit′lo) An infection involving the distal phalanx of a finger.

Humans are surrounded and inhabited by an enormous number of microorganisms. The ability of these organisms to cause disease depends on both the microorganism and the state of the body's defenses. The organism must be capable of causing disease, and the individual must be susceptible to the disease. Microorganisms are traditionally divided into those that produce disease (pathogenic) and those that do not (nonpathogenic). To cause disease the organism must gain access to the body, accommodate to growth in the human environment, and avoid multiple host defenses. These defense mechanisms include intact skin and mucosal surfaces, antimicrobial secretory and excretory products on the skin and mucosa, the competition among the components of the normal microflora, the inflammatory response, and the immune response.

Numerous infectious diseases can affect the tissues of the oral cavity. Bacterial, fungal, and viral infections are the most common; but even protozoan and helminthic infections, although extremely rare, have been reported.

The oral cavity can be the primary site of involvement of an infectious disease, or a systemic infection can have oral manifestations. These infections are transmitted from one individual to another by several different routes. Organisms can be transferred through the air on dust particles or water droplets. Some organisms require intimate and direct contact to be transferred. Some can be transferred on hands and objects, and others such as hepatitis B must be transferred from one person to another in blood or other body fluids. Microorganisms initially invading the oral tissues can cause a local infection, systemic infection, or both. Microorganisms circulating in the bloodstream can cause lesions in the oral cavity, and microorganisms causing infection in the lungs can be transferred to oral tissues when they are present in sputum. The oral cavity contains numerous microorganisms that make up the normal oral microflora. Changes such as a decrease in salivary flow, antibiotic administration, and immune system alterations affect the oral microflora so that organisms that are usually nonpathogenic are able to cause disease. This type of infection is called an **opportunistic infection.**

Microorganisms penetrating epithelial surfaces act as foreign material and stimulate the inflammatory response (see Chapter 2). The inflammatory response is a nonspecific response and results in edema and the accumulation of a large number of white blood cells at the site. The responses of the immune system are highly specific (see Chapter 3). Specific antibodies are formed in response to specific antigens; microorganisms are antigens.

Humoral immunity (immunity that is mediated by antibodies) is an effective defense against some microorganisms, and cell-mediated immunity (immunity in which T-lymphocytes are responsible for the respons) is the primary defense against others such as intracellular bacteria (tuberculosis), viruses, and fungi. Microbial infections are responsible for many more diseases than those included in this chapter. The diseases discussed here are common, cause specific oral lesions, and help to illustrate principles of infectious disease. Dental caries and periodontal disease clearly are infectious diseases that are important to dental hygienists. However, they are not included in this text because they are usually studied in courses other than oral pathology. The dental hygienist frequently encounters oral infectious diseases and must be able to recognize their clinical features and significance for control of infection.

BACTERIAL INFECTIONS

IMPETIGO

Impetigo is a bacterial skin infection caused primarily by *Staphylococcus aureus* and occasionally by *Streptococcus pyogenes.* Impetigo most commonly involves the skin of the face or extremities and is usually seen in young children. The organisms are present on skin, and nonintact skin is necessary for infection; areas of trauma such as cuts and abrasions and areas of dermatitis are likely sites of this infection. The lesions of impetigo are infectious. Direct contact is required for transmission. Impetigo presents as either vesicles that rupture, resulting in thick, amber-colored crusts, or longer-lasting bullae. Lesions may itch (**pruritus**), and regional lymphadenopathy may be present. Systemic manifestations such as fever and **malaise** generally do not occur with this infection. When impetigo affects the perioral skin, the lesions may resemble recurrent herpes simplex infection (Herpes simplex infection is discussed later in this chapter). However, recurrent herpes simplex infection is much less common than impetigo in small children. The diagnosis of impetigo is made on the basis of the clinical presentation or by identification of the bacteria from cultures of the lesions. Topical or systemic antibiotics are used for treatment.

TONSILLITIS AND PHARYNGITIS

Tonsillitis and **pharyngitis** are inflammatory conditions of the tonsils and pharyngeal mucosa. Many different organisms cause them, including streptococci, adenoviruses, influenza viruses, and Epstein-Barr virus. The clinical features include sore throat, fever, tonsillar hyperplasia, and erythema of the oropharyngeal mucosa and tonsils.

Streptococcal tonsillitis and pharyngitis are common bacterial infections that are spread by contact with infectious nasal or oral secretions. The appearance of streptococcal tonsillitis and pharyngitis (i.e., “strep throat”) closely resembles tonsillitis and pharyngitis caused by other infections such as viral infections. Specific laboratory tests, including a rapid antigen detection test, are available for diagnostic confirmation of streptococcal infection. Antibiotics are used to treat streptococcal infection.

Tonsillitis and pharyngitis caused by group A β-hemolytic streptococci are significant because of their relationship to scarlet fever and rheumatic fever. **Scarlet fever** usually occurs in children. In addition to fever, patients with scarlet fever develop a generalized red skin rash that is caused by a toxin released by the bacteria. In addition to streptococcal tonsillitis and pharyngitis, oral manifestations of scarlet fever include petechiae on the soft palate and an appearance of the tongue that has been called **strawberry tongue.** The fungiform papillae are red and prominent, with the dorsal surface of tongue exhibiting either a white coating or erythema. Throat culture is helpful in confirming the diagnosis of stretpcocally pharyngitis in a patient with scarlet fever.

Rheumatic fever is a childhood disease that follows a group A β-hemolytic streptococcal infection, usually tonsillitis and pharyngitis. Rheumatic fever is characterized by an inflammatory reaction involving the heart, joints, and central nervous system. Rheumatic fever may result in permanent damage to heart valves.

TUBERCULOSIS

Tuberculosis is an infectious chronic **granulomatous disease** usually caused by the organism *Mycobacterium tuberculosis.* The chief form of the disease is a primary infection of the lung. Inhaled droplets containing bacteria lodge in the alveoli of the lungs. After undergoing phagocytosis by macrophages, the organisms are resistant to destruction and multiply in the macrophages. They then disseminate in the bloodstream. After a few weeks dissemination ceases. The signs and symptoms of this lung infection include fever, chills, fatigue and malaise, weight loss, and persistent cough. The bacteria can be carried to widespread areas of the body and cause involvement of organs such as the kidneys and liver. This is called **miliary tuberculosis.** Involvement of the submandibular and cervical lymph nodes (usually as a result of ingesting the organism in nonpasteurized milk) causes enlargement of those nodes and is called **scrofula** or **tuberculous lymphadenitis.** The lung infection can occur at any age. Most commonly foci of infection in the lungs become completely walled off and heal by fibrosis and calcification. A reactivation of the primary lesion can occur years after the initial infection. This reactivation is usually a result of a compromised immune response.

Oral lesions associated with tuberculosis occur but are rare. They most likely appear when organisms are carried from the lungs in sputum and transmitted to the oral mucosa (Figure 4-1). The tongue and palate are the most common sites for oral lesions of tuberculosis, but they may occur anywhere in the oral cavity, even in bone as in osteomyelitis. Oral lesions appear as painful, nonhealing, slowly enlarging ulcers that can be either superficial or deep.

Diagnosis

Oral lesions of tuberculosis are identified by biopsy and microscopic examination of the tissue. The characteristic histopathologic lesions of tuberculosis are **granulomas.** The granulomas are composed of areas of necrosis surrounded by macrophages, multinucleated giant cells, and lymphocytes. Similar lesions occur in sarcoidosis, deep fungal infections, and foreign-body reactions. Staining the tissue to be examined microscopically with a special stain may reveal the organisms. Tissue culture to diagnose tuberculosis requires a specialized laboratory.

A skin test is used to determine if an individual has been exposed and infected with *M. tuberculosis.* An antigen called **purified protein derivative** is injected into the skin. If the individual's immune system has previously encountered the antigen, a positive inflammatory skin reaction occurs (a type IV delayed-hypersensitivity reaction). This skin reaction indicates previous infection with the bacteria but not necessarily active disease. When a skin test result is positive, chest radiographs are taken to determine if active tuberculosis disease is present.

Effective drug treatment for tuberculosis became available in the 1940s. In the United States most tuberculosis treatment centers had closed by the mid-1970s. State health departments reported a dramatic increase in new cases in the mid-1980s, particularly in densely populated urban areas. This increase was suggested to be related to human immunodeficiency virus infection and to noncompliance of patients with therapy. Recent public health efforts have focused on ensuring compliance with antituberculosis drug treatment; as a result the number of new cases reported has decreased.

Tuberculosis is an infectious disease that can be transmitted occupationally to dental health care personnel. Routine use of universal precautions, including eye protection, mask, or facial shield, is important in preventing the transmission of airborne droplet infections such as tuberculosis. However, for patients with active tuberculosis, routine dental treatment is deferred. When emergency dental treatment is needed, the use of a special mask is recommended to ensure prevention of transmission of the tuberculosis organism.

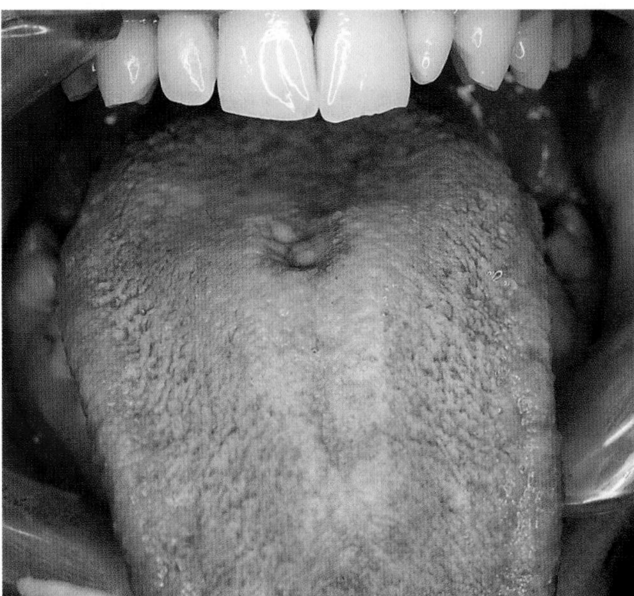

FIGURE 4-1 ■ Ulcer on tongue seen in tuberculosis.

Treatment and Prognosis

Oral lesions resolve with treatment of the patient's primary (usually pulmonary) disease. Several different combination medications, including isoniazid and rifampin, are used to treat tuberculosis. Treatment continues for many months and may continue for as long as 2 years. Patients usually become noninfectious shortly after treatment begins. Consultation with the patient's physician should confirm that treatment is ongoing and the patient is no longer infectious.

ACTINOMYCOSIS

Actinomycosis is an infection caused by a filamentous bacterium called *Actinomyces israelii.* These organisms were at one time thought to be fungi; therefore the name ends in the suffix "mycosis," which usually indicates a fungal infection.

The most characteristic form of the disease is the formation of abscesses that tend to drain by the formation of sinus tracts (Figure 4-2). The colonies or organisms appear in the pus as tiny, bright yellow grains and are called *sulfur granules* because of their yellow color. The organisms can also be identified by microscopic examination. These organisms are common inhabitants of the oral cavity. It is not clear why

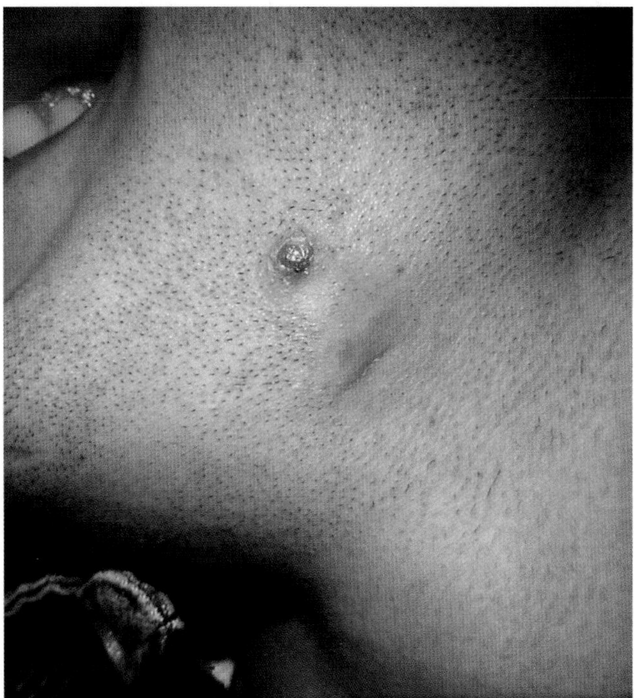

FIGURE 4-2 ■ Actinomycosis. Skin lesion over mandible. Incision and drainage site seen below lesion. "Sulfur granules" were noted in the laboratory report, and the condition was treated with long-term antibiotic therapy.

they only occasionally cause disease. Predisposing factors have not been identified. The infection is often preceded by tooth extraction or an abrasion of the mucosa.

Generally the clinician makes a diagnosis of actinomycosis by identifying the colonies in the tissue from the lesion. Actinomycosis is treated with long-term high doses of antibiotics.

SYPHILIS

Syphilis is a disease caused by the spirochete *Treponema pallidum.* The organism is transmitted from one person to another by direct contact. The spirochete, a corkscrewlike organism, can penetrate mucous membranes but requires a break in the continuity of the skin surface to invade through the skin. The organisms die quickly when exposed to air and changes in temperature. Syphilis is usually transmitted through sexual contact with a partner who has active lesions. It can also be transmitted by transfusion of infected blood or by transplacental inoculation of a fetus from an infected mother.

Table 4-1

Stages of syphilis

Stage	Oral Lesion
Primary	Chancre
Secondary	Mucous patch
Latent	None
Tertiary	Gumma

The disease occurs in three stages: (1) primary, (2) secondary, and (3) tertiary (Table 4-1). The lesion of the primary stage, called the **chancre,** is highly infectious and forms at the site at which the spirochete enters the body (Figure 4-3). Regional lymphadenopathy accompanies the chancre. The lesion heals spontaneously after several weeks without treatment, and the disease enters a latent period.

The secondary stage occurs about 6 weeks after the primary lesion appears. In the secondary stage diffuse eruptions of the skin and mucous membranes occur. The skin lesions have many forms. The oral lesions are called **mucous patches** and appear as multiple, painless, grayish-white plaques covering ulcerated mucosa. The lesions of secondary syphilis are the most infectious. They undergo spontaneous remission but can recur for months or years. After remission the disease may remain latent for many years.

The tertiary lesions occur years after the initial infection if the infection has not been treated. They chiefly involve the cardiovascular system and the central nervous system. The localized tertiary lesion is called a **gumma** and is noninfectious. A gumma can occur in the oral cavity; the most common sites are the tongue and palate. The lesion appears as a firm mass that eventually becomes an ulcer. The gumma is a destructive lesion and can lead to perforation of the palatal bone.

Congenital Syphilis

Syphilis can be transmitted from an infected mother to the fetus because the organism can cross the placenta and enter the fetal circulation. **Congenital syphilis** often causes serious and irreversible damage to the child such as facial and dental abnormalities. The developmental disorders that result from fetal and neonatal syphilis are described in Chapter 5.

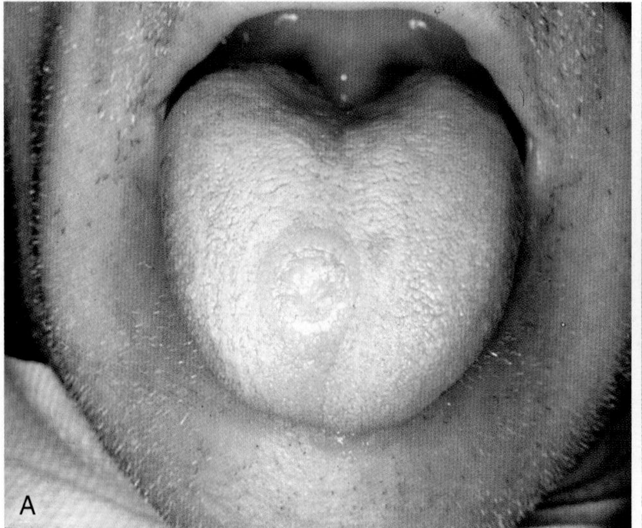

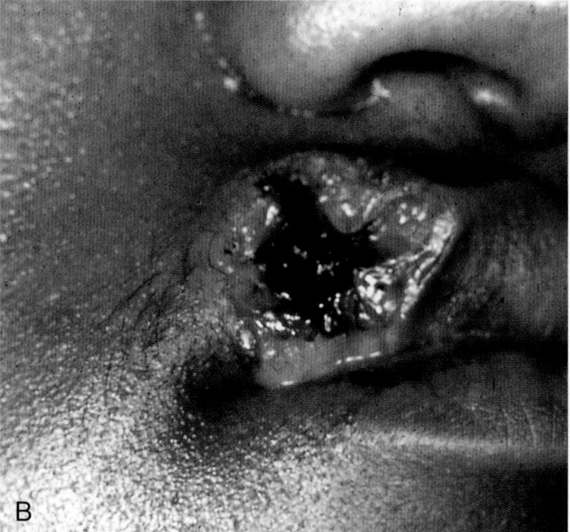

FIGURE 4-3 ■ **A,** Chancre on tongue seen in primary syphilis. **B,** Chancre on lip. (**A** courtesy Dr. Norman Trieger; **B** courtesy Dr. Edward V. Zegarelli.)

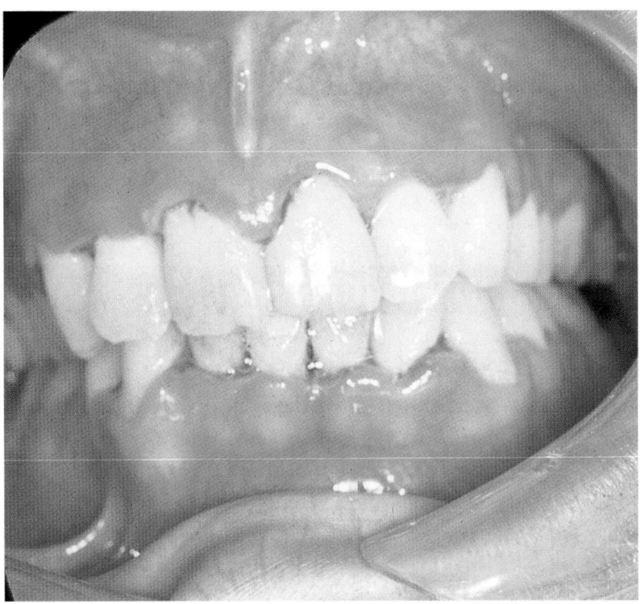

FIGURE 4-4 ■ Necrotizing ulcerative gingivitis.

Diagnosis and Treatment

The diagnosis of syphilitic lesions occurring on skin can be made using a special microscopic technique called a **dark-field examination** to identify the spirochetes. However, other spirochetes are present in the oral cavity; therefore this examination is not reliable for oral lesions. Two of the serologic (blood) tests that are commonly used to confirm the diagnosis of syphilis: (1) the Venereal Disease Research Laboratories (VDRL) test, and (2) the fluorescent treponemal antibody absorption test. These tests may produce negative results in primary syphilis because sufficient antibodies may not have formed for the test result to be positive.

Syphilis is generally treated with penicillin. The VDRL test is used again to evaluate the success of treatment. The antibody titer decreases if treatment has been successful.

NECROTIZING ULCERATIVE GINGIVITIS

Necrotizing ulcerative gingivitis (NUG) is also called **acute necrotizing ulcerative gingivitis (ANUG).** It is a painful erythematous gingivitis with necrosis of the interdental papillae (Figure 4-4). NUG is usually caused by a combination of a fusiform bacillus and a spirochete *(Borrelia vincentii)* and is associated with decreased resistance to infection.

The gingiva is painful and erythematous, with necrosis of the interdental papillae generally accompanied by a foul odor and metallic taste. The necrosis results in cratering of the interdental papillae area. Sloughing of the necrotic tissue presents as a pseudomembrane over the tissues. Systemic manifestations of infection such as fever and cervical lymphadenopathy may be present. Clinical features distinguish NUG from acute marginal gingivitis and the gingival component of acute primary herpes simplex infection (see Figure 4-17, *B*).

PERICORONITIS

Pericoronitis is an inflammation of the mucosa around the crown of a partially erupted, impacted tooth. The soft tissue around the mandibular third molar is the most common location for pericoronitis. The inflammation is usually the result of infection by bacteria that are part of the normal oral microflora, which proliferate in the pocket between the soft tissue and the crown of the tooth. Compromised host defenses, ranging from minor illnesses to immunodeficiency, are associated with an increased risk of pericoronitis. Trauma from an opposing molar and impaction of food under the soft tissue flap (operculum) covering the distal portion of the third molar may also precipitate pericoronitis.

Diagnosis

The diagnosis of pericoronitis is made on the basis of the clinical presentation. The tissue around the crown of a partially erupted tooth is swollen, erythematous, and painful.

Treatment and Prognosis

Treatment of pericoronitis includes mechanical débridement and irrigation of the pocket and systemic antibiotics. Extraction of the impacted molar is usually necessary to prevent recurrence.

ACUTE OSTEOMYELITIS

Acute osteomyelitis involves acute inflammation of the bone and bone marrow (Figure 4-5, *A*). Acute osteomyelitis of the jaws is most commonly a result of the extension of a periapical abscess. It may follow fracture of the bone or surgery and may also result from bacteremia.

Diagnosis

The diagnosis of the specific organism causing acute osteomyelitis is based on culture results, and treatment is based on antibiotic sensitivity testing. Microscopic examination shows nonviable bone, necrotic debris, acute inflammation, and bacterial colonies in the marrow spaces. No change is seen on the radiograph unless the disease has been present for more than 1 week.

Treatment and Prognosis

The treatment of acute osteomyelitis involves drainage of the area and the use of appropriate antibiotics.

CHRONIC OSTEOMYELITIS

Chronic osteomyelitis is a long-standing inflammation of bone. It may occur in inadequately treated acute osteomyelitis, long-term inflammation of bone with no recognized

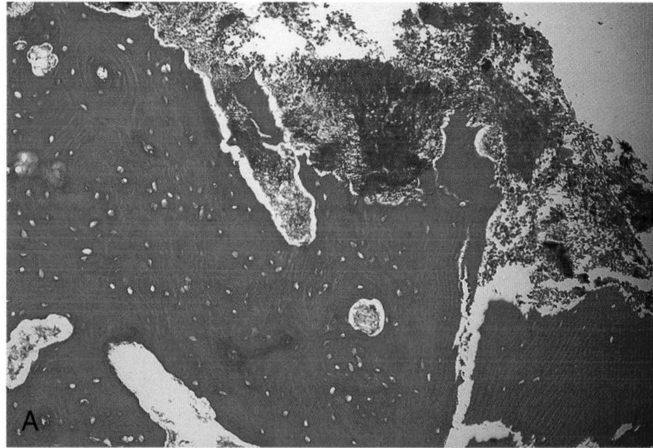

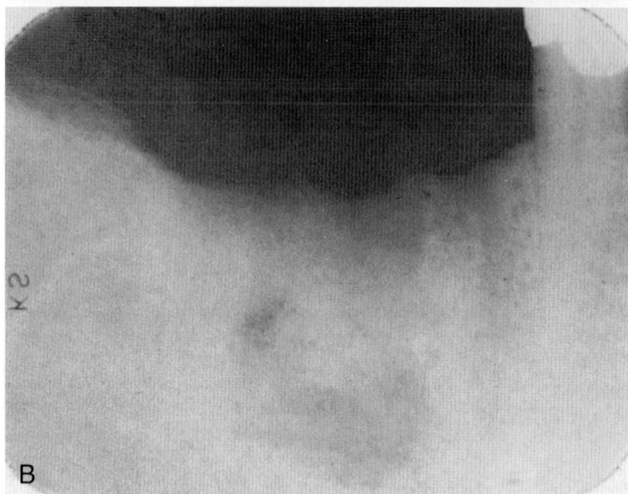

FIGURE 4-5 ■ **A,** Low-power microscopy of acute osteomyelitis showing nonviable bone. Bacterial colonies and inflammatory cells are seen between trabeculae of bone. **B,** Chronic osteomyelitis as seen radiographically.

acute phase, Paget disease, sickle cell disease, or bone irradiation that results in decreased vascularity. The involved bone is painful and swollen, and radiographic examination reveals a diffuse and irregular radiolucency that can eventually become radiopaque (Figure 4-5, *B*). When radiopacity develops, the condition is called **chronic sclerosing osteomyelitis.** Recently, cases of osteonecrosis of the mandible and maxilla have been reported in patients taking bisphosphonate medication. This may appear clinically similar to chronic osteomyelitis. Bisphosphonate associated osteonecrosis is described in Chapter 9.

Diagnosis

The diagnosis of chronic osteomyelitis is based on biopsy results and the histologic examination, which shows chronic inflammation of bone and marrow. Bacterial culture may be helpful, but bacteria may be difficult to identify.

Treatment

Treatment of chronic osteomyelitis involves débridement and administration of systemic antibiotics. In some patients the use of hyperbaric oxygen may be needed to successfully treat this condition.

FUNGAL INFECTIONS

CANDIDIASIS

Candidiasis, also called **moniliasis** and **thrush,** occurs as a result of an overgrowth of the yeastlike fungus *Candida albicans.* It is the most common oral fungal infection. This fungus is part of the normal oral microflora in many individuals, particularly those who wear dentures. Overgrowth of *Candida albicans* is associated with many different conditions, including the following:

- Antibiotic therapy
- Cancer chemotherapy
- Corticosteroid therapy
- Dentures
- Diabetes mellitus
- Human immunodeficiency virus infection
- Hypoparathyroidism
- Infancy (newborn)
- Multiple myeloma
- Primary T lymphocyte deficiency
- Xerostomia

Newborn infants are particularly susceptible to an overgrowth of this fungus because they do not have either an established oral microflora or a fully developed immune system. Pregnant women often have *Candida vaginitis,* and the organism is transmitted to the infant while passing through the birth canal. Antibiotics can alter the bacteria of the oral microflora, which can allow the overgrowth of *Candida albicans.* Systemic and topical corticosteroids, diabetes, and cell-mediated immune system deficiency are other factors that allow the overgrowth of this fungus. Candidiasis is one of the most common oral lesions that occur in association with immunodeficiency. Candidiasis generally affects the superficial layers of the epithelium; therefore, when it is present, the proliferating organisms are easily identified in a sample obtained by scraping the surface (mucosal smear) of the lesion.

Types of Oral Candidiasis

Several forms of oral candidiasis exist; recognition of their clinical features is important so that candidiasis is included in the differential diagnosis of a variety of clinical presentations. The types of oral candidiasis are:

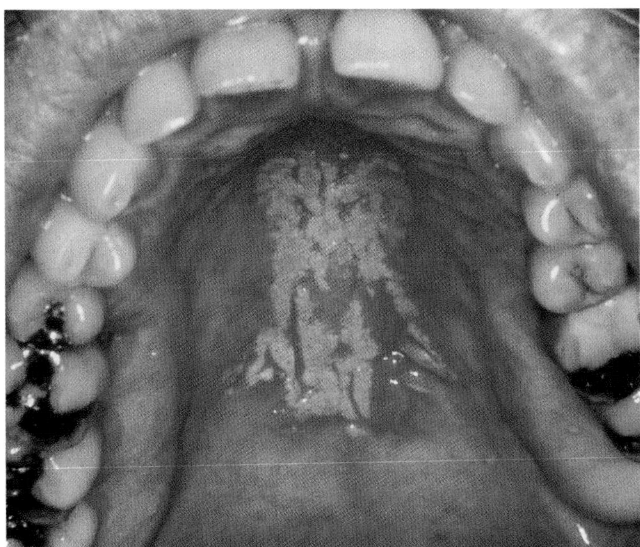

FIGURE 4-6 ■ Pseudomembranous candidiasis.

- Pseudomembranous
- Erythematous
- Denture stomatitis (chronic atrophic candidiasis)
- Chronic hyperplastic (candida leukoplakia)
- Angular cheilitis

Pseudomembranous Candidiasis

A white curdlike material is present on the mucosal surface in **pseudomembranous candidiasis** (Figure 4-6). The underlying mucosa is erythematous. Occasionally a burning sensation is felt, and the patient may complain of a metallic taste.

Erythematous Candidiasis

An erythematous, often painful, mucosa is the presenting complaint in **erythematous candidiasis** (Figure 4-7). This type of candidiasis may be localized to one area of the oral mucosa or be more generalized.

Denture Stomatitis

Denture stomatitis is the most common type of candidiasis affecting the oral mucosa. It is also called **chronic atrophic candidiasis** (Figure 4-8). This type of candidiasis also presents as erythematous mucosa, but the erythematous change is limited to the mucosa covered by a full or partial denture. The lesions may vary from petechiae-like to more generalized and granular. It is most common on the palate and maxillary alveolar ridge. Denture stomatitis is asymptomatic and is usually discovered by the dentist or dental hygienist during a routine oral examination.

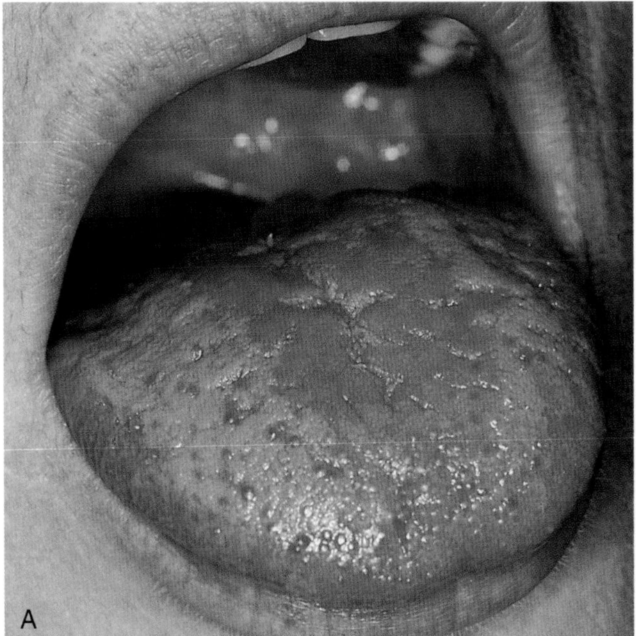

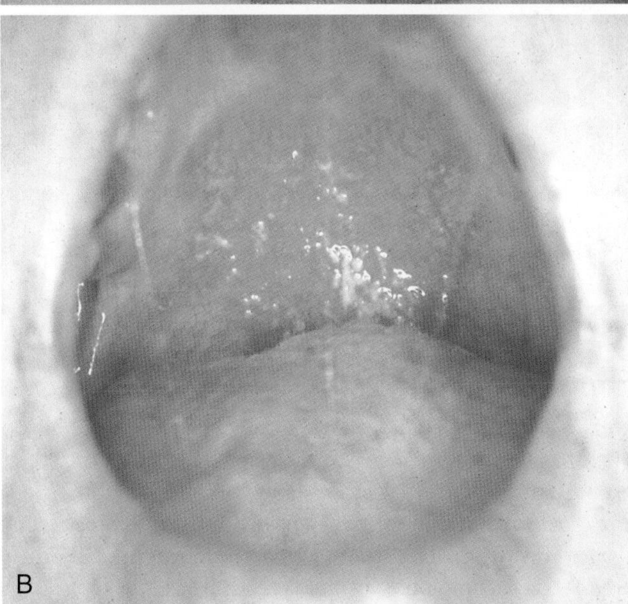

FIGURE 4-7 ■ Erythematous candidiasis. **A,** Recent-onset and erythematous lesions elsewhere in the oral cavity differentiate this from median rhomboid glossitis. **B,** Response to antifungal treatment confirmed the diagnosis of oral candidiasis in this patient.

Chronic Hyperplastic Candidiasis

Chronic hyperplastic candidiasis (Figure 4-9) appears as a white lesion that does not wipe off the mucosa. **Candidal leukoplakia** and **hypertrophic candidiasis** are other names for this type of oral candidiasis. An important diagnostic feature of this type of candidiasis is its response to antifungal medication: when leukoplakia is caused by candidiasis, it disappears when treated with antifungal medication (therapeutic diagnosis). If the lesion does not respond to antifungal therapy, biopsy should be considered to establish the diagnosis of the lesion.

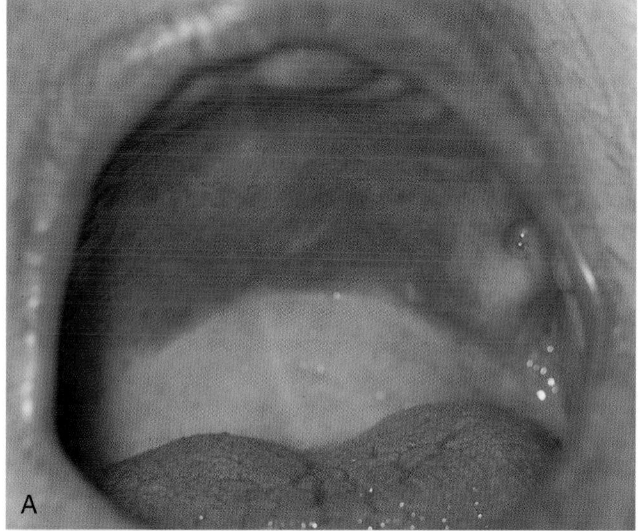

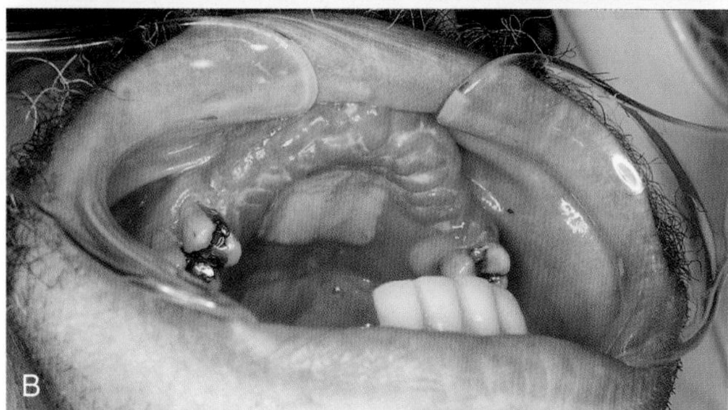

FIGURE 4-8 ■ Chronic atrophic candidiasis (denture stomatitis). **A,** Full denture. **B,** Partial denture.

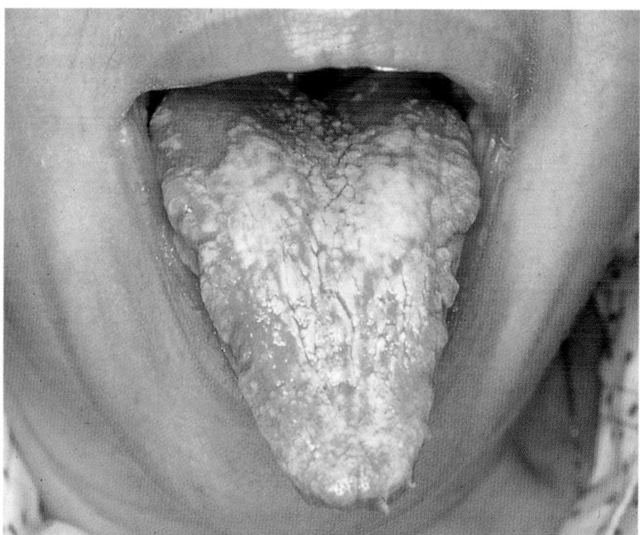

FIGURE 4-9 ■ Chronic hyperplastic candidiasis. The white appearance of the tongue did not wipe off, and it disappeared with antifungal treatment.

Angular Cheilitis

Candida organisms are often the cause of **angular cheilitis** (Figure 4-10). It appears as erythema or fissuring at the labial commissures. Angular cheilitis may be caused by other factors such as nutritional deficiency; however, it most commonly results from *Candida* infection. Angular cheilitis frequently accompanies intraoral candidiasis.

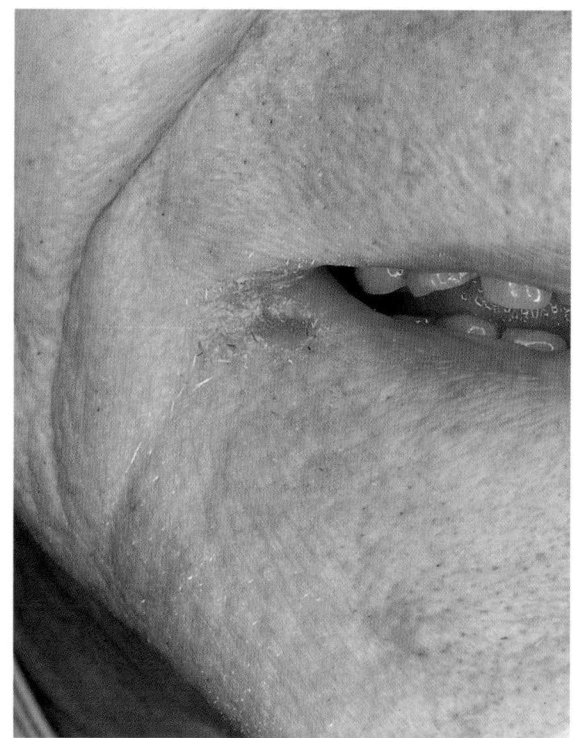

FIGURE 4-10 ■ Angular cheilitis.

Chronic Mucocutaneous Candidiasis

A severe form of candidiasis that usually occurs in patients who are severely immunocompromised is called **chronic mucocutaneous candidiasis.** The patient has chronic oral and genital mucosal candidiasis, skin as well as lesions. Oral involvement may appear as pseudomembranous, erythematous, or hyperplastic candidiasis; and angular cheilitis is common. The skin lesions usually involve the nails and skinfolds.

Median Rhomboid Glossitis

Several studies have reported an association between **median rhomboid glossitis** (Figure 4-11) and candidiasis. It appears as an erythematous, often rhombus-shaped, flat-to-raised area on the midline of the posterior dorsal tongue. *Candida* organisms have been identified in some lesions, and some lesions disappear with antifungal treatment. However, the response to antifungal treatment is not consistent; therefore, although this lesion has been associated with candidiasis, the cause is not yet clear.

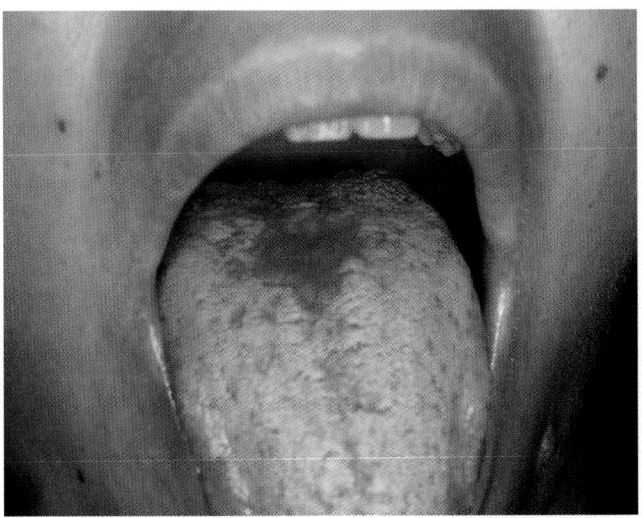

FIGURE 4-11 ■ Median rhomboid glossitis.

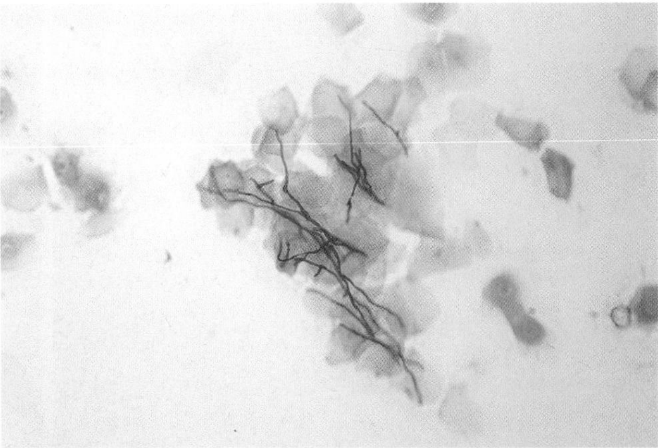

FIGURE 4-12 ■ Photomicrograph of a smear showing epithelial cells and *Candida* organisms.

Diagnosis and Treatment

Because *Candida* is part of the oral microflora in many individuals, a culture is not useful for diagnosis. A positive culture result indicates that the organisms are present but not that they are causing infection. The use of the mucosal smear (Figure 4-12) is usually more helpful. The surface of the lesion is scraped vigorously with a tongue blade, wooden spatula, or specially designed brush; and the scrapings are spread on a glass slide and fixed with alcohol. The slide is then sent to an oral pathology laboratory for staining and examination. In addition to the smear, the response of the lesion to antifungal treatment is important in confirming the diagnosis of candidiasis. Lesions caused by *Candida* should resolve with antifungal treatment. Both topical and systemic medications are used for candidiasis. However, in some patients, particularly those who are immunocompromised, candidiasis is persistent and recurrent.

Although the final diagnosis and management of a patient with oral candidiasis is the responsibility of the dentist, dental hygienists are often the first to recognize the oral changes characteristic of this condition. Recurrent oral candidiasis may be an early sign of a severe underlying medical problem.

DEEP FUNGAL INFECTIONS

Oral lesions occur in some deep fungal infections (e.g., histoplasmosis, coccidioidomycosis, blastomycosis, and cryptococcosis). They are all characterized by primary involvement of the lungs. Oral lesions are caused by implantation of the organism carried by sputum from the lungs to the oral mucosa.

Infections caused by these organisms are more common in certain areas of the United States than in others. Histoplasmosis is widespread in the midwestern United States, and coccidioidomycosis is more prevalent in parts of the western United States, particularly the San Joaquin Valley of California. Blastomycosis is common in the Ohio-Mississippi river basin area. Therefore oral lesions caused by these organisms are most likely seen in areas of the country in which the infection is most common.

Cryptococcosis is transmitted through inhalation of organisms contained in dust from bird droppings, particularly from pigeons. In addition to the regional distribution of these infections, reactivation, including the development of oral lesions, can also occur in patients who are immunocompromised.

Diagnosis

The initial signs and symptoms of these deep fungal infections are usually related to the primary lung infection. Oral lesions are preceded by pulmonary involvement. These oral lesions are chronic, nonhealing ulcers that can resemble squamous cell carcinoma. Diagnosis is made by biopsy and microscopic examination. Special staining of the tissue reveals the organisms, which can be identified by their microscopic appearance. The tissue can also be cultured; this is useful in establishing the diagnosis.

Treatment

Systemic antifungal medications such as amphotericin B or ketoconazole or itraconazole are used to treat these infections. However, latent infections may remain even after treatment and may reappear if the individual's immune system becomes deficient.

MUCORMYCOSIS

Mucormycosis, also called **phycomycosis,** is a rare fungal infection. The organism is a common inhabitant of soil and is usually nonpathogenic. However, infection with this

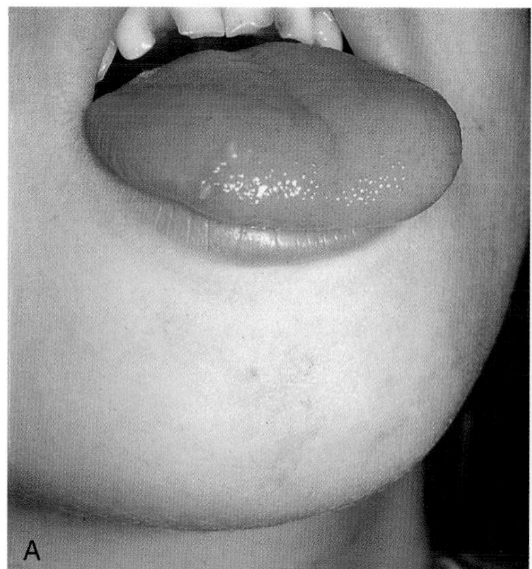

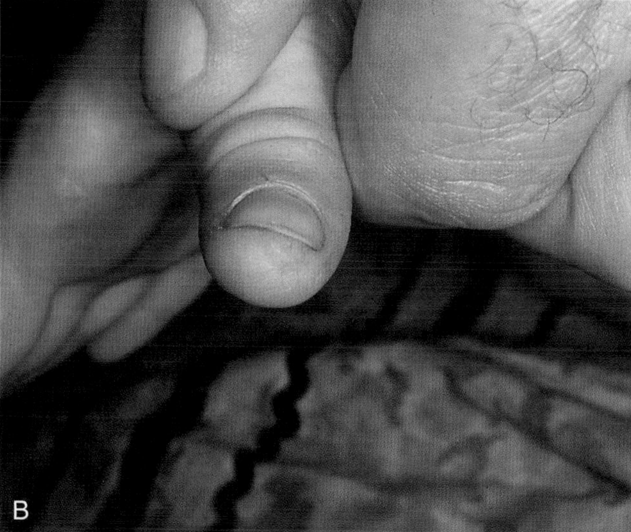

FIGURE 4-13 ■ **A** and **B**, Verruca vulgaris on the tongue of a child with a similar lesion on the thumb. (Courtesy Dr. Edward V. Zegarelli.)

organism occurs in diabetic and severely debilitated patients. The disease often involves the nasal cavity, maxillary sinus, and hard palate and can present as a proliferating or destructive mass in the maxilla. The diagnosis is made by biopsy and identification of the organisms in the tissue.

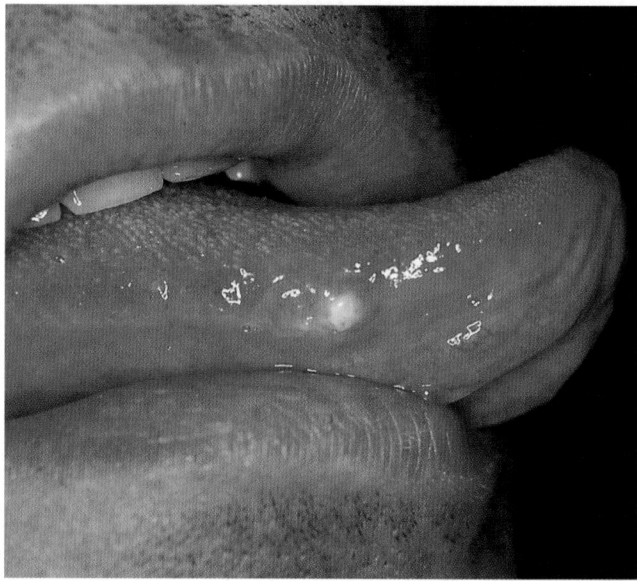

FIGURE 4-14 ■ Verruca vulgaris on the lateral aspect of the tongue in an adult.

VIRAL INFECTIONS

HUMAN PAPILLOMAVIRUS INFECTION

More than one hundred different types of the **human papilloma virus (HPV)** have been identified. Several have been identified in oral lesions, and some have been identified in normal oral mucosa. Human papilloma viruses have also been implicated in neoplasia.

Verruca Vulgaris

The **verruca vulgaris,** or common wart, is a papillary oral lesion caused by an human papilloma virus. It is a common skin lesion. Oral lesions are less common than skin lesions, but they do occur. The virus is inoculated by direct contact and may be transmitted from skin to oral mucosa. The lips are one of the most common intraoral sites for this lesion. Autoinoculation occurs through finger sucking or fingernail biting in patients with verrucae on the hands or fingers (Figure 4-13). The verruca vulgaris is usually a white, papillary, exophytic lesion (Figure 4-14) that closely resembles and is related to the benign tumor of squamous epithelium called the **papilloma** (see Chapter 7).

Histologically the verruca vulgaris consists of fingerlike projections of markedly keratotic, stratified squamous epithelium that exhibits a prominent granular cell layer; numerous cells with clear cytoplasm called koilocytes are present in the upper spinous layer of the epithelium. These cells contain the viral particles that are visible by electron microscopic examination. Each of the projections contains a central core of fibrous connective tissue containing many blood vessels. The vacuolated cells in the epithelium contain the viral particles.

Diagnosis

Biopsy and histologic examination reveal the light microscopic features of this lesion. Immunologic staining is also useful in identifying these viruses.

Treatment and Prognosis

Conservative surgical excision is the treatment of choice for verruca vulgaris. These lesions may recur. In addition, patients with skin lesions should be instructed to refrain from finger sucking or fingernail biting to prevent reinoculation and development of new lesions.

Condyloma Acuminatum

The **condyloma acuminatum** is a benign papillary lesion that is caused by another papilloma virus. The virus is generally transmitted by sexual contact and is most common in the anogenital region. It is transmitted to the oral cavity through oral-genital contact or self-inoculation.

Oral condylomas appear as papillary, bulbous masses and can occur anywhere in the oral mucosa (Figure 4-15). Multiple lesions may be present. They have been reported to occur on the tongue, buccal mucosa, palate, gingiva, and alveolar ridge. The oral condyloma tends to be more diffuse than the papilloma or verruca vulgaris and is generally not as well keratinized as the verruca vulgaris. The condyloma is pink, whereas the verruca vulgaris is usually white.

Histologically the condyloma acuminatum is composed of fingerlike (papillary) projections of epithelium covering cores of connective tissue. The epithelium is thickened, and cells with clear cytoplasm are seen throughout the epithelium. These clear cells contain viral particles that can be identified through immunologic staining.

When the condyloma acuminatum occurs in the oral cavity, it is generally treated by conservative surgical excision. However, recurrence is common, and multiple lesions make management difficult. Patients should be instructed to avoid oral-genital contact with an infected partner to prevent reinoculation.

Focal Epithelial Hyperplasia

Focal epithelial hyperplasia, also called *Heck disease,* is characterized by the presence of multiple whitish-to–pale pink nodules distributed throughout the oral mucosa (Figure 4-16). The disease is most common in children and was first described in Native Americans, but it has since been described in many different areas of the world. This disease is caused by another human papilloma virus. The lesions are generally asymptomatic and do not require treatment. They resolve spontaneously within a few weeks. Histologically the lesions show thickened epithelium with broad, connected rete ridges. Cells in the epithelium have clear cytoplasm, which is a common finding in lesions caused by a human papilloma virus.

HERPES SIMPLEX INFECTION

Two major forms of the herpes simplex virus exist: (1) type 1 and (2) type 2. Oral infections are generally caused by type 1, and genital infections are most commonly caused by type 2. Oral infection with the herpes simplex virus occurs in an initial (primary) form and a recurrent (secondary) form. The herpes simplex virus is one of a group of viruses called human herpes viruses (HHVs). Other herpes viruses include varicella-zoster virus (VZV), Epstein-Barr virus (EBV), cytomegalovirus (CMV), and kaposi sarcoma-associated herpes virus (KSHV human herpes virus 8). Herpes simplex viruses have the ability to persist in an individual in a clinically quiescent or latent state. The primary infection undergoes remission without the virus being completely eliminated.

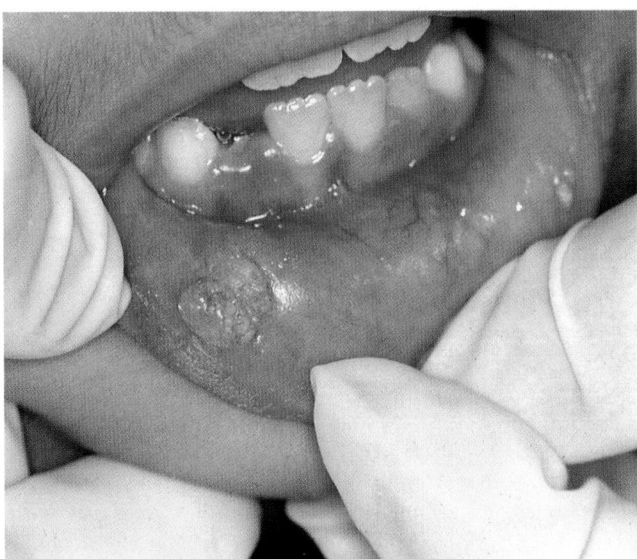

FIGURE 4-15 ■ Condyloma acuminatum. The presence of condyloma acuminatum in a child is strongly suggestive of sexual abuse. (Courtesy Dr. Sidney Eisig.)

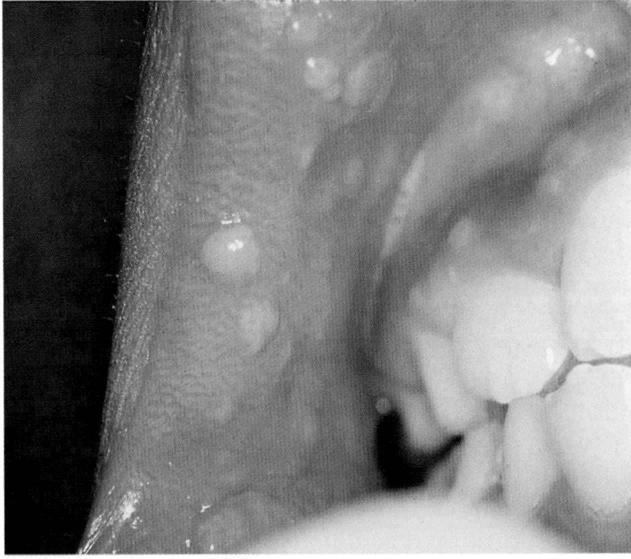

FIGURE 4-16 ■ Focal epithelial hyperplasia. (Courtesy Dr. Stanley Kerpel.)

Primary Herpetic Gingivostomatitis

The oral disease caused by initial infection with the herpes simplex virus is called **primary herpetic gingivostomatitis** (Figure 4-17). Painful, erythematous, and swollen gingiva and multiple tiny vesicles on the perioral skin, vermilion border of the lips, and oral mucosa characterize the disease. These vesicles progress to form ulcers. Systemic symptoms such as fever, malaise, and cervical lymphadenopathy generally occur first, followed by gingival involvement and the appearance of mucosal vesicles and ulcers. The disease most commonly occurs in children between the ages of 6 months and 6 years. However, it may occur at any age if an individual who has not been previously exposed to the virus comes into contact with it or if a sufficient level of antibodies has not developed to confer protection against reinfection. Because many more individuals have antibodies to herpes simplex than have a history of the disease, the majority of infections are thought to be subclinical. The disease is usually self-limited. The lesions heal spontaneously in 1 to 2 weeks.

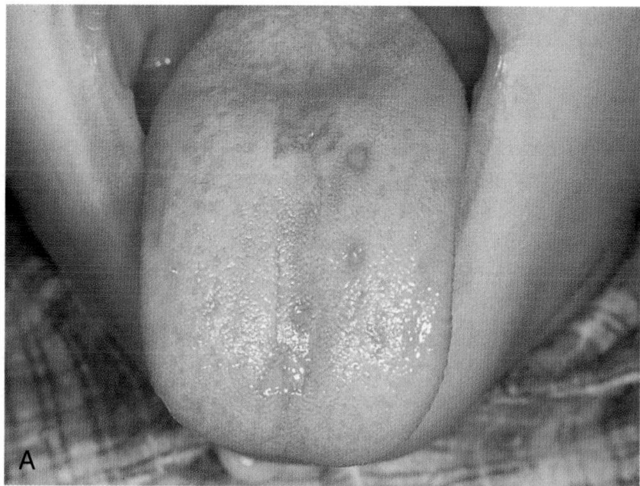

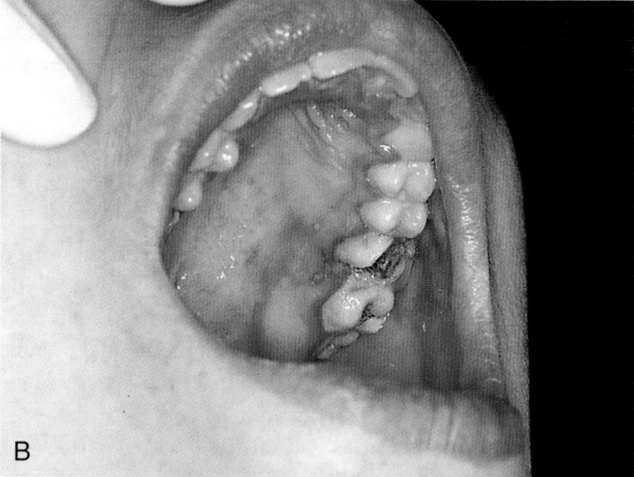

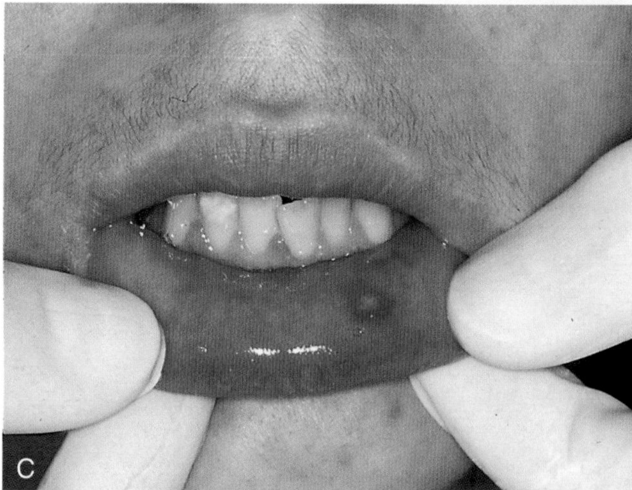

FIGURE 4-17 ■ **A,** Primary herpetic gingivostomatitis in a child. **B** and **C,** Primary herpetic gingivostomatitis in an adolescent. (**A** courtesy Dr. Edward V. Zegarelli.)

Recurrent Herpes Simplex Infection

The herpes simplex virus tends to persist in a latent state, usually in the nerve tissue of the trigeminal ganglion, and causes localized recurrent infections. It has been estimated that one third to one half of the population of the United States experience **recurrent herpes simplex infection**. The most common type of recurrent oral herpes simplex infection occurs on the vermilion border of the lips and is called **herpes labialis** (Figure 4-18), which is also called a **cold sore** or **fever blister.** Recurrent infections are often produced by certain stimuli such as sunlight, menstruation, fatigue, fever, and emotional stress. These stimuli are thought to trigger the viral replication and immunologic changes that result in clinical lesions.

Recurrent herpes simplex infection can also occur intraorally (Figure 4-19). The appearance and location of these lesions are important to distinguish them from aphthous ulcers (Table 4-2). Recurrent intraoral herpes simplex occurs on keratinized mucosa that is fixed to bone, most commonly the hard palate and gingiva. The lesions appear as painful clusters of tiny vesicles or ulcers that can coalesce to form a single ulcer with an irregular border. Usually patients experience prodromal symptoms such as pain, burning, or tingling in the area in which the vesicles develop. The lesions heal without scarring in 1 to 2 weeks. Episodes of recurrence vary from once a month in some individuals to once a year in others.

Herpes simplex virus is transmitted by direct contact with an infected individual, and the lesions of the primary infection occur at the site of inoculation. The herpes simplex virus can be isolated from both primary and recurrent lesions. The amount of virus present is highest in the vesicle stage. In some individuals the virus is present in the oral cavity, even when no lesions are present. Herpes simplex virus can cause a painful infection of the fingers called **herpetic whitlow** in dentists and dental hygienists (Figure 4-20). Herpetic whitlow can be either a primary or a recurrent infection. Herpes simplex can also cause eye infection (Figure 4-21). Routine

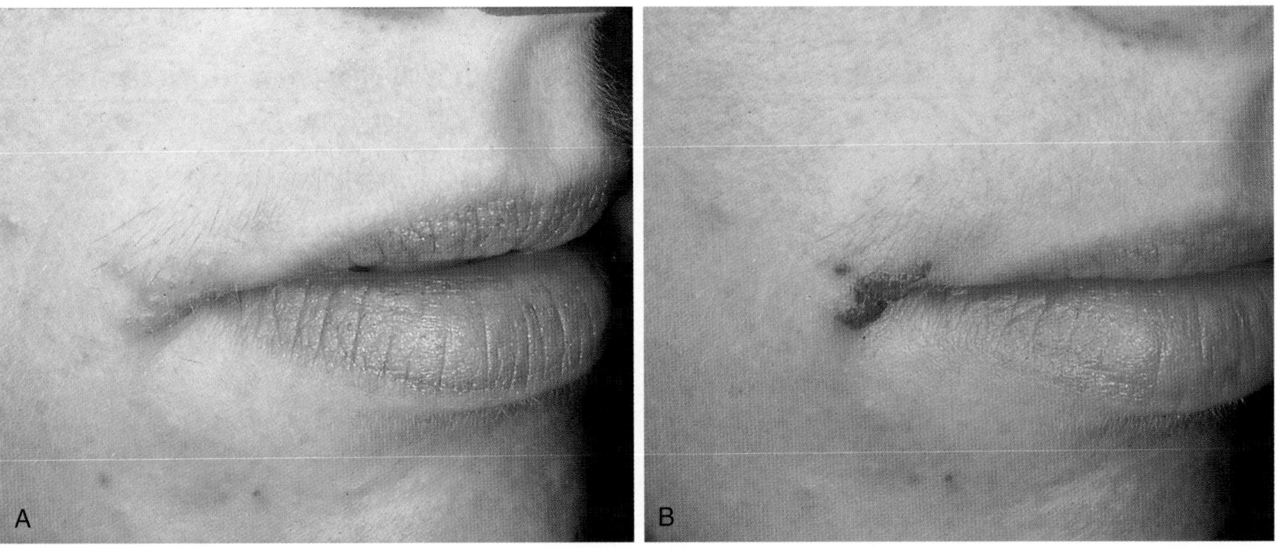

FIGURE 4-18 ■ Herpes labialis. **A,** Twelve hours after onset. **B,** Forty-eight hours after onset.

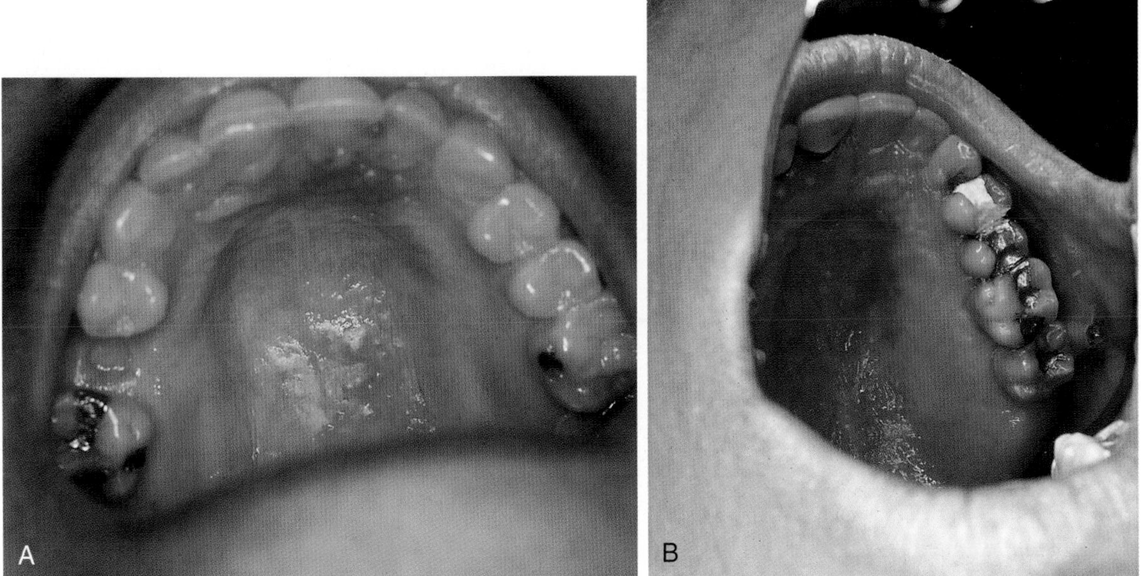

FIGURE 4-19 ■ **A** and **B,** Recurrent intraoral herpes simplex.

barrier infection control procedures (mask, eye protection, and gloves) are important in preventing the transmission of the herpes simplex virus to dental health care providers.

Diagnosis

The diagnosis of herpes simplex infection, both primary and recurrent, is generally based on the clinical characteristics of the disease (see Table 4-2). In immunocompromised patients the characteristic clinical features may be lacking. A viral culture can be performed to confirm the diagnosis. This procedure requires a special culture medium and at least 2 days before results are available.

Herpes simplex virus causes changes in epithelial cells that can be seen microscopically. These virally altered cells can be seen in tissue obtained by biopsy or on a smear taken by scraping the basal cells of the lesion and spreading them on a glass slide, fixing them with alcohol, and submitting them to a pathology laboratory for staining and examination (Figure 4-22). Smears of herpes simplex ulceration have been reported to be positive for virally altered cells only about 50% of the time.

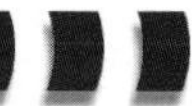

Table 4-2

Comparison of the clinical features of recurrent minor aphthous ulcers and recurrent herpes ulceration

Feature	Minor Aphthous Ulcers	Herpes Simplex Ulceration
Location	Nonkeratinized mucosa	Keratinized mucosa
Number	One to several	Multiple (crops)
Vesicle precedes ulcer	No	Yes
Pain	Yes	Yes
Size	<1 cm	1-2 mm
Borders	Round to oval	Crops of ulcers coalesce to form a large irregular ulcer
Recurrent	Yes	Yes

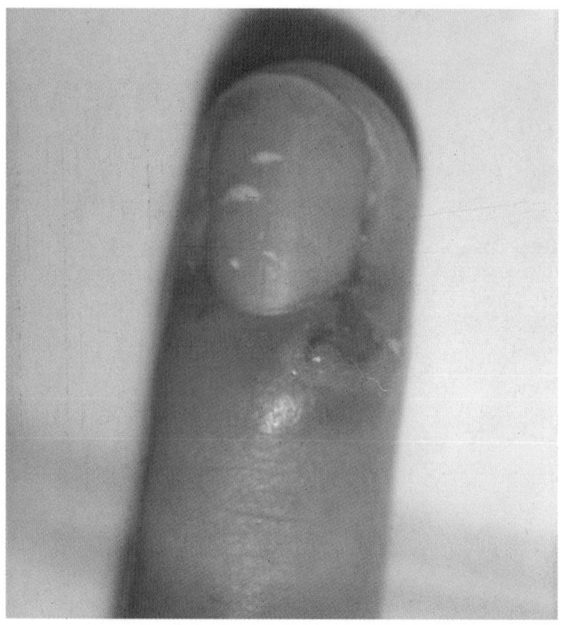

FIGURE 4-20 ■ Herpetic whitlow in a dental hygienist. (Courtesy Susan Rod Graham.)

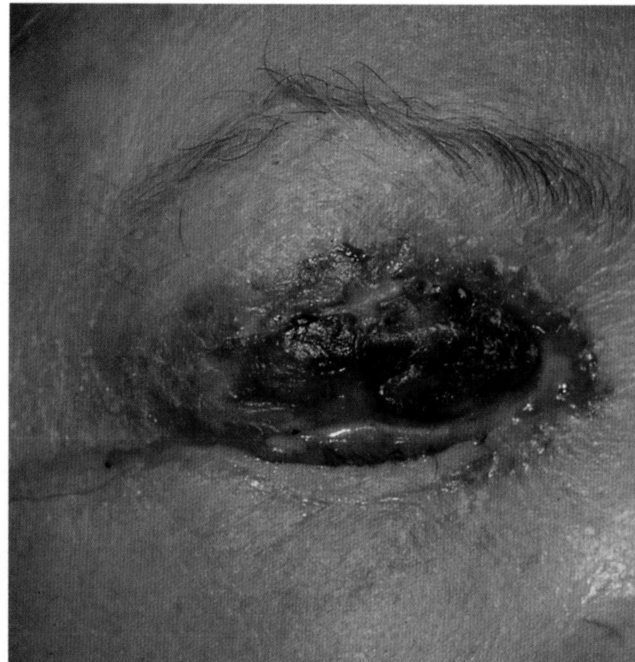

FIGURE 4-21 ■ Herpetic eye infection. (Courtesy Dr. Sidney Eisig.)

Treatment

Antiviral drugs such as acyclovir are available for the treatment of herpes simplex infection and are used for treating genital herpes simplex infection. Antiviral drugs have not been shown to be consistently effective in treating the intraoral lesions of herpes simplex infection except in immunocompromised patients. The use of sunscreens may prevent the development of herpes labialis. Systemic antiviral medication has been approved by the Food and Drug Administration for treating and preventing herpes labialis. Topical application of antiviral drugs may prevent or decrease the duration of herpes labialis when they are administered very early in the development of the lesion (prodrome) before epithelial damage has occurred.

VARICELLA-ZOSTER VIRUS

The **varicella-zoster virus (VZV)** causes both chickenpox (varicella) and shingles (herpes zoster). Respiratory aerosols and contact with secretions from skin lesions transmit the virus. Both chickenpox and herpes zoster are contagious.

Chickenpox

Chickenpox is a highly contagious disease that causes vesicular and pustular eruptions of the skin and mucous membranes, along with systemic symptoms such as headache,

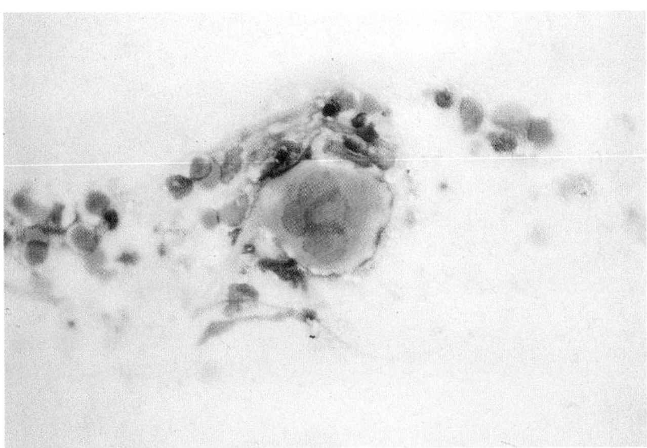

FIGURE 4-22 ■ Smear of virally altered cells resulting from herpes simplex. (Courtesy Dr. Harry Lumerman.)

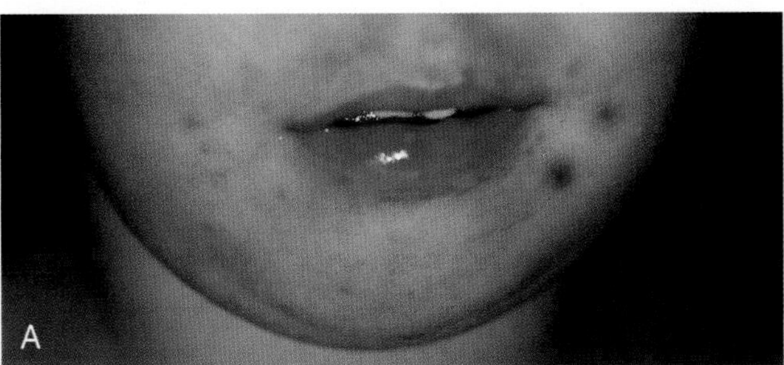

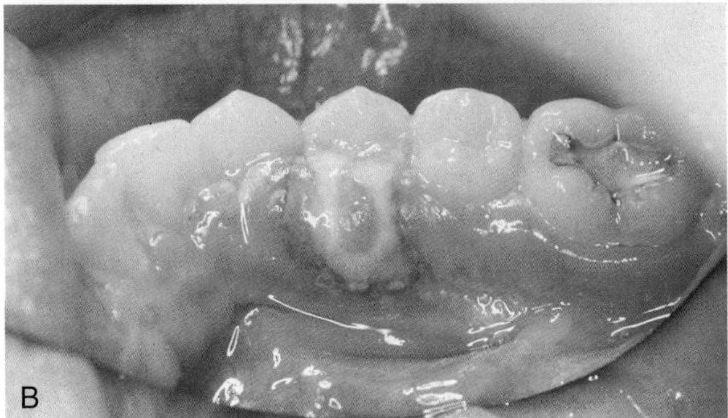

FIGURE 4-23 ■ Chickenpox. **A,** Skin lesions. **B,** Gingival lesion. (Courtesy Dr. Roger S. Kitzis.)

fever, and malaise (Figure 4-23). The **incubation period** is about 2 weeks. Chickenpox usually occurs in children; although oral lesions occur, they generally do not cause severe discomfort. Usually an individual has only a single episode of chickenpox; but second, milder forms have also been described. Recovery generally occurs in 2 to 3 weeks.

Herpes Zoster

Although chickenpox has been described in adults, the virus usually causes a different form of disease in this population. The form that usually occurs in adults is called **herpes zoster** or **shingles**. It is characterized by a unilateral, painful eruption

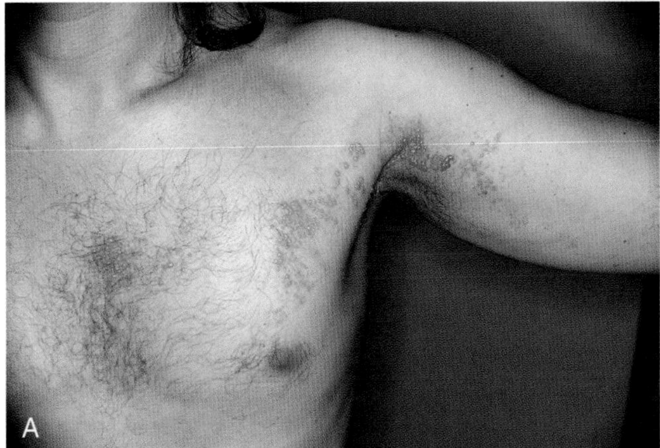

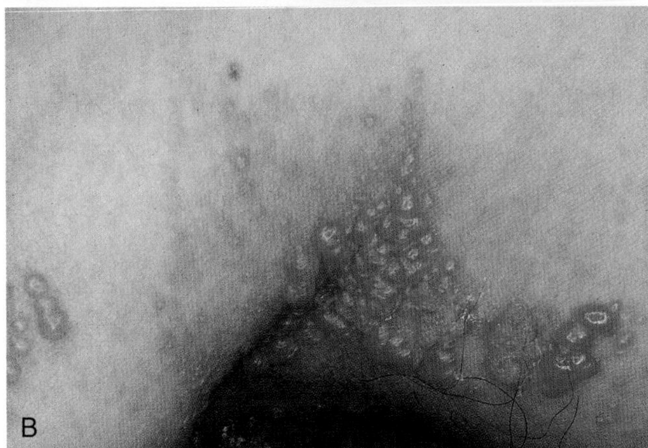

FIGURE 4-24 ■ Herpes zoster. **A,** Unilateral distribution of vesicles along the distribution of a sensory nerve. **B,** Many vesicles coalesce to form large lesions.

of vesicles along the distribution of a sensory nerve (Figure 4-24). Whether or not the varicella-zoster virus is harbored in the sensory ganglia (during the interval between chickenpox and herpes zoster) in a manner similar to that of the herpes simplex virus is not clear. However, herpes zoster often occurs in association with immunodeficiency or certain malignancies such as Hodgkin disease and leukemia. A vaccine is available to prevent varicella-zoster infections. The vaccine is given to children to prevent chickenpox and to older adults to prevent the recurrence of the infection as herpes zoster.

The depression of cell-mediated immunity (CMI) appears to be important in the development of herpes zoster. Any of the three branches of the trigeminal nerve may be affected: (1) the ophthalmic branch, (2) the maxillary branch, or (3) the mandibular branch (Figure 4-25). Oral lesions occur when the maxillary or mandibular branches are affected (Figure 4-26). The oral lesions, like the skin lesions, are characterized by their unilateral distribution. Prodromal symptoms of pain, burning, or **paresthesia** often precede the development of vesicles. Oral lesions are painful and begin as vesicles that progress to ulcers. The disease usually lasts for several weeks, and in some patients, neuralgia, which takes months to resolve, may follow the resolution of the lesions.

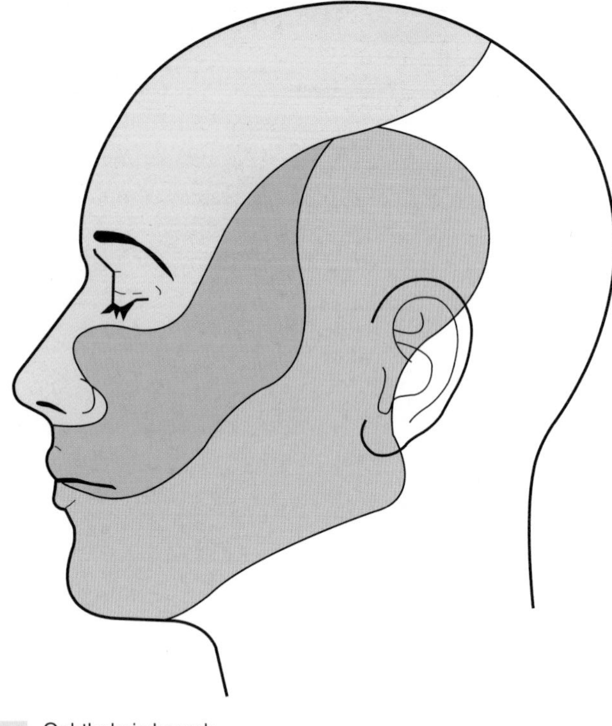

FIGURE 4-25 ■ Diagram of the branches of the trigeminal nerve.

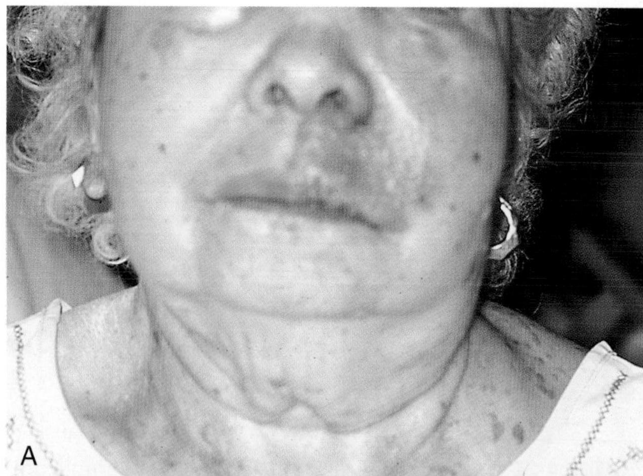

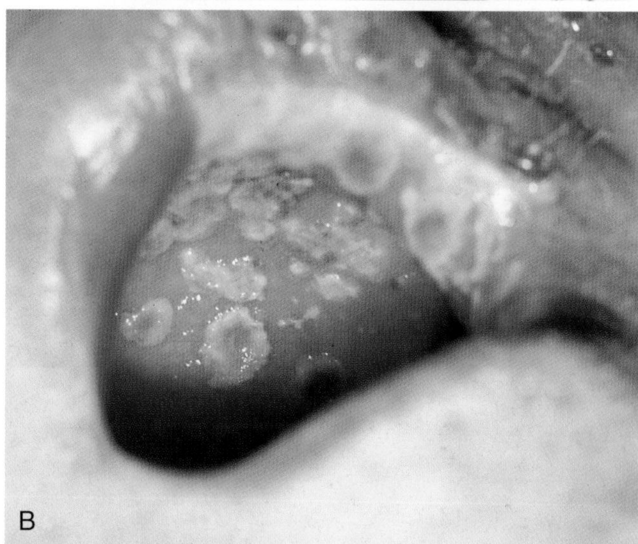

FIGURE 4-26 ■ Herpes zoster. **A,** Unilateral facial lesions occurring along the distribution of the maxillary branch of the trigeminal nerve. **B,** Intraoral lesions in the same patient illustrate the unilateral distribution of herpes zoster.

Diagnosis

The diagnosis of varicella and herpes zoster is generally made on the basis of the clinical features. Biopsy or a smear of the lesion may show the same type of virally altered epithelial cells that are seen in herpes simplex infection. Viral cultures may take weeks to grow.

Treatment

Varicella generally requires only supportive treatment. Antiviral drugs are used for immunocompromised patients and for patients with herpes zoster. In some patients corticosteroids have been used in an attempt to prevent the pain of postherpetic neuralgia.

EPSTEIN-BARR VIRUS INFECTION

The **Epstein-Barr virus** has been implicated in several diseases that occur in the oral region, including infectious mononucleosis, nasopharyngeal carcinoma, Burkitt lymphoma, and hairy leukoplakia. Nasopharyngeal carcinoma and Burkitt lymphoma are rare malignant neoplasms. Infectious mononucleosis and hairy leukoplakia are discussed here.

Infectious Mononucleosis

Infectious mononucleosis is an infectious disease caused by the Epstein-Barr virus (EBV). It is characterized by sore throat, fever, generalized lymphadenopathy, enlarged spleen, malaise, and fatigue. Palatal petechiae occur in infectious mononucleosis, usually appearing early in the course of the disease. The mechanism for the development of these petechiae is unclear. The diagnosis is confirmed by the identification in the blood of mononucleosis cells, which are atypical activated T lymphocytes. Severe complications such as hepatitis occur in some patients. In developed countries infectious mononucleosis occurs principally in late adolescence and young adults in upper socioeconomic classes. The virus is transmitted by close contact. Contact with saliva during kissing is a frequent route of transmission of Epstein-Barr virus. In most patients infectious

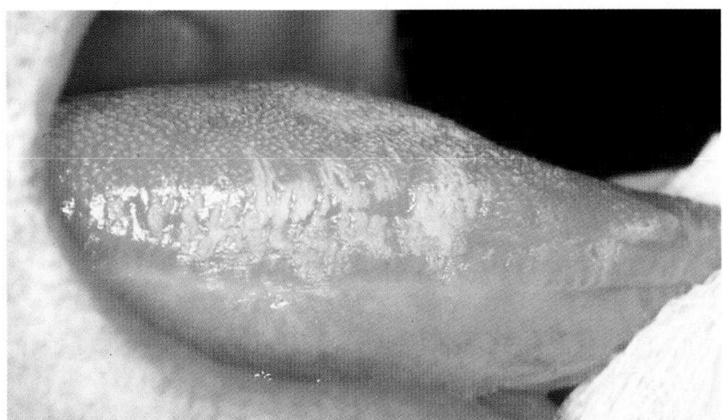

FIGURE 4-27 ■ Hairy leukoplakia.

mononucleosis is a benign, self-limited disease that resolves within 4 to 6 weeks. In some patients fatigue lasts much longer.

Hairy Leukoplakia

This irregular, corrugated white lesion most commonly occurs on the lateral border of the tongue (Figure 4-27). Epstein-Barr virus has been identified in the epithelial cells of **hairy leukoplakia** and is considered to be the cause of the lesion. Hairy leukoplakia was first identified in patients infected with HIV and occurs most commonly in these patients; it has also been reported in immunocompromized patients not infected with HIV.

COXSACKIEVIRUS INFECTIONS

The **coxsackieviruses,** named for the town in New York where the virus was first discovered, cause several different infectious diseases. Three of these have distinctive oral lesions and are discussed here. Fecal-oral contamination, saliva, and respiratory droplets can be the means of transmission.

Herpangina

Herpangina characteristically includes vesicles on the soft palate (Figure 4-28), along with fever, malaise, sore throat, and difficulty swallowing (dysphagia). An erythematous pharyngitis is also present. The disease is usually mild to moderate and resolves in less than 1 week without treatment.

Hand-Foot-and-Mouth Disease

Hand-foot-and-mouth disease usually occurs in epidemics in children younger than 5 years of age. Oral lesions are generally painful vesicles and ulcers that can occur anywhere in the mouth. Multiple macules or papules occur on the skin, typically on the feet, toes, hands, and fingers. Lesions resolve spontaneously within 2 weeks.

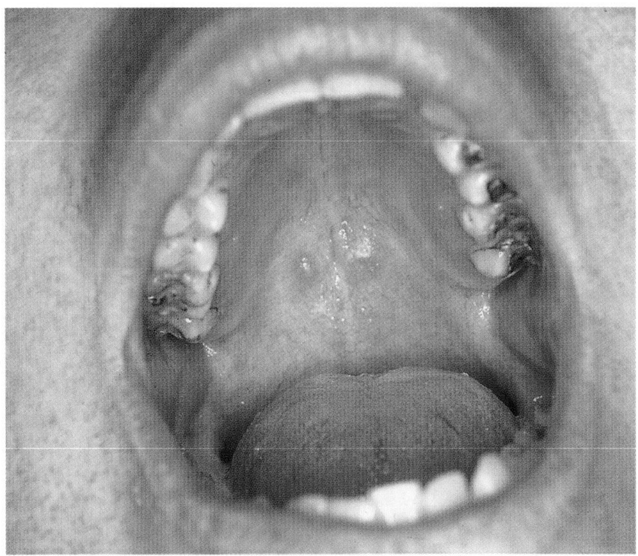

FIGURE 4-28 ■ Herpangina.

Diagnosis

Although the oral lesions may resemble herpes simplex infection, the distribution of the skin lesions and the mild systemic symptoms usually help to differentiate the two conditions. Viral culture and measurement of circulating antibodies to the type of coxsackievirus that causes hand-foot-and-mouth disease may help to confirm the diagnosis but generally are not necessary.

Treatment

The disease is generally mild and of short duration. Treatment usually is not required.

Acute Lymphonodular Pharyngitis

Acute lymphonodular pharyngitis is another coxsackievirus infection that is characterized by fever, sore throat, and mild headache. Hyperplastic lymphoid tissue of the soft palate or tonsillar pillars appears as yellowish or dark pink nodules. The disease generally lasts several days to 2 weeks and does not usually require treatment.

OTHER VIRAL INFECTIONS THAT MAY HAVE ORAL MANIFESTATIONS

Measles

Measles is a highly contagious disease causing systemic symptoms and a skin rash that results from a type of virus called a ***paramyxovirus.*** The disease most commonly occurs in childhood. Early in the disease, Koplik spots, which are small erythematous macules with white necrotic centers, may occur in the oral cavity.

Mumps

Mumps, or **epidemic parotitis,** is a viral infection of the salivary glands that is also caused by a paramyxovirus. The disease most commonly occurs in children and is characterized by painful swelling of the salivary glands, most commonly bilateral swelling of the parotid glands.

HUMAN IMMUNODEFICIENCY VIRUS AND ACQUIRED IMMUNODEFICIENCY SYNDROME

The virus associated with **acquired immunodeficiency syndrome (AIDS)** was identified in 1983; in 1986 it was designated as **human immunodeficiency virus (HIV).** The HIV virus is transmitted by sexual contact with infected persons, by contact with infected blood and blood products, and to infants of infected mothers. HIV infects cells of the immune system. The most important of the cells of the immune system that the virus infects is the CD4 T-helper lymphocyte. This lymphocyte is important both in CMI and in regulating the immune response. As the disease progresses, this lymphocyte becomes depleted. Other cells that may be infected with HIV include macrophages, Langerhans cells, dendritic cells, and cells of the nervous system.

THE SPECTRUM OF HUMAN IMMUNODEFICIENCY VIRUS

Many individuals experience an acute disease that occurs shortly after infection with HIV, whereas other individuals remain asymptomatic. The acute disease resolves, and infected individuals may have no signs or symptoms of disease for some time. In most patients infected with HIV, a progressive immunodeficiency eventually develops. As the immune system begins to fail, the number of CD4 lymphocytes decreases; nonspecific problems such as fatigue and opportunistic infections such as oral candidiasis may develop. As the immune system becomes profoundly deficient, life-threatening opportunistic infections and cancers occur. The most severe result of infection with HIV is AIDS.

DIAGNOSING AIDS

The diagnosis of AIDS is well defined. The definition of AIDS has been established by the Centers for Disease Control and Prevention (CDC) and is given in Box 4-1. Since it was identified in the early 1980s, this definition has been changed several times as knowledge of the disease has grown. The most recent definition of AIDS in adults and adolescents includes HIV infection with severe CD4 lymphocyte depletion (less than 200 CD4 lymphocytes per microliter [μl] of blood). The normal CD4 lymphocyte count is between about 550 and 1000 lymphocytes/μl blood. The revised definition continues to include a number of opportunistic diseases such as *Pneumocystis carinii* pneumonia, esophageal candidiasis, and Kaposi sarcoma. Also included is HIV-related wasting syndrome. In addition to including the CD4 lymphocyte count, the revised definition includes pulmonary tuberculosis, recurrent pneumonia, and invasive cervical cancer.

HUMAN IMMUNODEFICIENCY VIRUS TESTING

Tests that identify antibody to HIV are the tests generally used to determine if a person has been infected with HIV. Recently a rapid HIV test has been approved. This test identifies antibody to HIV either in oral fluid or in blood. The oral test uses a collector specially designed to obtain a sample of transudate through the oral mucosa. A positive oral test is confirmed by a blood test. A negative test does not require confirmation. Routine HIV testing generally uses a blood test that is an **enzyme-linked immunosorbent assay (ELISA).** When this test is positive twice, it is followed by a more specific test called the **Western blot test.** To be considered seropositive for HIV, a person must have two positive ELISA test results followed by a positive Western blot test result. Other tests such as the polymerase chain reaction (PCR) identify virus rather than antibody. In the United States different states have different laws concerning HIV testing. Informed consent by the patient and pretest counseling may be required before HIV testing can be done.

CLINICAL MANIFESTATIONS

As mentioned, the initial infection with HIV may be completely asymptomatic. However, early in HIV infection the amount of circulating virus is very high, and the risk of transmission to others may be very high. In some individuals lymphadenopathy may develop; in still others an acute illness resembling infectious mononucleosis and lasting 8 to 14 days can occur. When this acute illness develops, the patient may have sore throat, general malaise, myalgia, and arthralgia, lymphadenopathy, and fever. Patients with acute infection can also have a skin rash, nausea, and diarrhea. After this acute illness, some individuals have persistent lymphadenopathy, but many become completely asymptomatic.

The virus infects cells of the immune system; as a result this system stops protecting the individual against certain infections and tumors. In time, as the immune system becomes deficient, a variety of signs and symptoms can develop, signaling changes in the immune system. Several of these signs and symptoms occurring together are sometimes called *AIDS-related complex*. They include oral candidiasis, fatigue, weight loss, and lymphadenopathy. HIV can also infect cells of the nervous system, resulting in dementia in some patients.

Antibodies to HIV generally begin to be detectable in blood about 6 weeks after the initial infection. However, in some individuals antibodies may not be detectable for 6 months and occasionally for up to 1 year or more.

Box 4-1

Definition of Acquired Immunodeficiency Syndrome

Acquired immunodeficiency syndrome (AIDS) is an illness characterized by one or more of the following diseases or conditions.

Human Immunodeficiency Virus Laboratory Tests Not Performed or Results Inconclusive and the Patient Has No Other Cause of Immunodeficiency

1. Candidiasis of the esophagus, trachea, bronchi, or lungs
2. Cryptococcosis, extrapulmonary
3. Cryptosporidiosis with diarrhea persisting longer than 1 month
4. Cytomegalovirus disease of an organ other than liver, spleen, or lymph nodes in a patient older than 1 month of age
5. Herpes simplex virus infection causing a mucocutaneous ulcer that persists longer than 1 month or bronchitis, pneumonitis, or esophagitis for any duration affecting a patient older than 1 month of age
6. Kaposi sarcoma affecting a patient less than 60 years of age
7. Lymphoma of the brain affecting a patient less than 60 years of age
8. Lymphoid interstitial pneumonia, pulmonary hyperplasia, or both, affecting a child less than 13 years of age
9. *Mycobacterium avium* or *Mycobacterium kansasii* disease, disseminated
10. *Pneumocystis carinii* pneumonia
11. Progressive multifocal leukoencephalopathy
12. Toxoplasmosis of the brain affecting a patient older than 1 month of age

With Laboratory Evidence of Human Immunodeficiency Virus Infection

Less than 200 CD4+ T lymphocytes/µl or a CD4+ T-lymphocyte percentage of total lymphocytes less than 14

Any of the preceding diseases listed or those that follow:

1. Multiple bacterial infections of certain types affecting a child less than 13 years of age
2. Coccidioidomycosis, disseminated
3. Human immunodeficiency virus (HIV) encephalopathy (HIV dementia)
4. Histoplasmosis, disseminated
5. Isosporiasis with diarrhea persisting longer than 1 month
6. Lymphoma of the brain at any age
7. Kaposi sarcoma
8. Certain types of lymphoma
9. Mycobacterial disease other than tuberculosis, disseminated
10. Extrapulmonary tuberculosis
11. *Salmonella* septicemia, recurrent
12. HIV-related wasting syndrome
13. Pulmonary tuberculosis
14. Recurrent pneumonia
15. Invasive cervical cancer

Even if HIV laboratory test results are negative, if other causes of immunodeficiency are not ruled out, a diagnosis of AIDS can be made if certain of these diseases are diagnosed.

Adapted from Centers for Disease Control and Prevention: 1993 revised classification system for HIV infection and expanded surveillance case definition for AIDS among adolescents and adults, *MMWR Recomm Rep* 41(RR-17):1, 1992.

The spectrum of HIV infection includes the full range of problems that result from infection with this virus from asymptomatic infection to AIDS (Figure 4-29). AIDS represents terminal HIV infection in this spectrum. It is not yet known how many of the persons who become infected with HIV go on to experience immunodeficiency, opportunistic diseases, or dementia. Some patients who are HIV-seropositive appear to remain immunocompetent for many years. Cofactors that can contribute to the development of the immunodeficiency are being studied. Each year the results of natural history studies show an increase in the percentage of HIV-infected individuals in whom AIDS develops.

MEDICAL MANAGEMENT

Tests such as PCR are used to measure the amount of HIV circulating in serum. This is called viral load. Measurement of viral load along with the CD4 lymphocyte count is used to assess HIV infection. Patients with HIV infection are managed with combinations of different types of antiretroviral (anti-HIV) drugs and drugs that prevent and treat opportunistic diseases. The combination of drugs is called *highly active antiretroviral therapy* (HAART or ART). Measurement of viral load is used to evaluate the effectiveness of antiretroviral therapy. Management of HIV infection is continually changing in response to the results of ongoing clinical drug trials.

ORAL MANIFESTATIONS

Oral lesions are prominent features of AIDS and HIV infection (Box 4-2). Some of these lesions are known to be indicators of developing immunodeficiency and predictors of the development of AIDS in individuals who are HIV seropositive. The oral lesions that occur develop because of the deficiency in cell mediated immunity and the deregulation of immunologic responses that occurs when the T-helper cells ($CD4^+$ lymphocytes) become depleted. Oral lesions include opportunistic infections, tumors, and autoimmune-like diseases. As a result of management of HIV infection with antiviral

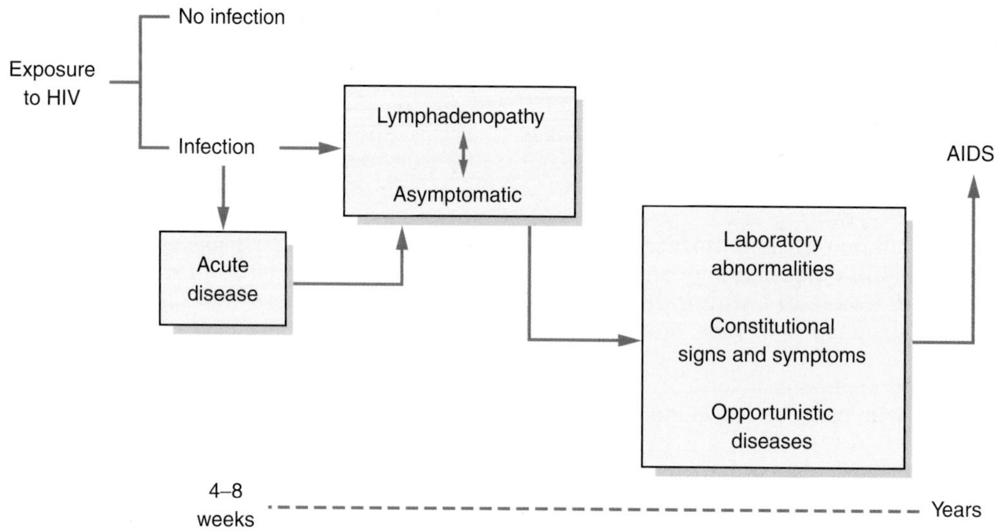

FIGURE 4-29 ■ Spectrum of human immunodeficiency virus disease.

Box 4-2

Oral Lesions Associated With Human Immunodeficiency Virus Infection

- Candidiasis
- Herpes simplex infection
- Herpes zoster
- Hairy leukoplakia
- Human papilloma virus lesions
- Atypical gingivitis and periodontitis
- Other opportunistic infections reported
    - *Mycobacterium avium, M. intracellulare*
    - Cytomegalovirus
    - *Cryptococcus neoformans*
    - *Klebsiella pneumoniae*
    - *Enterobacter cloacae*
    - *Histoplasma capsulatum*
- Kaposi sarcoma
- Non-Hodgkin lymphoma
- Aphthous ulcers
- Mucosal pigmentation
- Bacterial salivary gland enlargement and xerostomia
- Spontaneous gingival bleeding resulting from thrombocytopenia

therapy, oral manifestations of HIV are much less common than earlier in the history of this disease.

Oral Candidiasis

This oral lesion occurs frequently in individuals with cell-mediated immunodeficiency and is one of the most common oral lesions seen in persons with HIV infection (Figure 4-30). It is also called thrush. All of the different types of oral candidiasis described earlier in this chapter, including mucocutaneous candidiasis, can occur. It is important to remember that candidiasis can be associated with a variety of conditions other than HIV infection, such as uncontrolled diabetes, other immunodeficiency diseases, antibiotic treatment, and xerostomia. Both topical and systemic antifungal treatment can be used to control oral candidiasis in the patient with immunodeficiency caused by HIV infection. Recurrence is common.

In persons who are known to be infected with HIV, the development of oral candidiasis is worrisome because it generally signals the beginning of a progressively severe immunodeficiency. Persons with unexplained oral candidiasis should be referred to a physician for evaluation if the cause of the candidiasis cannot be determined. Studies have shown oral candidiasis to be a very early sign of developing immunodeficiency and predictive of the development of AIDS in a person who is infected with HIV. Oral lesions caused by other fungal infections such as histoplasmosis and coccidioidomycosis have also been reported in persons with HIV infection, but they are rare.

Herpes Simplex Infection

Ulcers caused by the herpes simplex virus occur in persons with HIV infection (Figure 4-31). Herpes labialis and lesions consistent with intraoral recurrent herpes simplex infection can also develop in persons with HIV infection. The clinical characteristics of these lesions are the same as those occurring in immunocompetent individuals. However, when the immune system, particularly cell mediated immunity, becomes deficient, HIV-infected individuals are at risk for the development of ulcers caused by the herpes simplex virus that do not have the same clinical characteristics as those seen in immunocompetent persons. These appear as persistent, superficial, painful ulcers that can be located anywhere in the oral cavity. Small, characteristic herpes simplex–like ulcers can be seen surrounding larger ulcers, but their presence cannot be depended on for

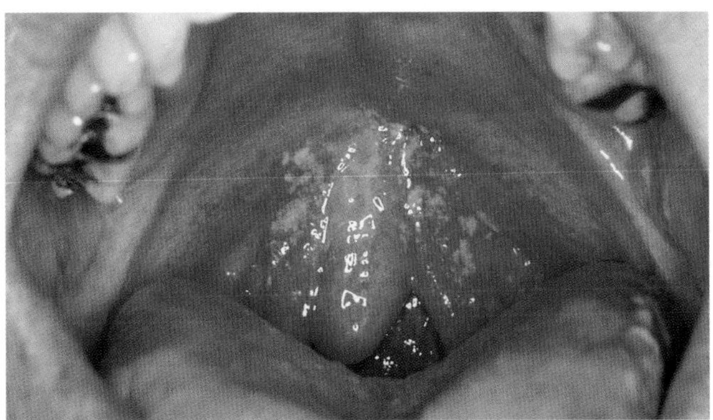

FIGURE 4-30 ■ Candidiasis in a patient with human immunodeficiency virus infection. Removable white plaques are present on the mucosa of the soft palate.

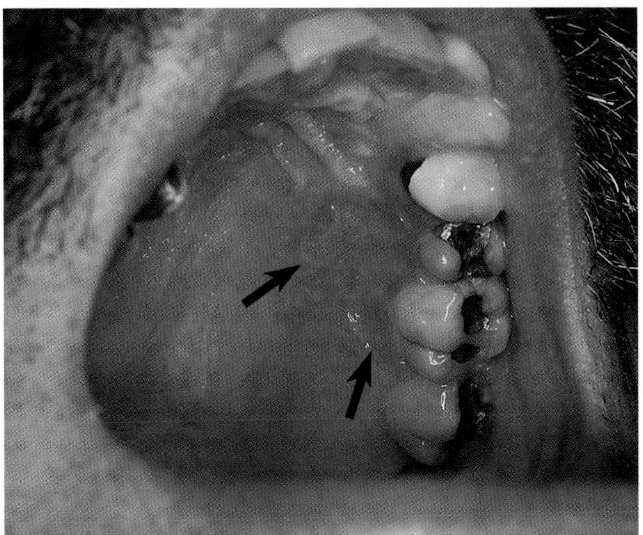

FIGURE 4-31 ■ Herpes simplex ulceration of the hard palate in a patient with human immunodeficiency virus infection. *Arrows* point to the periphery of the ulcer.

diagnosis. The diagnosis of these ulcers is made by several methods, including viral culture, cytologic smear, biopsy, and response to the antiviral medication acyclovir.

Ulceration of the oral mucosa from herpes simplex infection that has been present for more than 1 month is an oral lesion that meets the criteria for the diagnosis of AIDS. This can occur only when a person has profound immunodeficiency. Oral ulcers caused by cytomegalovirus may also occur in HIV-infected individuals who are severely immunodeficient. These ulcers are much rarer than those caused by herpes simplex virus.

Herpes Zoster

Herpes zoster is caused by the varicella-zoster virus and is described earlier in this chapter. When herpes zoster occurs in a person with HIV infection, it generally follows the usual pattern (see Figures 4-24 to 4-26). Although the infection can disseminate, most cases are self-limited. In the facial and oral area the lesions appear as distinctly unilateral ones following the distribution of one or more branches of the trigeminal nerve. The development of herpes zoster in a person infected with HIV is a sign of developing immunodeficiency.

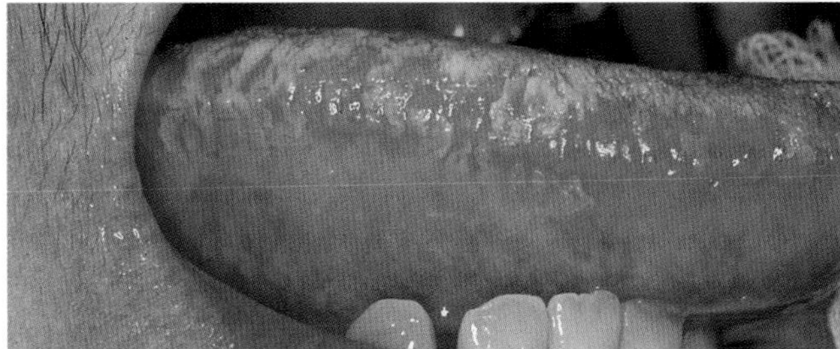

FIGURE 4-32 ■ Hairy leukoplakia.

Hairy Leukoplakia

Hairy leukoplakia is caused by Epstein-Barr virus and was discussed earlier in this chapter. It was first described in individuals with HIV infection; although it has been reported in HIV-negative individuals, most cases are an oral manifestation of HIV infection. It almost always occurs on the lateral borders of the tongue and may extend onto the dorsal and ventral tongue (see Figure 4-27; Figure 4-32). On the lateral tongue it appears as an irregular white lesion that has a corrugated surface. The corrugations may not be present when the lesions extend onto the dorsal or ventral tongue. Histologically this lesion shows hyperkeratosis (often with hairlike projections), epithelial hyperplasia, vacuolated epithelial cells, and little or no inflammatory infiltrate in the underlying connective tissue.

Other white lesions such as those resulting from chronic tongue chewing and hyperplastic candidiasis can resemble hairy leukoplakia clinically. Biopsy of the lesions can reveal a histologic appearance that is consistent with hairy leukoplakia. However, the most reliable method of diagnosis is identification of the Epstein-Barr virus in the lesion.

Generally hairy leukoplakia is not treated. Lesions may respond to antiviral medication such as acyclovir or zidovudine but recur when treatment is discontinued. Studies have shown hairy leukoplakia to be predictive of the development of AIDS in HIV-infected persons.

Papilloma Virus Infections

Lesions caused by papilloma viruses are described earlier in this chapter. Papillary oral lesions resulting from several different papilloma viruses have been described in persons with HIV infection. They have either normal color or slightly erythematous mucosa (Figure 4-33). These lesions may be persistent and may occur in multiple oral mucosal locations.

Results of studies have suggested that the prevalence of these human papilloma virus lesions has not decreased with antiretroviral therapy as has the prevalence of most other HIV-associated oral lesions. Diagnosis of these lesions is made by biopsy and histologic examination, with special tests to identify papillomavirus.

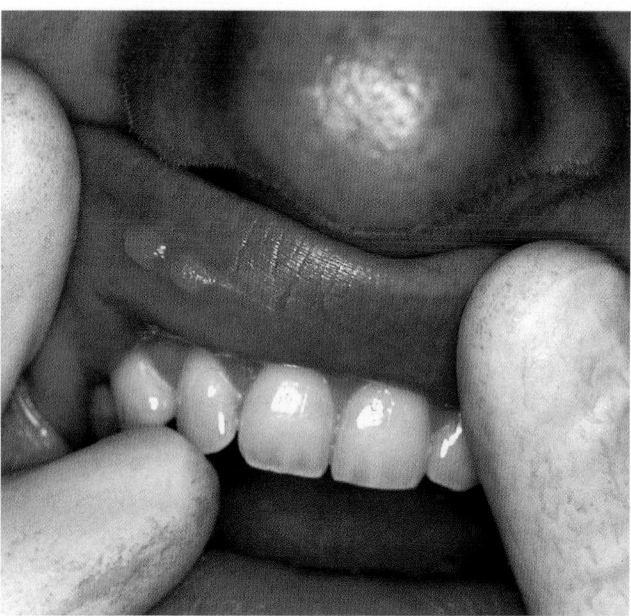

FIGURE 4-33 ■ Papillary lesion of the upper lip caused by human papilloma virus in a patient with human immunodeficiency virus infection.

Kaposi Sarcoma

Kaposi sarcoma is one of the opportunistic neoplasms that occur in patients with HIV infection. A herpes virus called human herpes virus (HHV-8) or kaposi sarcoma-associated herpes virus (KSHV) has been associated with this neoplasm. Oral lesions appear as reddish-purple, flat or raised lesions and are seen anywhere in the oral cavity. The most common locations are the palate and gingiva (Figure 4-34).

The diagnosis is made by biopsy. However, the clinical appearance of the lesion can be used when it is characteristic and the diagnosis of Kaposi sarcoma has been made at another site. At present no effective treatment for Kaposi sarcoma exists. Surgical excision to decrease the size of the lesion is sometimes attempted, as are radiation treatment and chemotherapy. Kaposi sarcoma is one of the intraoral lesions that may fulfill the criteria for the diagnosis of AIDS.

Lymphoma

Non-Hodgkin lymphoma is another of the malignant tumors that occur in association with HIV infection. It occasionally occurs in the oral cavity. Epstein-Barr virus has been associated with this neoplasm. These tumors have appeared as nonulcerated, necrotic, or ulcerated masses and have been surfaced by either ulcerated or normal-colored erythematous mucosa (Figure 4-35).

The diagnosis is made by biopsy and histologic examination. Treatment involves several different chemotherapeutic drugs. Oral lymphoma is another oral lesion that may meet the criteria for the diagnosis of AIDS.

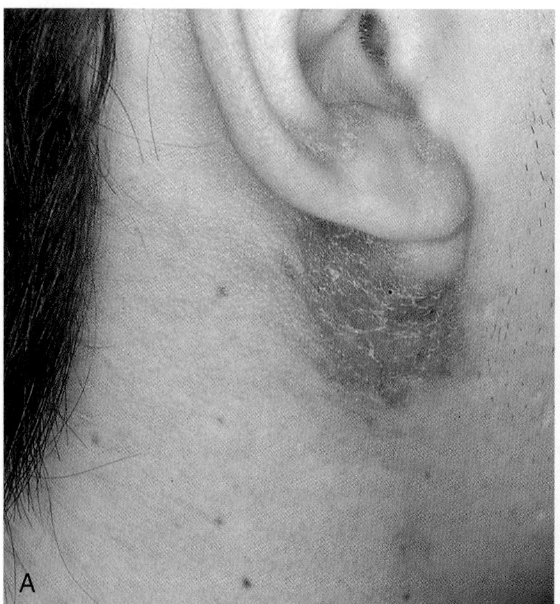

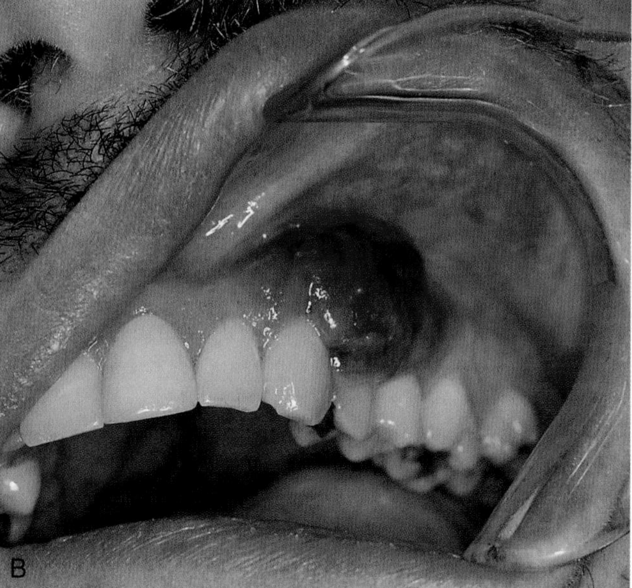

FIGURE 4-34 ■ Kaposi sarcoma in a patient with acquired immunodeficiency syndrome. **A,** Skin. **B,** Gingiva. (Courtesy Dr. Fariba Younai.)

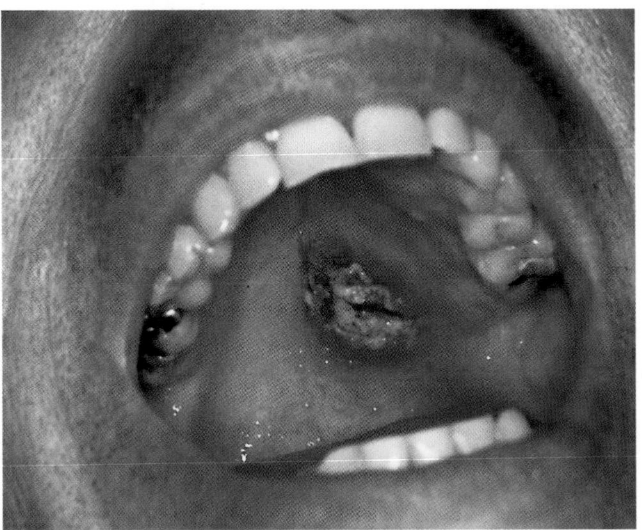

FIGURE 4-35 ■ Intraoral lymphoma in a patient with acquired immunodeficiency syndrome.

Gingival and Periodontal Disease

In patients with HIV infection unusual forms of gingival and periodontal disease can develop. These occur in HIV-infected individuals whose immune system has become deficient. These have been called **linear gingival erythema (LGE)** and **necrotizing ulcerative periodontitis (NUP).** A condition resembling necrotizing ulcerative gingivitis (NUG) also occurs in individuals with HIV infection.

Linear gingival erythema has three characteristic features: (1) spontaneous bleeding, (2) punctate or petechiae-like lesions on the attached gingiva and alveolar mucosa, and (3) a bandlike erythema of the gingiva that does not respond to therapy. Linear gingival erythema is different from typical gingivitis in that gingivitis is generally not characterized by spontaneous bleeding and the erythema of typical gingivitis responds within a few days to 1 week to scaling, root planing, and improvement of oral hygiene. Linear gingival erythema occurs independently of oral hygiene status.

Some patients experience gingivitis that resembles necrotizing ulcerative gingivitis, and it can be either generalized or localized to specific areas. Necrotizing ulcerative periodontitis resembles necrotizing ulcerative gingivitis in that patients experience pain, spontaneous gingival bleeding, interproximal necrosis, and interproximal cratering (Figure 4-36). Patients also experience intense erythema and, most characteristically, extremely rapid bone loss. **Necrotizing stomatitis** is characterized by extensive focal areas of bone loss along with the features of necrotizing ulcerative periodontitis.

The specific causes of these atypical gingival and periodontal diseases remain unclear. The microbiota associated with these diseases is being studied and have not been found to be distinctly different from those of inflammatory periodontal disease. These atypical gingival and periodontal conditions are not common in HIV-infected individuals and appear to occur in patients whose immune systems have become severely compromised.

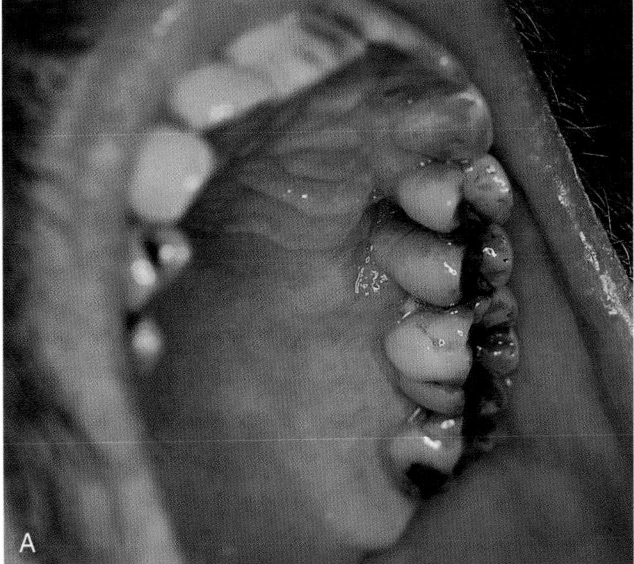

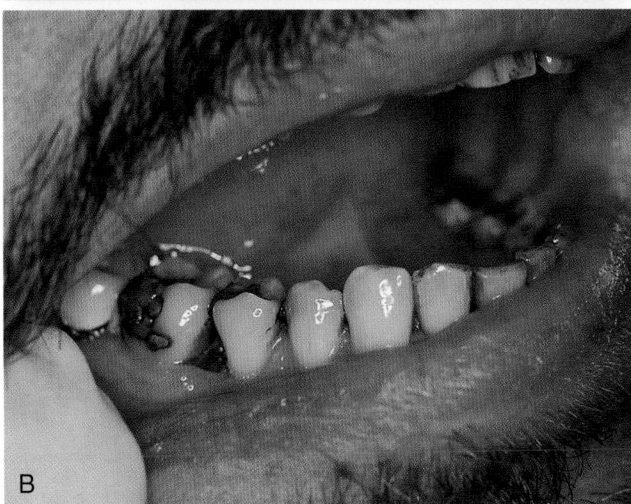

FIGURE 4-36 ■ **A** and **B,** Atypical periodontal disease in a patient with human immunodeficiency virus infection.

Treatment of HIV gingivitis and periodontitis involves scaling, root planing, and soft tissue curettage. In addition, intrasulcular lavage with povidone-iodine, use of chlorhexidine mouth rinse, and short-term systemic metronidazole administration have been helpful in the treatment of these conditions. Good oral hygiene, including the use of smaller toothbrushes and interproximal cleaning devices, has been a component of management.

Most HIV-infected patients do not have HIV-associated gingival and periodontal problems. However, recognition of early lesions is essential to prevent extensive bone loss, and frequent recall is helpful in early identification of gingival and periodontal disease. Lack of response to periodontal treatment is a clue to the recognition of HIV-associated gingivitis and periodontitis.

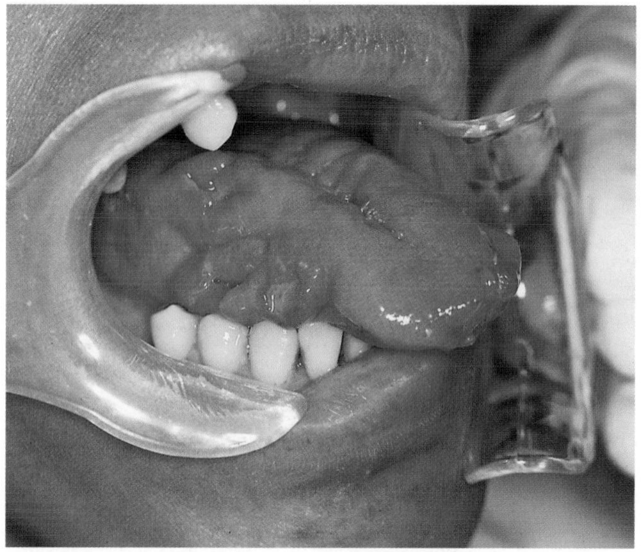

FIGURE 4-37 ■ Persistent, nonspecific (major aphthouslike) ulcers in a patient with human immunodeficiency virus infection. (Courtesy Dr. Sidney Eisig.)

Spontaneous Gingival Bleeding

A decrease in the number of platelets resulting from an autoimmune type of thrombocytopenic purpura is occasionally seen in patients with HIV infection. These patients can have bleeding gums or mucosal petechiae. Gingival bleeding not related to thrombocytopenia has also been described in linear gingival erythema and necrotizing ulcerative periodontitis. A platelet count and bleeding time should be considered before deep scaling procedures are performed.

Aphthous Ulcers

Characteristic minor aphthous ulcers occur in patients with HIV infection and AIDS. Studies have suggested that an increase in the incidence of these ulcers occurs in patients with HIV infection. The clinical appearance and behavior of minor aphthous ulcers in HIV-infected patients is the same as in other individuals (see Chapter 3). Minor aphthous ulcers are diagnosed on the basis of their clinical appearance.

Ulcers that resemble major aphthous ulcers also occur in patients with HIV infection (Figure 4-37). They appear as deep, persistent, painful ulcers and must be differentiated from infectious ulcers. Biopsy and histologic examination of these ulcers does not show any evidence of an infectious cause. These ulcers respond to topical and systemic corticosteroid therapy. Topical application of tetracycline and thalidomide has also been used in the management of these ulcers. Similar ulcers have been reported in the esophagus of patients with HIV infection.

Salivary Gland Disease

Bilateral parotid gland enlargement has been reported to occur in patients who are HIV positive (Figure 4-38). The histologic appearance is reported to be that of a benign lymphoepithelial lesion, often with a prominent cystic component. Xerostomia has been reported to be associated with HIV infection. The cause is not clear. It may be related to medication administration or salivary gland disease.

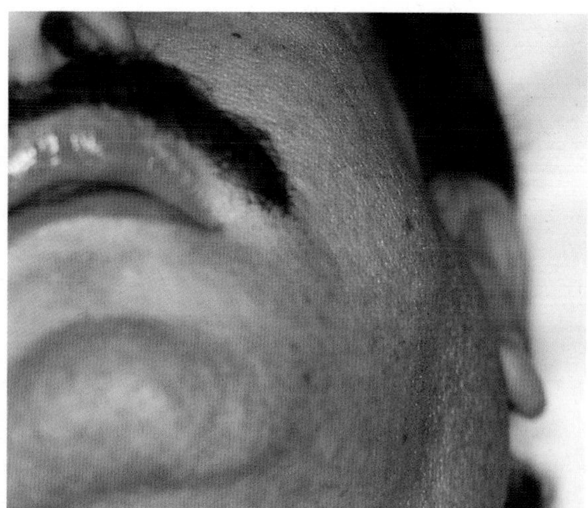

FIGURE 4-38 ■ Salivary gland enlargement was bilateral in this patient with human immunodeficiency virus infection.

Mucosal Melanin Pigmentation

Macular areas of melanin pigmentation of unknown cause also occur in patients with HIV infection. These do not require treatment, and the significance of these lesions is not known.

Selected References

Books

Kumar V et al: *Robbins basic pathology*, ed 8, Philadelphia, 2007, Saunders.

Neville BW et al: *Oral and maxillofacial pathology*, ed 3, St. Louis, 2009, Saunders.

New York State Department of Health AIDS Institute: http://www.hivguidelines.org (clinical guidelines).

Regezi JA, Sciubba JJ, Jordan RCK: *Oral pathology: clinical-pathologic correlations*, ed 5, Philadelphia, 2008, Saunders.

Journal Articles

Alves M. et al: Longitudinal evaluation of loss of attachment in HIV-infected women compared to HIV-uninfected women. *J. Periodont.* 77:773, 2006.

Baccaglini L et al: Management of oral lesions in HIV-positive patients, *Oral Surg Oral Med Oral Pathol Oral Radiol Endod* 103 Suppl:S50, 2000.

Depaola LG: Human immunodeficiency virus disease: natural history and management, *Oral Surg Oral Med Oral Pathol Oral Radiol Endod* 90:266, 2000.

Centers for Disease Control and Prevention: 1993 revised classification system for HIV infection and expanded surveillance case definition for AIDS among adolescents and adults, *MMWR Recomm Rep* 41(RR-17):1, 1992.

Challacombe SJ: Immunologic aspects of oral candidiasis, *Oral Surg Oral Med Oral Pathol* 78:202, 1994.

Eisen D: The clinical characteristics of intraoral herpes simplex virus infection in 52 immunocompetent patients, *Oral Surg Oral Med Oral Pathol Oral Radiol Endod* 86:432, 1998.

Eisenberg E, Krutchkoff D, Yamase H: Incidental oral hairy leukoplakia in immunocompetent persons, *Oral Surg Oral Med Oral Pathol* 74:332, 1992.

Eng H-L et al: Oral tuberculosis, *Oral Surg Oral Med Oral Pathol Oral Radiol Endod* 81:415, 1996.

Fotos PG, Vincent SD, Hellstein JW: Oral candidiasis: clinical, historical, and therapeutic features of 100 cases, *Oral Surg Oral Med Oral Pathol* 74:41, 1992.

Glick M, Muzyka BC: Alternative therapies for major aphthous ulcers in AIDS patients, *J Am Dent Assoc* 123:61, 1992.

Green TL et al: Oral lesions mimicking hairy leukoplakia: a diagnostic dilemma, *Oral Surg Oral Med Oral Pathol* 67:422, 1989.

Greenspan D et al: Incidence of oral lesions in HIV-1-infected women: reduction with HAART. *J Dent Res* 83:145, 2004.

Hodgson TA, Greenspan D, Greenspan JS: Oral lesions of HIV disease and HAART in industrialized countries, *Adv Dent Res* 19:57, 2006.

Harris AM, Van Wyk CW: Heck's disease (focal epithelial hyperplasia): a longitudinal study, *Community Dent Oral Epidemiol* 21:82, 1993.

Hernandez YL, Daniels TE: Oral candidiasis in Sjögren's syndrome: prevalence, clinical correlations, and treatment, *Oral Surg Oral Med Oral Pathol* 68:324, 1989.

Holbrook WP, Gunnlaugur TG, Ragnarsson KT: Herpetic gingivostomatitis in otherwise healthy adolescents and young adults, *Acta Odontol Scand* 59:113, 2001.

Holmstrup P, Westergaard J: Periodontal diseases in HIV-infected patients, *J Clin Periodontol* 21:270, 1994.

Iacopino AM, Wathen WF: Oral candidal infection and denture stomatitis: a comprehensive review, *J Am Dent Assoc* 123:46, 1992.

Jones AC, Gulley ML, Freedman PD: Necrotizing ulcerative stomatitis in human immunodeficiency virus–seropositive individuals: a review of the histopathologic, immunohistochemical, and virologic characteristics of 18 cases, *Oral Surg Oral Med Oral Pathol Oral Radiol Endod* 89:323, 2000.

Koorbusch GF, Fotos P, Terhark K: Retrospective assessment of osteomyelitis, *Oral Surg Oral Med Oral Pathol* 74:149, 1992.

Kulak-Ozkan Y, Kazazoglu E, Arikan A: Oral hygiene habits, denture cleanliness, presence of yeasts and stomatitis in elderly people, *J Oral Rehabil* 29:300, 2002.

Leigh JE, Kishore S, Fidel PL Jr: Oral opportunistic infections in HIV-positive individuals: review and role of mucosal immunity, *AIDS Patient Care* 18:443, 2004.

Leggott PJ: Oral manifestations of HIV infection in children, *Oral Surg Oral Med Oral Pathol* 73:187, 1992.

Lynch DP: Oral candidiasis: history, classification and clinical presentation, *Oral Surg Oral Med Oral Pathol* 78:189, 1994.

MacPhail LA et al: Recurrent aphthous ulcers in association with HIV infection: description of ulcer types and analysis of T-lymphocyte subsets, *Oral Surg Oral Med Oral Pathol* 71:678, 1991.

MacPhail LA et al: Differences in risk factors among clinical types of oral candidiasis in the Women's Interagency HIV Study, *Oral Surg Oral Med Oral Pathol Oral Radiol Endod* 93:45, 2002.

McKenzie CD, Gobetti JP: Diagnosis and treatment of orofacial herpes zoster: report of cases, *J Am Dent Assoc* 120:679, 1990.

Miller RL: The differential diagnosis of white lesions resembling oral hairy leukoplakia, *J Tenn Dent Assoc* 73:20, 1993.

Morrow DJ, Sandhu HS, Daley TD: Focal epithelial hyperplasia (Heck's disease) with generalized lesions of the gingiva: a case report, *J Periodontol* 64:63, 1993.

Narana N, Epstein JB: Classifications of oral lesions in HIV infection, *J Clin Periodontol* 28:137, 2001.

Pankhurst CL: Candidiasis (oropharyngeal), *Clin Evid* 15:1849, 2006.

Peterman TA et al: The changing epidemiology of syphilis, *Sex Transm Dis* 32: Supp S4, 2005.

Praetorius F: HPV-associated diseases of the oral mucosa, *Clin Dermatol* 15:399, 1997.

Rams TE et al: Microbiological study of HIV-related periodontitis, *J Periodontol* 62:74, 1991.

Redding SW, Luce EB, Boren MW: Oral herpes simplex virus infection in patients receiving head and neck radiation, *Oral Surg Oral Med Oral Pathol* 69:578, 1990.

Robinson JL, Vaudry WL, Dobrovolsky W: Actinomycosis presenting as osteomyelitis in the pediatric population, *Pediatr Infect Dis J* 24:365, 2005.

Ryder MI: An update on HIV and periodontal disease, *J Periodontol* 73:1071, 2002.

Samaranayake LP: Oral mycoses in HIV infection, *Oral Surg Oral Med Oral Pathol* 73:171, 1992.

Schiodt M: HIV-associated salivary gland disease, *Oral Surg Oral Med Oral Pathol* 37:164, 1992.

Shirlaw PJ et al: Oral and dental care and treatment protocols for the management of HIV-infected patients, *Oral Dis* 8(Suppl 2):136, 2002.

Siegel MA: Diagnosis and management of recurrent herpes simplex infections, *J Am Dent Assoc* 133:1245, 2002.

Soysa NS, Samaranayake LP, Ellepola AN: Diabetes mellitus as a contributory factor in oral candidosis, *Diabet Med* 23:455, 2006.

Swango PA, Kleinman D, Konzelman JL: HIV and periodontal health, *J Am Dent Assoc* 122:49, 1991.

Watkins P: Impetigo: aetiology, complications and treatment options, *Diabet Med* 19:51, 2005.

Williams CA et al: HIV-associated periodontitis complicated by necrotizing stomatitis, *Oral Surg Oral Med Oral Pathol* 69:351, 1990.

Zhu WY et al: Human papillomavirus DNA in the dermis of condyloma acuminatum, *J Cutan Pathol* 20:447, 1993.

REVIEW QUESTIONS

1. The most specific of the body's defense mechanisms against infection is:
   A. Intact skin.
   B. The immune response.
   C. Skin secretions.
   D. The inflammatory response.

2. Which statement is *false*?
   A. The primary lesion of syphilis is called a *chancre*.
   B. The secondary lesion of syphilis occurs at the site of inoculation with the organism.
   C. The tertiary lesion of syphilis is called a gumma.
   D. Syphilis is caused by the spirochete *Treponema pallidum*.

3. Perioral lesions of impetigo may resemble:
   A. Syphilis.
   B. Recurrent herpes simplex infection.
   C. Herpes zoster.
   D. Actinomycosis.

4. Which of the following is not associated with group A, β-hemolytic streptococcal infection?
   A. Tonsillitis
   B. Syphilis
   C. Scarlet fever
   D. Rheumatic fever

5. Oral candidiasis is caused by a:
   A. Bacterium.
   B. Yeastlike fungus.
   C. Spirochete.
   D. Protozoan.

6. Which statement is *false*?
   A. Angular cheilitis may be caused by *Candida albicans*.
   B. White lesions resulting from candidiasis may not rub off the mucosal surface.
   C. Erythematous candidiasis is usually completely asymptomatic.
   D. Denture stomatitis may be a form of oral candidiasis.

7. Which type of infection is involved when normal components of the oral microflora can cause disease?
   A. Chronic inflammatory
   B. Opportunistic
   C. Hyperplastic
   D. Granulomatous

8. The most characteristic clinical feature of herpes zoster is:
   A. Ulcer formation.
   B. Pain.
   C. Unilateral distribution of lesions.
   D. Abscesses that drain through fistulas.

9. A cytologic smear may be helpful in the diagnosis of:
   A. Coxsackievirus infection.
   B. Human papilloma virus infection.
   C. Tuberculosis.
   D. Candidiasis.

10. Which condition is *not* associated with the Epstein-Barr virus?
    A. Hairy leukoplakia
    B. Herpangina
    C. Nasopharyngeal carcinoma
    D. Infectious mononucleosis

11. Which of the following stages of syphilis is not infectious?
    A. Primary
    B. Secondary
    C. Tertiary
    D. All stages are equally infectious

12. Which of the following is not associated with syphilis?
    A. Mucous patch
    B. Venereal Disease Research Laboratories and fluorescent treponemal antibody
    C. Dark-field microscopy
    D. Hypodontia

13. Which of the following microorganisms causes tuberculosis?
    A. *Mycobacterium israelii*
    B. *Actinomycosis tuberculum*
    C. *Mycobacterium tuberculosis*
    D. *Treponema pallidum*

14. A positive skin reaction to PPD indicates:
    A. Active tuberculosis.
    B. Contagious tuberculosis.
    C. Infection with the tuberculosis bacteria.
    D. Need for antibiotic therapy.

15. A specific *clinical* characteristic found in actinomycosis is:
    A. Periapical radiolucency.
    B. Filamentous bacteria.
    C. Fungal infection.
    D. Sulfur granules present in exudates.

16. Which of the following is *not* a clinical characteristic of necrotizing ulcerative gingivitis?
    A. Painful gingiva
    B. Xerostomia
    C. Foul odor
    D. Metallic taste

17. Which of the following is associated with chronic osteomyelitis?
    A. Sickle cell anemia
    B. Paget disease
    C. Radiation treatment involving bone
    D. All of the above

18. Which of the following is *not* associated with the development of oral candidiasis?
    A. Antibiotic therapy
    B. HIV infection
    C. Xerostomia
    D. Herpangina

19. Verruca vulgaris:
    A. Clinically resembles an irritative fibroma.
    B. Is caused by a human papilloma virus.
    C. Is most commonly seen on the buccal mucosa.
    D. Clinically resembles a pyogenic granuloma.

20. Another name for a common wart is:
    A. Papilloma.
    B. Verruca vulgaris.
    C. Condyloma acumenatum.
    D. Fibroma.

21. Which of the following is caused by a papilloma virus and is considered a sexually transmitted disease?
    A. Actinomycosis
    B. Syphilis
    C. Condyloma acuminatum
    D. Infectious mononucleosis

22. Painful oral ulcers, gingivitis, fever, malaise, and cervical lymphadenopathy in a child younger than 6 years old would cause the hygienist to suspect which of the following diseases?
    A. Herpangina
    B. Heck disease
    C. Primary herpes simplex infection
    D. Herpetic whitlow

23. The most common form of recurrent herpes simplex infection is:
    A. Herpes zoster.
    B. Herpetic whitlow.
    C. Herpangina.
    D. Herpes labialis.

24. The primary infection with the varicella-zoster virus is called:
    A. Primary herpetic gingivostomatitis.
    B. Chickenpox.
    C. Shingles.
    D. Measles.

25. Herpangina is caused by:
    A. Coxsackievirus.
    B. Herpes simplex virus.
    C. Varicella zoster virus.
    D. Epstein-Barr virus.

26. Antibody testing to determine if a person has been infected with HIV includes which of the following tests?
    A. Schilling
    B. Complete blood count
    C. Prothrombin time and partial thromboplastin time
    D. Enzyme-linked immunosorbent assay and Western blot

27. Which one of the following oral conditions is an early sign of a deficiency in the immune system and is commonly found in patients with HIV infection?
    A. Geographic tongue
    B. Advanced periodontitis
    C. Candidiasis
    D. Histoplasmosis

28. Hairy leukoplakia most commonly occurs on the:
    A. Buccal mucosa.
    B. Dorsal tongue.
    C. Lateral tongue.
    D. Soft palate.

29. Which one of the following oral conditions is *not* a lesion associated with HIV or AIDS?
    A. Candidiasis
    B. Hairy leukoplakia
    C. Kaposi sarcoma
    D. Leukoedema

30. LGE has specific characteristics that include spontaneous bleeding, petechiae on the attached gingiva and alveolar mucosa, and a band of erythema at the gingival margin. Which one of the following statements is *true*?
    A. These tissues respond well to scaling and root planing.
    B. Excellent oral hygiene and home care techniques will eliminate these gingival conditions.
    C. This condition will automatically develop into advanced periodontal disease in all HIV patients.
    D. Linear gingival erythema patients do not respond to scaling or oral hygiene techniques; the gingival condition exists independently of the patient's oral hygiene status.

CHAPTER 4 Synopsis

Condition/Disease	Cause	Age/Race/Sex	Location
Infectious Disease			
Bacterial infections	*Staphylococcus aureus* or occasionally *Streptococcus pyogenes*	Most commonly seen in children	Skin
Impetigo			
Tonsillitis and Pharyngitis			
Tuberculosis	Infectious disease *Mycobacterium tuberculosis*	*	Primary infection of lung Bacteria can spread to other areas of the body
Actinomycosis	Infectious disease *Actinomyces israelii*	*	Skin/oral mucosa
Syphilis	Infectious disease *Treponema pallidum*	Usually seen in sexually active adults Congenital: infected mother to fetus (Chapter 5)	Primary: site of inoculation Secondary: diffuse lesions of skin and mucous membranes Tertiary: cardiovascular system Central nervous system: oral lesions may occur
Necrotizing Ulcerative Gingivitis (NUG)	Infectious disease *Borrelia vincentii* + fusiform bacillus	†	Gingiva
Pericoronitis	Inflammatory process, usually infection	More common in adolescents and young adults at the of eruption of third molars	Tissue around the crown of a partially erupted impacted tooth
Acute Osteomyelitis	Inflammation/Infection	*	Bone
Chronic Osteomyelitis	Infammation/infection	*	Bone

N/A, Not applicable.
*No significant information.
†Not covered in this text.

Clinical Features	Radiographic Features	Microscopic Features	Treatment	Diagnostic Process
Vesicles or crusted lesions	N/A	N/A	Topical or systemic antibiotics	Clinical Laboratory
Oral lesions: rare Painful, nonhealing, slowly enlarging, deep or superficial ulcer Most common locations are tongue and palate	N/A	Granulomas containing the causative organism	Combination antituberculosis agents	Laboratory Microscopic
Draining abscesses "Sulfur granules" in pus draining from abscess	N/A	Bacterial colonies in tissue from the lesion	Long-term, high dose of antibiotic therapy	Clinical Microscopic
Oral lesions Primary: chancre Secondary: mucous patches Tertiary: gumma	N/A	Skin: dark-field identification of spirochetes	Antibiotic agents (usually penicillin)	Clinical Laboratory
Painful, erythematous gingivitis with necrosis and cratering of the interdental papillae, foul odor, metallic Fever, cervical lymphadenopathy	N/A	N/A	Antibiotic agents Débridement of necrotic tissue Oral hygiene care	Clinical
Erythematous, painful swollen tissue around the crown of the partially erupted tooth	Impacted tooth can be seen on radiograph	N/A	Débridement and irrigation Antibiotic therapy Extraction of impacted tooth	Clinical
	No radiographic change unless present for more than 1 week	Nonviable bone Necrotic debris Acute inflammation Bacterial colonies	Antibiotic therapy Drainage of area	Clinical Laboratory
Involved bone is painful with swelling	Irregular radiolucency	Chronic inflammation of bone and bone marrow	Débridement Antibiotic therapy Hyperbaric oxygen	Clinical Radiographic Laboratory

Continued

CHAPTER 4 Synopsis (continued)

Condition/Disease	Cause	Age/Race/Sex	Location
Fungal Infections			
Oral Candidiasis	Opportunistic infectious disease *Candida albicans*	*	Oral mucosa
Deep Fungal Infections			
Histoplasmosis **Coccidioidomycosis** **Blastomycosis** **Cryptococcosis**	*Histoplasma capsulation* *Coccidioides immitis* *Blastomyces dermatitidis* *Cryptococcus neoformans*	*	Primary lung infection Secondary oral mucosal involvement
Mucormycosis	†	*	Nasal cavity Maxillary sinus Hard palate
Viral Infections			
Verruca Vulgaris	A human papilloma virus	†	Skin Lips: most common oral location
Condyloma Acuminatum	A human papilloma virus	†	Oral mucosa: any location
Focal Epithelial Hyperplasia	A human papilloma virus	Occurs in children	Oral mucosa

N/A, Not applicable.
*No significant information.
†Not covered in this text.

Clinical Features	Radiographic Features	Microscopic Features	Treatment	Diagnostic Process
Appearance depends on type Pseudomembranous Erythematous Chronic atrophic (denture stomatitis) Chronic hyperplastic Angular cheilitis Chronic mucocutaneous	N/A	*Candida* hyphae present on mucosal smear *Candida* hyphae in biopsy tissue	Antifungal therapy	Clinical Microscopic Therapeutic
Chronic nonhealing ulcers	Irregular radiolucency if bone involvement	Identification of causative organism	Appropriate antifungal agents	Microscopic Laboratory
Proliferating mass with destruction of bone	Irregular radiolucency if bone involvement	Identification of causative organism	Appropriate antifungal agent Management of underlying disease	Microscopic
White, papillary exophytic lesion resembling a papilloma	N/A	Fingerlike projection of keratotic squamous epithelium with central cores of well-vascularized fibrous connective tissue Cells with clear cytoplasm in the upper spinous layer	Surgical excision Immunologic staining to identify presence of papilloma virus May recur	Microscopic
Pink, papillary lesion usually more diffuse than papilloma or verruca vulgaris May be multiple lesions	N/A	Thickened epithelium with fingerlike projections covering cores of connective tissue Cells with clear cytoplasm seen throughout the epithelium	Surgical excision Recurrence is common	Microscopic
Multiple whitish-to-pale pink nodules distributed throughout the oral mucosa	N/A	Thickened epithelium with broad, connected rete bridges Cells with clear cytoplasm seen in the epithelium	Self-limited disease	Clinical Microscopic

Continued

CHAPTER 4 Synopsis (continued)

Condition/Disease	Cause	Age/Race/Sex	Location
Herpes Simplex Infection	Herpes simplex virus Most oral infections are type 1, some type 2		
Primary Herpetic Gingivostomatitis	Herpes simplex virus	Generally in children Less common in adolescents and adults	Lips, gingival, oral mucosa
Recurrent Herpes Simplex Infection	Herpes simplex virus	Usually seen in adolescents and adults	Herpes labialis: vermillion of lips Recurrent intraoral form: keratinized mucosa (hard palate gingiva)
Varicella-Zoster Virus Infection			
Chickenpox	Varicella-zoster virus	Usually seen in children Less common in adolescents and adults	Skin Mucous membranes
Herpes Zoster	Varicella-zoster virus	Occurs in adults	Skin Mucous membranes
Infectious Mononucleosis	Epstein-Barr virus	Usually occurs in adolescents and young adults	Systemic disease
Herpangina	A coxsackievirus	Usually young children and adults	Soft palate
Hand-Foot-Mouth-Disease	A coxsackievirus	Affects children under 5 years old	Oral mucosa Skin: feet, hands, fingers
Acute Lymphonodular Pharyngitis			
Measles	A paramyxovirus	Most commonly occurs in children	Primarily skin Oral mucosa: early lesions
Mumps	A paramyxovirus	Most commonly occurs in children	Salivary glands

N/A, Not applicable.
*No significant information.
†Not covered in this text.

Clinical Features	Radiographic Features	Microscopic Features	Treatment	Diagnostic Process
Multiple tiny vesicles that progress to form painful ulcers Painful, erythematous, swollen gingiva Fever, malaise, cervical lymphadenopathy	N/A	Virally altered epithelial cells in mucosal smear on biopsy tissue	Self-limited disease	Clinical Microscopic
Focal crops of tiny vesicles that coalesce to form a single ulcer Prodromal symptoms	N/A	Virally altered epithelial cells in mucosal smear or biopsy tissue	Self-limited disease	Clinical
Vesicular and pustular eruptions Oral lesions usually do not cause comfort	N/A	Virally altered epithelial cells in mucosal smear or biopsy tissue	Self-limited disease	Clinical
Unilateral distribution of painful vesicles: ulcers along a sensory nerve Prodromal symptoms	N/A	Virally altered epithelial cells in mucosal smear or biopsy tissue	Antiviral agents Corticosteroids	Clinical
Palatal petechiae Sore throat Fever Generalized lymphadenopathy Enlarged spleen Malaise Fatigue	N/A	Mononucleosis cells in blood	Usually self-limited disease	Laboratory
Fever Malaise Vesicles on the soft palate	N/A	N/A	Self-limited disease	Clinical
Dysphagia Oral lesions: vesicles anywhere in the mouth	N/A	N/A	Self-limited disease	Clinical
Oral mucosa: Koplik spots—erythematous macules with white necrotic centers	N/A	N/A	Self-limited disease	Clinical
Painful, usually bilateral enlargement of salivary glands	N/A	N/A	Self-limited disease	Clinical

Continued

CHAPTER 4 Synopsis (continued)

Condition/Disease	Cause	Age/Race/Sex	Location
HIV Infection/AIDS	Immune deficiency resulting from infection with the human immunodeficiency virus	Newborn infants to adults	Systemic disease

N/A, Not applicable.
*No significant information.
†Not covered in this text.

Clinical Features	Radiographic Features	Microscopic Features	Treatment	Diagnostic Process
Opportunistic diseases Oral manifestations include oral candidiasis, herpes simplex infection, herpes zoster, hairy leukoplakia, papillomavirus lesions, Kaposi sarcoma, lymphoma and atypical periodontal disease, major aphthouslike ulcers, salivary gland disease and xerostomia, and mucosal pigmentation Autoimmune type Thrombocytopenia may result in spontaneous gingival bleeding	Severe and rapid bone loss seen in atypical periodontal disease	Dependent on opportunistic disease	Combination antiretroviral agents Management of specific opportunistic disease	Laboratory Microscopic

chapter 5

Developmental Disorders

Olga A.C. Ibsen, Joen M. Iannucci

OBJECTIVES

After studying this chapter, the student will be able to:

1. Define each of the words in the vocabulary list for this chapter.
2. Define inherited disorders.
3. Recognize developmental disorders of the dentition.
4. Describe the embryonic development of the face, oral cavity, and teeth.
5. Define each of the developmental anomalies discussed in this chapter.
6. Identify (clinically, radiographically, or both) the developmental anomalies discussed in this chapter.
7. Distinguish between intraosseous cysts and extraosseous cysts.
8. Describe the differences between odontogenic and nonodontogenic cysts.
9. Name four odontogenic cysts that are intraosseous.
10. Name two odontogenic cysts that are extraosseous.
11. Name four nonodontogenic cysts that are intraosseous.
12. Name four nonodontogenic cysts that are found in the soft tissues of the head, neck, and oral region.
13. List and define three anomalies that affect the number of teeth.
14. List and define two anomalies that affect the size of teeth.
15. List and define five anomalies that affect the shape of teeth.
16. Define and identify each of the following anomalies affecting tooth eruption: impacted teeth, embedded teeth, and ankylosed teeth.
17. Identify the diagnostic process that contributes most significantly to the final diagnosis of each developmental anomaly discussed in this chapter.

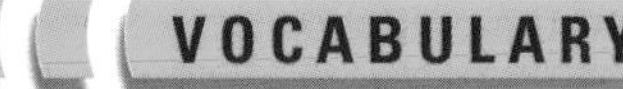

VOCABULARY

Ankyloglossia (ang″kĭ-lo-glos′e-ah) Extensive adhesion of the tongue to the floor of the mouth or the lingual aspect of the anterior portion of the mandible.

Ankylosed teeth (ang′kĭ-lōsd tēth) Teeth that are fused to the alveolar bone; a condition especially common with retained deciduous teeth.

Anodontia (an″o-don′she-ah) Congenital lack of teeth.

Anomaly (ah-nom′ah-le) Marked deviation from normal, especially as a result of congenital or hereditary defects.

Commissure (kom′ĭ-shūr) The site of union of corresponding parts (e.g., the corners of the lips) (labial commissure, commissural lip pits)

Concrescence (kon-kres′ens) In dentistry a condition in which two adjacent teeth become united by cementum.

Congenital (kon-jen′ĭ-tal) Present at and existing from the time of birth.

Cyst (sist) An abnormal sac or cavity lined by epithelium and enclosed in a connective tissue capsule.

Dens in dente (dens in den′te) "A tooth within a tooth"; a developmental anomaly that results when the enamel organ invaginates into the crown of a tooth before mineralization.

Dentinogenesis (den″tĭ-no-jen′ĕ-sis) The formation of dentin.

Differentiation (dif′er-en″she-a′shun) The distinguishing of one thing from another.

Dilaceration (di-las″er-a′shun) An abnormal bend or curve, as in the root of a tooth.

Fusion (fu′zhun) The union of two adjacent tooth germs.

Gemination (jem-ĭ-na′shun) "Twinning"; a single tooth germ attempts to divide, resulting in the incomplete formation of two teeth; the tooth usually has a single root and root canal.

Hypodontia (hi″po-don′she-ah) Partial anodontia; the lack of one or more teeth.

Impacted teeth (im-pakt′ed tĕth) Teeth that cannot erupt into the oral cavity because of a physical obstruction.

Macrodontia (mak″ro-don′she-ah) Abnormally large teeth.

Microdontia (mi″kro-don′she-ah) Abnormally small teeth.

Multilocular (mul-tĭ-lok′ū-ler) A radiographic appearance in which many circular radiolucencies exist; these can appear "soap bubble–like" or "honeycomb-like."

Nodule (nod′ūl) A small solid mass that can be detected through touch.

Predilection (prĕd-ĭ-lĕk′shun) A disposition in favor of something; preference.

Proliferation (pro-lif″ĕ-ra′shun) The multiplication of cells.

Stomodeum (sto″mo-de′um) The embryonic invagination that becomes the oral cavity.

Supernumerary (soo″per-nu′mer-ar″e) In excess of the normal or regular number, as in teeth.

The development of the human body is an extremely complex process that begins when an egg is fertilized by a sperm. It continues with a series of cell divisions, multiplications, and **differentiation** into various tissues and structures. A failure or disturbance that occurs during these processes may result in a lack, excess, or deformity of a body part. These disorders are called **developmental disorders,** or **developmental anomalies.**

Inherited disorders are different from developmental disorders in that they are caused by an abnormality in the genetic makeup (genes and chromosomes) of an individual and transmitted from parent to offspring through the egg or sperm (see Chapter 6).

A **congenital disorder** is one that is present at birth. It can be either inherited or developmental; however, the cause of most congenital abnormalities is unknown.

The complex process of **proliferation** and differentiation that takes place in the human body provides numerous possibilities for errors or defects in development. The head and neck region is a common location for such errors because of its intricate sequence and pattern of development. This chapter includes descriptions of developmental disorders of the face, oral cavity, and teeth with which the dental hygienist should be familiar.

Some of the developmental disturbances discussed in this chapter can be identified clinically, whereas others are identified by radiographic examination; still others require biopsy and histologic examinations. A thorough clinical examination, including examination of extraoral and intraoral structures, is an essential component. Dental radiographs are an important part of the examination. Any developmental anomalies observed either clinically or radiographically are documented in the patient's record even if no treatment is indicated. The patient is informed of all dental anomalies, their possible implications, and the treatment necessary, if any. In some instances referral to a specialist is indicated. To better understand these developmental disorders, a brief review of the embryonic development of the face, oral cavity, and teeth is included in this chapter.

EMBRYONIC DEVELOPMENT OF THE FACE, ORAL CAVITY, AND TEETH

FACE

Development of the face is a process of selective growth or proliferation and differentiation (Figures 5-1 and 5-2). During the third week of embryonic life, an invagination or infolding of the ectoderm forms the primitive oral cavity, which is called the **stomodeum.** Just above the stomodeum is a process called the **frontal process,** and just below it is a structure called the first **branchial arch.** Additional branchial arches form below the first branchial arch. All of the face and most of the structures of the oral cavity develop from either the frontal process or the first branchial arch. The first branchial arch divides into two **maxillary processes** and the **mandibular process.** The maxillary processes give rise to the upper part of the cheeks, the lateral portions of the upper lip, and part of the palate. The mandibular arch forms the lower part of the cheeks, the mandible, and part of the tongue.

As development continues, two pits (called **olfactory pits**) mark the future openings of the nose that develop on the surface of the frontal process. They divide the frontal process into three parts: (1) the **median nasal process,** (2) the **right lateral nasal process,** and (3) the **left lateral nasal process.** The lateral nasal processes form the sides of the nose, whereas the median nasal process forms the center and tip of the nose. Later the median nasal process grows downward between the maxillary processes to form a pair of bulges called the **globular process.** This continues to grow downward, forming the portion of the upper lip called the **philtrum.** Most of these

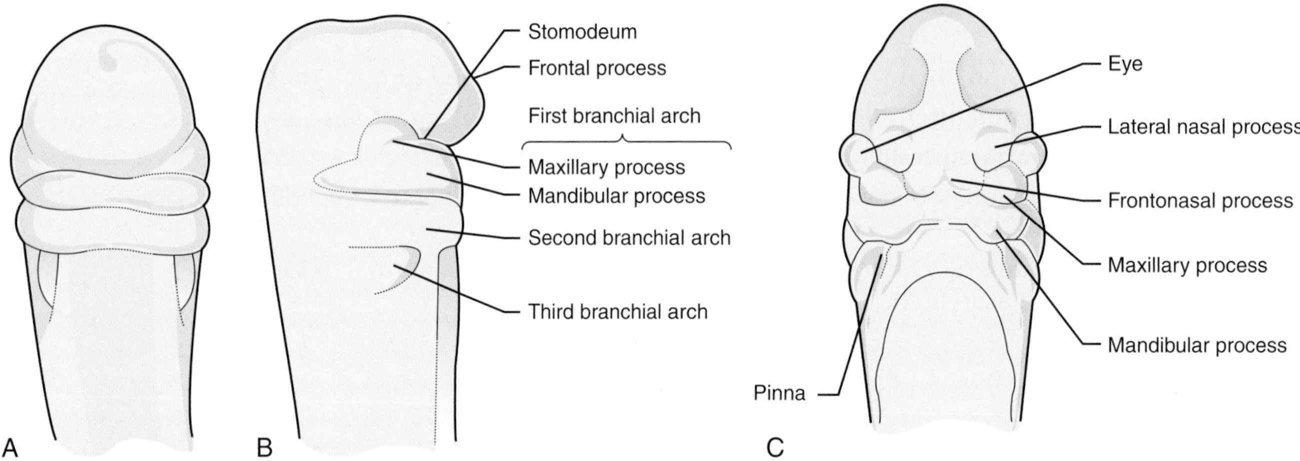

FIGURE 5-1 ■ In the third week of embryonic life an invagination or infolding of the ectoderm forms the primitive oral cavity called the stomodeum. **A** and **B,** As facial development continues, the first branchial arch divides into two maxillary processes. **C,** The fourth week of development.

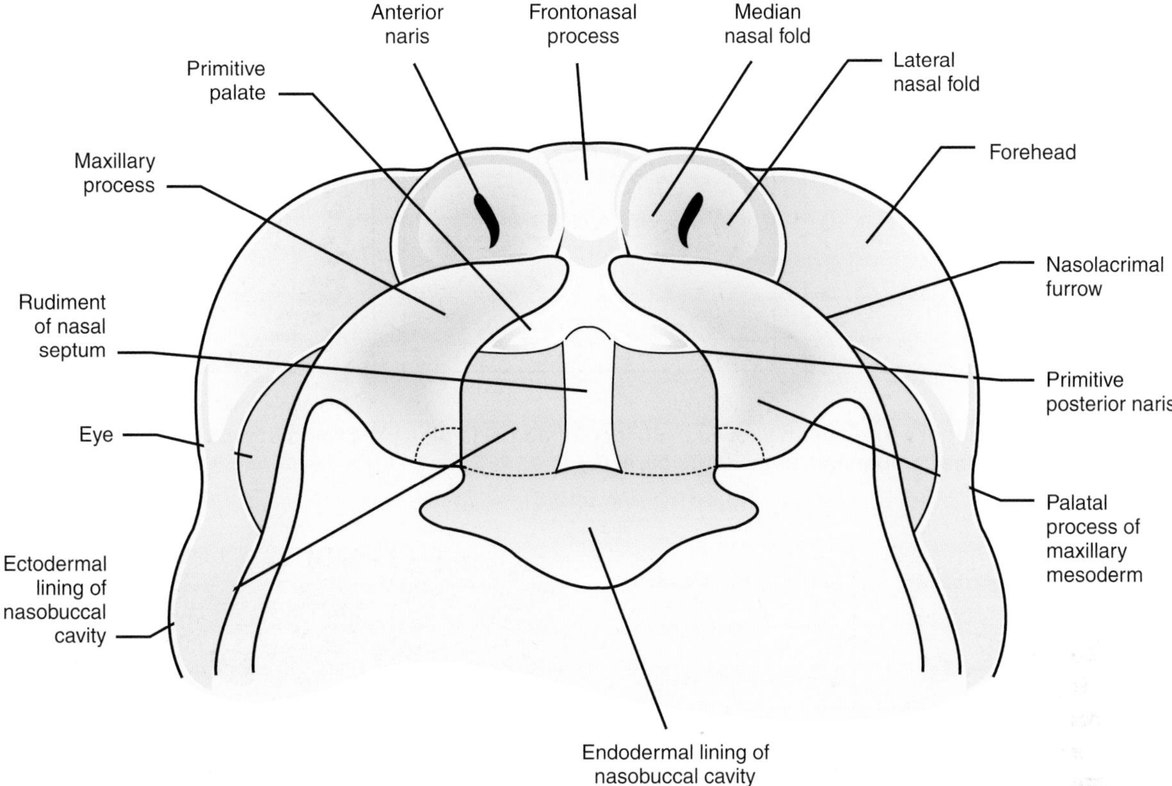

FIGURE 5-2 ■ The right and left palatine processes fuse to form the maxilla and premaxilla. A Y-shaped pattern results.

developments are completed by the end of the eighth week of embryonic life.

ORAL AND NASAL CAVITIES

The area of the palate called the **premaxilla** develops from the globular process. The **lateral palatine processes** (left and right) are formed from the maxillary processes. These lateral palatine processes then fuse with the premaxilla. The fusion creates a Y-shaped pattern (see Figure 5-2). The nasal septum arises from the median nasal process. The right and left maxillary processes fuse together with the nasal septum at the center of the palate.

The tongue develops from the first three branchial arches. The second and third branchial arches are located just below the first branchial arch (see Figure 5-1, *B*). The body of the tongue forms from the first branchial arch, and the base of the tongue forms from the second and third branchial arches.

TEETH

Tooth development, or **odontogenesis,** in the human embryo takes place at about the fifth week of embryonic life and involves both ectoderm and ectomesenchyme. The ectomesenchyme is derived from neural crest cells.

Odontogenesis begins with the formation of a band of ectoderm in each jaw called the **primary dental lamina**. Ten small knoblike proliferations of epithelial cells develop on the primary dental lamina in each jaw (Figure 5-3, *A*). Each of these proliferations extends into the underlying mesenchyme, becoming the early enamel organ for each of the primary teeth (Figure 5-3, *B*).

The tooth germ is composed of three parts: (1) the enamel organ, (2) the dental papilla, and (3) the dental sac or follicle (Figure 5-3, *C*). The enamel organ develops from ectoderm, and the dental papilla and dental sac or follicle develop from mesenchyme. Cell differentiation in the enamel organ progresses to produce ameloblasts, which form enamel. In the dental papilla odontoblasts are produced to form dentin. The permanent or **succedaneous** enamel organs form at the same time.

Formation of dental hard tissues occurs during the fifth month of gestation (Figure 5-4). **Dentinogenesis** is the formation of **dentin**. Dentin is the first mineralized tooth tissue to appear. When it begins to form, the mesenchymal tissue within the tooth germ is called the **dental papilla.** After dentin is produced, the dental papilla is called the dental pulp. **Enamel** is the product of the enamel organ. Enamel matrix begins to form shortly after dentin, and mineralization and maturation of enamel follow the formation of the matrix. **Amelogenesis** refers to the formation of enamel.

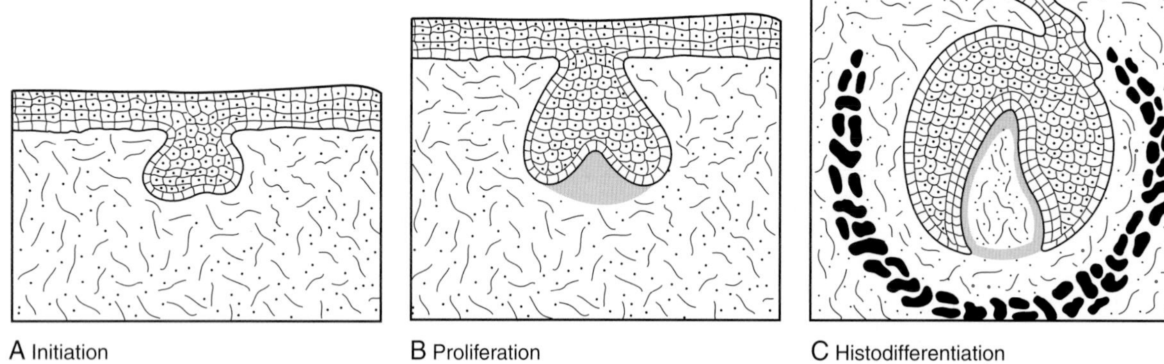

FIGURE 5-3 ■ Development of a tooth germ showing initiation of dental lamina **(A)**, proliferation of dental lamina **(B)**, and differentiation of the components of the tooth germ **(C)**.

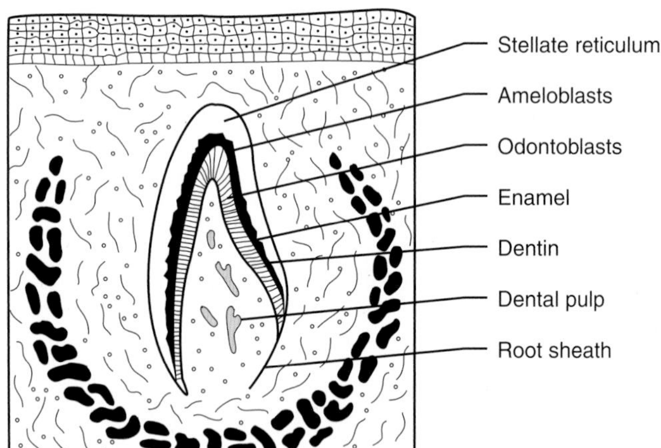

FIGURE 5-4 ■ Deposition of enamel and dentin.

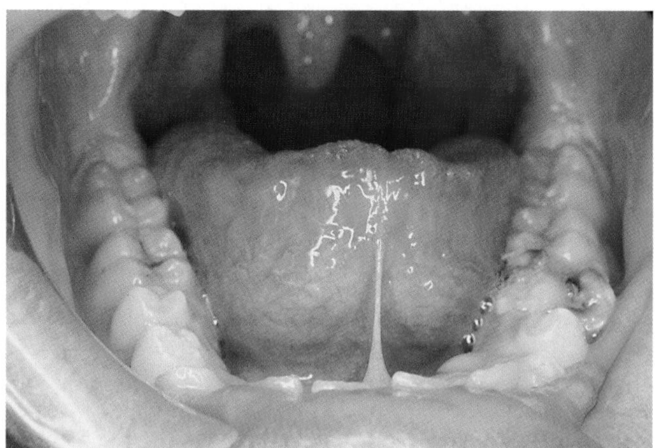

FIGURE 5-5 ■ Ankyloglossia. The short lingual frenum is attached near the tip of the tongue. (Courtesy Dr. George Blozis.)

The dental sac or follicle that surrounds the developing tooth germ provides cells that form cementum, the periodontal ligament, and alveolar bone. **Cementogenesis** (the formation of **cementum**) occurs after crown formation is complete. An epithelial structure called the ***Hertwig's epithelial root sheath*** proliferates to shape the root of the tooth and induces the formation of the root dentin. The cells of the Hertwig's epithelial root sheath must break up and pull away from the root surface before cementum can be produced. Very little cementum is produced until the tooth has erupted and is in occlusion and functioning. Root length is not completed until 1 to 4 years after the tooth erupts into the oral cavity.

DEVELOPMENTAL SOFT TISSUE ABNORMALITIES

ANKYLOGLOSSIA

Ankyloglossia is an extensive adhesion of the tongue to the floor of the mouth, which is often referred to as "tongue-tied." Ankyloglossia is derived from the Greek words "ankylos," meaning adhesion, and "glossa," meaning tongue. This adhesion results from the complete or partial fusion of the lingual frenum to the floor of the mouth. Total ankyloglossia is rare. Partial ankyloglossia appears clinically as a very short lingual frenum connecting the anteroventral portion of the tongue to the floor of the mouth (Figure 5-5). Patients with a short lingual frenum may exhibit no adverse effects, but some may have problems with speech. Gingival recession and bone loss can occur if the frenum is attached high on the lingual alveolar ridge. Surgical removal of a portion of the lingual frenum, known as **frenectomy,** is the usual treatment for ankyloglossia.

COMMISSURAL LIP PITS

Commissural lip pits are epithelium-lined blind tracts located at the corners of the mouth (commissures) (Figure 5-6). These tracts may be shallow, or they may be several millimeters deep. They are a relatively common developmental **anomaly**. The cause of commissural lip pits is not clear; both

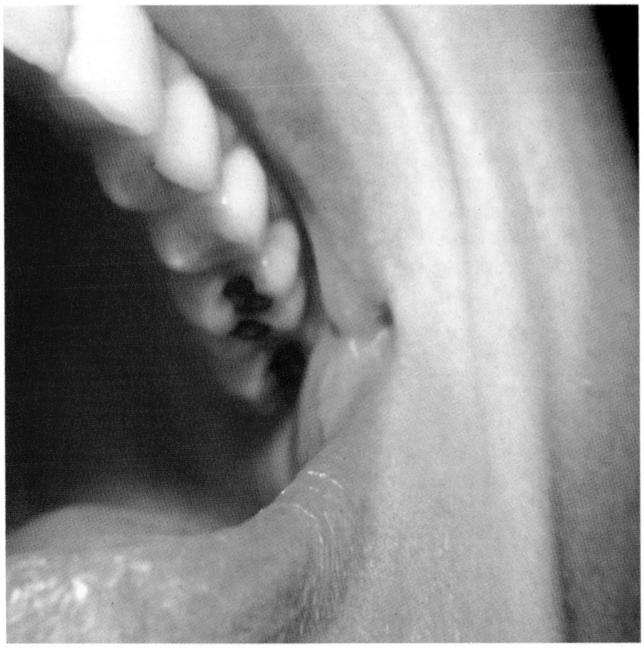

FIGURE 5-6 ■ Commissural lip pit. A deep depression is seen at the labial commissure.

the incomplete fusion of the maxillary and mandibular processes and the defective development of the horizontal facial cleft have been suggested. The commissural lip pit may be observed during examination.

Another lip pit that occasionally may be seen is the **congenital lip pit.** It occurs near the midline of the vermilion border of the lip and may appear as either a unilateral or a bilateral depression. No treatment is indicated for lip pits.

LINGUAL THYROID

Lingual thyroid, or **ectopic lingual thyroid nodule,** is a small mass of thyroid tissue located on the tongue away from the normal anatomic location of the thyroid gland. It is an uncommon developmental anomaly that results from the failure of the primitive thyroid tissue to migrate from its developmental location in the area of the foramen cecum on the posterior portion of the tongue to its normal position in the neck.

Clinically the lingual thyroid nodule appears as a smooth nodular mass at the base of the tongue posterior to the circumvallate papillae on or near the midline. It can be asymptomatic or can cause a feeling of fullness in the throat or difficulty in swallowing. Histologically the lingual thyroid is composed of immature or mature thyroid tissue.

On occasion the size of the lingual thyroid necessitates its removal. However, this nodule may be the patient's only functioning thyroid tissue. Therefore it is necessary to establish the presence of functioning thyroid tissue elsewhere before any nodular lesion located in the posterior aspect of the tongue is removed. If a normally located thyroid gland is lacking or nonfunctional, the lingual thyroid is not removed.

DEVELOPMENTAL CYSTS

A cyst is an abnormal, pathologic sac or cavity lined by epithelium and enclosed in a connective tissue capsule. Cysts occur throughout the body, including the oral region.

The cysts discussed in this chapter are all related to the development of the face, jaws, and teeth. Some have a distinctive histologic appearance, and a definitive diagnosis is based on microscopic examination of the tissue. Other cysts are lined by less distinctive epithelium. The diagnosis of these cysts is based on both the histologic appearance of the tissue and the location of the cyst.

The most common cyst observed in the oral cavity is caused by pulpal inflammation and is called the **periapical cyst,** (radicular cyst) (see Chapter 2). It develops from a preexisting periapical granuloma found at the apex of a non-vital tooth. The **residual cyst** is a periapical cyst that remains after extraction of the offending tooth. Because cysts are commonly observed in the jaws and surrounding soft tissues, the dental hygienist should understand their diagnostic criteria, pathogenesis, and prognosis. The preliminary identification of a cystic lesion is within the scope of dental hygiene practice.

Developmental cysts are classified as **odontogenic** (related to tooth development) and **nonodontogenic** (not related to tooth development). Cysts are also classified according to location, cause, origin of the epithelial cells, and histologic appearance (Box 5-1). Developmental cysts can vary in size from small, asymptomatic lesions to large lesions that can cause expansion of bone. Very large and long-standing lesions can resorb tooth structure or move teeth. Oral cysts that occur within bone are called **intraosseous cysts,** and cysts that occur in soft tissue are called **extraosseous cysts.**

Radiographically cysts within bone generally appear as well-circumscribed radiolucencies. All cysts may appear **unilocular,** but some are more likely to appear as multilocular radiolucencies. When cysts are found within soft tissue, usually no radiographic change occurs.

ODONTOGENIC CYSTS

Dentigerous Cyst

A **dentigerous cyst,** also called a **follicular cyst,** forms around the crown of an unerupted or developing tooth (Figure 5-7). It is the second most common odontogenic cyst after the periapical cyst. The epithelial lining originates from the reduced enamel epithelium after the crown has completely formed and calcified. Fluid accumulates between the crown and the reduced enamel epithelium. The reduced enamel epithelium results from remnants of the enamel organ. The most common location for the dentigerous cyst is around the crown of an unerupted or impacted mandibular third molar. However, a dentigerous cyst may form around the crowns of other unerupted or impacted teeth such as the maxillary

Box 5-1

Classification of Developmental Cysts

Odontogenic		Nonodontogenic	
Intraosseous	Extraosseous	Intraosseous	Extraosseous
▪ Dentigerous cyst	▪ Eruption Cyst	▪ Nasopalatine duct cyst	▪ Nasolabial cyst
▪ Primordial cyst		▪ Median palatal cyst	▪ Branchial Cleft Cyst (cervical lymphoepithelial cyst and intraoral lymphoepithelial cyst)
▪ Odontogenic keratocyst		▪ Globulomaxillary cyst	
▪ Lateral periodontal cyst	▪ Gingival Cyst	▪ Median mandibular cyst	
			▪ Epidermal cyst
			▪ Thyroglossal Tract cyst

cuspid or a supernumerary tooth. There is a higher incidence in males and this cyst is most often seen in young adults in their twenties and thirties. The size of these cysts can range from small and asymptomatic to very large. When large, it is capable of displacing teeth or causing a fracture of the mandible.

Radiographically the dentigerous cyst appears as a well-defined, unilocular radiolucency around the crown of an unerupted or impacted tooth (Figure 5-8, *A* and *B*). Histologically the lumen is most characteristically lined with cuboidal epithelium surrounded by a wall of connective tissue (Figure 5-8, *C*). It may also be lined with stratified squamous epithelium. The lumen may be filled with a watery or serous fluid.

Treatment of a dentigerous cyst involves the complete removal of the cystic lesion and usually the tooth involved. If it is not removed, the cyst wall continues to enlarge. In addition, a risk exists that a neoplasm (i.e., ameloblastoma) may develop (see Chapter 7).

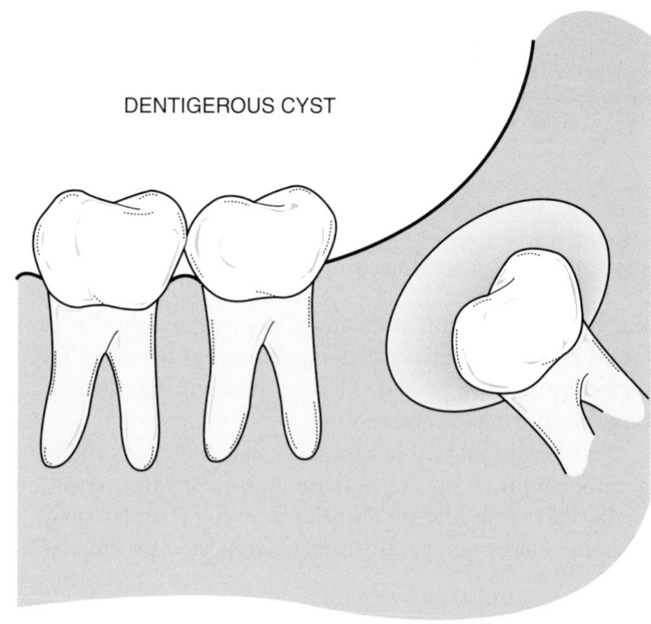

FIGURE 5-7 ▪ Schematic of a dentigerous cyst located around the crown of an unerupted or impacted tooth.

Eruption Cyst

An **eruption cyst** is similar to a dentigerous cyst. It is found in the soft tissue around the crown of an erupting tooth.

The eruption cyst can be seen in deciduous and permanent teeth, but it is most commonly associated with the first permanent molars and incisors.

Because the tooth erupts through the cyst, this condition usually does not require treatment. Occasionally the dome of the eruption cyst is removed to expose the crown. The tooth is allowed to erupt naturally.

Primordial Cyst

A **primordial cyst** develops in place of a tooth and is most commonly found in place of the third molar or posterior to an erupted third molar (Figure 5-9). It originates from remnants and degeneration of the enamel organ. A history that the tooth was never present is an essential component of the diagnostic process.

Primordial cysts are most often seen in the young adult; no sex **predilection** has been reported. Clinically the cyst usually is asymptomatic and is discovered on radiographic examination. Radiographically it is a well-defined, radiolucent lesion that can be either unilocular or multilocular. The histologic appearance and diagnosis of the primordial cyst may vary. Histologically the lumen is lined by stratified squamous epithelium surrounded by parallel bundles of collagen fibers. A layer of orthokeratin or parakeratin can cover the epithelium. The term *primordial cyst* simply refers to its development in place of a tooth. For this reason, biopsy and histologic examination of primordial cysts are essential. Histologically a primordial cyst can be an odontogenic keratocyst or a lateral periodontal cyst.

Treatment of a primordial cyst involves surgical removal of the entire lesion. The prognosis depends on the histology; the risk of recurrence depends on the histologic diagnosis. For example, if the cyst is histologically an odontogenic keratocyst, the risk of recurrence is greater than if the cyst is lined by nonkeratinized stratified squamous epithelium.

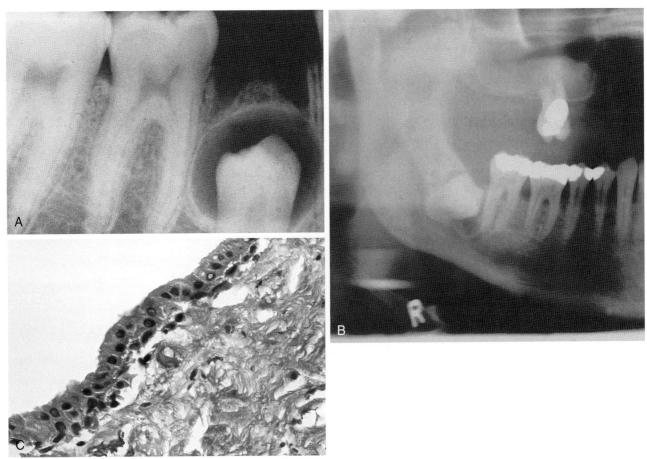

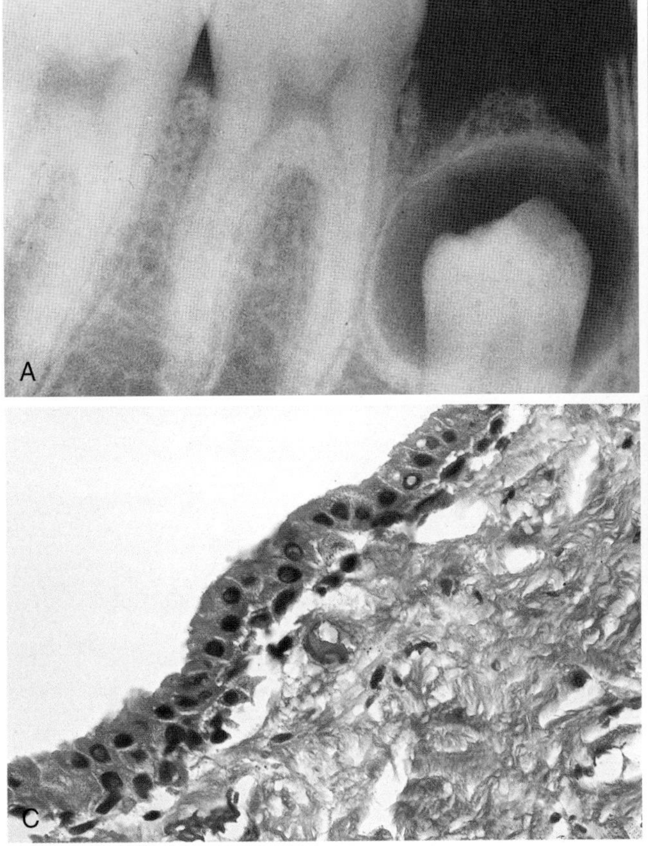

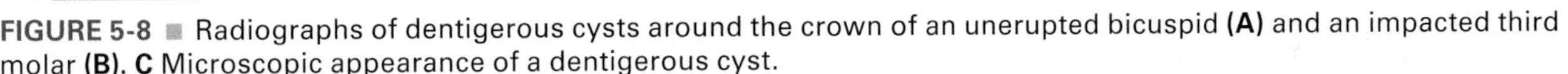

FIGURE 5-8 ■ Radiographs of dentigerous cysts around the crown of an unerupted bicuspid **(A)** and an impacted third molar **(B)**. **C** Microscopic appearance of a dentigerous cyst.

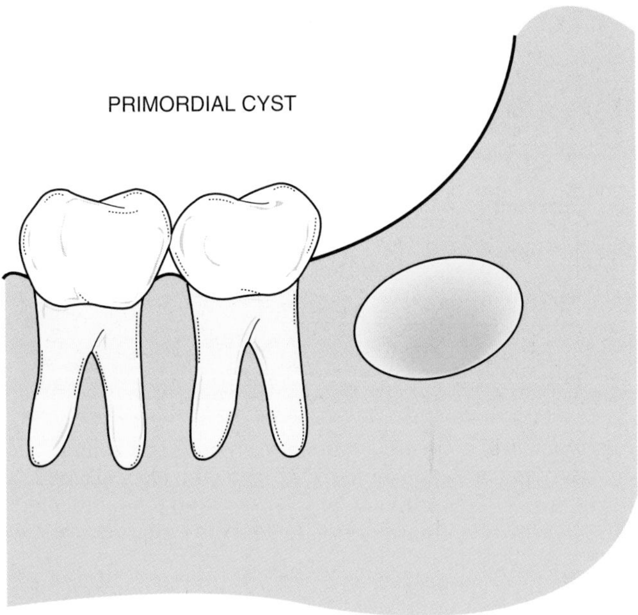

FIGURE 5-9 ■ Primordial cyst occurring in place of a tooth: the third molar, in this instance.

Odontogenic Keratocyst

An **odontogenic keratocyst (OKC)** is an odontogenic developmental cyst that is characterized by its unique histologic appearance and frequent recurrence. The lumen is lined by epithelium that is 8 to 10 cell layers thick and surfaced by parakeratin. The basal cell layer is palisaded and prominent; the interface between the epithelium and the connective tissue is flat (Figure 5-10, *A* and *B*).

These cysts are most often seen in the mandibular third molar region, and there is a slight predilection in males. Radiographically the odontogenic keratocyst frequently appears as a well-defined, multilocular, radiolucent lesion (Figure 5-10, *C*). Unilocular lesions may also occur. The radiographic appearance of an odontogenic keratocyst can be identical to that of an odontogenic tumor. The odontogenic keratocyst can move teeth and resorb tooth structure but does not usually cause expansion of bone. The OKC is also associated with nevoid basal cell carcinoma syndrome (Gorlin syndrome) (see Chapter 6).

Treatment of an odontogenic keratocyst is rather aggressive because of the high recurrence rate (Figure 5-10, *D* and *E*). The cyst generally extends beyond the borders that are seen on the radiograph because it extends between the

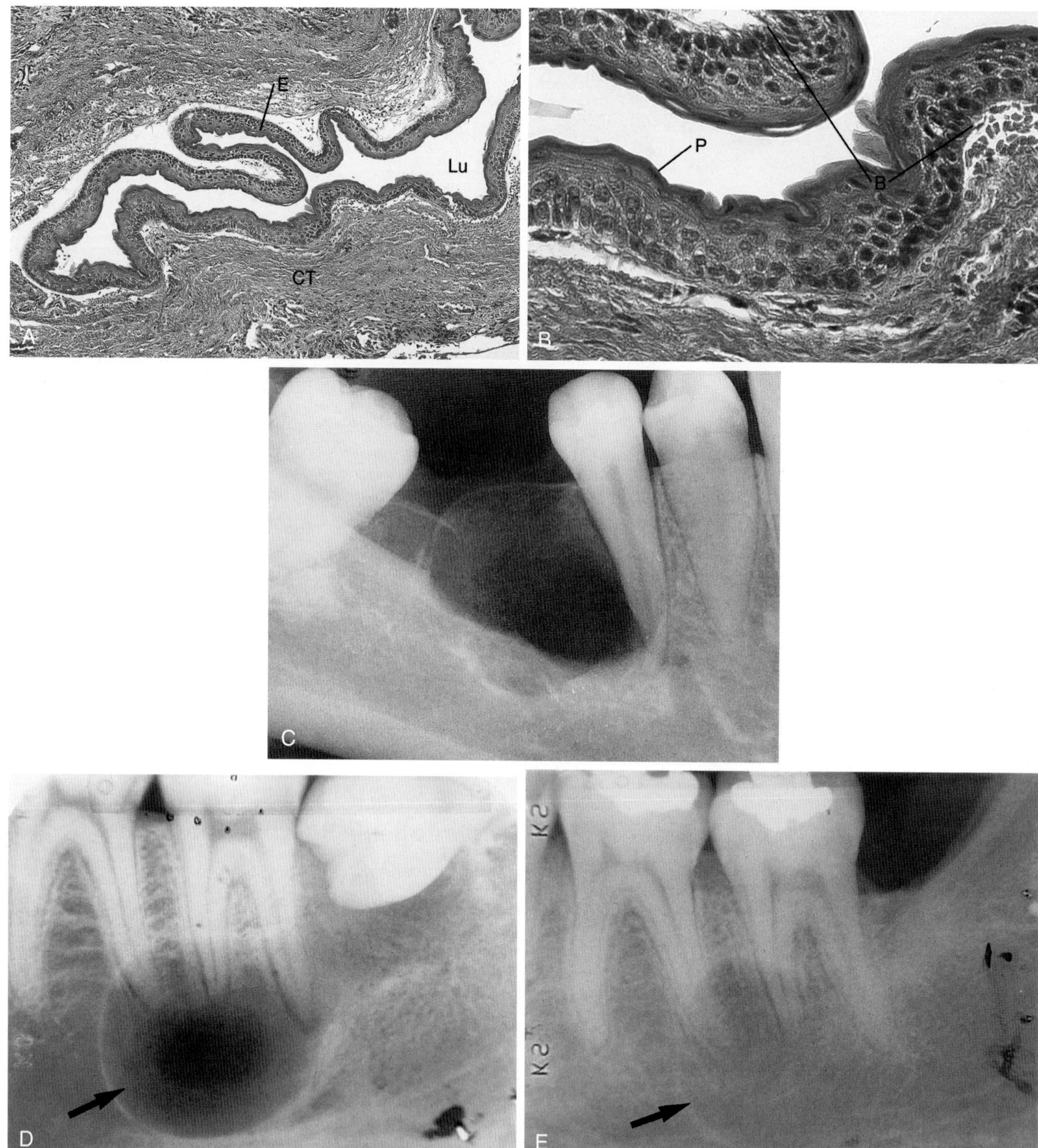

FIGURE 5-10 ■ **A,** Microscopic appearance of an odontogenic keratocyst (OKC) showing a thin uniform epithelial lining (low power). *Lu,* Lumen; *E,* epithelium; *CT,* connective tissue. **B,** Microscopic appearance of an OKC showing a corrugated parakeratotic surface *(P)* and a prominent basal cell layer *(B)* (high power). **C,** Radiograph of an OKC showing a multilocular radiolucency. **D,** Radiograph of an OKC extending to the third molar. **E,** Same patient in **D** 2 years later, showing recurrence of OKC. The reader should note that the third molar has been removed.

trabeculae of bone. Therefore thorough surgical excision and osseous curettage are recommended. Careful follow-up and evaluation are essential.

Calcifying Odontogenic Cyst

The **calcifying odontogenic cyst** (COC) is a developmental nonaggressive cystic lesion lined by odontogenic epithelium that closely resembles the epithelium of the odontogenic tumor called an *ameloblastoma*; in addition, it has a characteristic feature called *ghost cells*. Generally the cyst is treated conservatively and does not recur. A solid variant of the calcifying odontogenic cyst is called the odontogenic ghost cell tumor; it has been suggested that this solid variant represents a neoplasm rather than a cyst. Because of its histologic resemblance to the ameloblastoma, the calcifying odontogenic cyst is described in detail in Chapter 7.

Lateral Periodontal Cyst and Gingival Cyst

The **lateral periodontal cyst** is named for its location. It is seen most often in the mandibular cuspid and premolar area. It presents as an asymptomatic, unilocular or multilocular radiolucent lesion located on the lateral aspect of a tooth root (Figure 5-11, *A*). Histologically a thin band of stratified squamous epithelium that exhibits focal epithelial thickenings lines the cyst (Figure 5-11, *B*). The **gingival cyst** exhibits the same type of epithelial lining as the lateral periodontal cyst and is located in the soft tissue of the same area. The gingival

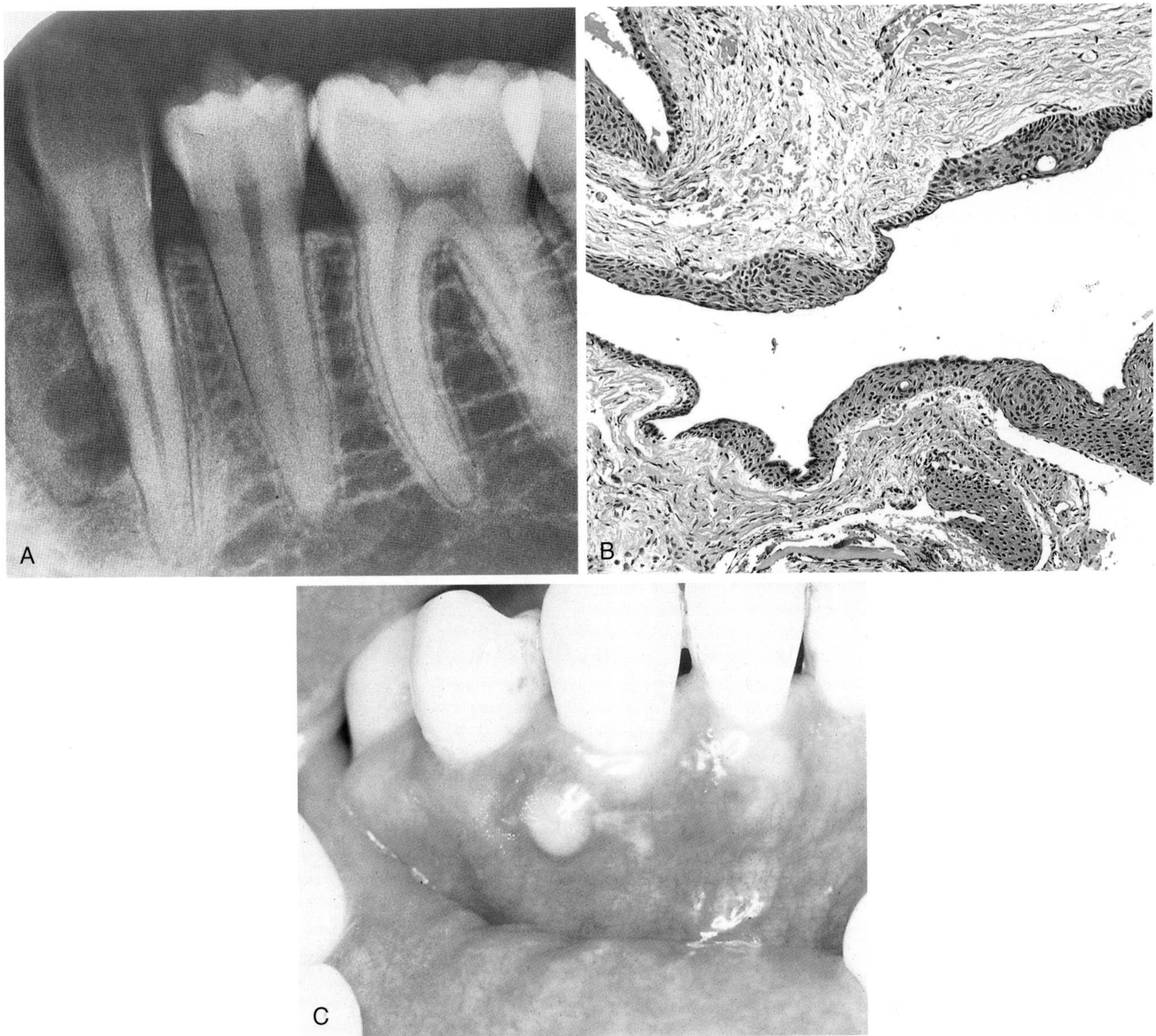

FIGURE 5-11 ■ **A,** Radiograph of a lateral periodontal cyst. This biloculated, well-defined radiolucency is located lateral to the tooth root. **B,** Microscopic appearance of a lateral periodontal cyst showing a thin epithelial lining with focal epithelial thickenings. **C,** Gingival cyst. (**C** courtesy Drs. Paul Freedman and Stanley Kerpel.)

cyst appears as a small bulge or swelling of the attached gingiva or interdental papillae (Figure 5-11, *C*).

The lateral periodontal cyst is found most often in males. No sex predilection has been reported for gingival cysts. Both the lateral periodontal cyst and the gingival cyst are treated by surgical excision. A few cases of recurrence of lateral periodontal cysts have been reported.

NONODONTOGENIC CYSTS

Nasopalatine Canal Cyst

A **nasopalatine canal cyst (incisive canal cyst)** is located within the nasopalatine canal or the incisive papilla. When found in the papilla, it is referred to as a **cyst of the palatine papilla.** This cyst arises from epithelial remnants of the embryonal nasopalatine ducts. The lesion is most commonly seen in adults between 40 and 60 years of age, and a strong predilection exists for males. The cyst is usually asymptomatic. There may be a small pink bulge near the apices and between the roots of the maxillary central incisors on the lingual surface. The adjacent teeth are usually vital.

Radiographically the nasopalatine canal cyst is a well-defined, radiolucent lesion that is often heart shaped (Figure 5-12, *A*), resulting from the anatomic Y shape of the canal. When it is heart shaped, it is evenly distributed to the right and left of the midline.

Histologically the cyst is lined by epithelium that varies from stratified squamous to pseudostratified ciliated columnar epithelium (Figure 5-12, *B*). The connective tissue wall contains nerves and blood vessels that are normally found in the area and may also contain inflammatory cells.

Treatment of a nasopalatine canal cyst is surgical enucleation. It is especially important that surgery take place in the edentulous patient before the fabrication of a prosthesis. Recurrence is rare.

Median Palatine Cyst

A **median palatine cyst** appears as a well-defined unilocular radiolucency and is located in the midline of the hard palate (Figure 5-13). The cyst is thought to be a more posterior form of a nasopalatine canal cyst. Histologically the median palatine cyst is lined with stratified squamous epithelium that is surrounded by dense fibrous connective tissue. The median palatine cyst is treated by surgical enucleation. The prognosis is good, and recurrence is rare.

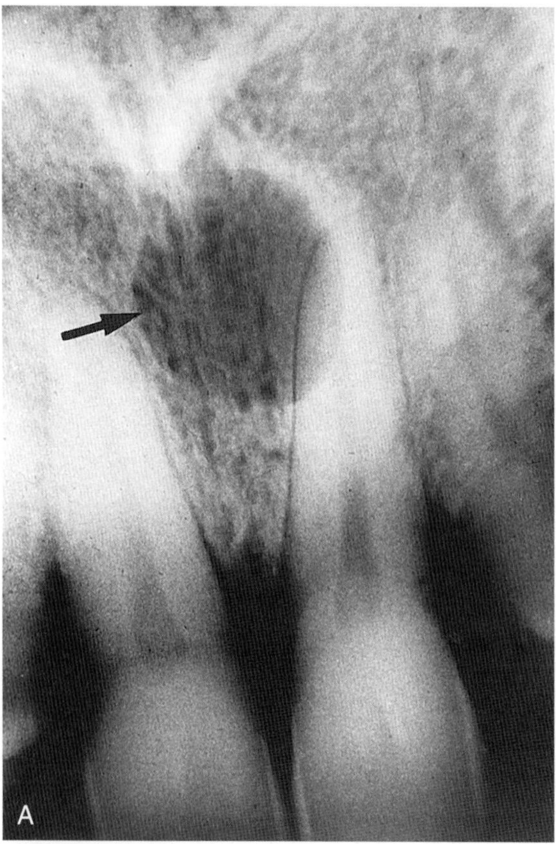

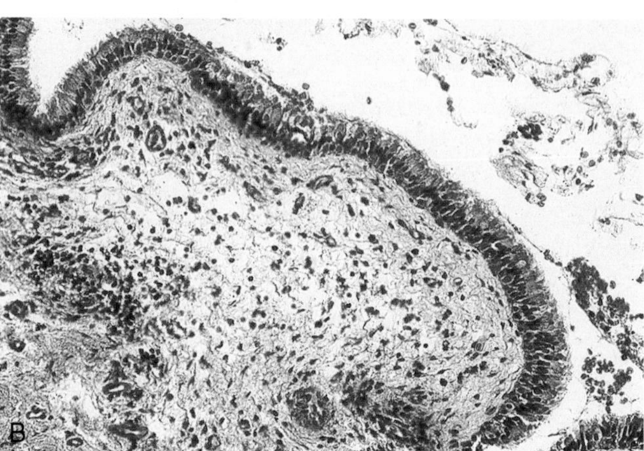

FIGURE 5-12 ■ **A,** An incisive canal cyst may be located in the anterior maxilla in either bone or soft tissue or both. This radiograph of an incisive canal cyst shows a well-circumscribed radiolucency between the maxillary central incisors. **B,** Microscopic appearance of an incisive canal cyst showing a pseudostratified, ciliated, columnar epithelial lining.

Globulomaxillary Cyst

Radiographically a **globulomaxillary cyst** is a well-defined, pear-shaped radiolucency found between the roots of the maxillary lateral incisor and cuspid (Figure 5-14). Although it was once thought to be a fissural cyst, it is now believed to be of odontogenic epithelial origin. Microscopic evaluation includes the central giant cell granuloma, OKC, and lateral periodontal cyst. The size of the lesion can vary; however, when it is large enough, a divergence of the roots can result. The adjacent teeth are usually vital. Pulp testing can rule out a periapical cyst or periapical granuloma. Surgical enucleation of the globulomaxillary cyst is recommended but determined by the microscopic diagnosis. The prognosis and recurrence also depend upon the final diagnosis.

Median Mandibular Cyst

A **median mandibular cyst** is a rare lesion. As its name indicates, it is located in the midline of the mandible. The origin of the median mandibular cyst is also unclear. Some believe it to be of odontogenic origin ranging from odontogenic cysts to tumors. Because no midline fusion occurs between the bony processes, there is no evidence of epithelial entrapment. The surrounding teeth are vital. Radiographically a well-defined radiolucency is seen below the apices of the mandibular incisors. A median mandibular cyst is treated by surgical removal, and prognosis is good.

Nasolabial Cyst

A **nasolabial cyst** is a soft tissue cyst with no alveolar bone involvement. The origin of this cyst is uncertain. At present it is thought to originate from the lower anterior portion of the nasolacrimal duct. The cyst is observed in adults 40 to 50 years of age; a strong predilection (4:1) exists for females.

Clinically there may be an expansion or swelling in the mucolabial fold in the area of the maxillary canine and the floor of the nose. Usually no radiographic change is associated with this cyst. However, when the lesion is large enough, expansive pressure can cause the resorption of bone (Figure 5-15). Histologically the cyst is lined with pseudostratified, ciliated columnar epithelium and multiple goblet cells. Treatment of a nasolabial cyst is surgical excision; prognosis is good, and recurrence is rare.

Branchial Cleft Cyst

A branchial cleft cyst (cervical **lymphoepithelial cyst**) is located on the lateral neck at the anterior border of the sternocleidomastoid muscle. It is composed of a stratified squamous epithelial lining surrounded by a well-circumscribed component of lymphoid tissue and connective tissue (Figure 5-16). It appears to arise from epithelium entrapped in a lymph node during development. When found intraorally, the lymphoepithelial cyst is most commonly seen on the floor of the mouth and the lateral borders of the posterior tongue.

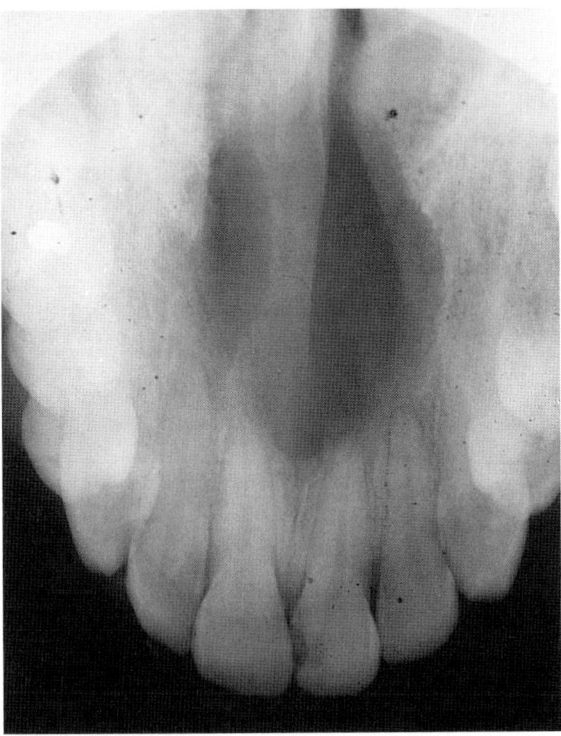

FIGURE 5-13 ■ Radiograph of a median palatine cyst showing a well-defined radiolucency located in the midline of the maxilla.

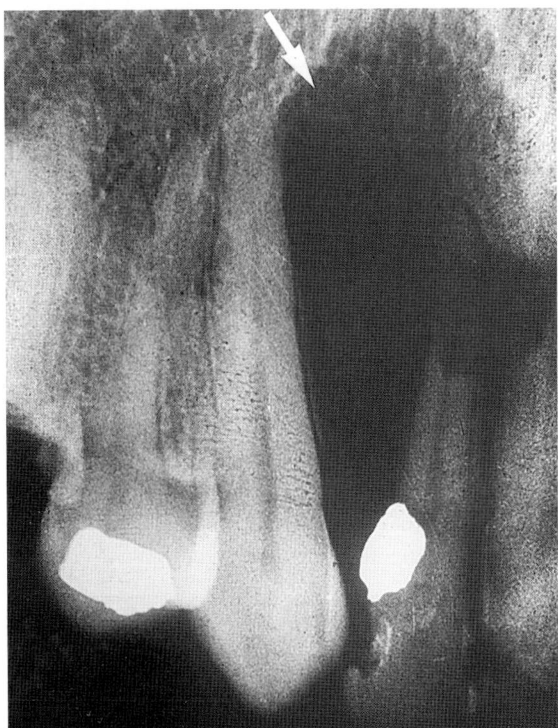

FIGURE 5-14 ■ Radiograph of a globulomaxillary cyst showing a characteristic pear-shaped radiolucency between the roots of the maxillary lateral incisor and cuspid.

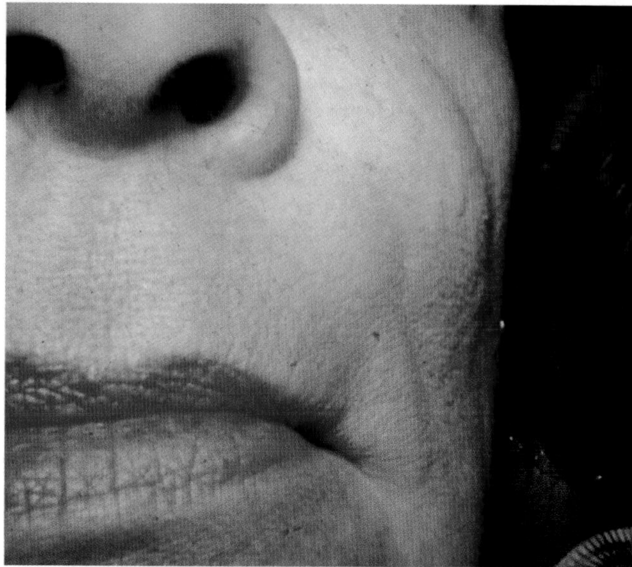

FIGURE 5-15 ■ Nasolabial cyst causing a swelling in the nasolabial fold area.

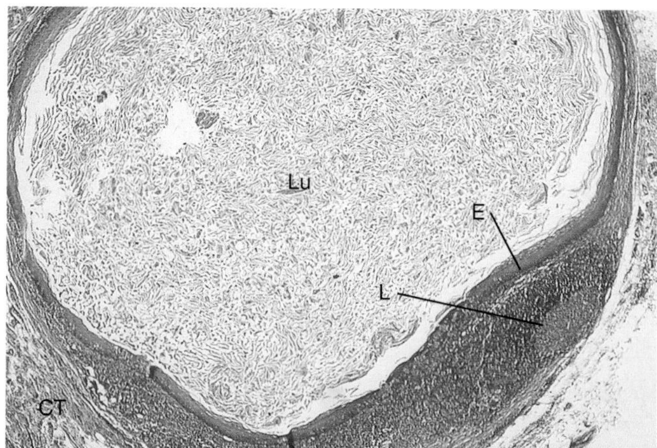

FIGURE 5-16 Microscopic appearance of a lymphoepithelial cyst showing lumen *(Lu)*, epithelial lining *(E)*, surrounding lymphocytes *(L)*, and connective tissue *(CT)* (low power).

The lymphoepithelial cyst appears as a pinkish-yellow, raised nodule when seen intraorally. Treatment of a branchial cleft cyst (cervical lymphoid cyst) and intraoral lymphoepithelial cyst consists of surgical excision, and prognosis is good.

Epidermal Cyst

An **epidermal cyst** presents as a raised nodule in the skin of the face or neck. Histologically the cyst is lined by keratinizing epithelium that resembles the epithelium of skin (epidermis). The cyst lumen is usually filled with keratin scales. Most epidermal cysts are thought to originate from the epithelium of the hair follicle. Occasionally when located in the skin of the cheek, the nodule may be noted intraorally from the buccal mucosal aspect and the skin. An epidermoid cyst is treated by surgical excision, and prognosis is good.

Dermoid Cyst and Benign Cystic Teratoma

A **dermoid cyst** is a developmental cyst that is often present at birth or noted in young children. It is more common in other parts of the body than in the head and neck. When the dermoid cyst occurs in the oral cavity, it is usually found in the anterior floor of the mouth. The cyst may cause displacement of the tongue and may have a doughlike consistency when palpated.

Histologically the dermoid cyst is lined by orthokeratinized, stratified squamous epithelium surrounded by a connective tissue wall. The lumen is usually filled with keratin. Hair follicles, sebaceous glands, and sweat glands may be seen in the cyst wall. A **benign cystic teratoma** has a cystic component that resembles the dermoid cyst. In addition, teeth, bone, muscles, and nerve tissue may be found in the wall of this lesion. Teeth are usually not found in the malignant form of the teratoma. Treatment of the dermoid cyst is surgical excision; prognosis is good, and malignant transformation is rare.

Thyroglossal Tract Cyst

A **thyroglossal tract (duct) cyst** forms along the same tract that the thyroid gland follows in development, from the area of the foramen cecum to its permanent location in the neck (Figure 5-17). Most of these cysts occur below the hyoid bone. The epithelial lining varies with location. Cysts above the hyoid bone are usually lined with stratified squamous epithelium, and those below the hyoid bone with ciliated columnar epithelium. Thyroid tissue may also be found within the connective tissue wall.

The thyroglossal tract cyst is most often found in young individuals under 20 years of age. There is no sex predilection. Clinically if this cyst is located below the hyoid bone, it presents as a smooth bulge or swelling in the area of the midline of the neck. If located on the posterior aspect of the tongue, a smooth, rather firm mass of tissue is present, which can vary in size from a few millimeters to several centimeters. The patient may complain of dysphagia (difficulty in swallowing) or difficulty when extending the tongue.

Treatment of a thyroglossal tract cyst consists of complete excision of the cyst and the tract, usually including a portion of the hyoid bone and muscle tissue along the thyroglossal tract. Generally prognosis is good, but a few cases of malignant transformation have been reported.

PSEUDOCYSTS

Static Bone Cyst

A **static bone cyst (lingual mandibular bone concavity** or **Stafne bone defect)** is not a true cyst because it is not a pathologic cavity and is not lined with epithelium. Therefore

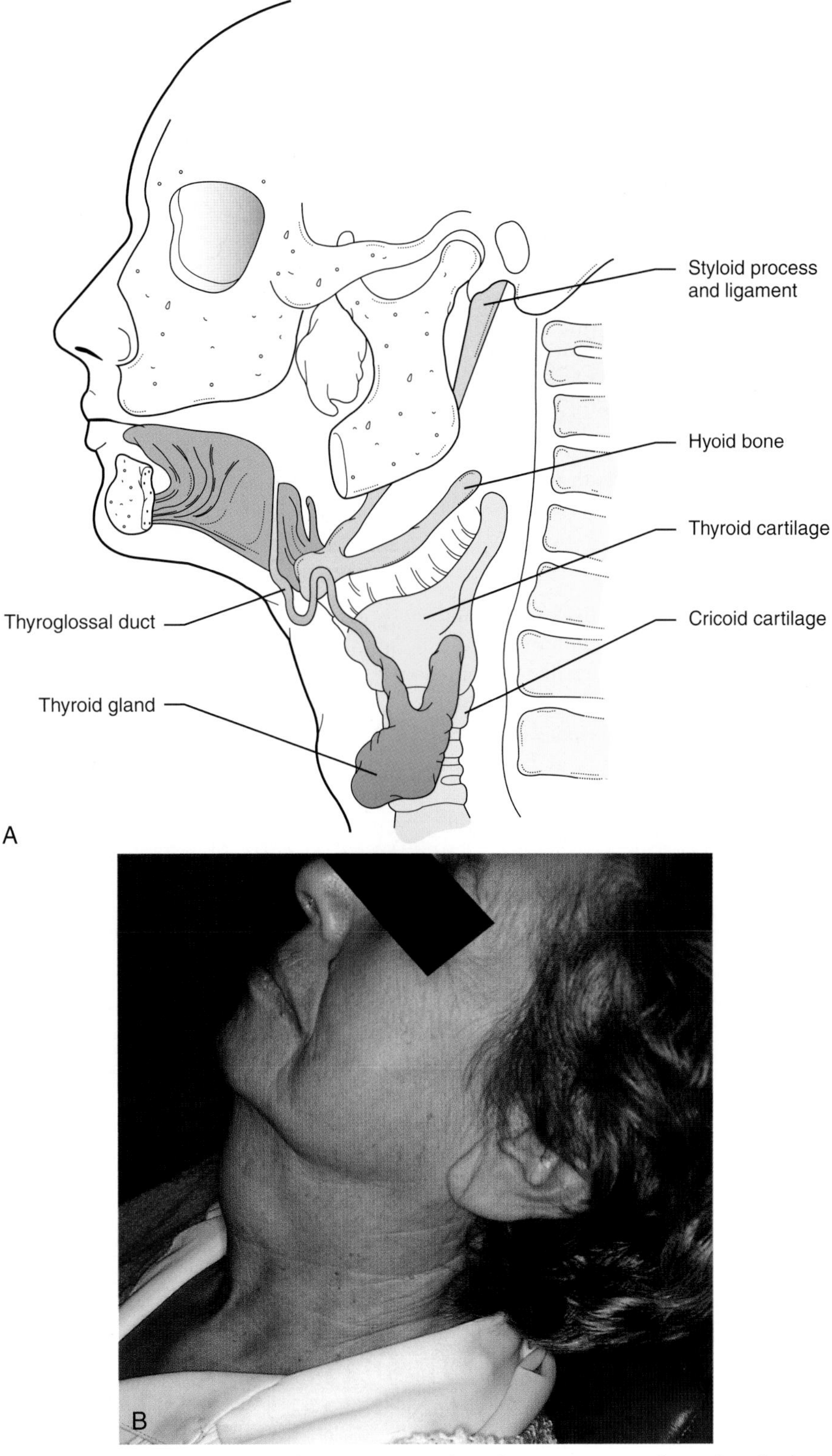

FIGURE 5-17 ■ **A,** The thyroglossal tract extends from the area of the foramen cecum lingual to the lower part of the neck. **B,** A thyroglossal tract cyst is the cause of this enlargement at the midline of the neck.

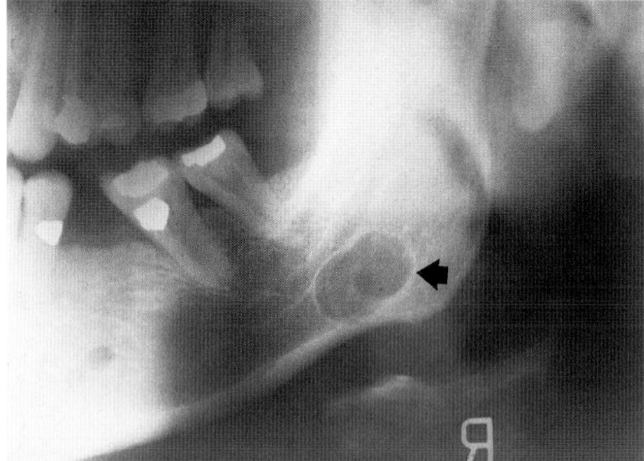

FIGURE 5-18 ■ Panoramic radiograph of a lingual mandibular bone concavity (Stafne bone cyst). *Arrow* points to a well-circumscribed radiolucency inferior to the mandibular canal.

it is often referred to as a *pseudocyst*. Clinically, an anatomic depression may be felt on the posterior lingual area of the mandible. Radiographically a well-defined cystlike radiolucency is observed in this posterior region of the mandible, inferior to the mandibular canal. The radiolucency is caused by the lingual depression in the mandible, which is filled with normal salivary gland tissue (Figure 5-18). The salivary gland tissue may be an extension of the sublingual gland. The lesion is usually asymptomatic. There is a predilection in men.

This developmental defect requires no treatment. A sialogram can be used to identify salivary gland tissue. If any question exists about the diagnosis, the patient is followed until it is determined that no enlargement of the radiolucency has occurred. If the radiolucency occurs above the mandibular canal, a biopsy may be indicated to establish the diagnosis and differentiate this pseudocyst from cysts and tumors having a predilection for that location.

Simple Bone Cyst

A **simple bone cyst (traumatic bone cyst)** is a pathologic cavity in bone that is not lined with epithelium. The cause is uncertain, although an association with trauma has been suggested. The lesion is found most often in young individuals, and there is no sex predilection The lesion is observed radiographically as a well-defined unilocular or multilocular radiolucent lesion that characteristically shows scalloping around the roots of teeth (Figure 5-19). It is usually asymptomatic and is discovered on routine radiographs. Surgical intervention reveals a void within the bone. A curettage is performed on the wall lining the void to establish bleeding. The void or space fills up with bone 6 months to 1 year after the surgical procedure. Prognosis is excellent, and recurrence is unusual.

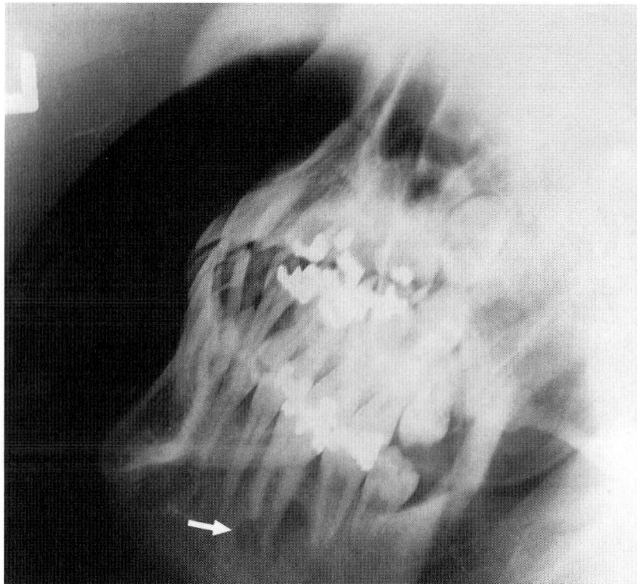

FIGURE 5-19 ■ Extraoral radiograph showing a simple (traumatic) bone cyst in the mandible with its unique radiolucent characteristic, scalloping around the roots. (Courtesy Dr. Edward V. Zegarelli.)

Aneurysmal Bone Cyst

An **aneurysmal bone cyst** is a pseudocyst that consists of blood-filled spaces surrounded by multinucleated giant cells and fibrous connective tissue (similar to the giant cell granuloma). There is no epithelial lining. The radiolucent lesion has a multilocular appearance that is often described as a "honeycomb" or "soap bubble." It is usually seen in individuals under 30 years of age, and a slight predilection is reported in females. When in the jaws, the clinical presentation may include expansion of the involved bone.

A previous history of trauma to the area has been reported in some cases, but no direct correlation exists. Other reports have noted an association between the aneurysmal bone cyst and other bone lesions. It has frequently been associated with fibrous dysplasia, central giant cell granuloma, chondroblastoma, and other primary bone lesions. These other lesions cause a change in vascularity that results in the aneurysmal bone cyst. Surgical excision and supplemental cryotherapy are the recommended treatments for an aneurysmal bone cyst.

DEVELOPMENTAL ABNORMALITIES OF TEETH

ABNORMALITIES IN THE NUMBER OF TEETH

Anodontia

Anodontia is the congenital lack of teeth. Total anodontia (lack of all teeth) is a rare condition that may affect either the deciduous or the permanent dentition. Because development

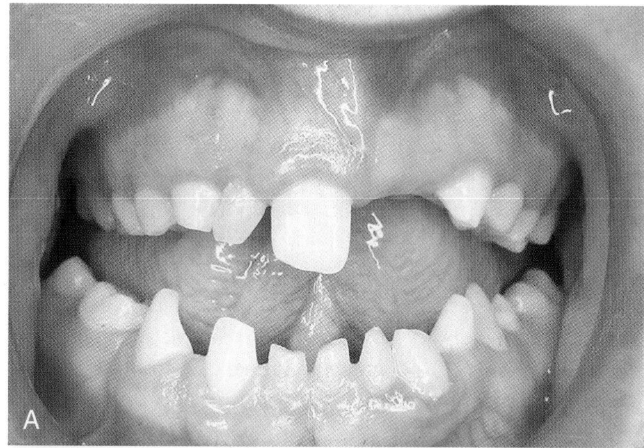

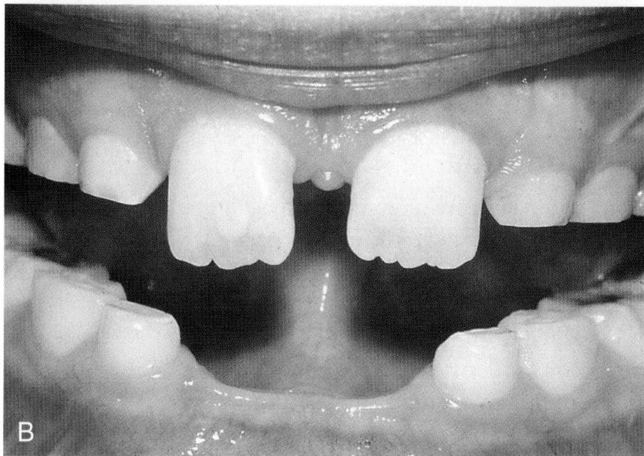

FIGURE 5-20 ■ **A** and **B**, Hypodontia. Teeth missing have not been extracted; they never developed. (**A** courtesy Dr. George Blozis; **B** courtesy Dr. Margot Van Dis.)

of both deciduous and permanent teeth begins before birth, their failure to develop is congenital. However, teeth may not be identified as missing until the time of normal eruption or initial radiographic examination. Total anodontia is often associated with the hereditary disturbance ectodermal dysplasia, which is described in Chapter 6. Missing teeth require prosthetic replacement.

Hypodontia

Hypodontia is the lack of one or more teeth. This developmental anomaly is rather common and may affect either deciduous or permanent teeth (Figure 5-20). Any tooth in either dentition may be missing. The permanent dentition is most commonly affected. The teeth most often missing are the maxillary and mandibular third molars, the maxillary lateral incisors, and the mandibular second premolars. Teeth are often missing bilaterally. The mandibular incisor is the tooth most commonly missing in the deciduous dentition. Teeth are identified as congenitally lacking by careful clinical and radiographic examination along with a thorough patient history.

Missing teeth tend to be **familial** (i.e., affecting more members of a family than would be expected by chance). In addition, factors such as jaw lesions in infancy and radiation therapy during tooth formation may result in the destruction of tooth germs and the subsequent lack of affected teeth.

Missing teeth may require prosthetic replacement. Their absence can also result in problems in occlusion caused by drifting or tipping of teeth. Orthodontic evaluation and treatment may be necessary. In addition, congenitally missing teeth may be a component of a syndrome. A syndrome is a group of findings that occur together. Patients with congenitally missing teeth should be evaluated for other abnormalities.

Supernumerary Teeth

Supernumerary teeth are extra teeth found in the dental arches (Figure 5-21). **Supernumerary** means more than the normal or regular number. Supernumerary teeth result from either the formation of extra tooth buds in the dental lamina or the cleavage of already existing tooth buds and may occur in either the deciduous or the permanent dentition. Extra teeth are most often seen in the maxilla and may occur singly or in multiples and unilaterally or bilaterally.

Typically the supernumerary tooth is smaller than a normal-size tooth and often does not erupt. Most are discovered on radiographs as incidental findings. A supernumerary tooth may or may not resemble a normal tooth in shape and position.

The most common supernumerary tooth is called the mesiodens, which is located between the maxillary central incisors at or near the midline. It is usually a small tooth with a conical crown and short roots (Figure 5-22). It may occur singly or in pairs and may be inverted when seen on a radiograph. The mesiodens can erupt or remain embedded or impacted.

The second most common supernumerary tooth is the maxillary fourth molar, which is also called a **distomolar** because it is located distal to the third molar (Figure 5-23 on p. 172). The distomolar can look like a miniature third molar or be of normal third molar size and shape. It rarely erupts into the oral cavity and is usually discovered on a radiograph.

Other supernumerary teeth include mandibular and maxillary premolars; maxillary lateral incisors; and the maxillary paramolar, a small rudimentary tooth that occurs buccal to the third molar. Erupted supernumerary teeth can cause crowding, malpositioning of adjacent teeth, or noneruption of normal teeth; therefore removal is often necessary. Nonerupted supernumerary teeth should be extracted because a risk exists for cyst development around the crown. Multiple supernumerary teeth may be a component of a syndrome such as cleidocranial dysplasia or Gardner syndrome. These syndromes are described in Chapter 6.

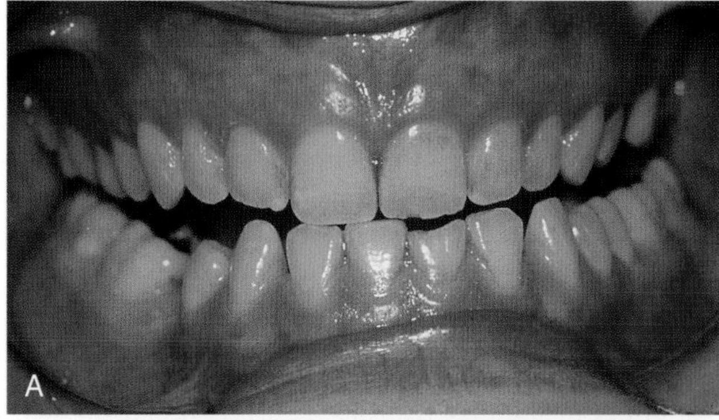

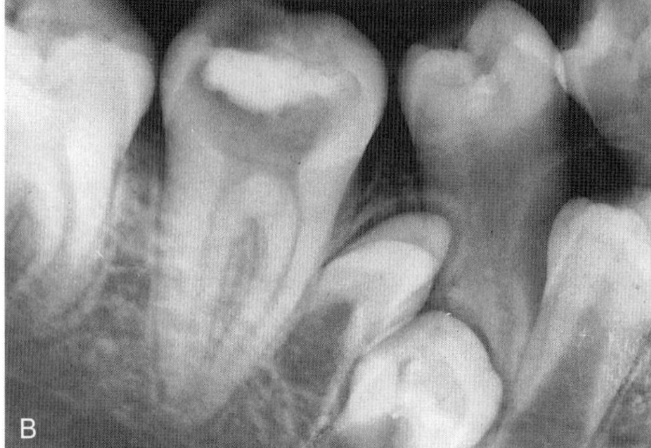

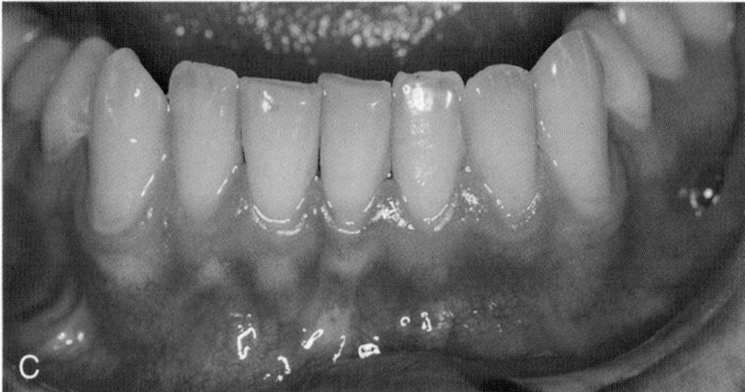

FIGURE 5-21 ■ **A,** Supernumerary teeth. This patient has four maxillary lateral incisors. **B,** Radiograph showing unerupted supernumerary teeth. **C,** Supernumerary mandibular incisor. (**A** courtesy Dr. Margot Van Dis; **B** courtesy Dr. George Blozis.)

ABNORMALITIES IN THE SIZE OF TEETH

Microdontia

Microdontia is a developmental anomaly in which one or more teeth in a dentition are smaller than normal. The term is derived from the Greek words "mikros," meaning small, and "odontos," meaning tooth. Microdontia is classified as true generalized microdontia, generalized relative microdontia, or microdontia involving a single tooth.

True generalized microdontia is seen in the pituitary dwarf and is extremely rare. All the teeth are smaller than normal. In generalized relative microdontia normal-size teeth appear small in large jaws. Heredity plays a role in generalized relative microdontia. For example, a child may inherit large jaws from one parent and normal-size teeth from the other, resulting in the illusion of small teeth. Microdontia involving a single tooth is far more common than true generalized microdontia or generalized relative microdontia. The maxillary lateral incisor and the maxillary third molar are the teeth most often affected (Figure 5-24 on p. 172). The maxillary lateral incisors often appear peg shaped, with the mesial and distal tooth surfaces converging toward the incisal edge. This "peg lateral" is smaller than normal, tends to occur bilaterally, has short roots, and is thought to be familial. The maxillary third molar microdont typically appears small but normally shaped. Microdonts are identified clinically if erupted or radiographically if unerupted. For cosmetic reasons erupted microdonts may be restored to resemble teeth of normal size and shape. Impacted microdonts should be surgically removed to prevent cyst formation.

Macrodontia

Macrodontia is an uncommon developmental anomaly in which one or more teeth in a dentition are larger than normal. The term is derived from the Greek words "makros," meaning large, and "odontos," meaning tooth. Macrodontia is classified in the same manner as microdontia: true generalized macrodontia, relative generalized macrodontia, and macrodontia involving a single tooth.

True generalized macrodontia is rare and is seen occasionally in cases of pituitary gigantism. Relative generalized macrodontia is seen in individuals with normal or slightly larger than normal teeth in small jaws and is generally caused by the patient's inheriting tooth size from one parent and jaw size from the other. Macrodontia affecting a single tooth is uncommon. Localized macrodontia affecting one side of the dental arches may be seen in a condition called **facial hemihypertrophy,** which involves the enlargement of half of the head with enlarged teeth on the involved side. No treatment is indicated for macrodontia.

ABNORMALITIES IN THE SHAPE OF TEETH

Gemination

Gemination is a developmental anomaly that occurs when a single tooth germ attempts to divide and results in the incomplete formation of two teeth. Geminate means paired or occurring in twos. The cause of this aborted twinning of a single tooth germ is unknown. Gemination is uncommon and is seen more frequently in the deciduous dentition, but occasionally it occurs in the permanent dentition. Gemination most often affects anterior teeth and is most often seen in the deciduous mandibular incisors and the permanent maxillary incisors.

Clinically gemination appears as two crowns joined together by a notched incisal area (Figure 5-25, *A* and *B* on

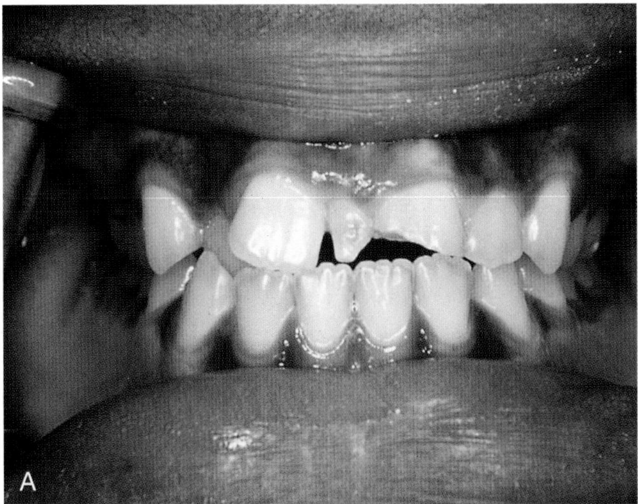

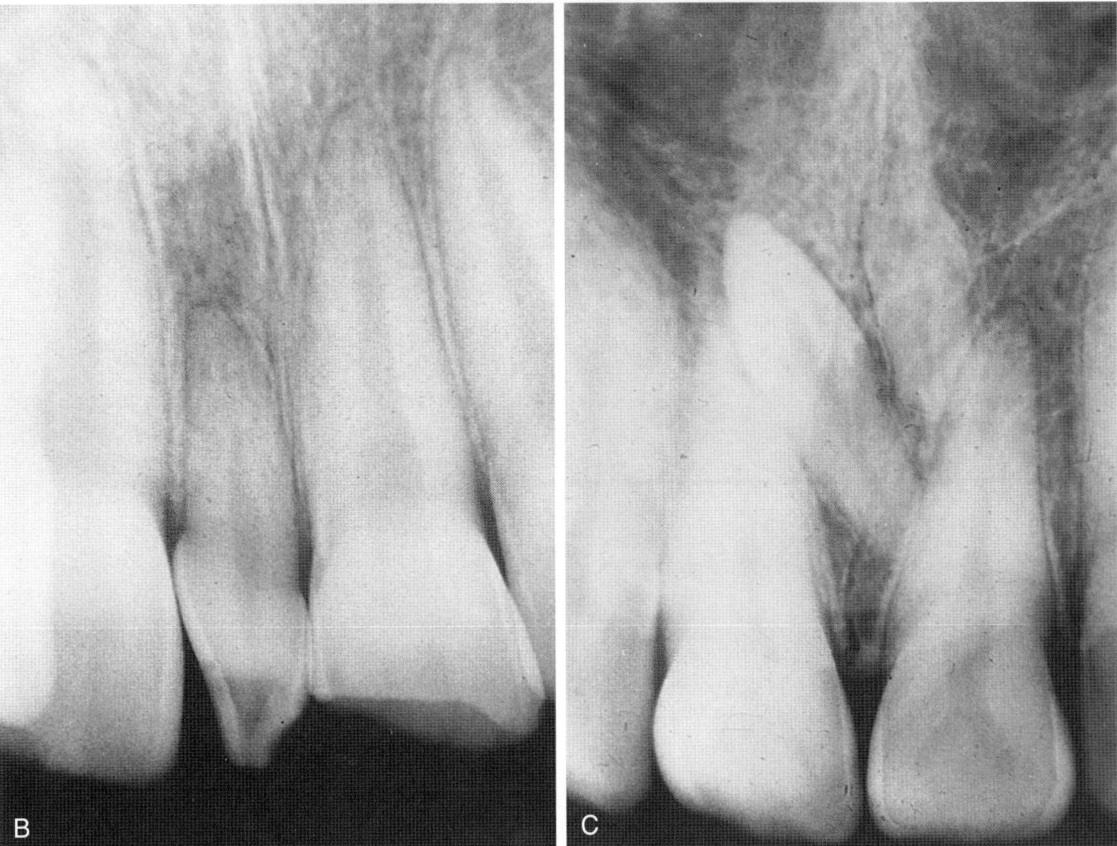

FIGURE 5-22 ■ **A,** Mesiodens seen between the maxillary central incisors. **B,** Radiograph of an erupted mesiodens. **C,** Radiograph showing a pair of inverted impacted mesiodens. (**A** and **B** courtesy Dr. George Blozis.)

p.173). Radiographically usually one single root and one common pulp canal exist (Figure 5-25, *C*). The patient has a full complement of teeth.

A geminated tooth poses an aesthetic problem, particularly when it occurs in the maxillary anterior region. It also poses a prosthetic challenge. Therefore treatment usually involves alteration of the tooth so that it resembles a normal tooth in size and shape.

Fusion

Fusion results from the union of two normally separated adjacent tooth germs. The cause of fusion is uncertain; heredity, external pressure, and crowding all have been suggested. Fusion of adjacent teeth can be complete or incomplete, depending on the stage of tooth development at the time of contact. Early contact of developing tooth germs can

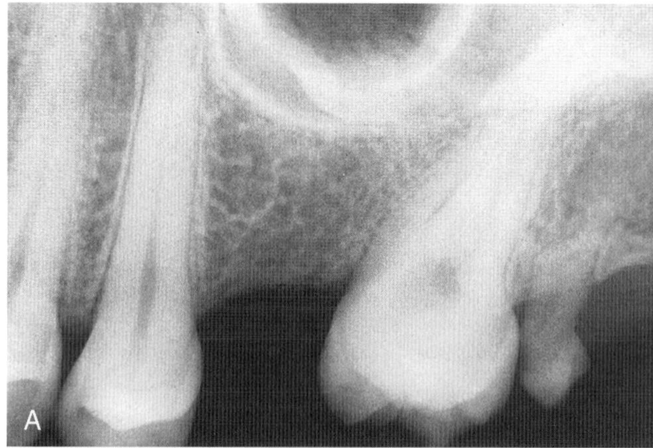

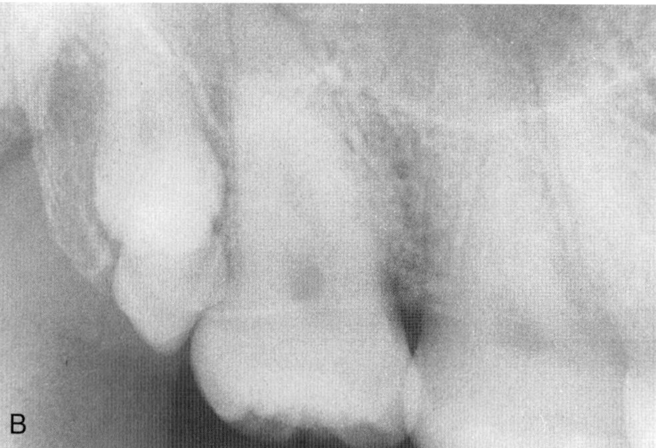

FIGURE 5-23 ■ **A,** Small erupted microdont distal to the maxillary second molar. **B,** Radiograph of a pair of distomolars located distal to the second molar. (**A** courtesy Dr. Margot Van Dis; **B** courtesy Dr. George Blozis.)

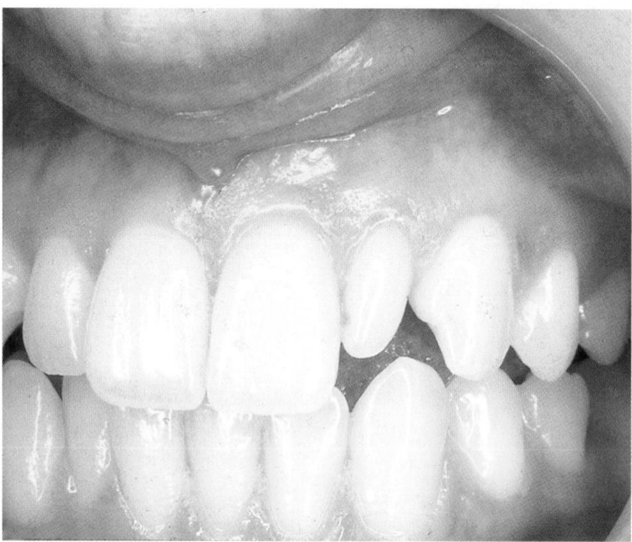

FIGURE 5-24 ■ Peg-shaped lateral incisor. (Courtesy Dr. George Blozis.)

result in a single large tooth; later contact can result in the union of crowns only or the union of roots only. True fusion always involves confluence of dentin. Fusion tends to occur in the anterior region, and the incisors are the teeth most often affected. Fusion of deciduous teeth occurs more often than fusion of permanent teeth.

Clinically fused teeth appear as a single large crown that occurs in place of two normal teeth and may exhibit an observable separation (Figure 5-26). Radiographically either separate or fused roots and root canals are seen. To differentiate fusion from gemination, the teeth must be counted. If the neighboring teeth of the tooth in question are present, the tooth is geminated; if a neighboring tooth is lacking, the tooth in question is fused. Fusion can occur between two adjacent normal teeth or between a normal tooth and a supernumerary tooth. It may be difficult to distinguish between a geminated tooth and the fusion of a normal tooth to a supernumerary tooth.

As with geminated teeth, fused teeth may present aesthetic and occlusal problems; they also pose a restorative challenge. Treatment involves alteration of the size and shape of the tooth and may involve replacement of one of the fused teeth.

Concrescence

In dentistry **concrescence** is a condition in which two adjacent teeth are united by cementum only. It is actually a form of fusion that takes place after tooth formation is complete and is usually discovered as an incidental radiographic finding (Figure 5-27). The cause of concrescence is thought to be crowding or trauma that results in the close approximation of adjacent tooth roots. Subsequent cementum deposition acts to fuse the two adjacent roots. Concrescence is most often seen in adjacent maxillary molars and adjacent supernumerary teeth and may involve erupted, unerupted, or impacted teeth.

Concrescence generally does not require treatment. If one of the teeth joined by cementum requires extraction, extraction of the fused neighbor is inevitable. However, the extraction of involved teeth is difficult, and excessive fracture of the associated alveolar bone may result.

Dilaceration

In dentistry **dilaceration** refers to an abnormal curve or angle in the root or, less frequently, the crown of a tooth (Figure 5-28 on p.175). This dental anomaly is thought to be caused by trauma to the tooth germ during root development. The position of the calcified portion of the tooth is changed, and the remainder of the tooth forms at an angle. A dilaceration can appear anywhere along the root portion of a tooth and can occur in any tooth in either the deciduous or the permanent dentition. A root dilaceration is usually discovered as an incidental radiographic finding.

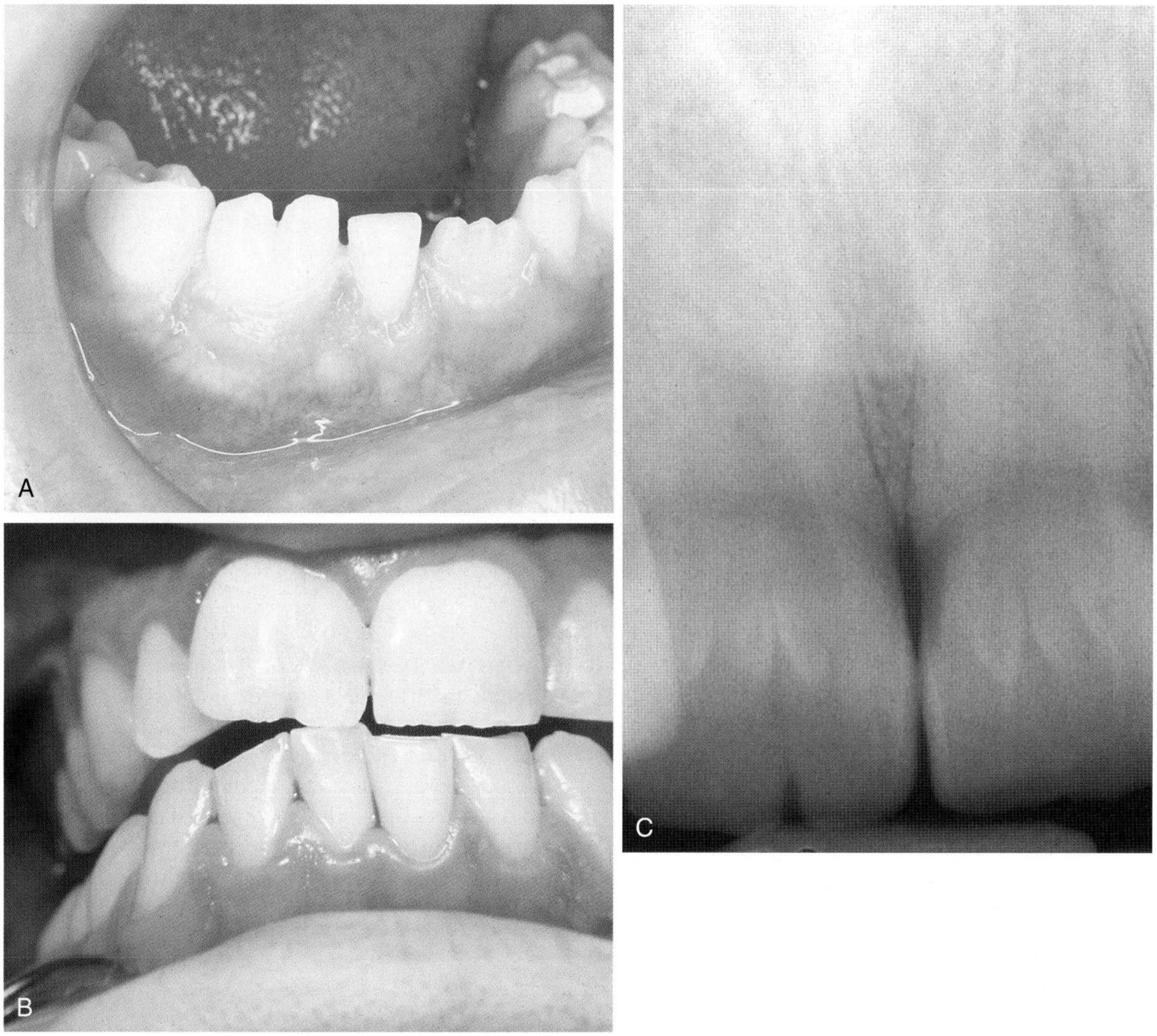

FIGURE 5-25 ■ **A,** Clinical picture of gemination in a mandibular cuspid. **B,** Gemination seen in a maxillary central incisor. **C,** Radiograph of the same maxillary central incisor. (**A** courtesy Dr. George Blozis.)

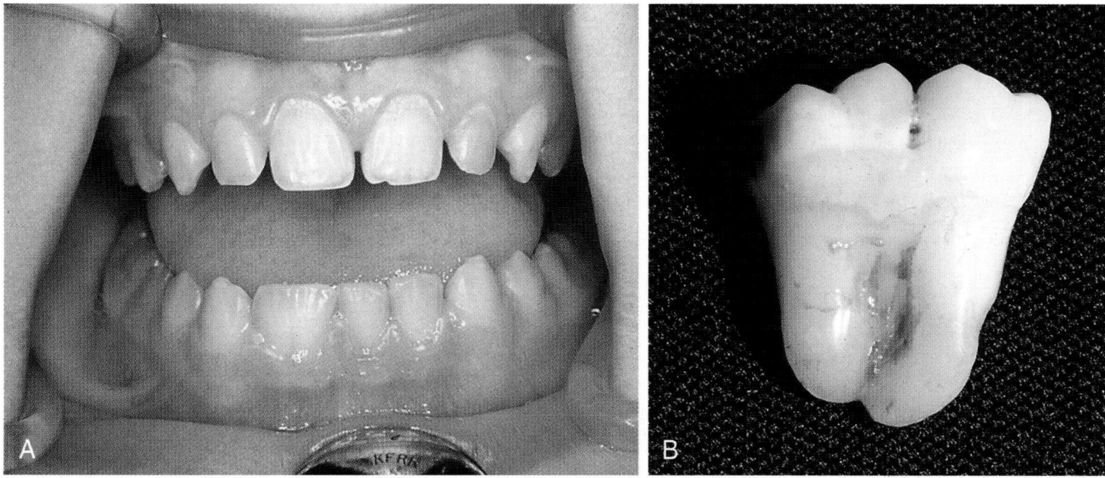

FIGURE 5-26 **A,** Clinical picture of fusion involving a permanent mandibular lateral incisor. **B,** Fusion of mandibular molars. (**A** courtesy Dr. George Blozis; **B** courtesy Dr. Rudy Melfi.)

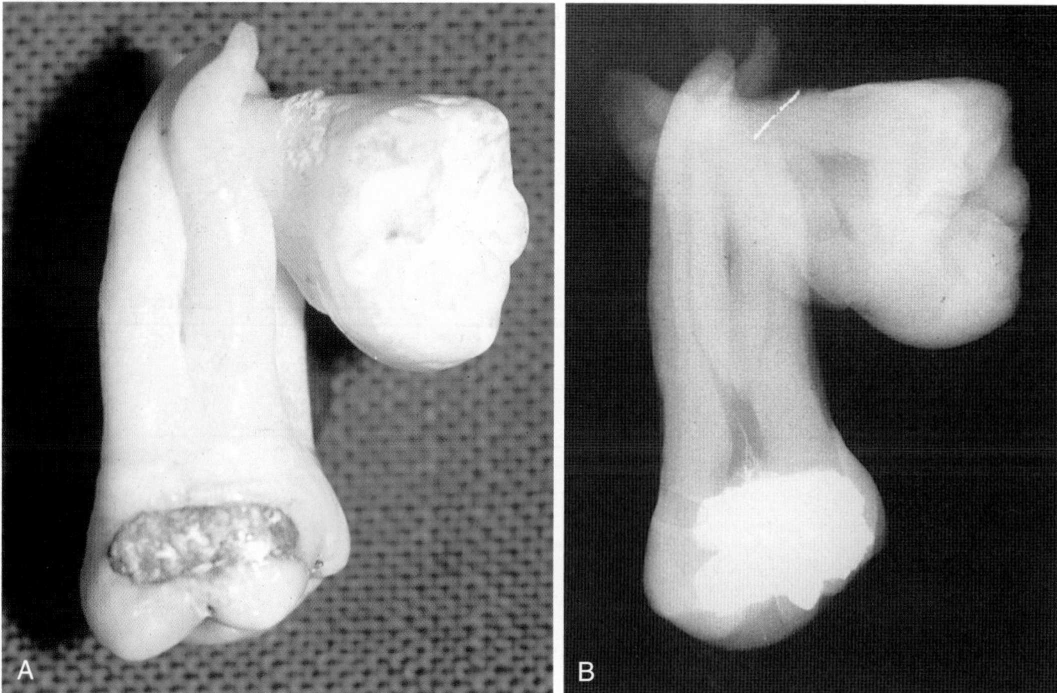

FIGURE 5-27 ■ Concrescence illustrated in a photograph **(A)** of extracted teeth and in a corresponding radiograph **(B)**. (Courtesy Dr. George Blozis.)

Dilacerations do not require treatment. However, they may cause problems if extraction or endodontic therapy becomes necessary. The importance of a preoperative radiograph is obvious.

Enamel Pearl

An **enamel pearl**, or **enameloma**, is a small, spheric enamel projection located on a root surface (Figure 5-29). This developmental anomaly is thought to occur as a result of the abnormal displacement of ameloblasts during tooth formation. The enamel pearl is usually found on maxillary molars. It is attached to cementum near the root bifurcation or trifurcation area. Occasionally it is located near the cementoenamel junction. The enamel pearl may consist of enamel only or enamel, dentin, and pulp.

The enamel pearl is an uncommon finding. It appears radiographically as a small, spheric radiopacity. Clinically the enamel pearl may be mistaken for calculus. Generally no treatment is necessary for this anomaly. Removal may be necessary if periodontal problems occur in the furcation area when an enamel pearl is present.

Talon Cusp

A **talon cusp** is an accessory cusp located in the area of the cingulum of a maxillary or mandibular permanent incisor (Figure 5-30 on p. 176). A talon is a claw of a predatory animal. The talon cusp is said to resemble an eagle's talon. It often projects lingually to the height of the incisal edge of the involved tooth. It is composed of normal enamel and dentin and contains a pulp horn. Frequently a caries-susceptible fissure is present between the cusps. Removal of the talon cusp is often indicated because it interferes with occlusion. Because of the presence of the pulp horn, endodontic therapy is necessary.

Taurodontism

Taurodontism is a term used to describe a developmental dental anomaly in which the teeth exhibit elongated, large pulp chambers and short roots (Figure 5-31). Taurodontism means "bull-like" teeth. The term was first used to describe teeth that resembled those of cud-chewing animals. Although the cause of taurodontism is uncertain, a variety of causes have been suggested, ranging from a primitive pattern of tooth development to the developmental failure of the Hertwig's epithelial root sheath to invaginate at the proper level.

Taurodontism is uncommon and seen in both the deciduous and the permanent dentitions; it usually affects a single molar tooth or several molars in the same quadrant. Taurodontism can occur unilaterally or bilaterally. The crown of the tooth appears clinically normal. A taurodont is identified by its characteristic radiographic appearance. The tooth tends to have a stretched appearance, and the pulp chamber is greatly enlarged and elongated without a constriction at the cementoenamel junction. The roots appear short, with the furcation located near the apices. No treatment is indicated for taurodontism.

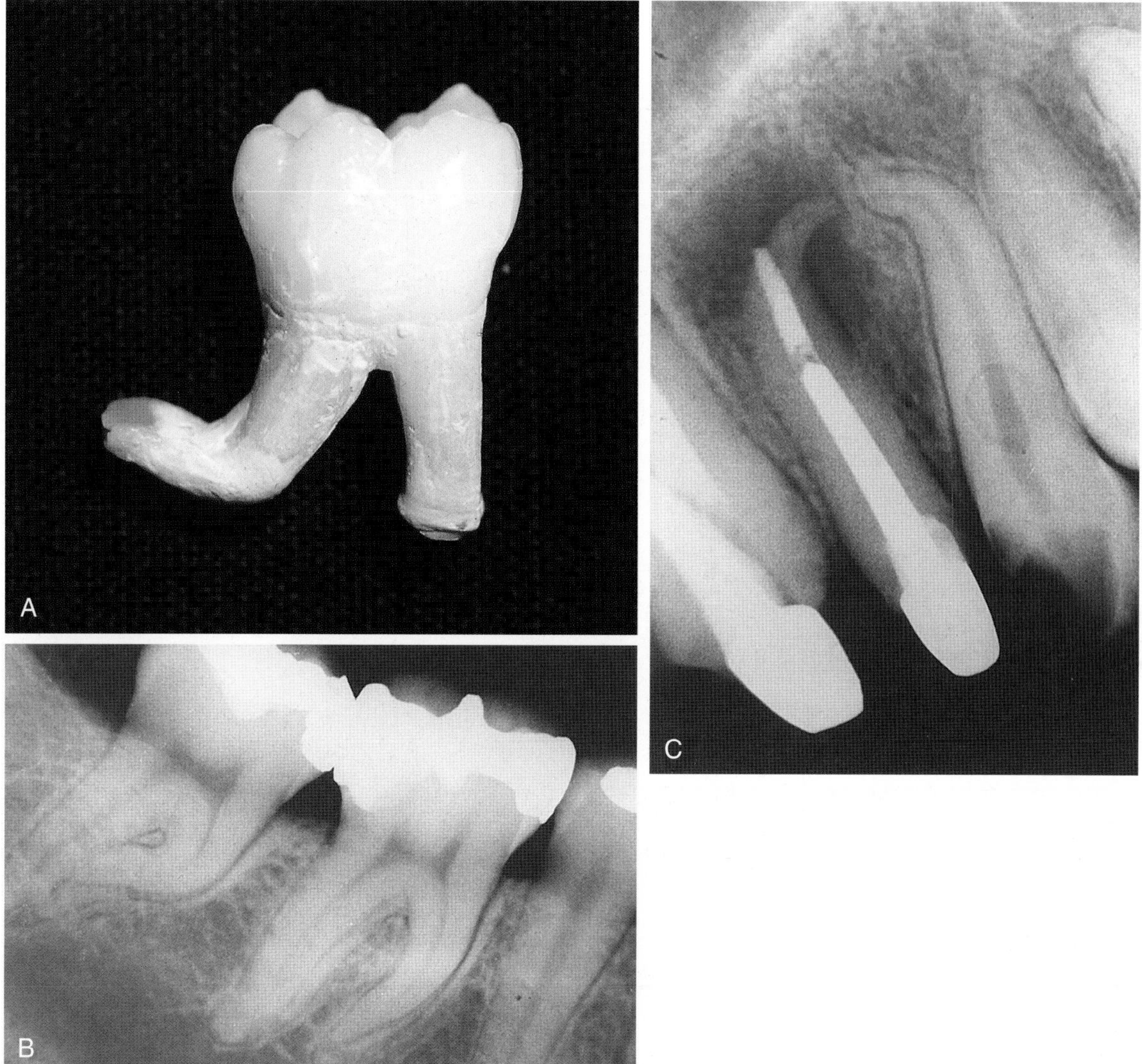

FIGURE 5-28 ■ **A,** Dilaceration on the distal root of an extracted tooth. **B,** Mesial root dilaceration on a mandibular second molar. **C,** Radiograph of root dilaceration in maxillary lateral and cuspid. (**A** courtesy Dr. Rudy Melfi.)

Dens in Dente

Dens in dente, also called **dens invaginatus,** is a developmental anomaly that results when the enamel organ invaginates into the crown of a tooth before mineralization (Figure 5-32 on p. 177). **Invaginate** means that one portion infolds into another portion of a structure. Radiographically a toothlike structure appears within the involved tooth. An elongated bulb or pear-shaped mass of enamel is seen in dentin surrounding a radiolucent area; hence the name *dens in dente,* or "tooth within a tooth." This defect typically is confined to the coronal third of the tooth, but in some cases it extends to include the entire root length. Clinically the dens in dente may appear as either a normally shaped or malformed crown that exhibits a deep pit or crevice in the area of the cingulum. The invaginated toothlike structure retains a communication with the outside of the tooth via the pit or crevice visible on the crown surface.

Dens in dente customarily affects a single tooth. Anterior teeth, particularly the maxillary and mandibular incisors, are more commonly affected than the posterior teeth. The maxillary lateral incisor is the most frequently affected tooth, and when affected it is often peg shaped.

The dens in dente is vulnerable to caries, pulpal infection, and necrosis as a result of the communication between the oral cavity and the invaginated area of the tooth. Consequently the dens in dente is often nonvital and is seen in association with a periapical lesion (periapical cyst, periapical granuloma, periapical abscess). If the dens in dente is detected shortly after eruption, a prophylactic restoration can be placed in the deep pit or crevice to prevent caries and subsequent pulpal necrosis. A nonvital dens in dente may be treated endodontically. A malformed crown can be restored with composite materials or a full-coverage crown.

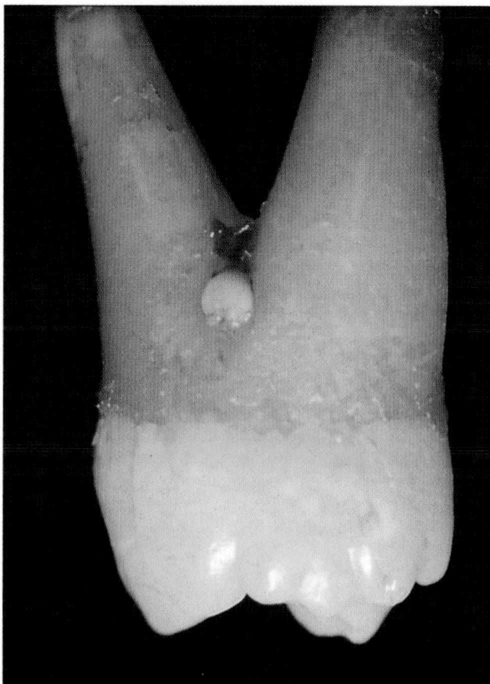

FIGURE 5-29 ■ Enamel pearl in the furcation area. (Courtesy Dr. Rudy Melfi.)

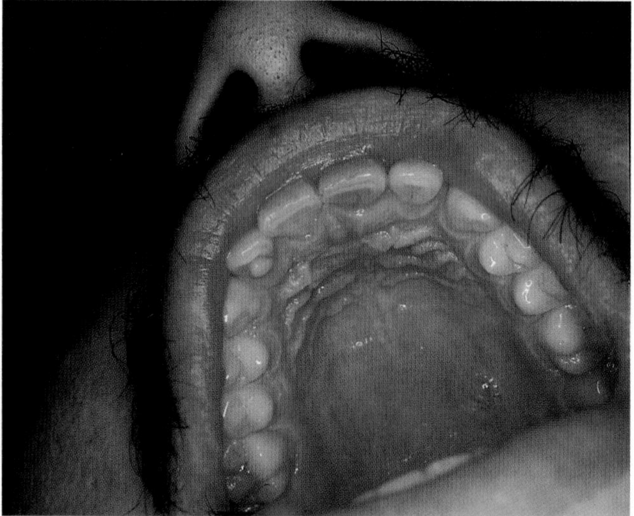

FIGURE 5-30 ■ Talon cusp on the lingual aspect of the maxillary right lateral permanent incisor.

Dens Evaginatus

Dens evaginatus is an accessory enamel cusp found on the occlusal tooth surface (Figure 5-33). This is a rare developmental anomaly that occurs most often on the mandibular premolars. When affected, they are called tuberculated premolars. Molars, cuspids, and incisors can also be affected. Dens evaginatus is thought to result from the proliferation and outpouching of enamel epithelium during tooth development.

Clinically the dens evaginatus appears as a small, rounded nodule on the occlusal surface of a mandibular premolar between the buccal and lingual cusps. A pulp horn may extend into this extra cusp. The dens evaginatus may not require treatment. However, it can cause occlusal problems, and removal may be necessary. Occlusal wear or fracture of this accessory cusp may result in pulp exposure, and endodontic treatment may be necessary.

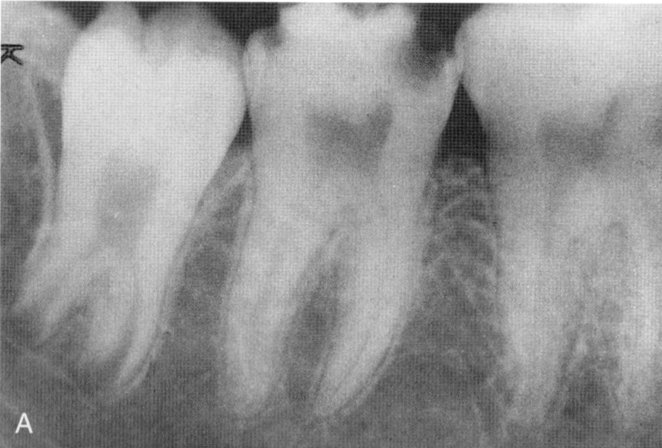

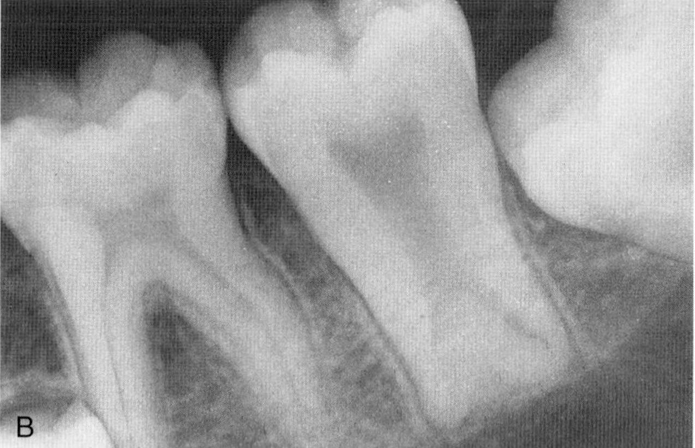

FIGURE 5-31 ■ **A,** Taurodont in the mandibular third molar. **B,** Taurodont in the mandibular second molar. (**A** courtesy Dr. Margot Van Dis; **B** courtesy Dr. George Blozis.)

Supernumerary Roots

Supernumerary roots (extra roots) can involve any tooth (Figure 5-34). No cause for this developmental anomaly has been identified. External pressure, trauma, and metabolic dysfunction during root development have been suggested. Supernumerary roots are not uncommon and tend to occur in teeth that exhibit root formation after birth. The multirooted teeth most often affected are the maxillary and mandibular third molars. The single-rooted teeth most often affected are the mandibular bicuspids and cuspids. Supernumerary roots may exhibit dilaceration and are diagnosed radiographically.

Generally no treatment is indicated for supernumerary roots. However, they become clinically significant if extraction of the involved tooth or endodontic therapy becomes necessary.

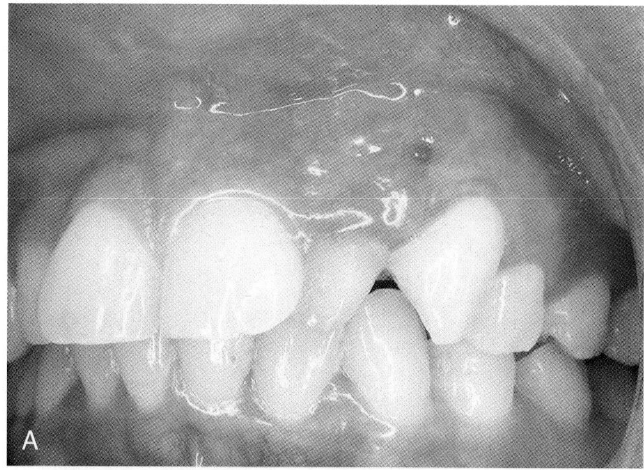

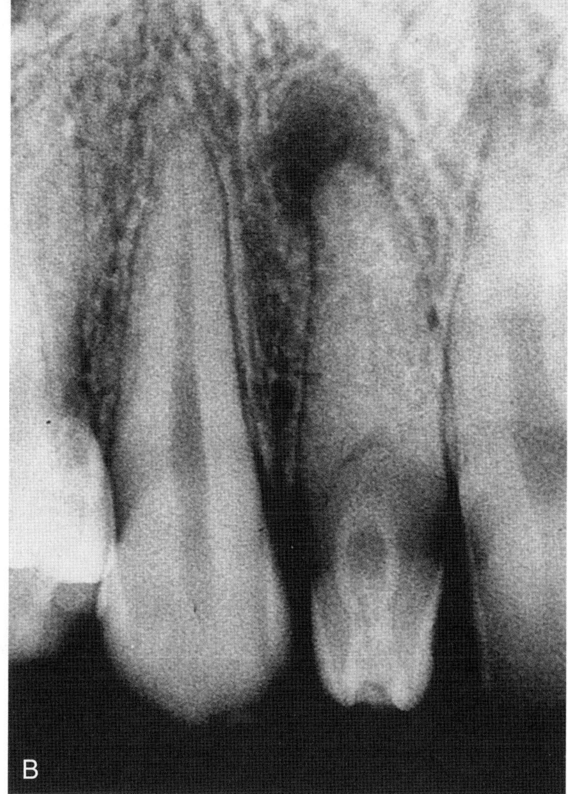

FIGURE 5-32 ■ **A,** Clinical illustration of dens in dente in maxillary lateral incisor. **B,** Radiograph of dens in dente in maxillary lateral incisor. (**A** courtesy Dr. George Blozis.)

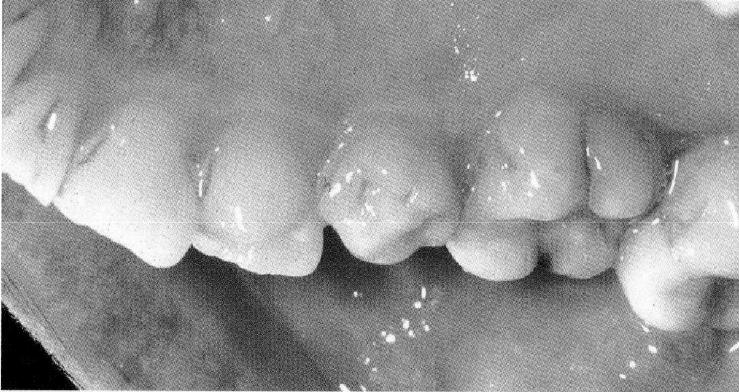

FIGURE 5-33 ■ Dens evaginatus of maxillary premolar. (Courtesy Dr. Margot Van Dis.)

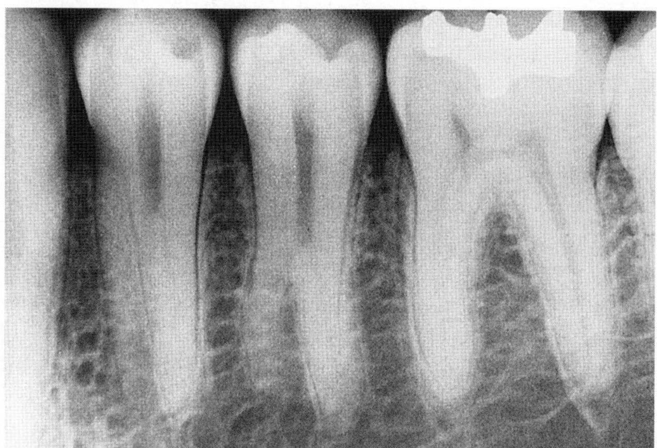

FIGURE 5-34 ■ Supernumerary roots in mandibular premolars.

ABNORMALITIES OF TOOTH STRUCTURE

Enamel Hypoplasia

Enamel hypoplasia is the incomplete or defective formation of enamel, resulting in the alteration of tooth form or color. **Hypoplasia** is defined as the incomplete development of an organ or tissue. Enamel hypoplasia results from a disturbance of or damage to ameloblasts during enamel matrix formation. Enamel hypoplasia can affect either the deciduous or the permanent dentition.

Numerous factors can cause enamel hypoplasia:

- Amelogenesis imperfecta
- Febrile illness (measles, chickenpox, scarlet fever)
- Vitamin deficiency (vitamins A, C, D)
- Local infection of a deciduous tooth
- Ingestion of fluoride
- Congenital syphilis
- Birth injury, premature birth
- Idiopathic factors

Enamel hypoplasia that is inherited is called **amelogenesis imperfecta** (see Chapter 6). The factors that cause enamel hypoplasia by injuring the sensitive ameloblasts during enamel formation are discussed in this chapter.

Enamel Hypoplasia Caused by Febrile Illness or Vitamin Deficiency

Ameloblasts are one of the most sensitive cell groups in the body. It is believed that any serious systemic disease or severe nutritional deficiency is capable of producing enamel hypoplasia. Febrile illnesses (measles, chickenpox, and scarlet fever) and vitamin deficiencies (vitamins A, C, and D) that

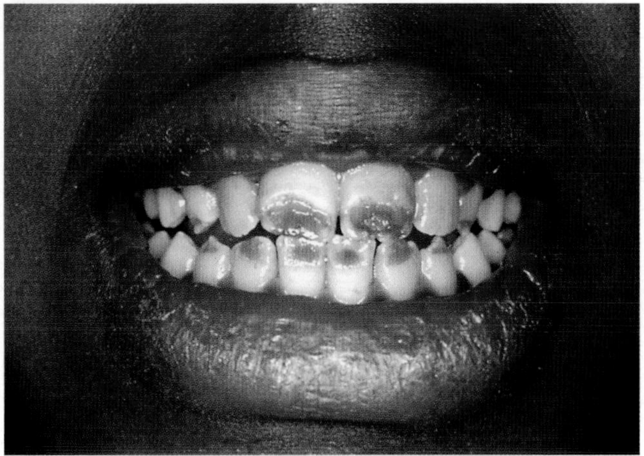

FIGURE 5-35 ■ Enamel hypoplasia. In this patient the enamel hypoplasia follows a pattern that is suggestive of a systemic problem such as a high fever.

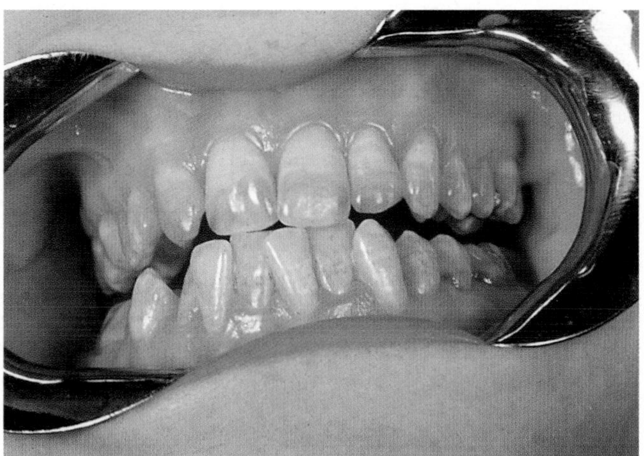

FIGURE 5-36 ■ Mottled enamel. The discoloration of the enamel in this patient occurred as a result of high fluoride intake.

occur during the time of tooth formation can result in a type of enamel hypoplasia characterized by pitting of the enamel. Only the crowns of teeth that are developing at the time of the febrile illness or vitamin deficiency are affected.

This type of hypoplasia usually involves the permanent central incisors, laterals, cuspids, and first molars, which are the teeth that form during the first year of life. One or more horizontal rows of tiny, deep pits are seen traversing the affected tooth surface. The number and rows of pits may vary, depending on the extent and severity of injury to the ameloblasts. These enamel pits tend to stain and appear unsightly (Figure 5-35).

Teeth affected with enamel hypoplasia of the pitting type may be restored with composites during childhood and later with porcelain veneers or full-crown coverage.

Enamel Hypoplasia Resulting from Local Infection or Trauma

Enamel hypoplasia of a permanent tooth may result from infection of a deciduous tooth. A single tooth is usually affected and is referred to as a **Turner tooth.** A carious deciduous tooth with periapical involvement can disturb the ameloblasts of the underlying permanent tooth. The severity of the defect depends on the severity of the deciduous tooth infection, the degree of periapical tissue involvement, and the stage of development of the underlying permanent tooth.

The teeth most often affected are the permanent maxillary incisors and the permanent mandibular premolars. The clinical appearance of the affected tooth depends on the extent of the injury. The color of the enamel of these teeth may range from yellow to brown, or severe pitting and deformity may be involved. These enamel defects can frequently be identified radiographically before the eruption of the involved tooth. An anterior Turner tooth may be restored to provide an improved aesthetic appearance; a posterior Turner tooth may require a restoration to provide improved function.

Enamel Hypoplasia Resulting from Fluoride Ingestion

Enamel hypoplasia resulting from fluoride ingestion, or **dental fluorosis**, occurs as a result of the patient ingesting high concentrations of fluoride during tooth formation, usually in drinking water. Affected teeth exhibit a mottled discoloration of enamel (Figure 5-36). Mottling refers to irregular areas of discoloration. The more fluoride ingested, the more severe the mottling. The optimum range of fluoride is 0.7 to 1.2 parts fluoride/million gallons of water. Ingestion of water with a fluoride concentration two to three times the recommended amount results in mild fluorosis that appears as white flecks and chalky opaque areas of enamel.

Ingestion of water containing four times the recommended amount of fluoride causes brown or black staining and a pitted or overall corroded enamel appearance.

All permanent teeth are involved in this type of enamel hypoplasia. The teeth affected by fluorosis are generally decay resistant. To improve the aesthetic appearance of these teeth, bleaching, bonding, composites, porcelain veneers, or full-coverage crowns can be used.

Enamel Hypoplasia Resulting from Congenital Syphilis

Syphilis is a contagious sexually transmitted disease caused by the spirochete *Treponema pallidum.* It is described in detail in Chapter 4. **Congenital syphilis** is transmitted from an infected mother to her fetus via the placenta. Children with congenital syphilis have numerous developmental anomalies and may be blind, deaf, or paralyzed. In utero infection by *T. pallidum* results in enamel hypoplasia of the permanent incisors and first molars. This is so rare that a lengthy discussion is not warranted.

The affected incisors are shaped like screwdrivers: broad cervically and narrow incisally, with a notched incisal edge

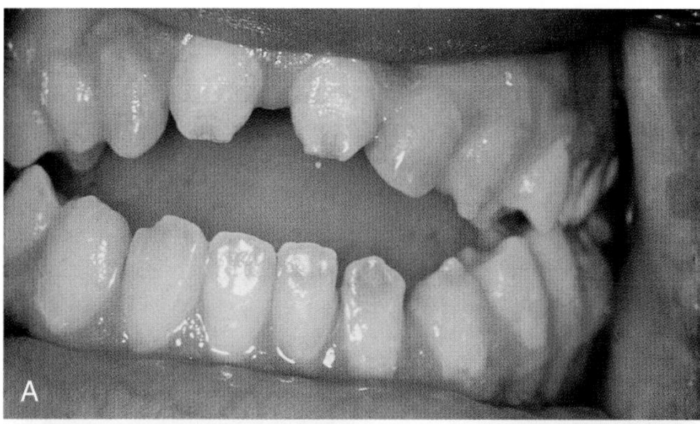

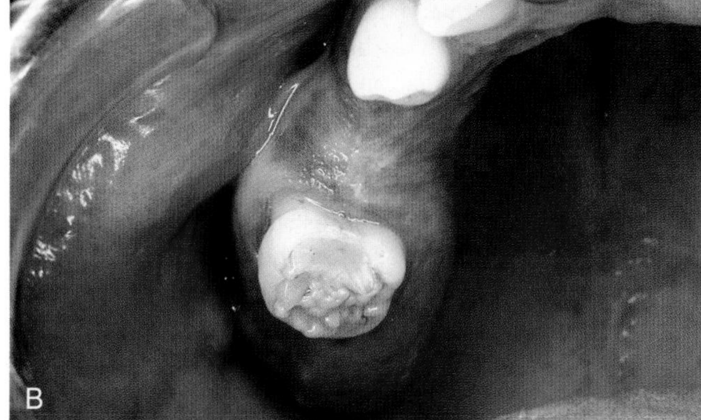

FIGURE 5-37 ■ **A,** Hutchinson incisors. **B,** Mulberry molars. (Courtesy Dr. George Blozis.)

(Figure 5-37, *A*). They are called **Hutchinson incisors.** First molars appear as irregularly shaped crowns made up of multiple tiny globules of enamel instead of cusps (Figure 5-37, *B*). Because of their berrylike appearance, these molars are called **mulberry molars.** Not every case of congenital syphilis exhibits these dental findings, and similarly shaped teeth may be seen in individuals without congenital syphilis.

Treatment to improve the aesthetic appearance of these teeth includes full-coverage crowns.

Enamel Hypoplasia Resulting from Birth Injury, Premature Birth, or Idiopathic Factors

Enamel hypoplasia can occur as a result of trauma or change of environment at the time of birth or in premature infants. In addition, many cases of enamel hypoplasia do not have an identifiable cause despite careful and thorough history taking. The ameloblast is a sensitive cell that is easily damaged. For this reason even a mild illness or systemic problem can result in enamel hypoplasia. Such illnesses may be so insignificant that they are not known to the patient or remembered by the patient's parents. To improve the aesthetic appearance of these teeth, composites, porcelain veneers, or full-coverage crowns can be used.

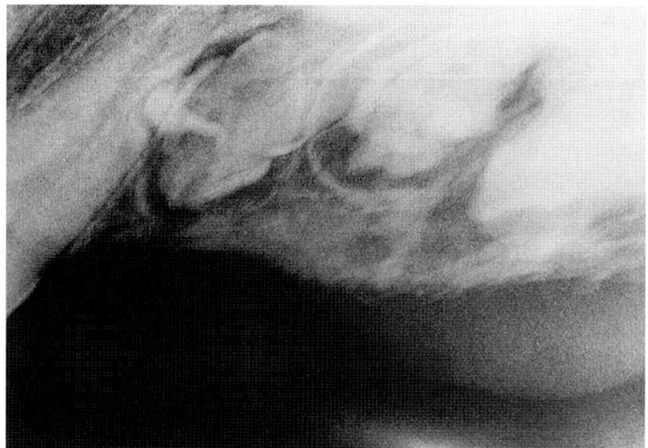

FIGURE 5-38 ■ Regional odontodysplasia.

Enamel Hypocalcification

Enamel hypocalcification is a developmental anomaly that results in a disturbance of the maturation of the enamel matrix. It usually appears as a localized, chalky white spot on the middle third of smooth crowns. The underlying enamel may be soft and susceptible to caries. The cause of enamel hypocalcification is uncertain; however, trauma during the maturation of enamel matrix has been suggested. Bleaching, composites, porcelain veneers, or full-coverage crowns can be used to improve the aesthetic appearance of these teeth.

Endogenous Staining of Teeth

Endogenous or **intrinsic staining of teeth** occurs as a result of the deposition of substances circulating systemically during tooth development. For example, ingestion of tetracycline during tooth development causes a yellowish-green discoloration of dentin that is visible through the enamel. At the time of eruption the teeth fluoresce under ultraviolet light. Later the tetracycline is oxidized, the color changes from yellowish to brown, and the teeth no longer fluoresce. Other conditions such as rhesus (Rh) incompatibility (erythroblastosis fetalis), neonatal liver disease, and congenital porphyria (an inherited metabolic disease) also cause endogenous staining of teeth.

Regional Odontodysplasia

Regional odontodysplasia, or **ghost teeth,** is an unusual developmental problem in which one or several teeth in the same quadrant radiographically exhibit a marked reduction in radiodensity and a characteristic ghostlike appearance (Figure 5-38). Very thin enamel and dentin are present. Occasionally the enamel is not visible on the radiograph. The pulp chambers of these teeth are extremely large. Either the teeth do not erupt, or eruption is incomplete. If ghost teeth erupt into the oral cavity, they are typically nonfunctional and malformed.

Regional odontodysplasia can affect either the deciduous or the permanent dentition. The maxilla, especially the anterior maxilla, is more often involved than the mandible. The cause of regional odontodysplasia is unknown. A vascular phenomenon has been suggested. Extraction usually is the treatment of choice for ghost teeth.

ABNORMALITIES OF TOOTH ERUPTION

Impacted and Embedded Teeth

Impacted teeth are teeth that cannot erupt because of a physical obstruction. **Embedded teeth** are those that do not erupt because of a lack of eruptive force. An impacted tooth is one of the most common developmental defects occurring in humans. Any tooth can be impacted. The most commonly impacted teeth are the maxillary and mandibular third molars, the maxillary cuspids, the maxillary and mandibular premolars, and supernumerary teeth. Impacted teeth are identified radiographically (Figure 5-39).

Third molar impactions are classified according to the position of the tooth: mesioangular, distoangular, vertical, and horizontal. The most common position of an impacted third molar is mesioangular. The crown of the third molar points in a mesial direction and is in contact with the second molar, which is preventing its eruption. In a distoangular impaction the crown of the third molar points in a distal direction toward the ramus, and the roots of the impacted tooth are adjacent to the distal root of the second molar. In a vertical impaction the crown of the third molar is in a normal position for eruption, but eruption is prevented by the distal aspect of the second molar or by the anterior border of the ramus. In a horizontal impaction the crown of the third molar is seen in a horizontal position relative to the inferior border of the mandible.

Teeth can be completely impacted in bone with no communication with the oral cavity, or they can be partially impacted. In a partial impaction the tooth lies partly in soft tissue and partly in bone. Partially impacted teeth often have a communication with the oral cavity and are susceptible to infections (see Pericoronitis, Chapter 4). For unknown reasons some completely impacted teeth undergo resorption. This resorption usually begins in the crown portion of the tooth, and the tooth is slowly replaced by bone. Radiographically this resorption should not be confused with caries. Caries of an impacted tooth is impossible unless communication with the oral cavity occurs.

Impacted teeth are surgically removed to prevent odontogenic cyst and tumor formation or damage (resorption) to adjacent teeth or because the bone (in some cases) may be more susceptible to fracture. Partially impacted third molars are removed to prevent infections. Studies have shown that the optimal time to extract impacted third molars is between the ages of 12 and 24 years. With increased age a greater incidence of nerve paresthesia exists.

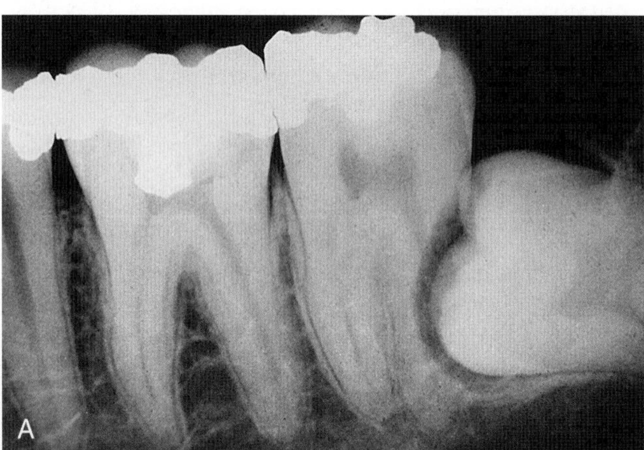

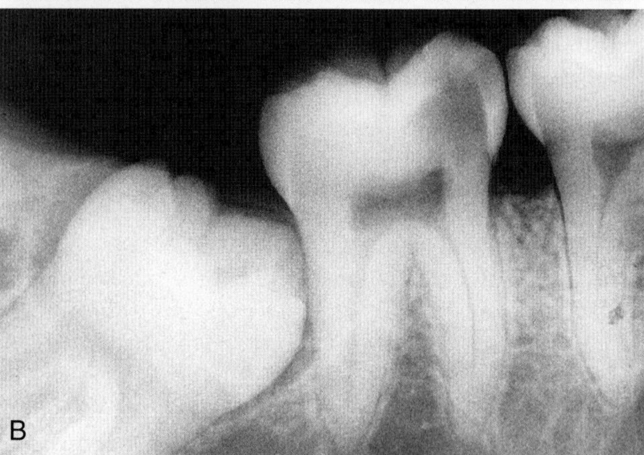

FIGURE 5-39 ■ **A,** Horizontal impaction of the third molar. **B,** Mesioangular impaction of the third molar.

Ankylosed Teeth

Ankylosed (or submerged) **teeth** are deciduous teeth in which bone has fused to cementum and dentin, preventing exfoliation of the deciduous tooth and eruption of the underlying permanent tooth (Figure 5-40). Deciduous molars are most often affected by ankylosis. The cause is unknown;

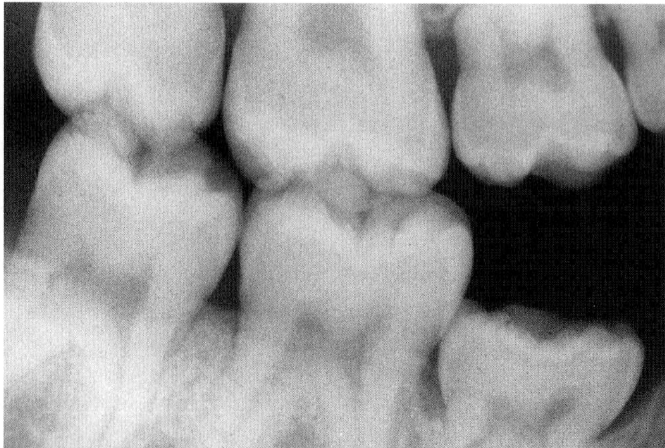

FIGURE 5-40 ■ Ankylosis of deciduous molar. (Courtesy Dr. Margot Van Dis.)

trauma and infection of the periodontal ligament have been suggested.

Initially the tooth erupts into the oral cavity into normal occlusion. The ankylosed tooth is not exfoliated. When the permanent teeth erupt, those adjacent to the ankylosed tooth have taller occlusocervical heights. Compared with the adjacent teeth, the ankylosed tooth appears submerged and has a different, more solid sound when percussed.

The presence of an ankylosed tooth is usually suspected on the basis of the clinical appearance and is confirmed radiographically. The periodontal ligament space is lacking or indistinct because of the union of bone and cementum, and the tooth usually exhibits root resorption. Ankylosis may be seen in permanent teeth that have been avulsed and reimplanted.

Extraction of ankylosed deciduous teeth is necessary to allow eruption of the underlying permanent tooth. Extraction of ankylosed permanent teeth is often necessary to prevent malocclusion, caries, and periodontal disease.

Selected References

Books

Alley KE, Melfi RC: *Permar's oral embryology and microscopic anatomy,* ed 10, Baltimore, 2000, Lippincott, Williams & Wilkins.

Darby M: *Mosby's comprehensive review of dental hygiene,* ed 6, St Louis, 2006, Mosby.

Langlais RP, Miller CS: *Color atlas of common oral diseases,* ed 3, Baltimore, 2003, Lippincott, Williams & Wilkins.

Miller BF: *Miller-Keane encyclopedia and dictionary of medicine, nursing, and allied health—revised reprint,* ed 7, Philadelphia, 2005, Saunders.

Neville BW, Damm DD, Allen CM: *Oral and maxillofacial pathology,* ed 3, St. Louis, 2009, Saunders.

Regezi JA, Sciubba JJ, Jordan RCK: *Oral pathology: clinical-pathologic correlations,* ed 5, St Louis, 2008, Saunders.

Regezi JA, Sciubba JJ, Pogrel MA: *Atlas of oral and maxillofacial pathology,* Philadelphia, 2000, Saunders.

Scheid RC: *Woelfel's dental anatomy: its relevance to dentistry,* ed 7, Baltimore, 2007, Lippincott, Williams & Wilkins.

Journal Articles

Alexander WN, Lilly GE, Irby WB: Odontodysplasia, *Oral Surg* 22:814, 1966.

Alfors E, Larson A, Sjögren S: The odontogenic keratocyst: a benign cystic tumor? *J Oral Maxillofac Surg* 42:10, 1984.

Al-Talabani NG, Smith CJ: Experimental dentigerous cysts and enamel hypoplasia: their possible significance in explaining the pathogenesis of dentigerous cysts, *J Oral Pathol* 9:82, 1980.

Baker BR: Pits of the lip commissures in Caucasoid males, *Oral Surg* 21:56, 1966.

Barker GR: A radiolucency of the ascending ramus of the mandible associated with invested parotid salivary gland material and analogous with a Stafne bone cavity, *Br J Oral Maxillofac Surg* 26:81, 1988.

Baum BJ, Cohen MM: Patterns of size reduction in hypodontia, *J Dent Res* 50:779, 1971.

Bodin I, Julin P, Thomsson M: Hyperdontia III: supernumerary anterior teeth, *Dentomaxillofac Radiol* 10:35, 1981.

Bodin I, Julin P, Thomsson M: Hyperdontia IV: supernumerary premolars, *Dentomaxillofac Radiol* 19:99, 1981.

Brannon RB: The odontogenic keratocyst—a clinicopathologic study of 312 cases. I. Clinical features, *Oral Surg* 42:54, 1976.

Brannon RB: The odontogenic keratocyst—a clinicopathologic study of 312 cases. II. Histologic features, *Oral Surg* 43:233, 1977.

Buchner A, Hansen LS: Lymphoepithelial cysts of the oral cavity: a clinicopathologic study of 38 cases, *Oral Surg* 50:441, 1980.

Burton DJ, Saffos RO, Scheffer RB: Multiple bilateral dens in dente as a factor in the etiology of multiple periapical lesions, *Oral Surg* 49:496, 1980.

Carter L, Carney Y, Perez-Pudlewski D: Lateral periodontal cyst: multifactorial analysis of a previously unreported series, *Oral Surg Oral Med Oral Pathol Oral Radiol Endod* 81:210, 1996.

Cavanha AO: Enamel pearls, *Oral Surg* 19:373, 1965.

Christ TF: The globulomaxillary cyst—an embryologic misconception, *Oral Surg Oral Med Oral Pathol* 30:515, 1970.

Conklin WW: Bilateral dens invaginatus in the mandibular incisor region, *Oral Surg* 45:905, 1978.

Dachi SF, Howell FV: A survey of 3874 routine full-mouth radiographs. II. A study of impacted teeth, *Oral Surg* 14:1165, 1961.

Darling AI, Levers BGH: Submerged human deciduous molars and ankylosis, *Arch Oral Biol* 18:1021, 1973.

Dean HT, Arnold FA: Endemic dental fluorosis or mottled teeth, *J Am Dent Assoc* 30:1278, 1943.

Dehlers FAC, Lee KW, Lee EC: Dens evaginatus (evaginated odontoma), *Dent Pract* 17:239, 1967.

Delany GM, Goldblatt LI: Fused teeth: a multidisciplinary approach to treatment, *J Am Dent Assoc* 103:732, 1981.

DiFiore PM, Hartwell GR: Median mandibular lateral periodontal cysts, *Oral Surg Oral Med Oral Pathol* 63:545, 1987.

Eisenbud LE et al: Aneurysmal bone cyst of the mandible, *Oral Surg Oral Med Oral Pathol* 64:202, 1987.

el-Mofty SK, Shannon MT, Mustoe TA: Lymph node metastasis in spindle cell carcinoma arising in an odontogenic cyst, *Oral Surg Oral Med Oral Pathol* 71:209, 1991.

Everett FG, Wescott WB: Commissural lip pits, *Oral Surg* 14:202, 1961.

Fantasia JE: Lateral periodontal cyst: an analysis of 46 cases, *Oral Surg* 48:237, 1979.

Freedman PD, Lumerman H, Gee JK: Calcifying odontogenic cyst, *Oral Surg* 40:93, 1975.

Gardner DG: An evaluation of reported cases of median mandibular cysts, *Oral Surg Oral Med Oral Pathol* 65:208, 1988.

Gardner DG: The dentinal changes in regional odontodysplasia, *Oral Surg* 38:887, 1974.

Gardner DG, Girgis SS: Taurodontism, shovel-shaped incisors and the Klinefelter syndrome, *J Can Dent Assoc* 8:372, 1978.

Gardner DG, Sapp JP: Regional odontodysplasia, *Oral Surg* 35:351, 1973.

Grahnen H, Granath LE: Numerical variations in primary dentition, *Odontol Revy* 12:342, 1961.

Grahnen H, Larsson PG: Enamel defects in deciduous dentition of prematurely born children, *Odontol Rev* 9:143, 1958.

Hamner JE III, Witko CJ, Metro PS: Taurodontism: report of a case, *Oral Surg* 18:409, 1964.

Henderson HZ: Ankylosis of primary molars: a clinical, radiographic, and histologic study, *J Dent Child* 46:117, 1979.

Hernandez GA et al: Aneurysmal bone cyst versus hemangioma of the mandible, *Oral Surg Oral Med Oral Pathol* 76:790, 1993.

Holt RD, Brook AH: Taurodontism: a criterion for diagnosis and its prevalence in mandibular first molars in a sample of 1115 British school children, *J Int Assoc Dent Child* 10:41, 1979.

Howell RE et al: CEA immunoreactivity in odontogenic tumors and keratocysts, *Oral Surg Oral Med Oral Pathol* 66:576, 1988.

Jasmin J, Ionesco-Benaiche N, Muller M: Latent fluorides: report of a case, *J Dent Child* 62:220, 1995.

Keith A: Problems relating to the teeth of the earlier forms of prehistoric man, *Proc R Soc Med* 6(part 3):103, 1913.

Kelly JR: Gemination, fusion, or both? *Oral Surg* 45:326, 1978.

King RC, Smith BR, Burk JL: Dermoid cyst in the floor of the mouth, *Oral Surg Oral Med Oral Pathol* 78:567, 1994.

Kitchin PC: Dens in dente, *J Dent Res* 15:1176, 1935.

Krolls SO, Donalhue AH: Double-rooted maxillary primary canines, *Oral Surg* 49:379, 1980.

Leamas R, Jimenez-Planas A: Taurodontism in premolars, *Oral Surg Oral Med Oral Pathol* 75:501, 1993.

Mathewson RJ, Siegel MJ, McCanna DL: Ankyloglossia: a review of the literature and a case report, *J Dent Child* 33:238, 1966.

Maurette PE, Jorge J, deMoraes M: Conservative treatment protocol of the odontogenic keratocyst. *J.Oral and Maxillofacial Surg* 64:379-383, 2006.

Mellor JK, Ripa LW: Talon cusp: a clinically significant anomaly, *Oral Surg* 29:224, 1970.

Milazzo A, Alexander SA: Fusion, gemination, oligodontia and taurodontism, *J Pedodontics* 6:194, 1982.

Mlynarczyk G: Enamel pitting: a common symptom of tuberous sclerosis, *Oral Surg Oral Med Oral Pathol* 71:63, 1991.

Morningstar CH: Effect of infection of deciduous molar on the permanent tooth germ, *J Am Dent Assoc* 24:786, 1937.

Partridge M, Towers JF: The primordial cyst (odontogenic keratocyst): its tumor-like characteristics and behavior, *Br J Oral Maxillofac Surg* 25:271, 1987.

Pendrys DG: Dental fluorosis in perspective, *J Am Dent Assoc* 122:63, 1991.

Ray GE: Congenital absence of permanent teeth, *Br Dent J* 90:213, 1951.

Reaume CE, Sofie VL: Lingual thyroid: review of the literature and a report of a case, *Oral Surg* 45:841, 1978.

Redman RS: Respiratory epithelium in an apical periodontal cyst of the mandible, *Oral Surg Oral Med Oral Pathol* 67:77, 1989.

Rushton MA: Invaginated teeth (dens in dente): contents of the invagination, *Oral Surg* 11:1378, 1958.

Rushton MA: Odontodysplasia: "ghost teeth," *Br Dent J* 119:109, 1965.

Sapp PJ, Stark M: Self-healing traumatic bone cysts, *Oral Surg Oral Med Oral Pathol* 69:597, 1990.

Shafer WG: Dens in dente, *NY Dent J* 19:220, 1953.

Suchina JA, Ludington JR Jr, Madden RM: Dens invaginatus of a maxillary lateral incisor: endodontic treatment, *Oral Surg Oral Med Oral Pathol* 68:467, 1989.

Tolson G et al: Report of a lateral periodontal cyst and gingival cyst in the same patient, *J Periodontol* 67:541, 1996.

Trope M: Root resorption of dental and traumatic origin: classification based on etiology, *Pract Periodontics Anesthet Dent* 10(4):515, 1998.

van Gool AV: Injury to the permanent tooth germ after trauma to the deciduous predecessor, *Oral Surg* 35:2, 1973.

Vorheis JM, Gregory GT, McDonald RE: Ankylosed deciduous molars, *J Am Dent Assoc* 44:68, 1952.

Weinmann JP, Svoboda JF, Woods RW: Hereditary disturbances of enamel formation and calcification, *J Am Dent Assoc* 32:397, 1945.

Yip WK: The prevalence of dens evaginatus, *Oral Surg* 38:80, 1974.

Yoshikazu S, Tanimoto K, Wada T: Simple bone cyst: evaluation of contents with conventional radiography and computed tomography, *Oral Surg Oral Med Oral Pathol* 77:296, 1994.

REVIEW QUESTIONS

1. Which term refers to a defect present at birth?
   A. Anomaly
   B. Inherited defect
   C. Congenital defect
   D. Developmental defect

2. Which term refers to the origin and tissue formation of teeth?
   A. Odontogenesis
   B. Dentinogenesis
   C. Amelogenesis
   D. Cementogenesis

3. Which term refers to the joining of teeth by cementum *only*?
   A. Fusion
   B. Gemination
   C. Twinning
   D. Concrescence

4. Which teeth are most often missing?
   A. Canines
   B. Deciduous second molars
   C. Third Molars
   D. Premolars

5. Which tooth is the most common supernumerary tooth?
   A. Mesiodens
   B. Distomolar
   C. Paramolar
   D. Hutchinson incisor

6. Which teeth most often appear smaller than normal?
   A. Mandibular premolars
   B. Maxillary lateral incisors
   C. Mandibular lateral incisors
   D. Mandibular third molars

7. Which term refers to the developmental anomaly that arises when a single tooth germ attempts to divide and results in the incomplete formation of two teeth?
   A. Fusion
   B. Gemination
   C. Concrescence
   D. Dilaceration

8. Which term refers to the developmental anomaly that arises from the union of two normally separated adjacent tooth germs?
   A. Twinning
   B. Gemination
   C. Fusion
   D. Dilaceration

9. Which term refers to an abnormal angulation or curve in the root or crown of a tooth?
   A. Fusion
   B. Gemination
   C. Concrescence
   D. Dilaceration

10. Which term refers to a developmental anomaly in which teeth exhibit elongated, large pulp chambers and short roots?
    A. Dens in dente
    B. Dens evaginatus
    C. Taurodontism
    D. Dilaceration

11. Which *developmental* anomaly is often associated with a nonvital tooth and periapical lesions?
    A. Dens in dente
    B. Dens evaginatus
    C. Taurodontism
    D. Talon cusp

12. Which of the following teeth most often exhibit supernumerary roots?
    A. Maxillary first premolars
    B. Maxillary third molars
    C. Mandibular first molars
    D. Maxillary first molars

13. Which one of the following describes the appearance of enamel hypoplasia resulting from a febrile illness or vitamin deficiency?
    A. Pitting defects
    B. Yellowish-brown discoloration
    C. Blackish-brown staining
    D. Chalky white spots

14. Which one of the following is associated with enamel hypoplasia resulting from congenital syphilis?
    A. Turner tooth
    B. Hutchinson incisors
    C. Taurodont
    D. Dens evaginatus

15. Which one of the following describes the appearance of enamel hypocalcification?
    A. Pitting defects
    B. Yellowish-brown discoloration
    C. Blackish-brown stains
    D. Chalky white spots

16. Which term describes a tooth that has not erupted because of the lack of eruptive force?
    A. Ankylosed
    B. Impacted
    C. Embedded
    D. Fused

17. Which teeth are most often impacted?
    A. Distomolars
    B. Maxillary and mandibular first molars
    C. Mandibular cuspids
    D. Mandibular third molars

18. Which term describes a tooth in which bone has fused to cementum and dentin and prevents the eruption of an underlying permanent tooth?
    A. Concrescence
    B. Embedded
    C. Ankylosed
    D. Fused

19. Which cyst is *not* an odontogenic cyst?
    A. Dentigerous cyst
    B. Primordial cyst
    C. Median palatal cyst
    D. Lateral periodontal cyst

20. The most common cause of the periapical cyst is:
    A. Caries
    B. Trauma
    C. Malignant infiltration
    D. Food impaction

21. Which cyst is an odontogenic intraosseous cyst that forms around the crown of a developing tooth?
    A. Coronal cyst
    B. Dentigerous cyst
    C. Lateral periodontal cyst
    D. Eruption cyst

22. Which cyst develops in place of a tooth?
    A. Dentigerous cyst
    B. Primordial cyst
    C. Follicular cyst
    D. Odontogenic keratocyst

23. Which cyst is characterized by its unique histologic appearance and frequent recurrence?
    A. Residual cyst
    B. Stafne bone cyst
    C. Odontogenic keratocyst
    D. Eruption cyst

24. The lateral periodontal cyst is defined by its location. In which area is the lateral periodontal cyst most commonly found?
    A. Mandibular third molar area
    B. Maxillary tuberosity area
    C. Between the maxillary premolars
    D. Between the mandibular cuspid and first premolar

25. The teeth are vital with all of the following cysts except:
    A. Nasopalatine canal cyst
    B. Cyst of the palatine papilla
    C. Dentigerous cyst
    D. Periapical cyst

26. Which cyst is characteristically pear shaped?
    A. Globulomaxillary cyst
    B. Median palatal cyst
    C. Incisal canal cyst
    D. Median mandibular cyst

27. Which cyst is a periapical cyst that was left behind after the extraction of the offending tooth?
    A. Periodontal cyst
    B. Gingival cyst
    C. Odontogenic cyst
    D. Residual cyst

28. With which cyst may the patient complain of dysphagia?
    A. Thyroglossal tract cyst
    B. Median palatal cyst
    C. Static bone cyst
    D. Traumatic bone cyst

29. Which cyst is considered a pseudocyst?
    A. Odontogenic keratocyst
    B. Traumatic bone cyst
    C. Lymphoepithelial cyst
    D. Primordial cyst

30. In addition to the odontogenic keratocyst, which lesion would the hygienist suspect if a radiograph revealed a multilocular radiolucency?
    A. Globulomaxillary cyst
    B. Aneurysmal bone cyst
    C. Stafne bone cyst
    D. Periapical cyst

31. Which term refers to the adhesion of the tongue to the floor of the mouth?
    A. Ankylosis
    B. Ankyloglossia
    C. Anodontia
    D. Amelogenesis

32. Which location is the most common for lip pits?
    A. Commissure
    B. Philtrum
    C. Nasolabial groove
    D. Labiomental groove

33. Which term refers to an ectopic mass of thyroid tissue located on the dorsal tongue?
    A. Thyroid cyst
    B. Thyroid tumor
    C. Lingual tonsil
    D. Lingual thyroid

34. Which term refers to the total absence of all teeth?
    A. Anodontia
    B. Hypodontia
    C. Hyperdontia
    D. Microdontia

35. Which term refers to the lack of one or more teeth?
    A. Anodontia
    B. Hypodontia
    C. Hyperdontia
    D. Microdontia

36. Which tooth is the second most common supernumerary tooth?
    A. Taurodont
    B. Mesiodens
    C. Paramolar
    D. Distomolar

37. Which term refers to abnormally small teeth?
    A. Taurodontia
    B. Macrodontia
    C. Microdontia
    D. Hypodontia

38. Which term refers to abnormally large teeth?
    A. Taurodontia
    B. Acromegaly
    C. Macrodontia
    D. Hypodontia

39. Which location is the most likely for an enamel pearl?
    A. Maxillary molars
    B. Maxillary second premolar
    C. Mandibular premolars
    D. Mandibular molars

40. Which location is the most likely for a talon cusp?
    A. Canines
    B. Incisors
    C. Molars
    D. Premolars

41. Which term refers to an accessory cusp located on the occlusal surface of a tooth?
    A. Mulberry cusp
    B. Talon cusp
    C. Dens invaginatus
    D. Dens evaginatus

42. Which term refers to the enamel hypoplasia of a permanent tooth that results from infection of a deciduous tooth?
    A. Hutchinson tooth
    B. Talon tooth
    C. Turner tooth
    D. Gorlin tooth

43. Which term refers to the irregular areas of discoloration that result from fluoride ingestion?
    A. Pitting defects
    B. Developmental defect
    C. Mottling defect
    D. Extrinsic staining

44. Which term refers to teeth that appear ghostlike on a dental radiograph?
    A. Taurodontism
    B. Enamel hypocalcification
    C. Regional odontodysplasia
    D. Enamel hypoplasia

45. Which term refers to teeth that cannot erupt because of physical obstruction?
    A. Fused
    B. Ankylosed
    C. Embedded
    D. Impacted

CHAPTER 5 Synopsis

Condition/Disease	Cause	Age/Race/ Sex	Location	Clinical Features
Ankyloglossia	Developmental	*	Tongue/floor of mouth	Complete or partial fusion of the lingual frenum of the tongue to the floor of the mouth
Commissural Lip Pits	Developmental	*	Commissures of the lip (corners of the mouth)	Tiny blind tracts are present in the corner of the lips
Lingual Thyroid	Developmental	*	Posterior, dorsal tongue	A mass of tissue at the midline posterior to the circumvallate papillae
Dentigerous Cyst	Developmental	Young adults	Around the crown of an unerupted, impacted, or developing tooth	When larger, can displace teeth
Eruption Cyst	Developmental	Children	Soft tissue around the crown of an erupting tooth	Swelling at the site of erupting tooth
Primordial Cyst	Developmental	Young adults	Develops in place of a tooth Mandibular third molar area most common site	Asymptomatic
Odontogenic Keratocyst	Developmental (dental lamina)	Most common ages 20-30	Posterior mandible most common site	When large, may cause buccal expansion
Lateral Periodontal Cyst	Developmental (dental lamina)	Affects men more than women Median age 50-60	Lateral aspect of tooth root Mandibular cuspid–premolar area	Asymptomatic
Gingival Cyst	Developmental (dental lamina)	Median age 50-60	Soft tissue of mandibular cuspid-premolar area	Bulge or swelling of gingival papilla or alveolar mucosa
Nasopalatine Canal Cyst (Incisal Canal Cyst)	Developmental	Affects men more than women Ages 40-60	Anterior maxilla Nasopalatine canal incisive papillae	Asymptomatic Pink bulge at the incisive papillae area

N/A, Not Applicable.
*Specific information not included in text.

Radiographic Features	Microscopic Features	Treatment	Diagnostic Process
N/A	N/A	Surgical removal of a portion of the lingual frenum	Clinical
N/A	N/A	None	Clinical
N/A	Normal thyroid tissue	Usually none, may be the individual's only functioning thyroid tissue Removal may be indicated if the mass is large	Clinical Laboratory (to identify thyroid tissue)
Well-defined unilocular radiolucency	Cyst lined by cubodial to squamous epithelium	Removal of cyst and associated tooth	Radiographic Microscopic
N/A	Cyst lined by cubodial to squamous epithelium	Usually none Tooth erupts though cyst	Radiographic Microscopic (erupting tooth)
Well-defined radiolucency	Cyst lined by cubodial to squamous epithelium	Surgical removal of the cyst	Radiographic
Well-defined, usually multilocular radiolucency	Cyst lined by thin corrugated parakeratotic squamous epithelium 8-10 cell layers thick Prominent, palisaded basal cell layer with flat interface between the epithelium and connective tissue	Surgical removal of the cyst with peripheral osseous curettage (recurrence high)	Microscopic
Unilocular or multilocular radiolucency	Cyst lined by thin nonkeratinized squamous epithelium with focal thickenings	Surgical removal	Microscopic Radiographic
N/A	Cyst lined by thin nonkeratinized squamous epithelium that may have focal thickenings	Surgical removal	Clinical Microscopic
Well-circumscribed radiolucency between the maxillary central incisors Open heart shaped	Cyst lined by squamous or respiratory epithelium Blood vessels and small nerves in cyst wall	Surgical removal	Radiographic Microscopic

Continued

CHAPTER 5 Synopsis (continued)

Condition/Disease	Cause	Age/Race/ Sex	Location	Clinical Features
Median Palatine Cyst	Developmental	*	Midline of hard palate posterior to the palatine papilla	If large, swelling at midline of hard palate
Globulomaxillary Cyst	Unclear	*	Between maxillary lateral and cuspid	Asymptomatic
Median Mandibular Cyst	Unknown	*	Midline of mandible	Asymptomatic If very large, may cause expansion of lingual aspect of mandible
Nasolabial Cyst	Developmental	Ratio of women to men: 4:1 Adults ages 40-50 years	Soft tissue of face Nasolabial fold area (maxillary canine, floor of the nose area)	Expansion or swelling in nasolabial fold area or in mucolabial fold area
Branchial Cleft Cyst (Cervical Lymphoepithelial Cyst) and Intraoral Lymphoepithelial Cyst	Developmental epithelium (entrapped in lymph node)	*	Lateral neck at the anterior boarder of the sternocleidomastoid muscle Intraoral: lateral border of the posterior tongue and floor of mouth	Branchial cyst appears as a bulbous area on the lateral neck Intraoral: pink-yellow well-delineated raised nodule
Epidermal Cyst	Epithelium of hair follicle	*	Skin of the face and neck	Localized, firm movable swelling
Dermoid Cyst	Developmental	Present at birth or young child	Anterior floor of mouth	If large, can displace tongue Doughlike consistency
Thyroglossal Tract Cyst	Developmental	Under 20 years of age	Along the thryroglossal tract from the foramen cecum to the normal location of the thyroid gland below the hyoid bone	If below the hyoid bone, bulge or swelling in the midline of the neck

N/A, Not Applicable.
*Specific information not included in text.

Radiographic Features	Microscopic Features	Treatment	Diagnostic Process
Unilocular radiolucency	Cyst lined by stratified squamous epithelium surrounded by dense fibrous connective tissue	Surgical removal	Radiographic Microscopic
Pear-shaped radiolucency	Cyst lining varies from squamous to cubodial to respiratory epithelium	Surgical removal	Radiographic Microscopic
Well-circumscribed radiolucency below the apices of the mandibular incisors	Cyst lined by squamous epithelium	Surgical removal	Radiographic Microscopic
N/A	Cyst lined by respiratory epithelium (pseudostratified ciliated columnar epithelium with goblet cells)	Surgical removal	Clinical Microscopic
N/A	Cyst lined by stratified squamous epithelium surrounded by lymphoid tissue	Surgical removal	Microscopic
N/A	Cyst lined by keratinized stratified squamous epithelium Lumen filled with keratin scales	Surgical removal	Microscopic
N/A	Cyst lined by stratified squamous epithelium surrounded by a connective tissue wall Hair follicles and glands seen in cyst wall	Surgical removal	Microscopic
N/A	Cyst lined by epithelium Thyroid tissue in connective tissue wall of cyst	Surgical removal Complete excision of cyst and tract	Microscopic

Continued

CHAPTER 5 Synopsis (continued)

Condition/Disease	Cause	Age/Race/Sex	Location	Clinical Features
Static Bone Cyst (Stafne bone defect)	Developmental depression on the lingual aspect of the posterior mandible. Can be unilateral or bilateral	Predilection in men	Anterior to angle of ramus Inferior to the mandibular canal	Asymptomatic
Simple Bone Cyst (Traumatic Bone Cyst)	Unclear Trauma suggested as possible cause	Age: teenage and young adults	Mandible	Usually asymptomatic Occasionally enlargement of bone
Aneurysmal Bone Cyst	Unclear Often associated with other bone lesions	Age: <30 yr Affects women more than men	Posterior maxilla or mandible	Expansion of involved bone
Anodontia	Developmental	*	Throughout arches	Absence of all primary or permanent teeth
Hypodontia	Developmental	*	Maxillary third molars Mandibular third molars Maxillary lateral incisors Mandibular second premolars	Absence of one or more teeth
Supernumerary Teeth	Developmental	*	Maxilla>mandible	Presence of one or more extra teeth; usually smaller than normal; may be erupted or unerupted
Mesiodens	Developmental	*	Near/at midline between maxillary central incisors	Most common extra tooth; may be erupted or unerupted/impacted Usually appear conical and small
Distomolar	Developmental	*	Distal to third molars	Second most common supernumerary tooth May be erupted (appears small) or impacted
Microdontia	Developmental	*	Maxillary lateral incisors Peg lateral is the most common Maxillary third molars	Affected tooth appears smaller than normal One or more teeth may be affected

N/A, Not Applicable.
*Specific information not included in text.

Radiographic Features	Microscopic Features	Treatment	Diagnostic Process
Well-circumscribed radiolucency in the mandible below the inferior alveolar canal	Not a true cyst (pseudocyst) Normal salivary gland tissue found within depression	No treatment	Radiographic
Radiolucency Characteristic scalloping around the roots of teeth	Not a true cyst (pseudocyst) Space in bone not lined by epithelium	Surgical intervention	Surgical
Multilocular radiolucency "Honeycomb soap bubble" appearance	Not a true cyst Blood-filled spaces surrounded by multinucleated giant cells and cellular connective tissue	Surgical removal and supplemental cryotherapy	Microscopic
All teeth absent	N/A	Prosthetic replacement of missing teeth	Clinical Radiographic
Absence of one or more teeth	N/A	Prosthetic replacement of missing teeth	Clinical Radiographic
One or more extra teeth	N/A	Extraction may be necessary	Clinical Radiographic
Extra tooth seen at the midline of the anterior maxilla	N/A	Extraction No treatment	Clinical Radiographic
Extra tooth distal to third molar	N/A	No treatment Extraction	Clinical Radiographic
Tooth smaller than normal	N/A	If erupted, restore to resemble a normal-size tooth	Clinical Radiographic

Continued

CHAPTER 5 Synopsis (continued)

Condition/Disease	Cause	Age/Race/Sex	Location	Clinical Features
Macrodontia	Developmental	*	Any tooth	Affected tooth appears larger than normal One or ore teeth may be affected
Gemination	Developmental	*	Primary>permanent Anterior>posterior	Tooth appears larger than normal Large crown (appears bifid) Normal number of teeth present
Fusion	Developmental	*	Primary>permanent Anterior>posterior Incisors	Adjacent teeth appear fused together Large crown seen
Concrescence	Developmental	*	Maxillary molars	Cannot observe clinically
Dilaceration	Developmental	*	Any tooth	Cannot observe clinically
Enamel Pearl	Developmental	*	Maxillary molars (furcation area)	Cannot observe clinically
Talon Cusp	Developmental	*	Molars	Crown appears normal
Dens in Dente	Developmental	*	Anterior>posterior Maxillary and mandibular incisors Maxillary lateral incisors	Tooth may appear normal or peg shaped
Dens Evaginatus	Developmental	*	Mandibular premolars, molars, cuspids, incisors	Accessory enamel cusp seen on occlusal surface
Supernumerary Roots	Developmental	*	Maxillary and mandibular third molars, mandibular premolars, and cuspids	Cannot observe clinically

N/A, Not Applicable.
*Specific information not included in text.

Radiographic Features	Microscopic Features	Treatment	Diagnostic Process
Tooth larger than normal	N/A	No treatment	Clinical Radiographic
Appears as a single tooth with a bifid crown and one common root canal	N/A	If esthetic problems, alteration of tooth to resemble normal-size tooth	Clinical Radiographic
Appears as a single large crown with separate or fused roots and root canals	N/A	If esthetic problem, alteration of tooth to resemble normal-size tooth	Clinical Radiographic
Appears as though the roots of adjacent teeth are connected	N/A	No treatment	Radiographic
Appears as a sharp bend in a tooth root	N/A	No treatment	Radiographic
Appears as a small sphere of enamel on a tooth root	N/A	No treatment	Radiographic
Appears as a tooth with abnormally short roots and low furcation area Pulp chamber is abnormally large	N/A	Removal of cusp and restoration of tooth if cusp interferes with occlusion	Clinical
Enamel invagination noted with crown of involved tooth	N/A	If tooth is vital, placement of a prophylactic restoration If nonvital, root canal therapy	Clinical Radiographic
May see pulp horn extending in accessory cusp	N/A	No treatment	Clinical
Visible extra root(s)	N/A	No treatment	Radiographic

Continued

CHAPTER 5 Synopsis (continued)

Condition/Disease	Cause	Age/Race/ Sex	Location	Clinical Features
Enamel Hypoplasia	Febrile illness or vitamin deficiency during tooth development	*	Permanent central and lateral incisors, cuspids, first molars	Crowns have one or more rows of tiny deep pits and stains
	Local infection or trauma during tooth development		Permanent maxillary incisor and mandibular premolars	Crowns have a yellowish brown color; pitting and enamel deformity may be present
	Fluoride ingestion during tooth development		All permanent teeth	Crowns have a mottled discoloration ranging from chalky white spots to brown-black staining
	Congenital syphilis		Permanent incisors and molars	Hutchinson incisors are screwdriver shaped
	Birth injury, premature birth, idiopathic factors		Any teeth	Mulberry molars resemble berries
Enamel Hypocalcification	Trauma to enamel during maturational phase	*	Any teeth	Crowns may have pitting, grooves, or staining Crowns have chalk white spots on the middle third
Endogenous Staining of Teeth	Ingestion of tetracycline or systemic disturbance during tooth development	*	Any teeth	With tetracycline staining, crowns appear yellowish-green or brownish-gray
Regional Odontodysplasia	Developmental	*	Several teeth in the same quadrant Primary or permanent teeth Maxilla>mandible	Affected teeth do not erupt or eruption is incomplete
Impacted Teeth	Developmental	*	Maxillary and mandibular third molars Maxillary cuspids	Teeth do not erupt
Ankylosed Teeth	Developmental	*	Most common deciduous molars	A primary ankylosed tooth prevents the eruption of the permanent tooth

N/A, Not Applicable.
*Specific information not included in text.

Radiographic Features	Microscopic Features	Treatment	Diagnostic Process
N/A	N/A	If necessary, restoration can be placed to improve appearance	Clinical
N/A	N/A	If necessary, restoration can be placed to improve appearance	Clinical
N/A	N/A	Restoration or bleaching can be used to produce a more aesthetic appearance	Clinical
N/A	N/A	Full-coverage crowns	Clinical
N/A	N/A		Clinical
N/A	N/A	If necessary, restoration can be placed to improve appearance If necessary, restoration can be placed to improve appearance	Clinical
N/A	N/A	If necessary, restoration can be used to improve appearance	Clinical
Reduced radiodensity of involved teeth Teeth appear "ghostlike" with large pulp chambers and thin enamel	*	Extraction	Clinical Radiographic
Impacted teethe are surround by bone	N/A	Surgical removal	Clinical Radiographic
Ankylosed teeth do not exhibit a periodontal ligament space	N/A	Extraction	Clinical Radiographic

chapter 6 Genetics

Heddie O. Sedano

OBJECTIVES

After studying this chapter, the student will be able to:

1. Define each of the words listed in the vocabulary for this chapter.
2. State the purpose of mitosis.
3. State the purpose of meiosis.
4. Explain what is meant by the Lyon hypothesis and give an example of its clinical significance.
5. Explain what is meant by a gross chromosomal abnormality and give three examples of syndromes that result from gross chromosomal abnormalities.
6. List the four inheritance patterns.
7. Explain what is meant by X-linked inheritance.
8. State the inheritance pattern and describe the oral manifestations and, if appropriate, the characteristic facies for each of the following: cyclic neutropenia, Papillon-Lefèvre syndrome, cherubism, Ellis–van Creveld syndrome, mandibulofacial dysostosis (Treacher Collins syndrome), osteogenesis imperfecta, hereditary hemorrhagic telangiectasia (Osler-Rendu–Parkes Weber syndrome), Peutz-Jeghers syndrome, white sponge nevus (Cannon disease), hypohidrotic ectodermal dysplasia, hypophosphatasia, and hypophosphatemic vitamin D—resistant rickets.
9. State the inheritance pattern, the oral or facial manifestations, and the type and location of the malignancy associated with each of the following syndromes: Gardner syndrome; nevoid basal cell carcinoma syndrome (Gorlin syndrome); multiple mucosal neuromas, medullary carcinoma of the thyroid gland, and pheochromocytoma syndrome (multiple endocrine neoplasia type 2B [MEN 2B]); and neurofibromatosis of von Recklinghausen.
10. State the location and malignant potential of the intestinal polyps in Peutz-Jeghers syndrome and Gardner syndrome.
11. List the four types of amelogenesis imperfecta.
12. Briefly compare and contrast dentinogenesis imperfecta, amelogenesis imperfecta, and dentin dysplasia, including the inheritance patterns, the clinical manifestations, and the radiographic appearance of each.

VOCABULARY

Alleles (ah-lēlz') Genes that are located at the same level or locus in the two chromosomes of a pair and that determine the same functions or characteristics.

Amino acid (ah-me'no as'id) Organic compound containing the amino group NH_2; amino acids are the main component of proteins.

Autosomes (aw'to-sōmz) (adjective, autosomal) Nonsex chromosomes, which are identical for men and women.

Barr body (bahr bod'e) Condensed chromatin of the inactivated X chromosome, which is found at the periphery of the nucleus of cells in women.

Carrier (kar'e-er) In genetics a heterozygous individual who is clinically normal but who can transmit a recessive trait or characteristic; also, a person who is homozygous for an autosomal-dominant condition with low penetrance.

Centromere (sen'tro-mēr) Constricted portion of the chromosome that divides the short arms from the long arms.

Chromatid (kro'mah-tid) Either of the two vertical halves of a chromosome that are joined at the centromere.

Chromatin (kro'mah-tin) General term used to refer to the material (deoxyribonucleic acid [DNA]) that forms the chromosomes.

Codon (ko'don) Vertical sequence of three bases in DNA that codes for an amino acid.

Consanguinity (kon"san-gwinĭ-te) Blood relationship; in genetics the term is generally used to describe a mating or marriage between close relatives.

Deoxyribonucleic acid (DNA) (de-ok"se-ri"bo-nu-kle'ik as'id) A substance composed of a double chain of polynucleotides; both chains coiled around a central axis form a double helix; it is the basic genetic code or template for amino acid formation.

Diploid (dip'loid) Having two sets of chromosomes; the normal constitution of somatic cells.

Dominant (dom'ĭ-nant) In genetics a trait or characteristic that is manifested when it is carried by only one of a pair of homologous chromosomes.

Expressivity (eks"pres-siv'ĭ-te) Degree of clinical manifestation of a trait or characteristic.

Facies (fa'she-ēz) Appearance of the face.

Gamete (gam'ēt) Spermatozoon or ovum.

Genetic heterogeneity (je-net'ik het"er-o-jē-ne'ĭ-te) Having more than one inheritance pattern.

Haploid (hap'loid) Cell with a single set of chromosomes; a gamete is haploid.

Heterozygote (het"er-o-zi'gōt) (adjective, heterozygous) Individual with two different genes at the allele loci.

Homozygote (ho"mo-zi'gōt) (adjective, homozygous) Individual having identical genes at the allele loci.

Hypohidrosis (hi'po-hĭ-dro'sis) Abnormally diminished secretion of sweat.

Hypotrichosis (hi'po-trĭ-ko'sis) Presence of less than the normal amount of hair.

Karyotype (kar'e-o-tĭp) Photomicrographic representation of a person's chromosomal constitution arranged according to the Denver classification.

Locus (lo'kus) (plural, loci) Position occupied by a gene on a chromosome.

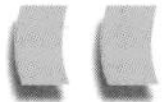

VOCABULARY (continued)

Meiosis (mi-o'sis) Two-step cellular division of the original germ cells, which reduces the chromosomes from 4nDNA to 1nDNA.

Metaphase (met'ah-fāz) Phase of cellular division in which the chromosomes are lined up evenly along the equatorial plane of the cell and in which they are most visible.

Mitochondria (mi″to kon'dre-ĕ) Cytoplasmic organelles that have their own DNA in a circular chromosome.

Mitochondrial DNA (mi″to kon'dre-ĕl DNA) Unique DNA that is maternally inherited.

Mitosis (mi-to'sis) Way in which somatic cells divide so that the two daughter cells receive the same number of identical chromosomes.

Mutation (mū-ta'shun) Permanent change in the arrangement of genetic material.

Oogenesis (o″o-jen'ĕ-sis) Process of formation of female germ cells (ova).

Ovum (o'vum) (plural, ova) Egg; mature feminine germ cell.

Penetrance (pen'ĕ-trans) Frequency with which a heritable trait is exhibited by individuals carrying the gene or genes that determine that trait.

Phenotype (fe'noh-tīp) Entire physical, biochemical, and physiologic makeup of an individual; genotype is the genetic composition, and phenotype is its observable appearance.

Recessive (re-ses'iv) Trait or characteristic that shows clinically when a double-gene dose (homozygous) exists in autosomic chromosomes or a single-gene dose exists in males if the trait is X linked.

Ribonucleic acid (RNA) (ri″bo-noo-kle'ik as'id) Single strands of polynucleotides found in all cells; different types of RNA have different functions in the production of proteins by the cell.

Ribosome (ri'bo-sōm) Cytoplasmic organelles in which proteins are formed on the basis of the genetic code provided by RNA.

Spermatogenesis (sper″mah-to-jen'ĕ-sis) Process of formation of spermatozoa (sperm).

Spermatozoon (sper″mah-to-zo'on) (plural, spermatozoa) Mature male germ cell.

Syndrome (sin'drōm) Set of signs or symptoms (or both) occurring together.

Translocation (trans″lo-ka'shun) Portion of a chromosome attached to another chromosome.

Trisomy (tri'so-me) Pair of chromosomes with an identical extra chromosome.

Genetics is the science that studies inheritance and the expression of inherited traits. The main objectives of this chapter are to introduce some of the basic concepts of genetics and present the clinical manifestations of some inherited oral disorders of interest to the dental hygienist. The descriptions of many syndromes are included. As explained in previous chapters, a **syndrome** is a distinctive association of signs and symptoms occurring together in the same patient. The syndromes included in this chapter are inherited. However, other syndromes such as acquired immunodeficiency syndrome (AIDS) are acquired, not inherited. In addition, the fact that an alteration is found as part of a syndrome does not mean that it cannot also occur independently. For example, cleft lip and palate occur as components of several syndromes and can also occur independently. The classification of syndromes is difficult because they are composed of several associated anomalies and the anomalies that compose the syndrome may not be present consistently in all patients with the same syndrome.

The term **phenotype** is used often in this chapter. It refers to the physical, biochemical, and physiologic traits of an individual. A phenotype can occur as a result of genetic factors or from a combination of genetic factors and environmental influences.

In this chapter, as in previous chapters, basic concepts are discussed first. These concepts are followed by descriptions of specific inherited disorders.

CHROMOSOMES

The hereditary units that are transmitted from one generation to another are called **genes.** They are found on **chromosomes,** which are located in the nucleus of the cell. Using a microscope, one can see chromosomes clearly only when the nucleus and cell are dividing (Figure 6-1). At other times the genetic material is dispersed in the nucleus (see Figure 6-1). Each cell of the human body, with the exception of mature germ cells (ova and spermatozoa), has 46 chromosomes. Half of these chromosomes are derived from the father, and the other half from the mother.

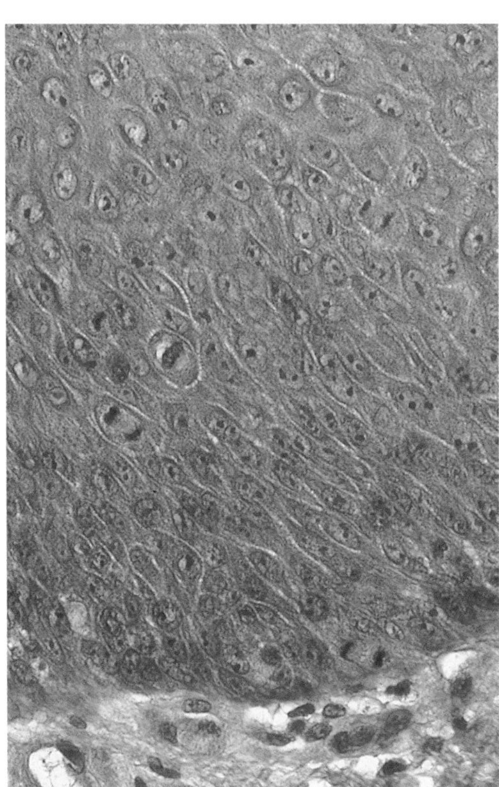

FIGURE 6-1 ■ High-power photomicrograph shows a dividing cell with visible chromosomes and nuclei of cells with scattered chromatin.

Chromosomes contain deoxyribonucleic acid (DNA), which directs the production of **amino acids**, polypeptides, and proteins by the cell. In addition, DNA has the ability to duplicate itself (self-replication). It creates exact copies of itself; and through the process of cell division cells identical to the original cell are formed.

NORMAL CELL DIVISION

MITOSIS

All cells in the body, with the exception of ova and spermatozoa, are called **somatic cells.** Cellular division is achieved by **mitosis** during a part of the life span of the somatic cell, called the **mitotic cycle.** The function of mitosis is to create an exact copy of each chromosome and, through division of the original cell, distribute an identical set of chromosomes to each daughter cell. After each cell division is completed and before the next division can occur, the cell enters the **gap 1 (G_1) phase**, which is followed by the **S phase,** in which replication of the DNA takes place. The **gap 2 (G_2) phase** follows the S phase and ends when mitotic division begins. The cell cycle is illustrated in Figure 6-2.

Stages of Mitosis

Mitosis is composed of four stages: (1) prophase, (2) metaphase, (3) anaphase, and (4) telophase. In each of these four stages, the chromosomes are distributed in a specific arrangement. In **metaphase** the chromosomes stain intensely and are arranged almost symmetrically at both sides of the center, or equatorial plane, of the cell. The appearance of a metaphase chromosome resembles the letter *X* (Figure 6-3), having a pair of "long arms" also known as *q arms* (see Figure 6-3, *3*) and a pair of "short arms" also known as *p arms* (see Figure 6-3, *1*). The size of the chromosome at metaphase and the length of the long and short arms vary from chromosome to chromosome. The constriction present in all chromosomes, which joins the short and long arms, is called the **centromere** (see Figure 6-3, *2*). During metaphase chromosomes are actually formed by two identical vertical halves, each composed of either left or right short and long arms and half of the centromere. Each of these identical halves is called a **chromatid** (see Figure 6-3, *4*). At metaphase each chromatid contains one molecule of DNA; therefore the DNA content of each chromosome is doubled (Figure 6-4). When cell division takes place, each chromosome splits vertically at the centromere; 46 chromatids (which now become chromosomes) form one daughter cell, and the other 46 chromatids form a second daughter cell. During prophase the chromosomes are lining up toward metaphase; in anaphase and telophase the chromatids are in the process of splitting.

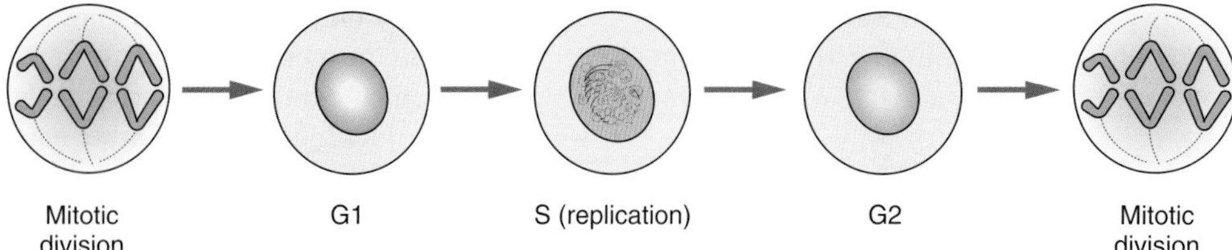

FIGURE 6-2 ■ The mitotic cycle shows the end of mitosis, followed by the G_1, S, and G_2 phases and the next mitosis.

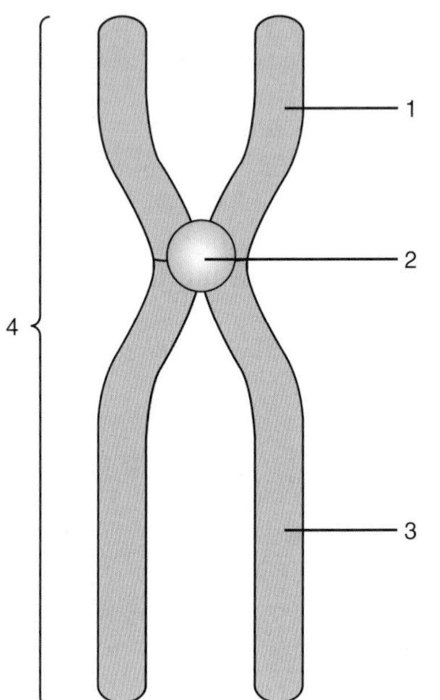

FIGURE 6-3 ■ Autosomal chromosome at metaphase shows *(1)* short arm, *(2)* centromere, *(3)* long arm, and *(4)* chromatid.

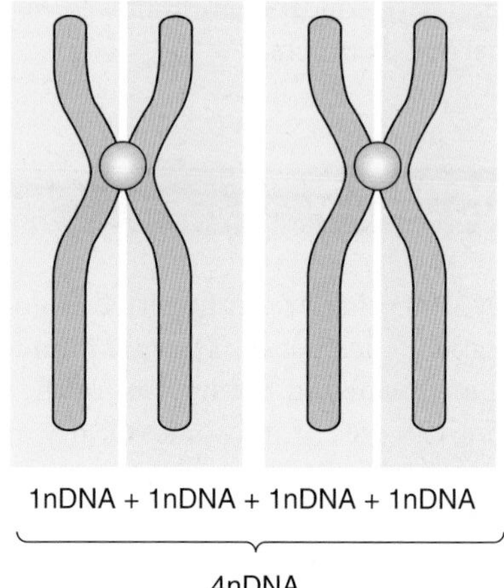

FIGURE 6-4 ■ Pair of autosomal chromosomes at metaphase. Each chromatid represents 1nDNA.

MEIOSIS

Primitive germ cells (oogonia, spermatogonia) have 46 chromosomes. Mature germ cells (ova, spermatozoa) have 23 chromosomes. **Meiosis** is a two-step special type of cell division in which the primitive germ cells reduce their chromosome number by half and become mature germ cells. The primitive germ cells have two chromosomes for each pair and are called **diploid**. The suffix *ploid* refers to the number of sets of chromosomes, and its prefix refers to the degree of ploidy. In diploid *di* indicates two. The mature germ cells (or **gametes**) have half the number of chromosomes and are called **haploid**. During the period in which the cell is not in division, the DNA content of diploid cells is designated 2nDNA; in metaphase it is double or 4nDNA. After the two stages of meiosis have been completed, the 4nDNA is reduced to 1nDNA. The two steps are called **first meiosis** and **second meiosis.** This reduction is necessary to maintain the normal number of human chromosomes. A new embryo must have 46 chromosomes per cell as did its parents. Therefore the union of germ cells needs to result in 46 chromosomes. If two cells with 46 chromosomes were combined, the resulting cell would have 92 chromosomes.

First Meiosis

Before the first meiosis in the primitive germ cells, a replication of DNA occurs that is similar to that observed in the S phase of somatic cells. After replication the members of each pair of chromosomes line up next to each other in an intimate point-by-point relationship (Figure 6-5, *A*). This pairing does not occur in mitosis. After pairing, the two chromosomes establish actual contact at different locations. These contacts are known as **chiasmata** (meaning X shaped) and determine points of crossing over (Figure 6-5, *B*). This crossing over achieves the exchange of chromosome segments between a chromatid of one chromosome and a chromatid of the other chromosome of a pair (between homologous chromosomes) (Figure 6-5, *C*). This special aspect of the first meiosis takes place at metaphase. After metaphase of the first meiotic division, the chromosomes separate from each other, but no splitting of the centromere occurs. The chromosomes remain intact, and each member of the pair migrates to one of the new cells, each of which contains 23 chromosomes but twice the final amount of DNA. During this migration chromosomes of the paternal and maternal lines segregate at

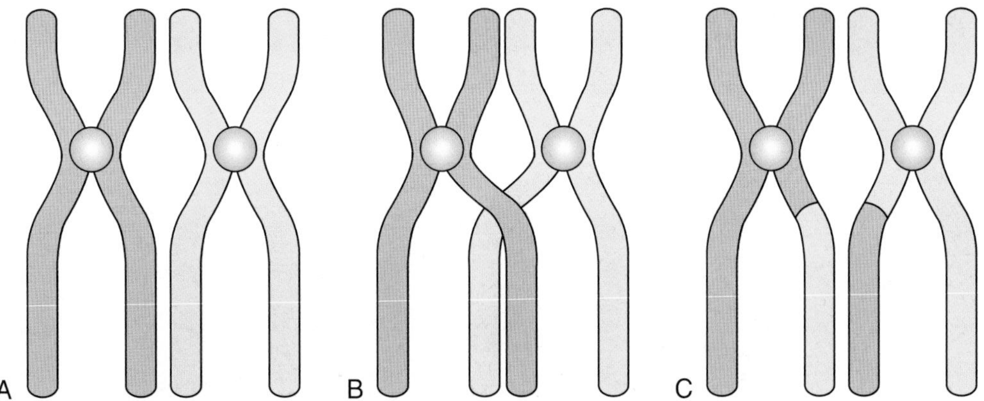

FIGURE 6-5 ■ Homologous autosomal chromosomes line up in first meiosis **(A)**, cross over during metaphase of first meiosis **(B)**, and exchange segments after crossing over **(C)**.

random, thus ensuring diversity of the species by creating a new combination of chromosomes.

Occasionally the chromosomes that were crossing over do not separate, and both migrate to the same cell. This is known as nondisjunction and results in the formation of a germ cell with an extra chromosome. If this occurs and that cell (either an **ovum** or a **spermatozoon**) participates in the formation of an embryo, three chromosomes (**trisomy**) instead of two result. An example of this type of abnormality is **Down syndrome,** also called **trisomy 21,** in which three of chromosome 21 are found instead of two. Trisomy has been reported for several different chromosomes.

In a female embryo **oogenesis** (ovum development) starts around the third month of prenatal life, and the future ova remain suspended crossing over from about the time of birth until the time ovulation starts. At the beginning of ovulation the first meiosis is completed. Nondisjunction is more prevalent in female oogenesis than in male **spermatogenesis**. This is probably because of the period of prolonged crossing over; therefore the older the woman, the greater the chance of shedding a trisomic ovum and of bearing a child with Down syndrome or other trisomy.

Second Meiosis

The second stage of meiosis is essentially a mitotic division in which each chromosome splits longitudinally. No replication of DNA occurs before the second meiosis. After the splitting two cells are formed, each containing the right amount of DNA (1nDNA) (Figure 6-6).

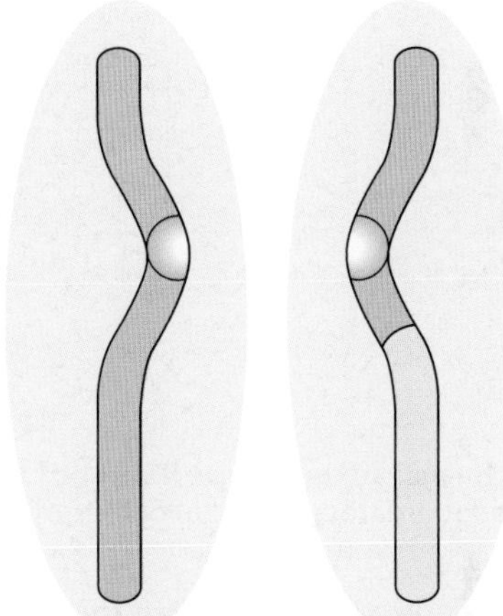

FIGURE 6-6 ■ Two haploid cells after second meiosis, each having 1nDNA.

Nondisjunction can occur during the first and second meiosis. If it occurs in second meiosis, a chromosome does not split, and one daughter cell has a full chromosome, and the other has none.

Immediately after fertilization the chromosomes of the ovum and spermatozoon, each having 1nDNA, condense independently and form round structures, each known as a pronucleus. The DNA in these pronuclei replicates, forming a set of 23 full chromosomes for each, the maternal and paternal pronuclei. When the membranes of these pronuclei break, the 46 chromosomes mix at random, initiating the first cellular division (mitosis) that starts the development of the new embryo.

LYON HYPOTHESIS

The sex chromosomes are designated XX in women and XY in men. During the early period of embryonic development (possibly by the end of the second week), the genetic activity of one of the X chromosomes in each cell of a female embryo is inactivated. The inactivation is a random process affecting either the X chromosome derived from the mother or the X chromosome derived from the father. Activated chromosomes are dispersed in the nucleus. The inactivated

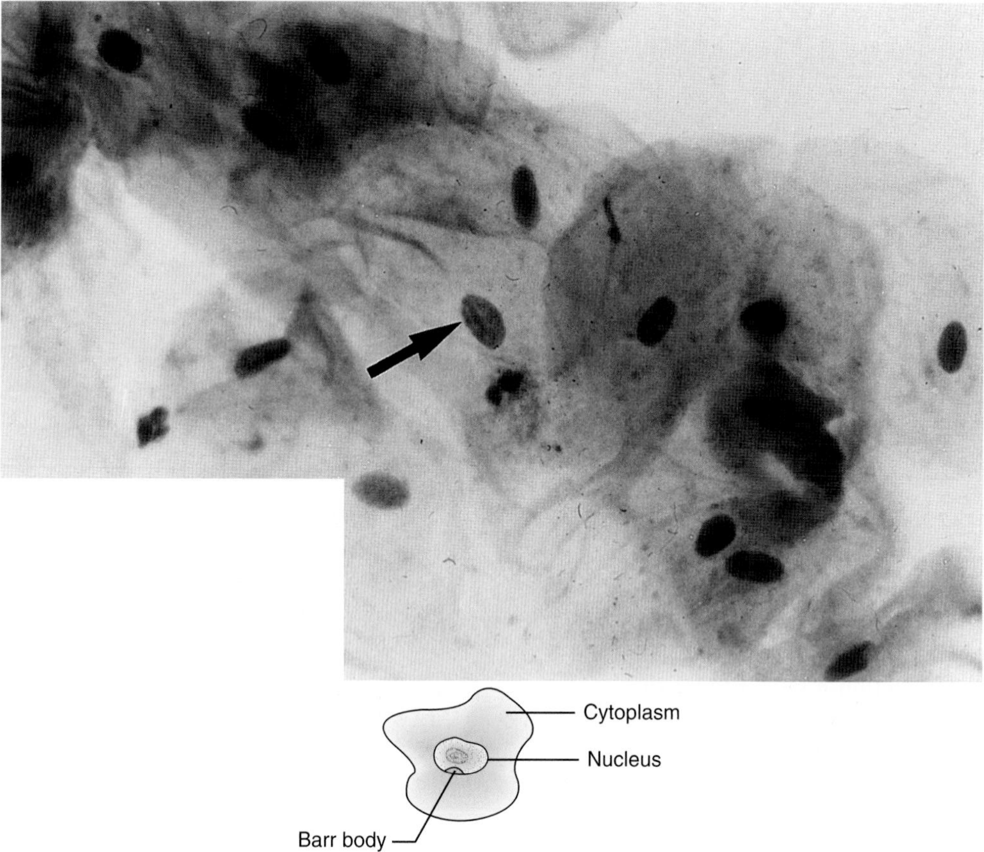

FIGURE 6-7 ■ Buccal smear shows Barr body (*arrow* points to small dark dot on nuclear membrane) at the periphery of the nucleus of a desquamated epithelial cell from a woman's buccal mucosa. (Courtesy Dr. Carl J. Witkop.)

chromosome remains contracted when the cell is not dividing and forms a structure known as the **Barr body**.

In female cells the Barr body can be seen easily under the light microscope, especially in cytologic smears, including those obtained from the oral mucosa. The Barr body appears as a dark dot at the periphery of the nucleus (Figure 6-7).

This inactivation of one of the X chromosomes in a female embryo was postulated by Mary Lyon and is known as the **Lyon hypothesis.** This hypothesis has interesting clinical implications for female **carriers** of conditions caused by genes located on the X chromosome, which are explained later in this chapter.

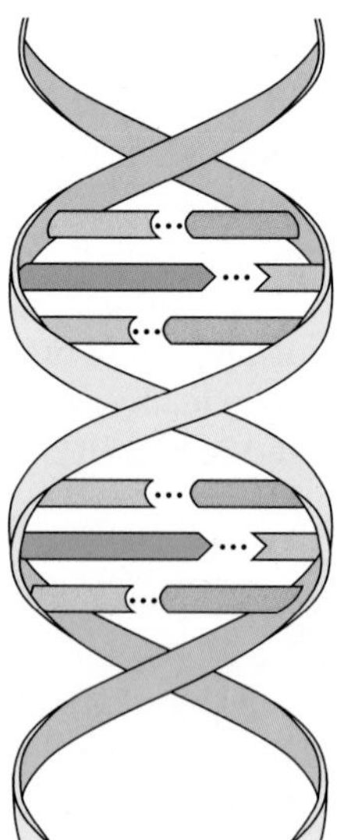

FIGURE 6-8 ■ DNA double helix.

MOLECULAR COMPOSITION OF CHROMOSOMES

DEOXYRIBONUCLEIC ACID

Chromosomes contain **deoxyribonucleic acid (DNA)**. DNA contains the basic code or template that carries all genetic information. The basic unit of DNA is called a **nucleotide,** which is formed by a nitrogen-containing base, a five-carbon sugar (deoxyribose), and a phosphate. Four bases are found in DNA: adenine (A), guanine (G), thymine (T), and cytosine (C). These chains of polynucleotides are coiled to form a structure called a **double helix** (Figure 6-8). In DNA the base adenine is always bound to the base thymine, and guanine is always bound to cytosine. This is a constant arrangement and is identical in all species from bacteria to humans, with just a few exceptions. Therefore the ratio of adenine to thymine (A/T) is always equal, and the same is true for the ratio of guanine to cytosine (G/C). In humans G/C pairs are about four times greater than A/T pairs. The polynucleotide chains run vertically in opposite directions. Therefore a sequence of adenine, guanine, and cytosine (AGC) is always matched by the sequence of thymine, cytosine, and guanine (TCG).

In the linear representation shown the number 1 indicates the nucleotide of one chain, and the number 2 indicates the nucleotide of the other chain. A molecule of hydrogen (H) binds both nucleotides. This arrangement is repeated horizontally to form the polynucleotide double spiral staircase (or helix) appearance of DNA (see Figure 6-8).

The vertical sequence of three bases is called a **codon**. It codes for an amino acid. Several amino acids form a polypeptide, and one or more polypeptides form a protein. A gene is often equated with the unit that forms a polypeptide.

DNA has the unique capability of self-replication, which is achieved by unwinding its double chain like the plaits of a braid. Each separated chain serves as a blueprint for another chain.

Mitochondrial DNA is found in the circular chromosome of the **mitochondria**, and it is maternally inherited. This is the DNA present in the cytoplasmic mitochondrial organelles of the ovum. Mitochondrial DNA is passed from the mother to all her offspring, regardless of sex.

RIBONUCLEIC ACID

To produce amino acids, polypeptides, and proteins, the genetic code contained in the DNA is transcribed into **ribonucleic acid (RNA)**, which differs from DNA in that it is a single strand (in its simplest form), its sugar is a ribose (the sugar in DNA is deoxyribose), and the base uracil (U) replaces the thymine (T) in DNA.

Types of Ribonucleic Acid

The four types of RNA are (1) messenger RNA (mRNA), (2) transfer RNA (tRNA), (3) ribosomal RNA (rRNA), and (4) heterogeneous RNA (hnRNA). RNA can be found in both the nucleus and the cytoplasm of a cell.

The first type of RNA, **mRNA,** is a blueprint of the genetic DNA for the coding of proteins. It carries the message for the DNA to **ribosomes** in the cytoplasm, in which proteins are produced. The second type of RNA, **tRNA,** transfers amino acids from the cytoplasm to the mRNA, positioning amino acids in the proper sequence to form polypeptides and hence proteins. The third type of RNA, **rRNA,** combines with several polypeptides to form ribosomes. The fourth type of RNA, **hnRNA,** is found within the nucleus and is the precursor of mRNA.

In the production of a protein (Figure 6-9) the mRNA carries the genetic code for the formation of that protein to the ribosomes. The tRNA brings amino acids to the ribosomes from the cellular cytoplasm. The amino acid sequence forms proteins according to the genetic code, and these proteins exit the ribosomes as they are formed.

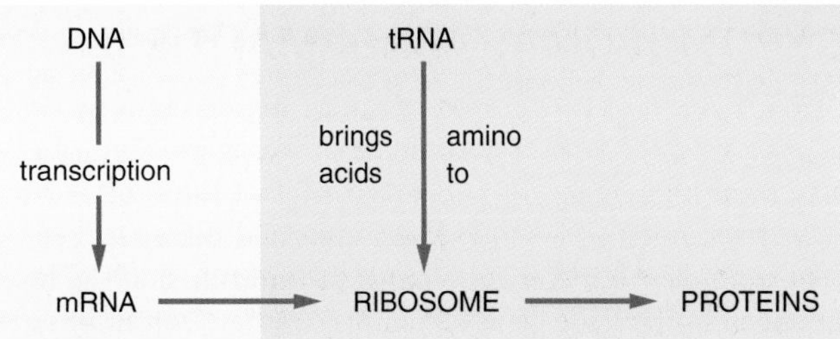

FIGURE 6-9 ■ Production (synthesis) of protein from DNA.

GENES AND CHROMOSOMES

Genes in a chromosome are located in a vertical linear manner. The genes in both members of a pair of chromosomes (homologous chromosomes) govern the same functions or dictate the same characteristics. The genes that are located at the same level (or **locus**) in homologous chromosomes and that dictate the same functions or characteristics are called **alleles**.

The manifestations (phenotype) of a gene action are not necessarily the same from one individual to another. This is best explained with the ABO blood group system. The locus can be occupied by either the factor that determines the blood group A or the factor that determines the blood group B. If it is empty, it results in the blood group O. The locus is always the same, and the three genes govern the same function; however, the clinical result is different. In this situation the trait or condition is said to have multiple alleles. For example, if both loci are AA or if they are AO, the person is said to have blood group A. If both loci are BB or BO, the person is said to have blood group B. If the loci are AB or BA, the person is said to have blood group AB. Only if both the loci are empty does the person have blood group O. The locus always controls blood group, but the group depends on the alleles that are present or lacking in each person.

When the allelic genes are identical, the person is said to be homozygous for that gene, or a **homozygote**. Using the ABO blood group system again as an example, a person with AA, BB, and OO would be homozygous. When the genes are different (for example, AB, AO, or BO), the person is said to be heterozygous for that gene, or a **heterozygote**. If a gene can express its effect clinically with a single dose (heterozygous), as in the combination AO = blood group A, the characteristic is said to be **dominant**. If the gene needs a double dose to exhibit its action (homozygous), the resulting characteristic or function is said to be **recessive**. For example, only the combination OO results in the blood group O.

CHROMOSOMAL ABNORMALITIES

Abnormalities of chromosomes can be divided into two categories: (1) molecular abnormalities and (2) gross abnormalities. Molecular alterations occur at the DNA level and are not detectable microscopically. Most inherited disorders represent examples of molecular changes (**mutations**) at the level of one or both allelic genes. Examples of these conditions are presented later in this chapter.

Gross chromosomal alterations can be observed in a karyotype. A **karyotype** (Figures 6-10 and 6-11) is a photographic representation of a person's chromosomal constitution. Clinicians can create a karyotype by culturing cells from blood, skin, or other tissues. One method uses peripheral blood by placing it in a test tube with heparin to avoid coagulation and centrifuging it. After centrifugation the white blood cells (leukocytes) are deposited at the bottom of the tube. The leukocytes are removed and placed in a culture medium containing phytohemagglutinin, which is a substance that enhances mitosis. Because chromosomes are best observed when cell division is arrested at metaphase, colchicine is added to the culture after 72 hours of culture at 37° C to stop mitosis at metaphase. This also prevents the centromere from dividing. A hypotonic solution is then added to the culture to make the cells swell. The cells are then fixed (preserved) and stained and observed under the microscope. Examples of well-defined mitoses are chosen and photographed. The photograph is enlarged, and each chromosome is cut out of the photographic print. When stained, the chromosomes have a bandlike appearance that allows an accurate identification of each. These cutouts are then pasted on a special chart to construct the karyotype.

GROSS CHROMOSOMAL ABNORMALITIES

Alterations in Number and Structure of Chromosomes

Gross chromosomal abnormalities are caused by either alterations in chromosome number, which are almost always a result of nondisjunction (explained earlier), or alterations in structure, which develop because of chromosomal breaks or abnormal rearrangements. The following illustrate alterations in number:

- **Euploid:** A complete second set of chromosomes, the total number being 92. This is incompatible with life.
- **Polyploid:** Three (triploid) or four (tetraploid) complete sets of chromosomes. This has been described occasionally in humans and is incompatible with life.
- **Aneuploid:** Any extra number of chromosomes that do not represent an exact multiple of the total chromosome complement (e.g., trisomy [a pair with an identical extra chromosome] and monosomy [a missing chromosome from a pair]).

Examples of structural abnormalities include the following:

- **Deletion:** The loss of part of a chromosome
- **Translocation:** A portion of a chromosome is attached to another chromosome.
- **Inversion:** A portion of a chromosome is upside-down.
- **Duplication:** A chromosome is larger than normal; the extra segment is identical to a segment of the normal chromosome.

Clinical Syndromes Resulting From Gross Chromosomal Abnormalities

Trisomy 21

This condition, also known as Down syndrome, is the most frequent of the trisomies. Ninety-five percent of cases of Down syndrome are the result of nondisjunction, mostly associated with late maternal age at the time of conception.

Slanted eyes characterize the **facies** (the appearance of the face). Patients are generally shorter than normal, and heart abnormalities are present in more than 30% of individuals with trisomy 21. The intelligence level varies from near normal to marked handicap.

Fissured tongue is frequently seen in patients with trisomy 21. Premature loss of teeth, especially the mandibular central incisors, caused by alveolar bone loss is seen frequently. Gingival and periodontal disease has been reported in 90% of affected individuals. Hypodontia (fewer teeth than normal), abnormally shaped teeth, and anomalies in eruption with malposition and crowding of teeth are common findings. Dental hygienists play an important role in the maintenance of oral health in these patients.

Trisomy 13

This disorder is characterized by multiple abnormalities in various organs. Seventy percent of live-born infants die within the first 7 months of life. Characteristic clinical findings include bilateral cleft lip and palate, microphthalmia or anophthalmia (small eyes or no eyes), superficial hemangioma of the forehead or nape of the neck, growth retardation, severe mental handicap, polydactyly of hands and feet (supernumerary digits), clenching of the fist with the thumb under the fingers, rocker-bottom feet, heart malformations, and several anomalies of the external genitals. The facial appearance is quite striking because of the cleft lip, cleft palate, and ocular abnormalities (Figure 6-12).

Turner Syndrome

Patients with Turner syndrome have a female phenotype, and in the majority of cases the karyotype has the normal 44 autosomic chromosomes and only one X chromosome. A normal female would have two X chromosomes: one from the

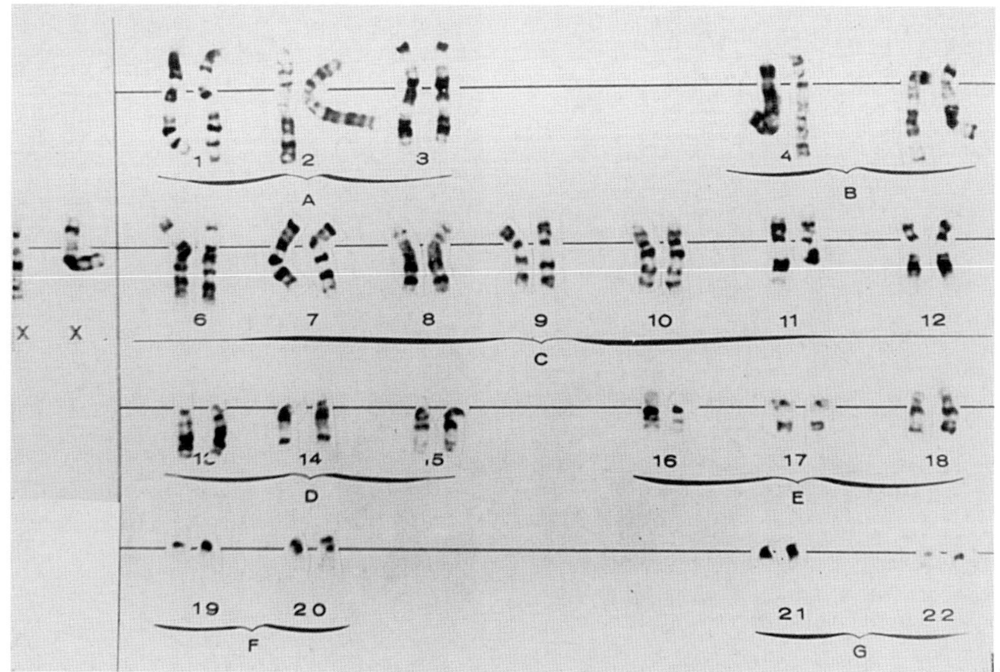

FIGURE 6-10 ■ Karyotype from a female shows the 22 pairs of autosomal chromosomes and the pair of X chromosomes. (Courtesy Dr. Jaroslav Cervenka.)

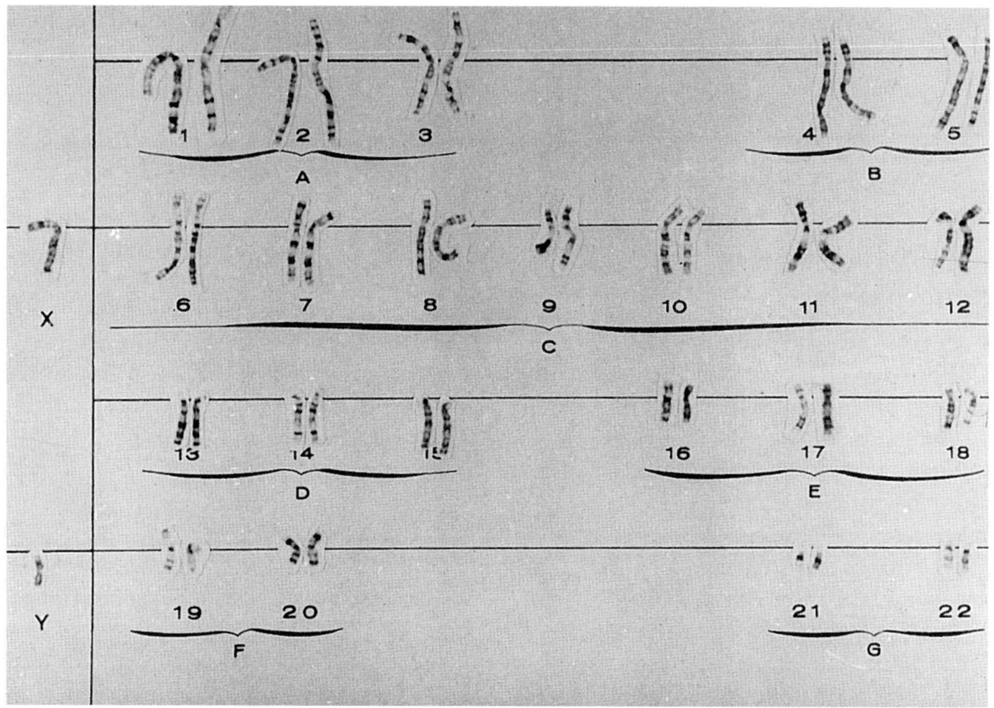

FIGURE 6-11 ■ Karyotype from a male shows the 22 pairs of autosomal chromosomes and the X and Y chromosomes. (Courtesy Dr. Jaroslav Cervenka.)

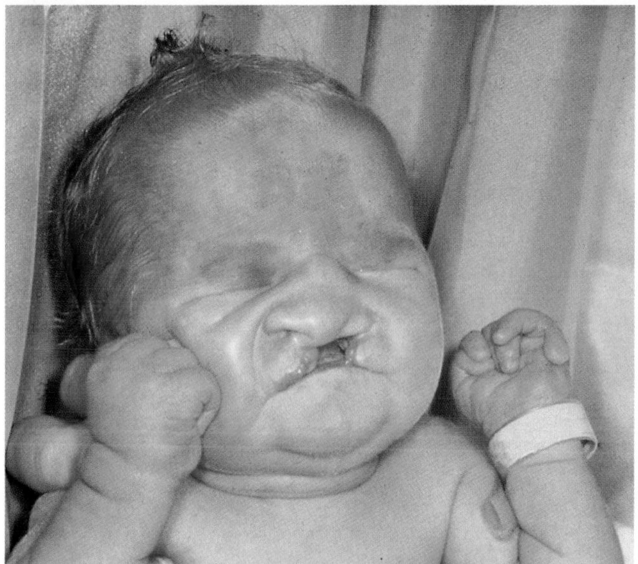

FIGURE 6-12 ■ Newborn with trisomy 13. Cleft lip, frontal hemangioma, and abnormal position of fingers should be noted.

mother and one from the father. Most cases of Turner syndrome are the result of nondisjunction of the X chromosome in the paternal gamete. Clinically these women are of short stature and have webbing of the neck and edema of the hands and feet (Figure 6-13). They frequently exhibit a low hairline on the nape of the neck. The chest is broad with wide-spaced nipples. The aorta frequently is abnormal, and body hair is sparse. The external genitals appear infantile, and generally the ovaries are not developed; therefore these individuals have primary amenorrhea (abnormal temporary or permanent cessation of the menstrual cycle). Smears taken from the oral mucosa demonstrate the lack of Barr bodies.

Klinefelter Syndrome

This condition occurs when an ovum carrying two X chromosomes is fertilized by a spermatozoon with a Y chromosome; therefore the fertilized ovum will have two X chromosomes plus a Y chromosome. The majority of cases result from nondisjunction of the X chromosome, generally in the ova of older women. Affected individuals have a male phenotype, and the condition cannot be detected until after puberty. These patients are taller than normal and have wide hips and a female pubic hair distribution. About 50% have gynecomastia (development of female breasts), and intelligence levels are lower than normal in 10% of affected individuals. The penis appears normal, but the testes are smaller and harder than normal and lack seminiferous tubules.

The maxilla is slightly hypoplastic (underdeveloped). Buccal smears reveal the presence of one Barr body.

Variations of Klinefelter syndrome also occur; they are represented by karyotypes containing XXXY or XXXXY. The greater the number of X chromosomes, the more pronounced the clinical manifestations, and the lower the level of intelligence. The maxilla becomes increasingly hypoplastic with increasing number of X chromosomes. Buccal smears show one Barr body for each extra X chromosome.

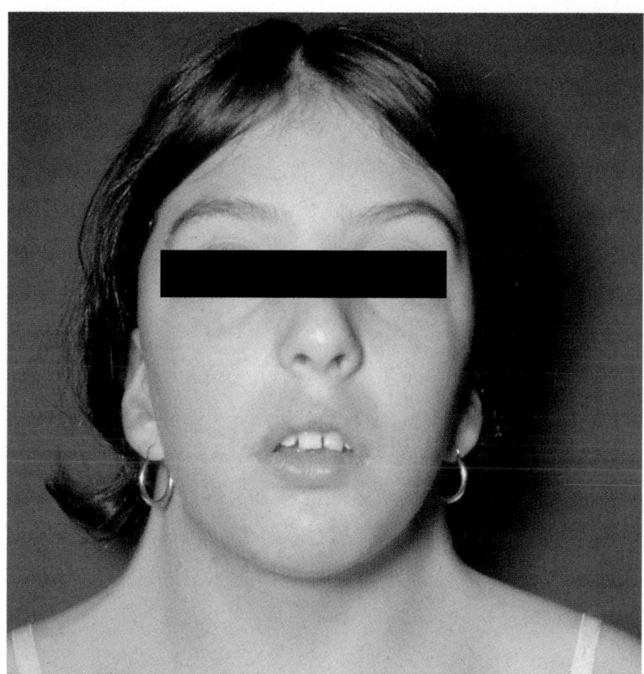

FIGURE 6-13 ■ Patient with Turner syndrome. Note the webbing of the neck.

Cri du chat (Cat Cry) Syndrome and Wolf-Hirschhorn Syndrome

These syndromes are examples of abnormalities caused by deletions. The cri du chat syndrome results from a deletion on the short arm of chromosome 5, and the Wolf-Hirschhorn syndrome results from a deletion on the short arm of chromosome 4. Newborns with a chromosome 5 deletion exhibit a catlike cry at birth and are mentally retarded. No oral abnormalities occur. Most newborns with the deletion in the short arm of chromosome 4 have a cleft palate and intelligence quotients of less than 30.

PATTERNS OF INHERITANCE

Because loci are present in both **autosomal** and X chromosomes and because of a double- and single-dose effect, four possible inheritance patterns exist. Dominant genes need only a single dose, and recessive genes need a double dose. The inheritance patterns are autosomal dominant, autosomal recessive, X-linked dominant, and X-linked recessive. Autosomal chromosomes include all chromosomes except those that determine sex (X and Y). The Y chromosome participates only in the differentiation of the masculine gonads.

Autosomal-Dominant Inheritance

A condition having autosomal-dominant inheritance is transmitted vertically from one generation to the next. Males and females are equally affected. When a person has a gene for the condition, the risk of having an affected offspring is 50% for each pregnancy. Genetic risk is always a mathematical estimate of probability governed by chance. Therefore none, less than half, half, more than half, or all of the offspring could be affected by a condition that is transmitted by autosomal-dominant inheritance.

An individual can carry a gene with a dominant effect without presenting any clinical manifestations. This is referred to as **lack of penetrance.** This situation can be explained partially by the presence of modifying genes in the same or other chromosomes. The clinical manifestations in autosomal-dominant disorders frequently vary among affected individuals. This is known as variable expressivity. **Penetrance** refers to the number of individuals affected, and **expressivity** pertains to the degree to which an individual is affected.

Autosomal-Recessive Inheritance

As stated previously, individuals exhibiting an autosomal-recessive trait must be homozygous for the gene. Clinically normal parents of affected children are heterozygous, and both are carriers of the trait. They are not generally recognized as carriers until after the birth of an affected child. If the enzymatic defect is known, carriers can be recognized before the birth of a child by assessing levels of the responsible enzyme in clinically normal members of a family with the trait. For parents who are carriers of the same recessive trait, the risk of having an affected child is 25%, the risk of having a homozygotic normal child is 25%, and the chance of having a heterozygotic carrier is 50% for each pregnancy. As in other inheritance patterns, risk is a mathematical estimate of the probability of an event occurring. If both parents are homozygous (have two of the genes of the trait) for a recessive trait, they would be expected to be affected, and all their children would be affected equally because they would also be homozygous (have two of the same genes) for the trait. In humans this type of situation is quite rare because individuals affected by the same recessive trait usually do not mate.

In genetics **consanguinity** means a familial relationship and is generally used to describe matings or marriages between close relatives, usually including first cousins. In the United States marriage or mating between very close relatives (parent-offspring, brother-sister, uncle-niece, aunt-nephew) is illegal, and in most states marriage of first cousins is also illegal. However, consanguineous matings occur sporadically. The chance of having deleterious genes in common increases between close relatives. When consanguinity exists between the members of a family, the chance of the offspring being homozygous for a deleterious gene increases. The closer the degree of consanguinity, the greater the risk.

X-Linked Inheritance

Women have two X chromosomes and therefore can be either heterozygous or homozygous for a gene that is located on the X chromosome. Thus in women X-linked traits can be dominant or recessive. Men have only one X and one Y chromosome. If a deleterious gene occurs on the X chromosome in a male, the condition or trait will be seen clinically, regardless of the dominant or recessive behavior of the same gene in women. The man's X chromosome is transmitted to all of his daughters and to none of his sons. The X chromosome in his sons comes from the mother. Consequently no male-to-male (from father to son) transmission of X-linked traits occurs. Some X-linked dominant traits are lethal in males. Females probably survive because of the action of the allelic normal gene on the second X chromosome. All offspring, male and female, of a woman homozygotic for a dominant X-linked condition will be affected with the condition. This is because all of her X chromosomes contain that gene (and all offspring receive an X chromosome). Because the gene is dominant, only one of the genes is necessary for that condition to occur. A mother who is a carrier of an X-linked recessive trait has a 50% risk of having an affected son and a 50% risk of having a carrier daughter. This is because both daughters and sons have a 50% risk of getting the X chromosome with the gene for that condition. Again the reader should remember that risk is a mathematical prediction. A male affected with an X-linked trait will have no affected sons because he does not give the X chromosome to his sons. All of his daughters will be carriers or affected, depending on the recessive or dominant nature of the trait, because all daughters will receive his X chromosome.

Lyon Hypothesis and X-linked Recessive Traits

As discussed previously, according to the Lyon hypothesis, one of the X chromosomes in the female is genetically cancelled at an early stage of embryonic development. This cancellation affects X chromosomes from both maternal and paternal lines. If a female embryo is a carrier of an X-linked recessive trait, half of the X chromosomes have the normal gene, and the other half have the abnormal gene (allele) for the given trait before cancellation occurs. Classic hemophilia (hemophilia A) is a good example. Hemophilia A is inherited as an X-linked recessive condition. In this disorder blood does not coagulate because of the low or almost nonexistent levels of factor VIII (antihemophilic globulin) in circulating blood. Males with the abnormal gene have a severe coagulation defect. In the female carrier some of the cancelled X chromosomes have the abnormal gene, and others have the normal one. The female carrier is a mosaic (i.e., she has both normal and abnormal X chromosomes). Because cancellation is random, the number of X chromosomes that remain genetically active and contain the normal or abnormal gene will vary. The female carrier's levels of factor VIII are often reduced; however, this reduction and the length of coagulation time vary, depending on the number of X chromosomes that contain the abnormal gene and remain genetically active. Although female carriers of the gene for hemophilia do not have as severe a problem as males, they tend to bleed more than usual after extraction of teeth or scaling and curettage. The variation in the bleeding problem in female carriers of the gene for hemophilia reflects the Lyon hypothesis. Other inherited disorders that reflect this hypothesis are described in detail later in this chapter. They include the X-linked type of amelogenesis imperfecta and hypohidrotic ectodermal dysplasia.

Genetic Heterogeneity

The term **genetic heterogeneity** is used when a condition has more than one inheritance pattern and differences in the degree of clinical manifestations for each of the inherited varieties. Amelogenesis imperfecta (described later in the chapter) is a condition that illustrates genetic heterogeneity.

In general, alterations in structural proteins (complex substances formed by one or more polypeptide) are inherited as a dominant trait, whereas alterations in enzymatic proteins (a protein inducing changes in other body substances) are inherited in a recessive manner; however, exceptions to this rule are seen.

Physical characteristics can be inherited as either dominant or recessive traits. The term **recessive** does not mean deleterious or abnormal. Instead it means that the individual must be homozygous for the trait for it to be seen. For example, in the ABO blood group system blood group O is recessive, whereas groups A and B are dominant. However, no blood group is abnormal.

Genes can be codominant. Again a good example is the ABO blood group. A and B are dominant over O, but when A and B are allelic, the result is blood group AB, in which both genes are exhibited. This is called **codominance**.

The four inheritance patterns refer to the characteristics that are governed by the action of one gene. This is called **single-gene inheritance. Oligogenic inheritance** refers to characteristics or traits that are inherited by the participation of several genes. These conditions show greater clinical variation than do those inherited through single-gene action. Characteristics such as tooth shape and form and eye color are determined by oligogenic inheritance. Most physical characteristics are oligogenic. The various genes that participate in determining a trait or condition can be located in the same chromosome or in different chromosomes.

Examples of Molecular Chromosomal Abnormalities

All of the inherited disorders in this section include oral and dental alterations and are discussed by location—gingiva and periodontium, jawbones and facies, oral mucosa, and teeth. Patients affected with these genetic abnormalities should receive routine dental hygiene care to maintain oral health. Specific dental hygiene management considerations are included only if they are unique to the disorder described.

Inherited Disorders Affecting the Gingiva and Periodontium

Most of the disorders included here are rare. However, they exhibit severe gingival or periodontal alterations (or both); therefore the dental hygienist should be aware of the disorders and their clinical manifestations.

Cyclic Neutropenia. The inheritance pattern of **cyclic neutropenia** is autosomal dominant; the responsible gene has been identified and is called ELA-2 (neutrophil elastase gene). This gene is located on the short arm of chromosome 19. In the chromosome mapping system its location is designated as 19p13.3. The disorder is characterized by a cyclic decrease in the number of circulating neutrophilic leukocytes (neutrophils); a decrease in the number of circulating neutrophils is called **neutropenia**. The cycles usually occur in intervals of 21 to 27 days, but in some patients the interval may be extended to several months. These episodes of neutropenia generally persist for 2 to 3 days.

The clinical manifestations are related to the decrease in neutrophils. Systemic manifestations of cyclic neutropenia include fever, malaise, sore throat, and occasional cutaneous infections. Oral manifestations consist of severe ulcerative gingivitis or gingivostomatitis (Figure 6-14). In addition to the gingiva, areas of ulceration can also occur on the tongue and surfaces of the oral mucosa. The ulcers are of variable size and have a craterlike appearance. They are very painful and have a bleeding base. Generally the oral lesions are infected secondarily. When neutrophils return to normal, the oral lesions tend to improve.

Patients with cyclic neutropenia are usually managed by first determining the frequency of the cycles through periodic neutrophil counts and then instituting preventive antibiotic therapy to protect against secondary opportunistic infections. Over time episodes of neutropenia and associated ulcerative gingivitis lead to severe periodontal disease, with loss of alveolar bone, tooth mobility, and exfoliation of teeth. Treatment should be initiated when the circulating neutrophil count is normal to reduce the risk of complications such as gingival hemorrhage and secondary infection. Dental hygiene care, including frequent appointments for removal of local irritants and maintenance of optimal oral hygiene, reduces the risk of opportunistic infections in patients with cyclic neutropenia.

Patients with cyclic neutropenia are treated with periodic granulocyte colony-stimulating factor (G-CSF) that reduces the symptoms and results in substantial clinical improvement.

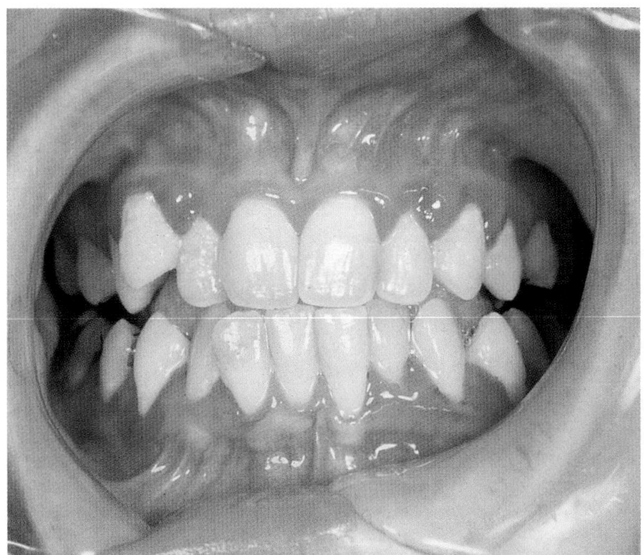

FIGURE 6-14 ■ Hypertrophic gingivitis with areas of gingival recession is exhibited in a patient with cyclic neutropenia.

Chronic neutropenia, also known as *Kostmann syndrome*, is another variety of neutropenia that is inherited as an autosomal recessive. The intraoral manifestations are similar to those of the cyclic variety but are constant. The responsible gene is still unknown, and it is also treated with periodic G-CSF.

Papillon-Lefèvre Syndrome. **Papillon-Lefèvre syndrome** has an autosomal-recessive inheritance pattern and is composed of marked destruction of the periodontal tissues (periodontoclasia) of both dentitions with premature loss of teeth and hyperkeratosis of the palms of the hands and soles of the feet (palmar and plantar hyperkeratosis).

The gene for this syndrome has been mapped to the long arm of chromosome 11 regions 14-21 (11q14-21). These patients are normal at birth except for a reddening of the palms of the hands and soles of the feet. Teeth erupt in normal sequence, position, and time. At about 1½ to 2 years of age, a marked gingivoperiodontal inflammatory process develops characterized by edema, bleeding, alveolar bone resorption, and mobility of teeth with consequent exfoliation. A red, scaly keratosis develops on the palms and soles concurrent with these oral lesions and occasionally extends to the dorsal surfaces of the hands and feet. The oral lesions are complicated by superimposed inflammation, and radiographs reveal marked alveolar bone resorption with vertical pockets. Teeth are lost in the same sequence in which they erupted. When the last tooth is lost, the gingiva regains a normal appearance.

The lesions on the hands and feet remain as reddish-white, scaly, thick areas of hyperkeratinization (Figure 6-15). The permanent dentition begins to erupt at the proper time. At about 8 or 9 years of age the gingivoperiodontal destruction is repeated in the same manner as occurred in the primary dentition (Figure 6-16). All permanent teeth are lost before 14 years of age. The gingiva again resumes a normal appearance.

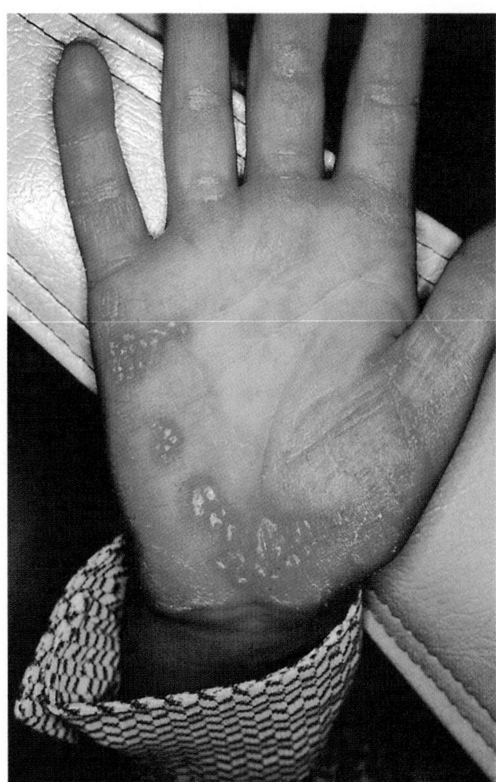

FIGURE 6-15 ■ Areas of hyperkeratinization of the palms are exhibited in a patient with Papillon-Lefèvre syndrome. (From Sedano HO, Sauk JJ, Gorlin RJ: *Oral manifestations of inherited disorders,* Boston, 1977, Butterworth. Used with permission.)

Peripheral blood neutrophil is depressed in all patients with Papillon-Lefèvre syndrome. This suggests that the neutrophils may be an important factor in the pathogenesis of severe periodontal disease in these patients. Retinoid therapy markedly improves the skin condition but has no effect on the periodontal disease in patients with this syndrome. To date all therapeutic attempts at preventing the gingival and periodontal destruction and subsequent loss of teeth have been unsuccessful. The basic defect that causes the condition is unknown. Peripheral blood neutrophil chemotaxis has been reported to be depressed in patients with Papillon-Lefèvre syndrome. This decreased chemotaxis suggests that neutrophils may play a role in periodontal destruction in patients with this syndrome. Current research suggests bacterial and viral involvement as the initiating factors for the periodontal destruction. It has been suggested that the genetic component of Papillon-Lefèvre syndrome is a predisposition rather than the main determinant of periodontal disease.

The skin manifestations remain for life, but treatment with retinol (oral etretinate) has proven somewhat effective in controlling the hyperkeratinization. These patients do not have any other abnormalities.

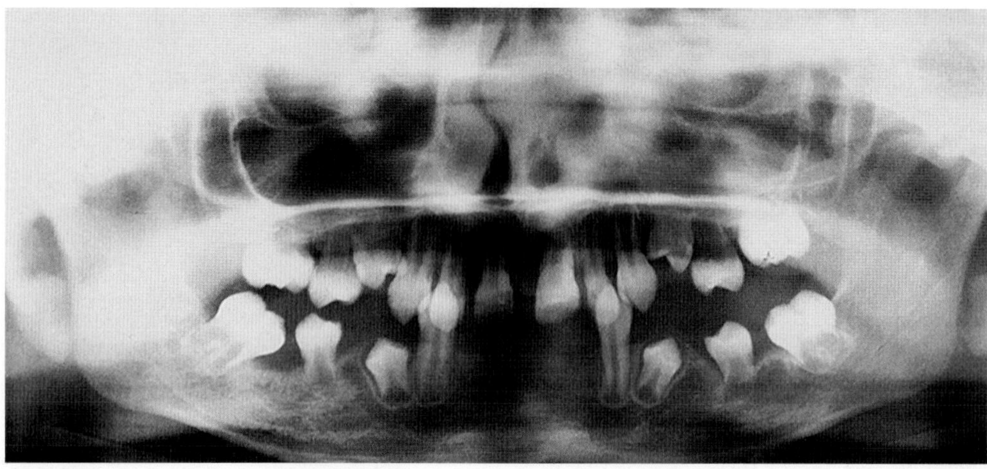

FIGURE 6-16 ■ Panoramic radiograph shows marked periodontal destruction with alveolar bone resorption in the patient in Figure 6-15. (From Sedano HO, Sauk JJ, Gorlin RJ: *Oral manifestations of inherited disorders,* Boston, 1977, Butterworth. Used with permission.)

Focal Palmoplantar and Gingival Hyperkeratosis. Areas of hyperkeratinization of the palms and soles and marked hyperkeratinization of the labial and lingual gingiva characterize **focal palmoplantar** and **gingival hyperkeratosis.** This syndrome has an autosomal-dominant inheritance pattern. The palmar and plantar hyperkeratosis starts at the tips of the fingers and toes and extends to the surface of the palms and soles. This process increases with age and also becomes localized, with calluses forming on the weight-bearing areas.

The oral hyperkeratinization is bandlike and a few millimeters in width (Figure 6-17). It follows the normal festooned contour of the gingiva. The free gingiva is not affected. Palatal and lingual mucosa occasionally can be affected with areas of hyperkeratinization. These changes start in childhood and increase with age. The rest of the oral cavity is normal.

Gingival Fibromatosis. **Gingival fibromatosis** is a component of several inherited syndromes. The gingival hypertrophy generally develops early in life, and within a few years the teeth are completely covered. The fibromatosis is composed of very firm tissue with a granular corrugated surface. Generally the color is paler than that of the normal gingiva and results from the marked collagenization of the fibrous connective tissue. The extensive gingival enlargement leads to protrusion of the lips.

In addition to isolated gingival fibromatosis (Figure 6-18), which has an autosomal-dominant inheritance pattern and no other associated abnormalities, gingival fibromatosis is a component of a number of syndromes. Because of the gingival involvement, several of these syndromes, although rare, are described here. However, only those that are well known and occur most frequently are included.

Dental hygiene care can reduce the risk of secondary inflammation and infection in patients with gingival fibromatosis.

Laband Syndrome. The inheritance pattern of **Laband syndrome** is autosomal dominant. In addition to gingival fibromatosis, patients have dysplastic or absent nails and malformed nose and ears because of soft and pliable cartilage formation, hepatosplenomegaly (enlarged liver and spleen), and hypoplasia of terminal phalanges of the fingers and toes with a resultant froglike appearance.

Gingival Fibromatosis With Hypertrichosis, Epilepsy, and Mental Retardation Syndrome. **Gingival fibromatosis with hypertrichosis, epilepsy, and mental retardation syndrome** has an autosomal-dominant inheritance pattern. Hypertrichosis (excessive growth of hair), especially of the eyebrows, extremities, genitals, and sacral region, characterize gingival fibromatosis with hypertrichosis, epilepsy, and mental retardation. Epilepsy and mental retardation can also occur in this syndrome but are inconsistent features.

Gingival Fibromatosis With Multiple Hyaline Fibromas. **Gingival fibromatosis with multiple hyaline fibromas** has an autosomal-dominant inheritance pattern and is also known as the *Murray-Puretíc Drescher syndrome.* In addition to gingival fibromatosis, it is characterized by hypertrophy of the nail beds and multiple hyaline fibrous tumors developing on the nose, chin, head, back, fingers, thighs, and legs. These tumors on the extremities can produce contractures of various joints, including hips, knees, shoulders, and elbows.

Inherited Disorders Affecting the Jaw Bones and Facies

Cherubism. The inheritance pattern of **cherubism** is autosomal dominant with marked penetrance (when the gene is present, the clinical manifestations are usually seen)

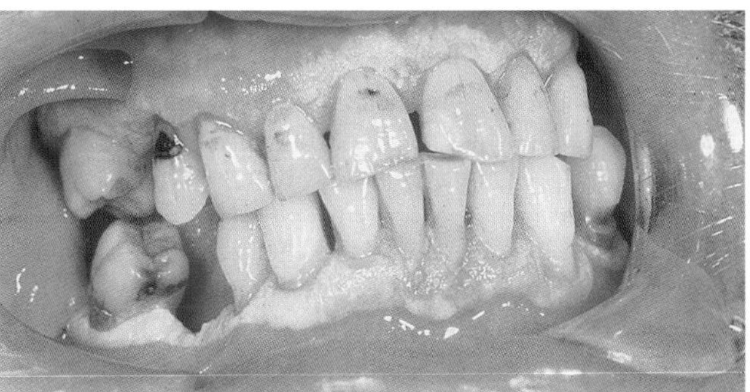

FIGURE 6-17 ■ Marked hyperkeratosis follows the normal contour of the gingiva in focal palmoplantar and gingival hyperkeratosis. (From Sedano HO, Sauk JJ, Gorlin RJ: *Oral manifestations of inherited disorders,* Boston, 1977, Butterworth. Used with permission.)

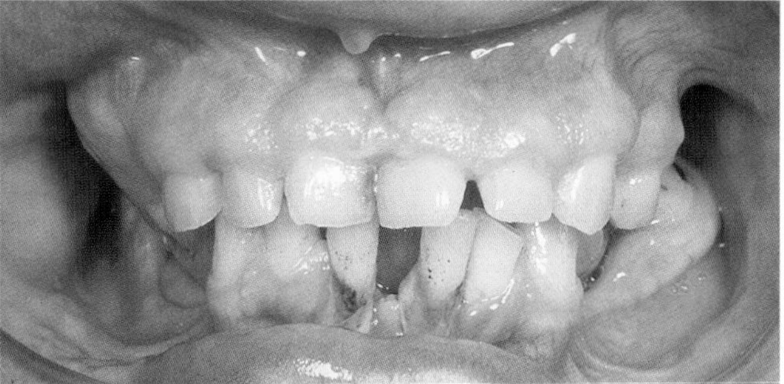

FIGURE 6-18 ■ Gingival hypertrophy is shown in a patient with isolated gingival fibromatosis.

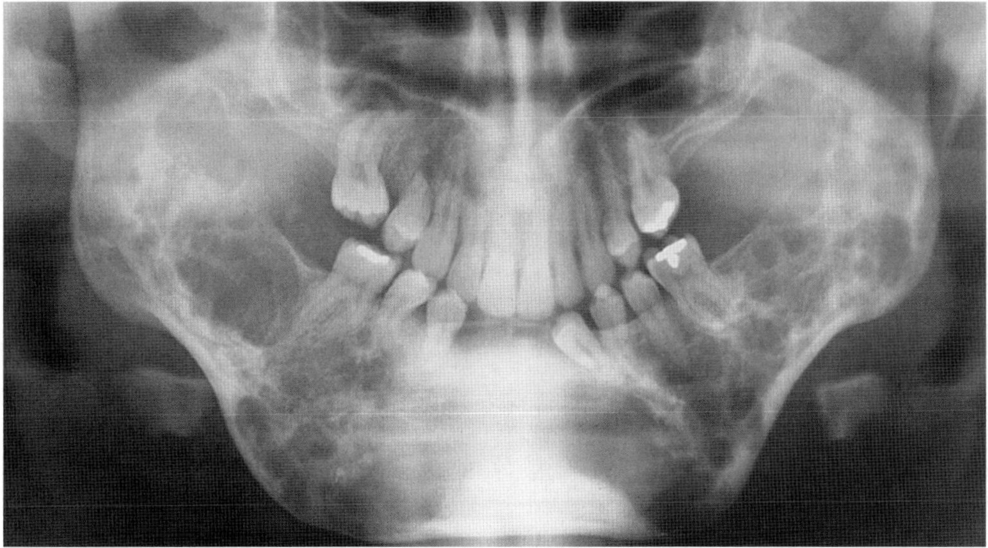

FIGURE 6-19 ■ Panoramic radiograph of the jaws shows typical bilateral soap-bubble image in a patient with cherubism. (From Young WG, Sedano HO: *Atlas of oral pathology,* Minneapolis, 1981, University of Minnesota Press. Used with permission.)

in males and variable expressivity and incomplete penetrance in females. The gene for cherubism has been mapped to the short arm of chromosome 4 region 16 (4p16). The first clinical manifestation is a progressive bilateral facial swelling that appears when the patient is between 1½ and 4 years of age. This change can affect either the mandible or the maxilla, but involvement of the mandible is most common. Displacement of the eyes is evident when the maxilla is affected. This, added to the bilateral deformity, produces the characteristic cherubic facial appearance that is responsible for the name of the syndrome. Increased distance between the eyes (ocular hypertelorism) is always present in affected patients. Radiographs of the jaws show a typical "soap-bubble" or multilocular appearance (Figure 6-19), which usually occupies the ascending ramus of the mandible and extends into the molar and premolar areas. Severe cases can involve the full mandible, but the condyle is always spared. When the maxilla is affected, the changes are observed at the level of the tuberosity and involve the antrum.

These areas of bone radiolucency are occupied by fibrous connective tissue containing multinucleated giant cells. The microscopic appearance resembles the central giant cell granuloma (described in Chapter 2). The bone lesions interfere with tooth development and eruption. Most of these patients have pseudoanodontia (teeth falsely appear to be lacking), especially of molars and premolars, because of delayed eruption.

The size of the jaws tends to increase rapidly until about puberty and then generally remains stable. After the individual reaches age 20 or 30 years, radiographs show an almost normal bone appearance, with a few areas of increased bone density. The facial deformity remains for life, and in some patients it can be quite striking.

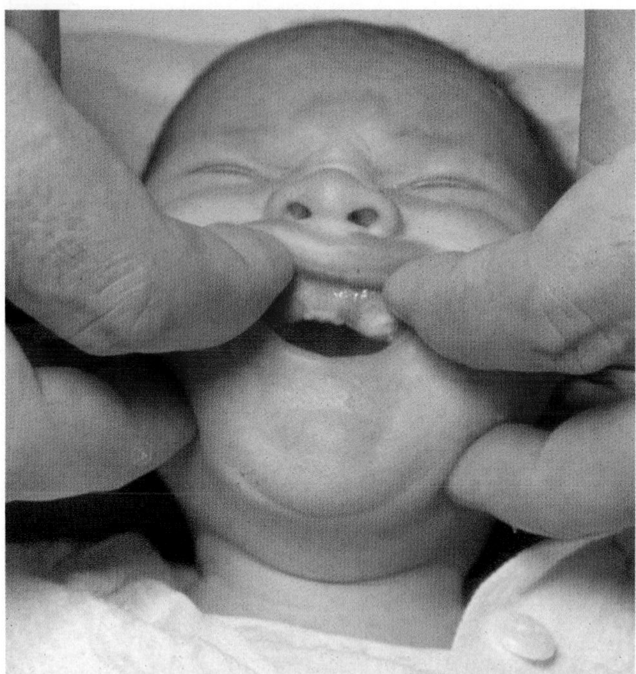

FIGURE 6-20 ■ Infant with Ellis–van Creveld syndrome (chondroectodermal dysplasia). The anterior maxillary vestibular sulcus is absent.

Ellis–Van Creveld Syndrome. **Ellis–van Creveld syndrome** has an autosomal-recessive inheritance pattern. The gene for this has been mapped to the short arm of chromosome 4 region 16 (4p16). Affected individuals are dwarfs because of distal shortening of the extremities. One third of these patients are mildly mentally handicapped. The hands show polydactyly (supernumerary digits) on the ulnar side, and fingernails and toenails are hypoplastic and deformed. Other skeletal anomalies include curvature of the legs and feet. Fifty percent of affected individuals have congenital heart defects. Anomalies of the external genitals, especially in males, are also observed.

The oral manifestations are constant and characteristic and include fusion of the anterior portion of the maxillary gingiva to the upper lip from canine to canine. Thus the anterior maxillary vestibular sulcus is lacking (Figure 6-20). This anomaly induces a V-notch appearance in the midline of the upper lip. The anterior lower alveolar ridge presents a serrated appearance caused by thick frenula, which start at the vestibular sulcus and traverse the alveolar ridge. The central incisors of both maxilla and mandible are generally lacking and are replaced by a centrally located abnormal tooth. Most of the teeth have a conical shape and exhibit enamel hypoplasia. More than 50% of newborns with this syndrome have natal teeth.

Cleidocranial Dysplasia. The inheritance pattern of **cleidocranial dysplasia** is autosomal dominant; however, about half of the cases are isolated examples caused by either spontaneous mutation or a gene with poor penetrance. The gene for this syndrome has been mapped to the short arm of chromosome 6 region 21 (6p21). The cranium develops a mushroom shape because the fontanelles remain open. This makes the face appear small. Frontal, parietal, and occipital enlargement is quite noticeable. Skull radiographs reveal the open fontanelles, which are often open for life. The paranasal sinuses are lacking or hypoplastic. The neck is long and narrow because of unilateral or bilateral aplasia (lack of development) or hypoplasia of the clavicles. Affected individuals are able to approximate their shoulders to the midline because of this clavicular alteration. Various other bone anomalies can also be present.

The premaxilla is generally underdeveloped, resulting in pseudoprognathism. These patients have many supernumerary teeth, sometimes even simulating a third dentition (Figure 6-21). They are crowded in the jaws and do not erupt. They also interfere with the eruption of normal teeth, resulting in pseudoanodontia. A lack of cellular cementum has been reported in patients with this syndrome. Multiple cysts can develop in association with the impacted teeth. About 1% of affected patients have cleft lip, cleft palate, or both.

Gardner Syndrome. **Gardner syndrome**, also known as *familial colorectal polyposis*, has an autosomal-dominant inheritance pattern with variable expressivity and marked penetrance. The adenomatous polyposis coli gene is responsible for Gardner syndrome and is located on the long arm of chromosome 5 regions 21-22 (5q21-22). One of the basic components is the presence of osteomas in various bones, especially the frontal bones, mandible, and maxilla. When they expand, osteomas of the facial skeleton obliterate the sinuses and induce facial asymmetry. Osteomas can also occur in the long bones of the skeleton but with less frequency than in the bones of the face.

In addition to osteomas, multiple odontomas can occur in the jawbones, especially the mandible (Figure 6-22). Teeth can exhibit hypercementosis and fail to erupt.

The most serious component of this syndrome is the presence of intestinal polyps, which become malignant at age 30 and after. Polyposis primarily affects the colon and rectum and generally develops before puberty. Some authors advocate intestinal resection when the polyps appear because their malignant transformation into adenocarcinoma is invariable, especially with increasing age.

Mandibulofacial Dysostosis. The inheritance pattern of **mandibulofacial dysostosis** is autosomal dominant with incomplete penetrance and variable expressivity. The gene for this syndrome has been mapped to the long arm of chromosome 5 regions 32-33.1 (5q32-33.1). The facies shows downward sloping of the palpebral fissures, a hypoplastic nose, hypoplastic malar bones with hypoplasia or absence of the zygomatic process, abnormal and misplaced ears, and a receding chin. The mouth appears fishlike, with downward sloping of the lip commissures. The lower eyelids show a cleft (coloboma) of the outer third, with a lack of lashes medial to it. The ears may exhibit tags, which on occasion can also be seen near the angle of the mouth.

Deafness is a constant feature resulting from a lack of otic ossicles. Mental development is within normal limits; difficulty in learning arises from deafness. Oral manifestations include a markedly hypoplastic mandible with flattened condyles and coronoid processes and an obtuse mandibular angle. Teeth are malposed, and malocclusion with open bite is quite evident. The palate is high, or a cleft is present in about 30% of affected patients (Figure 6-23). Gingival disease is common and is related to the dental abnormalities.

Nevoid Basal Cell Carcinoma Syndrome. The **nevoid basal cell carcinoma syndrome,** also known as *Gorlin syndrome,* has an autosomal-dominant inheritance pattern with high penetrance and variable expressivity. The gene for this syndrome maps to the long arm of chromosome 9 region 22.3 (9q22.3). The facies is characterized by mild hypertelorism (increased distance between the eyes) and mild prognathism, with frontal and parietal enlargement and a broad nasal root.

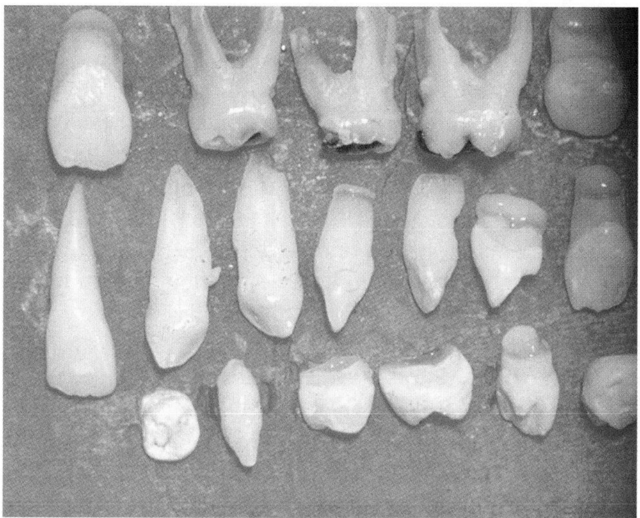

FIGURE 6-21 ■ Multiple extracted supernumerary teeth from a patient with cleidocranial dysplasia.

The cutaneous manifestations, which are called nevi, typically are basal cell carcinomas. The term **nevus** (plural, **nevi**), as defined here, is a congenital lesion characterized by skin pigmentation. These basal cell carcinomas appear early in life and continue to develop over the nose, eyelids, cheeks, neck, arms, and trunk. They can be flesh colored or pale brown and develop singly or in clusters. Histologically they are basal cell carcinomas. The palms and soles show small pits that become filled with dirt and appear as dark spots on those surfaces.

The oral manifestations of this syndrome consist of multiple cysts of the jaws (Figure 6-24) that (histologically) are odontogenic keratocysts (see Chapter 5). These cysts vary in size; they can be very large and have a marked tendency to recur after surgical removal. Occasionally an ameloblastoma arises in these cysts as part of this syndrome. The cysts develop as early as 5 to 6 years of age in some affected patients and interfere with normal development of the jawbones and teeth.

A great variety of skeletal anomalies have been reported in association with the nevoid basal cell carcinoma syndrome, the most constant being bifurcation or splaying of one or more ribs. Other frequent abnormalities of bone include shortening of the metacarpals, spina bifida occulta (defective closure of the bone encasement of the spinal cord), and kyphoscoliosis (a combination of scoliosis, which is a lateral curving of the spine, and kyphosis, which is an abnormal vertical curvature of the spine or "hunchback").

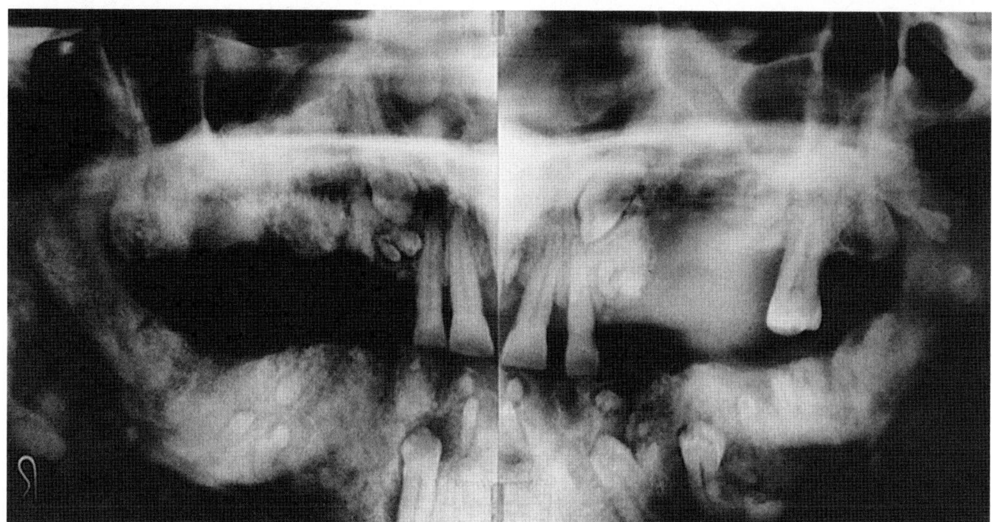

FIGURE 6-22 ■ Panoramic radiograph of a patient with Gardner syndrome shows multiple osteomas and odontomas. (Courtesy Dr. Carl J. Witkop.)

Many different neoplasms have been reported in association with this syndrome. Medulloblastoma (brain tumor) has been seen in many cases. Children surviving the medulloblastoma eventually present other manifestations of the syndrome. Other less frequent findings include calcified ovarian fibromas and mesenteric cysts.

Osteogenesis Imperfecta. **Osteogenesis imperfecta** is known to have an autosomal-dominant inheritance pattern with variable expressivity. However, only 30% of patients have a family history of this condition. The remaining 70% represent sporadic cases and cases suggesting autosomal-recessive inheritance. The basic defect is produced by different mutations affecting the genes that encode for type I collagen, resulting in abnormally formed bones that fracture easily. The genes responsible for the inherited varieties of osteogenesis imperfecta are mapped as follows: collagen type I alpha 2 is in the long arm of chromosome 7 region 22.1 (7q22.1); collagen type I alpha 1 is in the long arm of chromosome 17 region 21.31-22.05 (17q21.31-22.05). Osteogenesis imperfecta occurs in about 1 in 20,000 births, and major syndromes have been classified in four types: I, II, III, and IV.

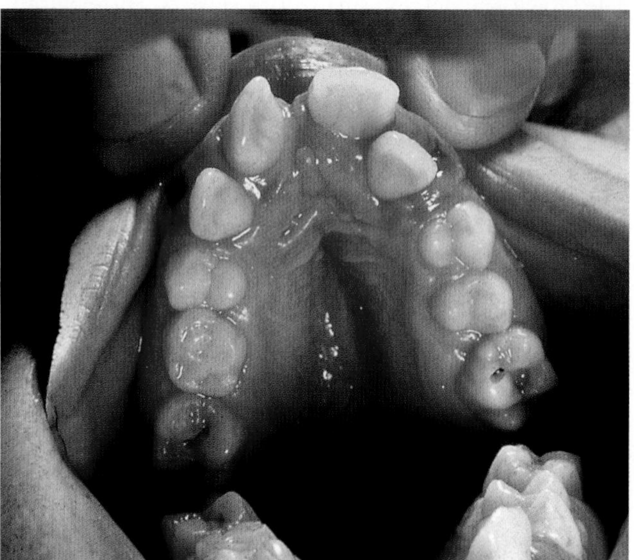

FIGURE 6-23 ■ Markedly high-arched palate and malpositioned teeth in a patient with mandibulofacial dysostosis.

The clinical manifestations vary markedly from patient to patient. The sporadic cases tend to be more severe than those with an autosomal-dominant inheritance pattern. The basic defect involves collagen and results in abnormally formed bones that fracture easily. Multiple bone fractures are the main clinical complication of this syndrome. In the congenital form newborns can have several fractured bones at birth. Infants with this condition have experienced fractures just by being moved. In the most severe cases all bones can be affected, presenting a plethora of abnormalities, including bowing of the legs, curvature of the spine (kyphosis and scoliosis), deformity of the skull, shortening of arms and legs, and other abnormalities. In the mildest cases individuals show only blue sclerae (a blue appearance of the white of the eye).

The oral manifestation of this syndrome is a dentinogenesis imperfecta–like condition (a description of dentinogenesis imperfecta follows later in this chapter). Primary teeth are affected in 80% of patients, whereas permanent teeth are affected in only 35% of these individuals (Figure 6-25). The crowns, roots, and pulp chambers generally are smaller than normal. Teeth appear opalescent or translucent at time of eruption, but they darken with age. The enamel is lost because the abnormal dentin cannot provide adequate support.

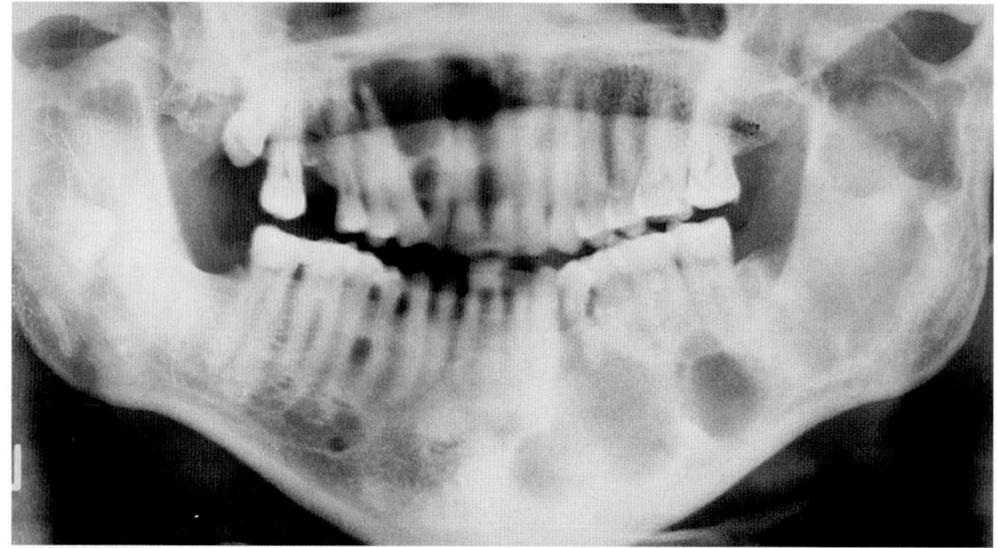

FIGURE 6-24 ■ Multiple mandibular radiolucencies in a patient with nevoid basal cell carcinoma syndrome. These lesions are odontogenic keratocysts.

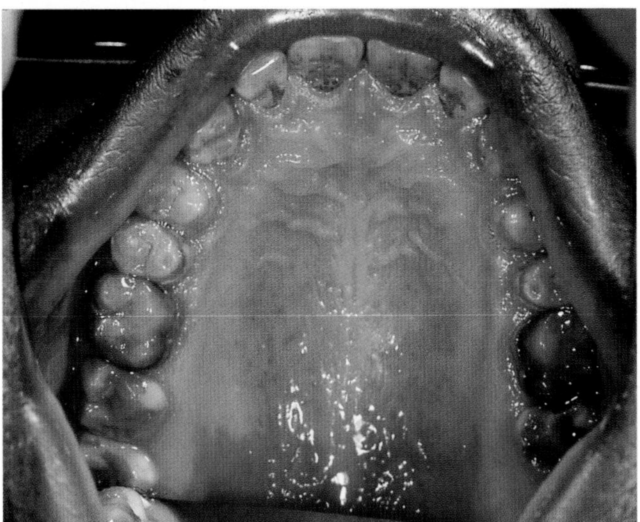

FIGURE 6-25 ■ Patient with osteogenesis imperfecta. Teeth are yellowish with chipped enamel.

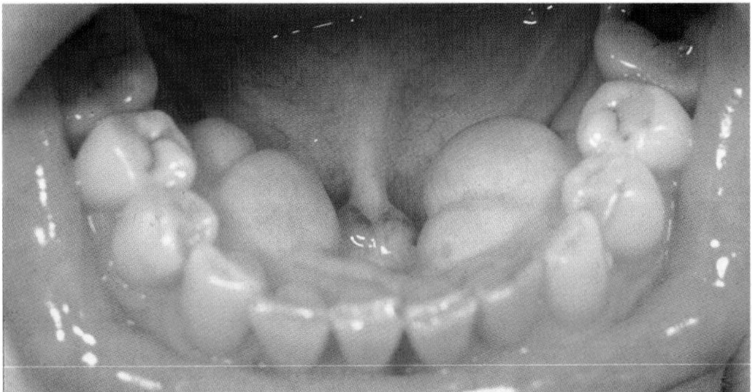

FIGURE 6-26 ■ Bilateral lobulated mandibular tori.

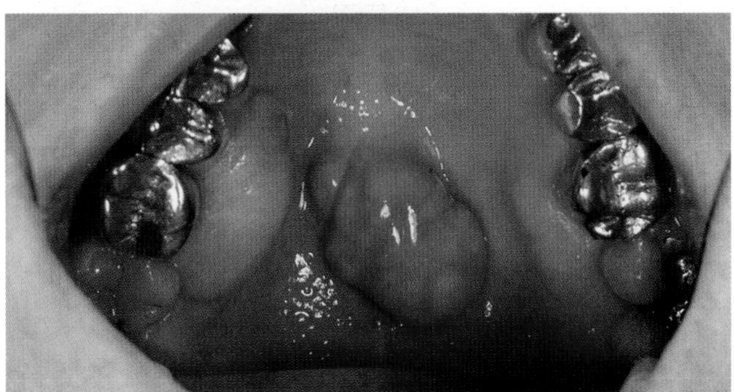

FIGURE 6-27 ■ Torus palatinus.

Torus Mandibularis. Mandibular tori (singular, torus) have an autosomal-dominant inheritance pattern with variable expressivity and marked penetrance. This anomaly can be unilateral or bilateral. These tori occur on the lingual aspect of the mandible in the area of the premolar teeth (Figure 6-26). Occurrence before age 15 years is extremely rare. The size of the torus is variable, and occasionally it can be multilobulated. Mandibular tori are symptomless and generally require no treatment. Surgical removal may be necessary if the patient needs a denture. Intraoral radiographs usually show a radiopacity in the area of the mandibular premolars if mandibular tori are present. (Mandibular tori are also discussed in Chapters 1 and 7.)

Torus Palatinus. Autosomal dominance with variable expressivity and almost 100% penetrance characterizes torus palatinus. A bony overgrowth occurs at the midline of the hard palate (Figure 6-27). A marked predilection exists for women (2:1), and a higher prevalence exists among Native Americans, including Inuits. Torus palatinus becomes evident around the time of puberty and is only rarely seen in children younger than 14 years of age. The size of this anomaly varies from nearly undetectable to large masses that occupy almost the entire hard palate. Some palatal tori are multilobular. Torus palatinus is symptomless. However, the surface mucosa is thin and easily traumatized. The torus may need to be removed if the patient needs a full denture. (Torus palatinus is also described in Chapters 1 and 7.)

Maxillary Exostosis. Exostoses have an autosomal-dominant inheritance pattern. **Maxillary exostoses** represent tori that generally develop on the buccal aspect of the maxillary alveolar ridge, usually in the molar and premolar area (Figure 6-28). They are generally symptomless unless traumatized. They may be single, multiple, unilateral, and bilateral and occur less frequently than either palatal or mandibular tori. (Exostoses are also described in Chapter 7.)

Inherited Disorders Affecting the Oral Mucosa

Isolated Cleft Palate and Cleft Lip With or Without Cleft Palate. The majority of cases of facial clefting are multifactorial in origin; they occur in about 1 in 800 births. A large number of inherited syndromes can include cleft lip and palate or isolated cleft palate as a component. When clefting is part of an inherited syndrome, its occurrence within affected families will be in accordance with the inheritance pattern of the syndrome. Most of these syndromes are very rare. **Cleft lip-palate** and **congenital lip pits** (Van der Woude syndrome) is the syndrome that is considered to occur most frequently; therefore it is the only one described here. It has an autosomal-dominant inheritance pattern with 80% penetrance for any of its components. In the majority of cases the gene has been mapped to the long arm of chromosome 1 regions 32 to 41 (1q32-41). The labial pits (Figure 6-29) are bilateral and are located near the midline of the vermilion border of the lower lip. They may be 3 mm or more in diameter and generally finish in a blind end. Occasionally they exude saliva because of their association with a labial minor salivary gland. These pits are rarely unilateral, and the clefting is bilateral in about 80% of patients. Some patients without clefting have agenesis (lack of

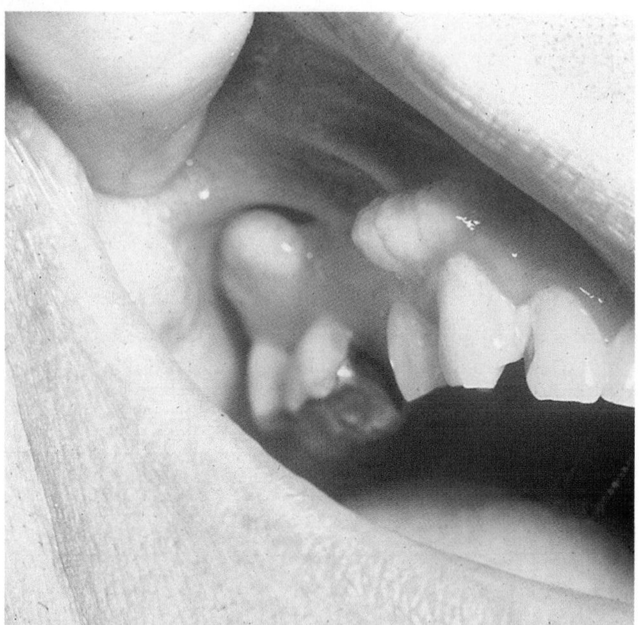

FIGURE 6-28 ■ Maxillary exostoses are inherited as autosomal dominant.

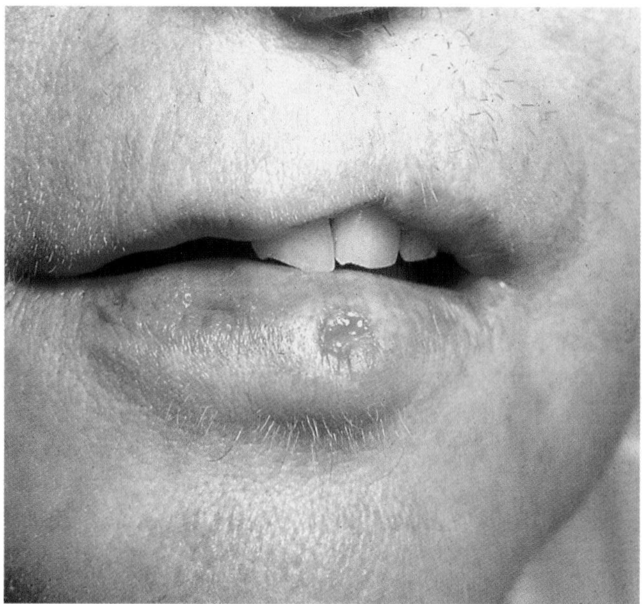

FIGURE 6-29 ■ Paramedial pits in the lower lip. Note the scar of the repaired cleft of the left upper lip

development) of the maxillary lateral incisors or peg lateral incisors. Other oral findings that have been seen include fibrous adhesions between the maxilla and mandible, a cleft uvula, and ankyloglossia.

Hereditary Hemorrhagic Telangiectasia. The inheritance pattern of **hereditary hemorrhagic telangiectasia,** also known as *Osler-Rendu–Parkes Weber syndrome,* is autosomal dominant. Recent studies indicate that this syndrome may have two different responsible loci: one at the long arm of chromosome 9 (9q3) and the other in chromosome 12. It is characterized by multiple capillary dilations of the skin and mucous membranes (Figure 6-30). The skin of the face shows numerous pinpoint and spiderlike telangiectases, especially on the lips, eyelids, and around the nose. The scalp and ears are also affected. Similar lesions are present in the nasal mucosa and are responsible for frequent and sometimes serious nosebleeds **(epistaxis)** that can last for several days. Any organ or mucous membrane can be the site of telangiectasia.

Telangiectases of the oral mucosa are especially prominent on the tip and anterior dorsum of the tongue. The palate, gingiva, and buccal mucosa are often affected but to a lesser degree. Hemorrhage from sites in the oral cavity, mainly the lips and tongue, is second in frequency to epistaxis. Gingival bleeding has been reported and is a possible complication of dental hygiene treatment. The risk of gingival hemorrhage should be a concern of the dental hygienist when treating a patient with this syndrome.

Multiple Mucosal Neuroma Syndrome. The combination of multiple mucosal neuromas, medullary carcinoma of the thyroid gland, and pheochromocytoma is identified as multiple endocrine neoplasia, type 2B (MEN 2B). The inheritance pattern is autosomal dominant with decreased penetrance. This syndrome is the result of mutations in the receptor tyrosine kinase that maps to chromosome 10q11.2. Patients are tall with characteristic thick, large lips and often everted upper eyelids. The mucosal neuromas are prominent on the lips and anterior dorsal surface of the tongue (Figure 6-31). They generally appear in the first few years of life. In addition, neuromas can occur on the buccal mucosa and the eyelids. The mucosal neuromas are seen as multiple, mobile, firm lumps covered by normal mucosa. Histologically they are aggregates of nerve tissue.

Medullary carcinoma of the thyroid has been diagnosed in more than 75% of patients with this syndrome; it generally develops in the second decade of life. Metastatic lesions develop frequently, and about 20% of patients die as a consequence of metastasis. The thyroid carcinoma produces calcitonin (a hormone normally produced by the C cells of the thyroid gland). The carcinoma can be detected by evaluating plasma levels of this hormone.

Pheochromocytoma is a benign neoplasm that generally develops in ganglia around the adrenal glands. The tumor is often bilateral and is responsible for night sweats, high blood pressure, and episodes of severe diarrhea. It generally develops in the second or third decade of life. The pheochromocytoma induces increased urinary levels of epinephrine and other substances. Other findings in this syndrome have included cutaneous pigmentation and a host of skeletal abnormalities.

Early diagnosis of this syndrome is imperative because of the high malignant potential of the thyroid carcinoma.

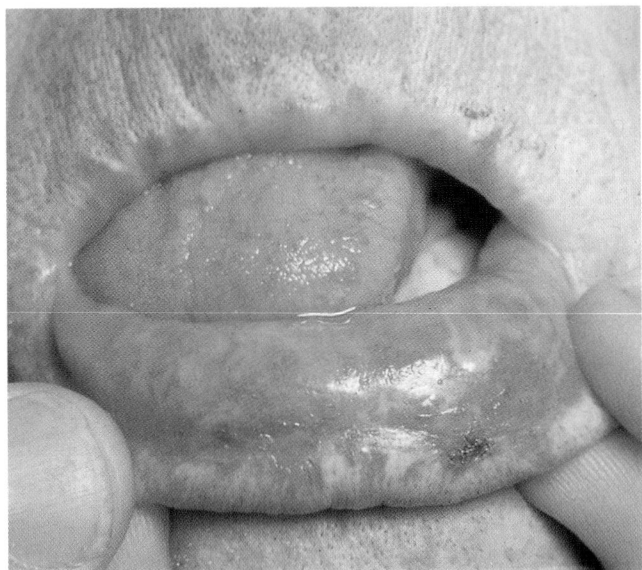

FIGURE 6-30 ■ Multiple telangiectases of lips and tongue in a patient with hereditary hemorrhagic telangiectasia. Gingival bleeding can be profuse in cases like this. (From Sedano HO, Sauk JJ, Gorlin RJ: *Oral manifestations of inherited disorders,* Boston, 1977, Butterworth. Used with permission.)

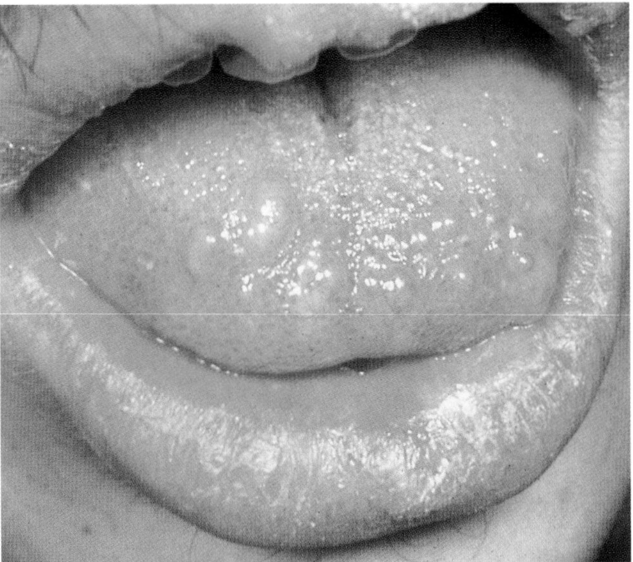

FIGURE 6-31 ■ Patient with MEN 2B syndrome with multiple mucosal neuromas on the tip of the tongue and upper lip. (From Sedano HO, Sauk JJ, Gorlin RJ: *Oral manifestations of inherited disorders,* Boston, 1977, Butterworth. Used with permission.)

Some authors recommend preventive thyroidectomy when this syndrome is diagnosed so that the development of carcinoma is avoided. The neuromas of the oral mucosa may be the earliest visible manifestation of this syndrome.

Neurofibromatosis of Von Recklinghausen. **Neurofibromatosis of von Recklinghausen,** also called *von Recklinghausen disease,* has an autosomal-dominant inheritance pattern and is probably a disorder of neural crest origin. The gene for this syndrome maps to the long arm of chromosome 17 region 11.2 (17q11.2). Several varieties exist; however, only the classic form is described here.

Multiple neurofibromas, which appear as papules and growths of various sizes, are seen on the facial skin, especially the eyelids. The tumors can arise anywhere, including the oral cavity, and can be present at birth or develop early in life, increasing in number and size at puberty. Malignant transformation of the neurofibromas occurs in an estimated 3% to 15% of patients with neurofibromatosis. Neurofibromas also develop in the central nervous system, eyes, ears, viscera, and intraosseous locations. Mental disability is observed occasionally, and multiple skeletal anomalies are common.

Oral involvement is seen in about 10% of patients and is characterized by single or multiple tumors at any location in the oral mucosa, the most frequent being the lateral borders of the tongue. Gingival neurofibromas can also occur in these patients (Figure 6-32), and intramandibular neurofibromas have been reported and present as radiolucencies in the mandible.

Café au lait (the color of coffee with milk) pigmentation of skin is present from the first decade of life in 90% of patients with neurofibromatosis. This pigmentation is quite marked in the axilla and can also affect other areas of the skin. Café au lait skin pigmentation generally precedes the development of the neurofibromas.

Peutz-Jeghers Syndrome. Autosomal-dominant inheritance characterizes the **Peutz-Jeghers syndrome**. The gene for this syndrome maps to the short arm of chromosome 19 region 13.3 (19p13.3). It consists of multiple melanotic macular pigmentations of the skin and mucosa, which are associated with gastrointestinal polyposis. The pigmentations occur around the eyes, nose, and mouth (Figure 6-33). These macules are a few millimeters in diameter and vary in number and degree of pigmentation. They tend to diminish with age. Intraorally larger areas of pigmentation are observed on the lips and buccal mucosa of about 98% of affected patients.

Pigmentation of the hands, nasal mucosa, and eyes can also occur. The intestinal polyps are hamartomas (an abnormal growth of normal tissue in its normal location). They develop mostly in the small intestine; only rarely do they undergo malignant transformation.

White Sponge Nevus. Autosomal-dominant inheritance with complete penetrance characterizes **white sponge nevus** (also called *Cannon disease,* or *familial white folded mucosal dysplasia*). The cause of white sponge nevus is a mutation in the mucosal keratin pair K4 or K13. The disorder can be present at birth or develop around puberty. Clinically it is characterized by a white, corrugated, soft, folding oral mucosa. The buccal mucosa is always affected, and in most

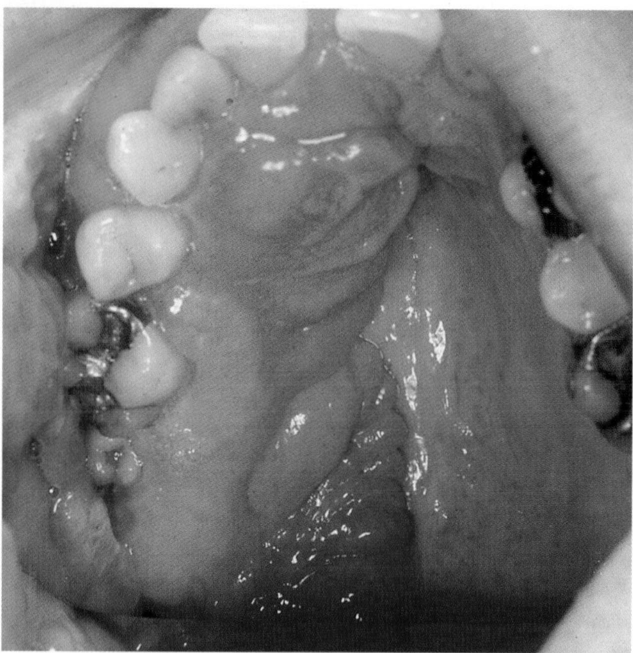

FIGURE 6-32 ■ Multiple neurofibromas of the maxillary gingiva and palate in a patient with neurofibromatosis of von Recklinghausen.

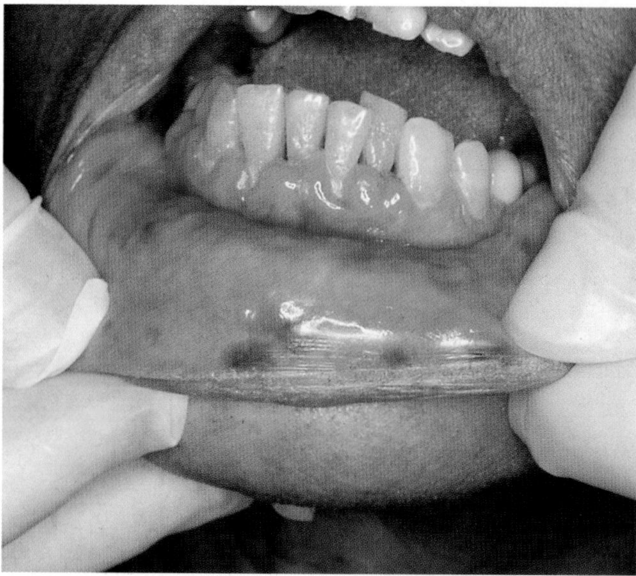

FIGURE 6-33 ■ Multiple small- to medium-size pigmented macules on the labial mucosa of a patient with Peutz-Jeghers syndrome.

patients the lesions are bilateral. A thick layer of keratin, which at times desquamates and leaves a raw mucosal surface, produces the whitening. Other areas of the oral mucosa can also be affected, but the free gingiva is spared.

Inherited Disorders Affecting the Teeth

Amelogenesis Imperfecta. A group of inherited conditions affecting the enamel of teeth and having no associated systemic defects characterizes **amelogenesis imperfecta**. Witkop and Sauk classified amelogenesis imperfecta into four types:

- Type I: Hypoplastic amelogenesis imperfecta
- Type II: Hypocalcified amelogenesis imperfecta
- Type III: Hypomaturation amelogenesis imperfecta
- Type IV: Hypoplastic-hypomaturation amelogenesis imperfecta

The *hypoplastic type* of amelogenesis imperfecta is characterized by tooth enamel that does not develop to a normal thickness because of failure of the ameloblasts to lay down enamel matrix properly. On radiographs the abnormal enamel contrasts normally with dentin. Several varieties of this type of amelogenesis imperfecta are further classified according to their clinical presentation: pitted, local, smooth, rough, and enamel agenesis. Combined with the clinical appearance, the classification also includes the inheritance pattern. Thus an autosomal-dominant and an autosomal-recessive variety exist for the local hypoplastic type. Among this group of enamel defects, the most frequent one is the pitted autosomal-dominant variety (Figure 6-34), which is characterized by teeth that have random pits on the enamel. The size of these pits varies from pinpoint to pinhead, and the pits are observed mostly on the labial and buccal surfaces of the permanent teeth. The pits are frequently arranged in rows or columns or both. Occasionally more than one tooth has a normal clinical appearance. The gene for the local hypoplastic autosomal-dominant type of amelogenesis imperfecta maps to the long arm of chromosome 4 (4q11-13).

An enamel of normal thickness that is poorly calcified characterizes the *hypocalcified type* of amelogenesis imperfecta (Figure 6-35). Two varieties of hypocalcified amelogenesis imperfecta exist: (1) an autosomal-dominant variety, and (2) an autosomal-recessive variety. The autosomal-recessive pattern is more severe in its clinical manifestations. At eruption teeth present yellow-to-orange enamel that is very soft and rapidly lost, leaving exposed dentin. On radiographs the enamel has a moth-eaten appearance and is less radiopaque than dentin. Cervical enamel is better calcified and generally remains on the crown. This type of amelogenesis imperfecta is frequently associated with an anterior open bite.

An enamel of mottled appearance but normal thickness characterizes the *hypomaturation type* of amelogenesis imperfecta. This type of amelogenesis imperfecta is composed of large amounts of enamel matrix; therefore the enamel is softer than normal. With pressure the tip of an explorer will penetrate the enamel. The basic defect seems to be in the enamel rod sheath. The enamel chips easily from the crown. On radiographs it has almost the same radiodensity as dentin. Four varieties of the hypomaturation type of amelogenesis imperfecta exist; however, only the snowcapped type is discussed here.

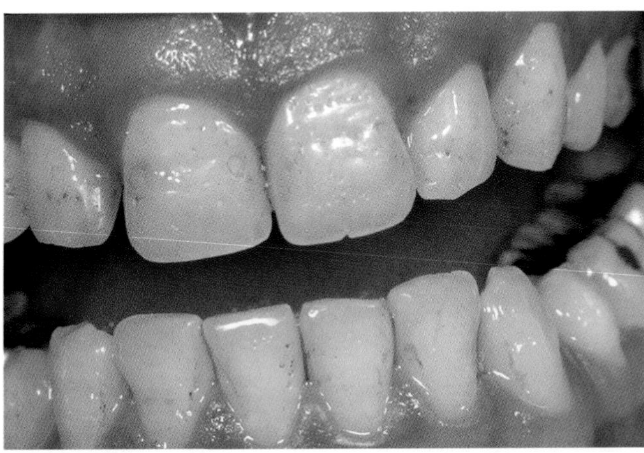

FIGURE 6-34 ■ Pitted autosomal-dominant amelogenesis imperfecta. Multiple pits on the labial surface of the teeth should be noted. Some of the pits have been filled with composite. (From Young WG, Sedano HO: *Atlas of oral pathology,* Minneapolis, 1981, University of Minnesota Press. Used with permission.)

A type of hypomaturation amelogenesis imperfecta, called *snow-capped amelogenesis imperfecta*, apparently has an X-linked recessive inheritance pattern in some families and an autosomal-dominant pattern in others. Clinically both varieties are identical and are characterized by a hypomaturation of the surface enamel of the occlusal third of all the teeth of both dentitions. The maxillary teeth are more severely affected with this whitish discoloration (Figure 6-36). The enamel in these areas is of regular hardness and smooth. It does not fracture or chip from the crown.

Its association with taurodontic teeth (described later in this chapter and also in Chapter 5) characterizes the *hypoplastic-hypomaturation type* of amelogenesis imperfecta. The thin enamel is yellow to brown and pitted. On radiographs the enamel has a radiodensity similar to dentin, and single-rooted teeth have large pulp chambers.

It is generally not easy to diagnose the exact type of amelogenesis imperfecta clinically because of the frequent similarity among different varieties. The mode of inheritance must be kept in mind, and an accurate family history should always be taken. Recently different mutations in several genes have been identified as responsible for some types of amelogenesis imperfecta; the genes are: AMELX, AMELY, ENAM, AMELOBLASTIN, TUFTELIN, ENAMELYSIN, KALLIKREIN, and DLX3.

The prevalence of all forms of amelogenesis imperfecta in the United States has been estimated at 1:15000.

Dentinogenesis Imperfecta. **Dentinogenesis imperfecta** is usually subdivided into three types. Type one is dentinogenesis imperfecta associated with osteogenesis imperfecta (previously described in this chapter). The other two types are not associated with osteogenesis imperfecta. The teeth in all three types have a similar clinical appearance.

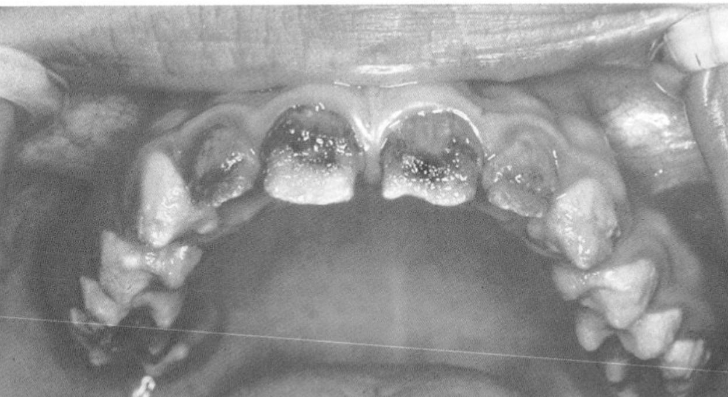

FIGURE 6-35 ■ Loss of enamel is exhibited in the teeth of a patient with hypocalcified amelogenesis imperfecta.

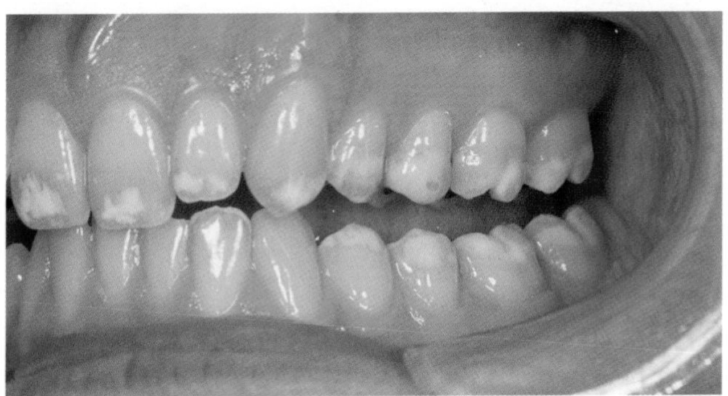

FIGURE 6-36 ■ Uniform whitening of incisal edges and occlusal cusps is exhibited in a case of snow-capped amelogenesis imperfecta.

Dentinogenesis imperfecta type II is also known as hereditary opalescent dentin. The inheritance pattern is autosomal dominant, and the gene maps to the long arm of chromosome 4 (4q13-21). Teeth have bulbous crowns with a color that varies from opalescent brown to brownish-blue (Figure 6-37). The primary teeth are usually affected more severely than the permanent teeth. Twenty percent of patients have enamel hypoplasia as well. The dentin is very soft, which produces chipping of enamel that results in tooth attrition. Occasionally this attrition can cause the teeth to be worn down to the alveolar process. Radiographically no pulp chambers or root canals are seen (Figure 6-38). Roots are short and thin with periapical radiolucencies. Patients may lose teeth prematurely because of complications produced by the attrition and the short roots. The basic defect lies with the odontoblasts, which lay down an abnormal matrix and then degenerate. Cells derived from the dental pulp, which lay down abnormal dentin, later replace these odontoblasts.

Dentin Dysplasia. **Dentin dysplasia** is subdivided into type I (radicular dentin dysplasia) and type II (coronal dentin dysplasia).

Radicular Dentin Dysplasia. Teeth with normal crowns, abnormal roots, and an autosomal-dominant inheritance pattern characterize this condition. The basic defect seems to lie in a disturbance in Hertwig's epithelial root sheath, which guides the formation of the root. Radiographs show total or partial lack of pulp chambers and root canals (Figure 6-39). Primary and secondary dentitions are affected equally. The color of the teeth is normal. Because of the short roots, the teeth generally are exfoliated prematurely, especially in the event of even minor trauma. The pulp chambers of the permanent teeth generally are not obliterated fully and have a half-moon appearance on the radiograph. Occasionally periapical cysts can be associated with this condition.

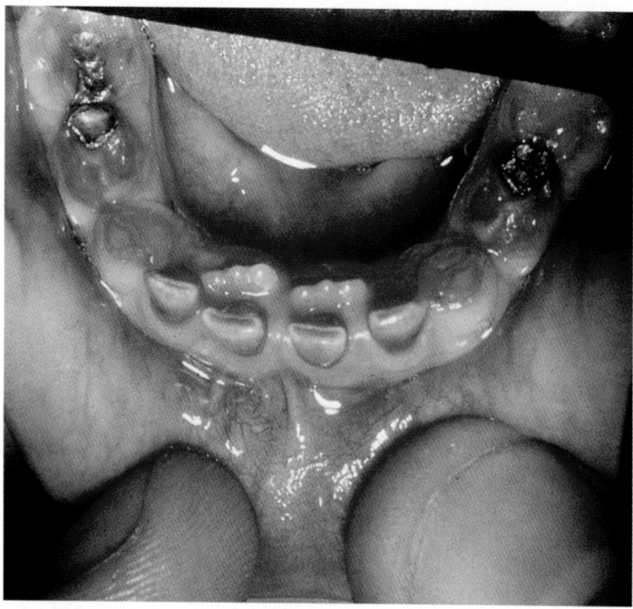

FIGURE 6-37 ■ Opalescent bluish hue in the anterior teeth typical of dentinogenesis imperfecta. The yellow color seen in the molars is from exposed abnormal dentin due to loss of enamel.

Coronal Dentin Dysplasia. Dentin dysplasia type II has an autosomal-dominant inheritance pattern. The basic defect in this condition is a mutation in the gene termed *dentin sialophosphoprotein* (DSPP) that maps to the long arm of chromosome 4 (4q13-21). Recently it has been shown that dentinogenesis imperfecta type II and dentin dysplasia type II share the DSPP gene loci and the proteins encoded by that gene. Translucent teeth with an amber color characterize the primary dentition. Radiographs show a lack of pulp chambers and small root canals. Primary teeth are quite similar to those observed in dentinogenesis imperfecta. Permanent teeth present normal crown formation with normal color. Radiographs show thistle-shaped pulp chambers in single-rooted teeth and a bow-tie appearance of the pulp chambers of permanent molars (Figure 6-40). Permanent teeth may or may not have pulp stones.

Hypohidrotic Ectodermal Dysplasia. **Hypohidrotic ectodermal dysplasia** represents a genetic heterogeneity. Although in the majority of families it is inherited as an X-linked recessive trait, in some families it is inherited as an autosomal-recessive trait. The clinical manifestations for both the X-linked and autosomal-recessive forms are identical. The gene for the X-linked variety of this syndrome maps to the long arm of the X chromosome region 12-13.1

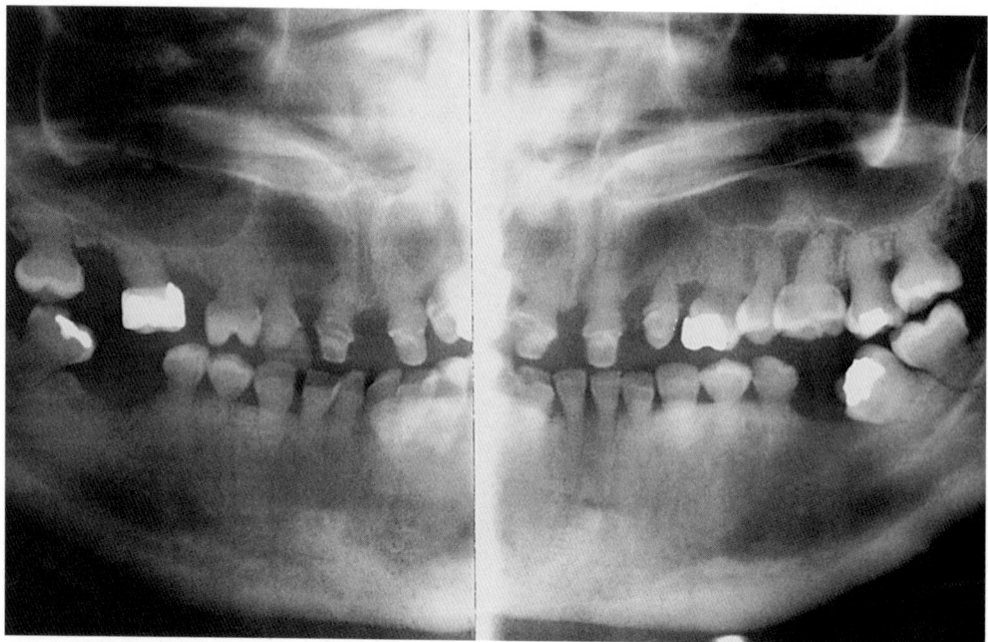

FIGURE 6-38 ■ Panoramic radiograph of a patient with dentinogenesis imperfecta shows marked short roots and almost complete lack of pulp chambers. (From Young WG, Sedano HO: *Atlas of oral pathology,* Minneapolis, 1981, University of Minnesota Press. Used with permission.)

(Xq12-13.1). The autosomal-recessive variety maps to the long arm of chromosome 2 (2q11-q13).

This entity represents the most severe form of ectodermal dysplasia. Its major components are hypodontia (partial anodontia), **hypotrichosis** (less than the normal amount of hair), and **hypohidrosis** (abnormally diminished secretion of sweat). Affected children are born without lanugo (body hair present at birth), and many have episodes of fevers of unknown causes because of the almost complete lack of sweat glands. Some patients die of hyperthermia (greatly increased body temperature) after prolonged exposure to the sun or heavy exercise. The clinical characteristics may not be apparent until the second year of life.

The facies is quite typical, with marked frontal bossing, depressed nasal bridge (saddle nose), protuberant lips, and almost complete lack of scalp hair. The hair that is present is usually blond, short, fine, and stiff. The skin is soft, thin, and very dry. Sebaceous glands are also lacking. Linear wrinkles and increased pigmentation are seen around the eyes and mouth. The eyelashes and eyebrows are often missing entirely. After puberty the beard generally is normal, but axillary and pubic hair is scanty.

The oral manifestations of hypohidrotic ectodermal dysplasia consist of hypodontia or rarely anodontia. When present, incisors and canines have small, conical crowns (Figure 6-41). The alveolar bone is formed only when teeth are

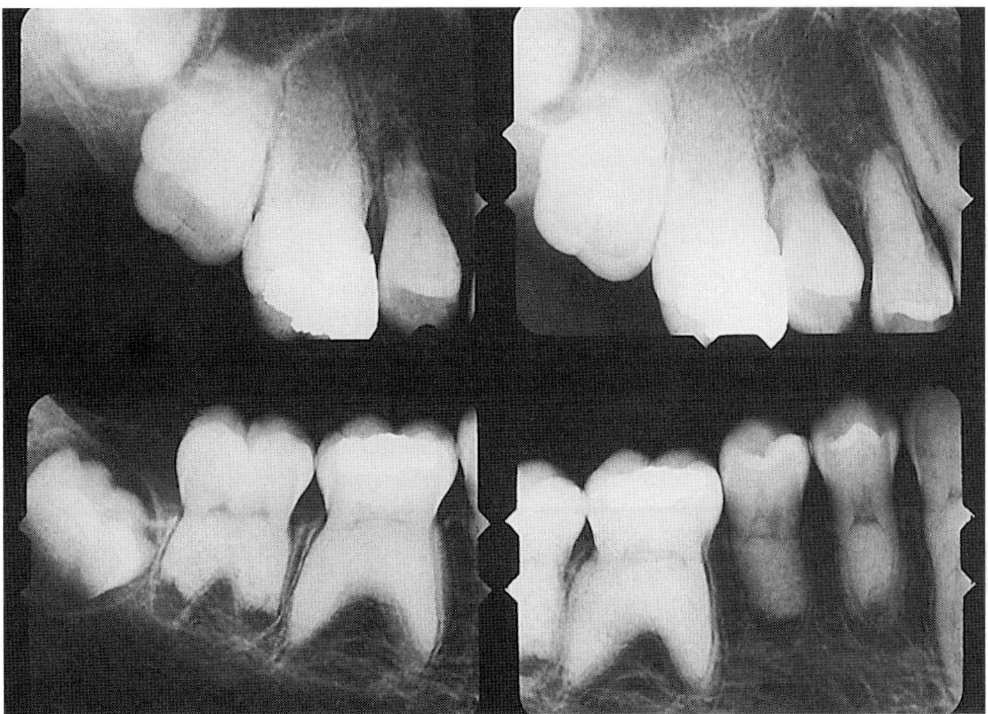

FIGURE 6-39 ■ Radiographs of a patient with radicular dentin dysplasia shows blunted and short tooth roots. The few remaining pulp chambers have a half-moon appearance. (Courtesy Dr. Carl J. Witkop.)

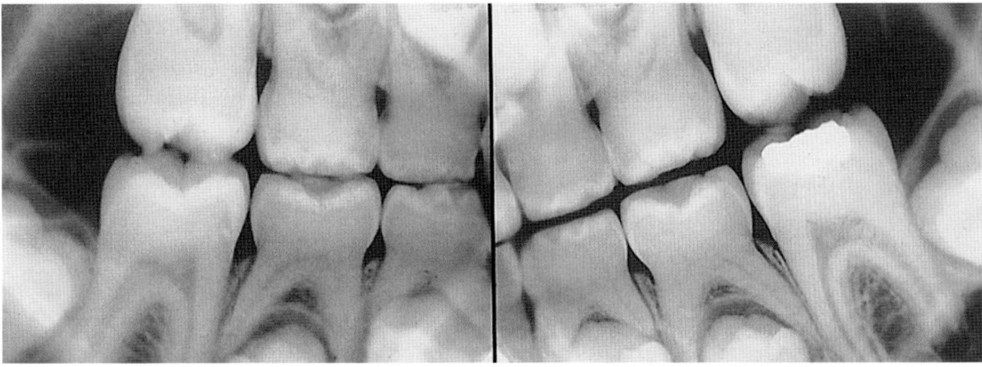

FIGURE 6-40 ■ Obliteration and partial lack of coronal pulp chambers and small root canals can be seen in teeth of a patient affected with coronal dentin dysplasia. (Courtesy Dr. Carl J. Witkop.)

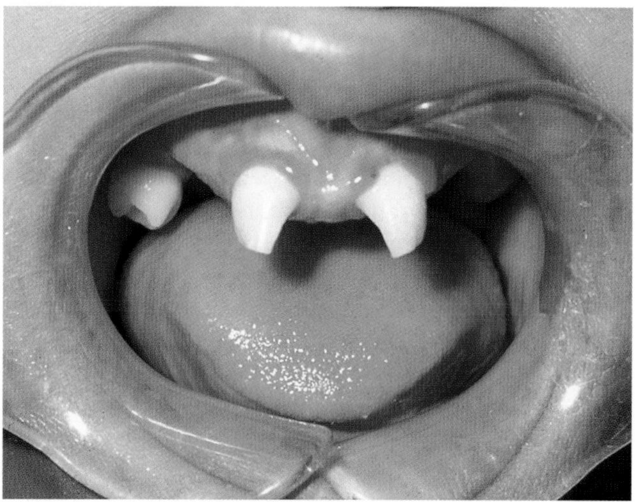

FIGURE 6-41 ■ Patient with hypohidrotic ectodermal dysplasia has only three abnormally shaped teeth.

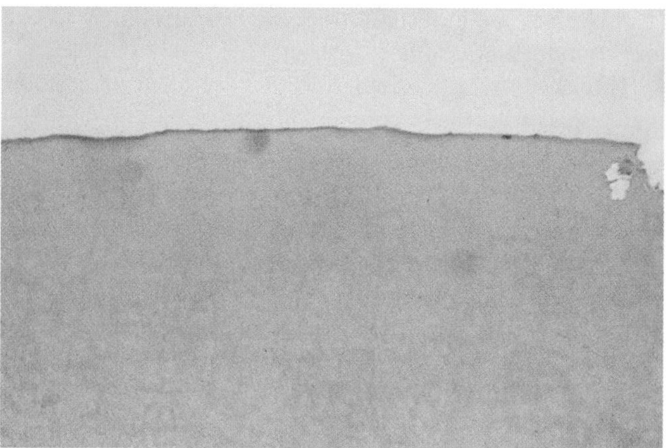

FIGURE 6-42 ■ Histologic section of a tooth from a patient with hypophosphatasia shows only dentin. Cementum is entirely lacking.

present; therefore patients lacking alveolar processes have loss of vertical dimension with markedly protruding lips. There may also be partial lack and aplasia of minor salivary glands in the buccal, labial, and lower respiratory tract mucosa.

Female carriers of the X-linked form of hypohidrotic ectodermal dysplasia have minor clinical manifestations such as thin and slightly sparse hair, cone-shaped teeth, hypodontia, and variable degrees of reduced sweating. This is in accordance with the Lyon hypothesis of variability of expression.

Hypophosphatasia. The inheritance pattern of **hypophosphatasia** is autosomal recessive. The gene for this syndrome maps to the short arm of chromosome 1 regions 36.1-34 (1p36.1-34). The basic defect in this condition is a decrease in serum alkaline phosphatase levels with increased urinary and plasma levels of phosphoethanolamine. Alkaline phosphatase participates in the process of calcification of bone and cementum; therefore these two tissues will be altered in patients with hypophosphatasia. Agenesis or abnormal formation of cementum in these patients leads to spontaneous premature shedding of primary teeth, especially mandibular incisors (Figure 6-42). Teeth are exfoliated without evidence of periodontal or gingival disease. The primary molars and permanent teeth are rarely if ever affected, which is probably associated with the greater mechanical fixation resulting from the larger size of their roots. The total lack of cementum observed in exfoliated teeth implies a lack of periodontal fiber attachment, with consequent exfoliation of single-rooted teeth. The most important alteration in this syndrome is the improper formation of mature bone. Therefore individuals who survive the neonatal period experience rachitic-like changes such as bowing of legs and multiple fractures.

Hypophosphatemic Vitamin D–Resistant Rickets. **Hypophosphatemic vitamin D–resistant rickets**, which is quite common, has an X-linked dominant inheritance pattern and is the result of a mutation in the PHEX gene. It consists of low serum levels of phosphorus, which are produced by low absorption of inorganic phosphate in the renal tubules, rickets or osteomalacia, resistance to treatment with usual doses of vitamin D, and a lack of other abnormalities. Affected individuals generally are of short stature and have bowlegs, especially if the condition is present from childhood. Adult-onset forms also exist, and the clinical manifestations in these patients are minor or even lacking, with the exception of low serum levels of inorganic phosphate.

The characteristic radiographic oral findings are large pulp chambers with very long pulp horns. In addition, the dentin exhibits pronounced cracks that extend to the dentinoenamel junction. These cracks induce fracture of the enamel with microexposure of the pulp and subsequent pulpal infection. Eventually, with the progress of the infectious inflammatory pulpal disease, periapical abscess formation occurs. Gingival abscesses are also frequent. Regional lymphadenitis accompanies these processes.

Pegged Or Absent Maxillary Lateral Incisors. The inheritance pattern of **pegged** or **absent maxillary lateral incisors** is generally autosomal dominant with variable expressivity. The lateral incisor can be small, peg shaped, or congenitally lacking, either unilaterally or bilaterally (Figure 6-43). Both primary and secondary dentitions can be affected, but mostly the latter. This condition has a prevalence of 1% to 3% in the white population and about 7% in Asians. In addition, the premolar teeth are congenitally lacking in 10% to 20% of affected individuals.

Taurodontism. **Taurodontism** is a genetic heterogeneous condition with dominant and recessive inheritance. It is characterized by very large, pyramid-shaped molars with large pulp chambers (Figure 6-44). (Taurodontic teeth [bull teeth] are also described in Chapter 5.) Taurodontism is most frequent among Native Americans, including Inuits. The

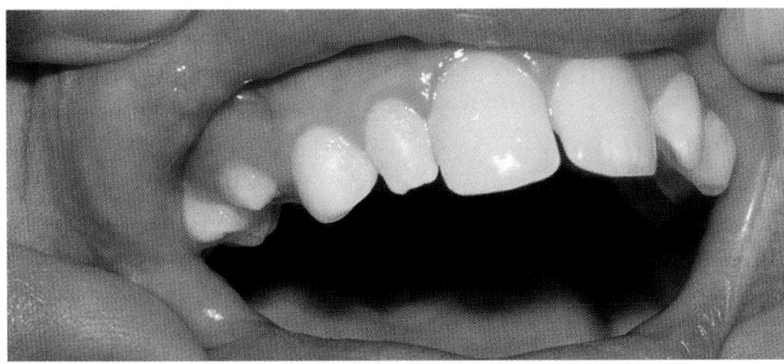

FIGURE 6-43 ■ Pegged maxillary lateral incisor. The conical shape should be noted.

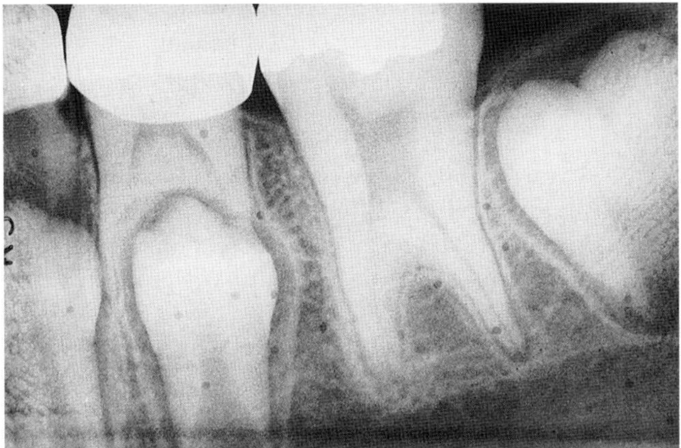

FIGURE 6-44 ■ Intraoral radiograph of taurodontic teeth shows large pulp chambers and low bifurcation of the roots in this pyramid-shaped molar.

furcation of the roots is displaced apically, and these teeth are classified according to the degree of furcation displacement. It is frequently found in Klinefelter syndrome (XXY) and is associated with many other syndromes as well.

Selected References

Books

Cummings MR: *Human heredity: principles and issues,* ed 7, Stamford, Conn, 2006, Brooks/Cole-Cengage Learning.

Fitzgerald MJT, Fitzgerald M: *Human embryology,* London, 1994, Saunders.

Gorlin RJ, Cohen MM, Hennekam RCM: *Syndromes of the head and neck,* ed 4, New York, 2001, Oxford University Press.

Neussbaum RL, McInnes RR, Willard HF: *Thompson and Thompson genetics in medicine,* ed 7, Philadelphia, 2007, Saunders.

Sadler TW: *Langman's medical embryology,* ed 10, Philadelphia, 2006, Lippincott, Williams & Wilkins.

Sapp JP, Eversole LR, Wisocki GP: *Contemporary oral and maxillofacial pathology,* ed 2, St Louis, 2004, Mosby.

Witkop CJ Jr, Sauk JJ Jr: *Dental and oral manifestations of hereditary disease,* Washington, DC, 1971, American Academy of Oral Pathology (monograph).

Witkop CJ Jr, Sauk JJ Jr: Heritable defects of enamel. In Stewart RE, Prescott GH, editors: *Oral facial genetics,* St Louis, 1976, Mosby.

Young WG, Sedano HO: *An atlas of oral pathology,* Minneapolis, 1981, University of Minnesota Press.

Journal Articles

Barnet ML, Friedman D, Kastner T: The prevalence of mitral valve prolapse in patients with Down's syndrome: implications for dental management, *Oral Surg Oral Med Oral Pathol* 66:445, 1988.

Bozzo L, Scully C, Aldred MJ: Hereditary gingival fibromatosis, *Oral Surg Oral Med Oral Pathol* 78:452, 1994.

Chadwick B et al: Laband syndrome: report of two cases, review of the literature, and identification of additional manifestations, *Oral Surg Oral Med Oral Pathol* 78:57, 1994.

Crawford PJM, Aldred MJ: Clinical features of a family with X-linked amelogenesis imperfecta mapping to a new locus (AIH3) on the long arm of the X chromosome, *Oral Surg Oral Med Oral Pathol* 76:187, 1993.

Ghaffar KA et al: Papillon-Lefèvre syndrome, *Oral Surg Oral Med Oral Pathol Oral Radiol Endod* 88:320, 1999.

Koury ME, Stella JP, Epker BN: Vascular transformation in cherubism, *Oral Surg Oral Med Oral Pathol* 76:20, 1993.

O'Connell AC, Marini JC: Evaluation of oral problems in an osteogenesis imperfecta population, *Oral Surg Oral Med Oral Pathol Oral Radiol Endod* 87:189, 1999.

Szilágyi A et al: Oral manifestations of patients with Turner syndrome, *Oral Surg Oral Med Oral Pathol Oral Radiol Endod* 89:577, 2000.

Yuasa K et al: Computed tomography of the jaws in familial adenomatosis coli, *Oral Surg Oral Med Oral Pathol* 76:251, 1993.

REVIEW QUESTIONS

1. The constriction present in all chromosomes, which joins the short and long arms, is called the:
   A. Equatorial plate.
   B. Chromatid.
   C. Centromere.
   D. Chiasmata.

2. The process by which a primitive germ cell becomes a gamete is called:
   A. Meiosis.
   B. S phase.
   C. Haploid.
   D. Mitosis.

3. Trisomy is defined as:
   A. Three extra chromosomes.
   B. A pair of chromosomes with an identical extra chromosome.
   C. The presence of two extra X chromosomes in a male.
   D. One extra chromosome in each pair.

4. The Lyon hypothesis is applied to:
   A. Autosomal-dominant traits.
   B. Autosomal-recessive traits.
   C. X-linked dominant traits.
   D. X-linked recessive traits.

5. Barr bodies are seen at the:
   A. Periphery of the cytoplasm in all human cells.
   B. Nuclear periphery of cells in women.
   C. Nuclear periphery of all human cells.
   D. Periphery of the cytoplasm in all cells from women.

6. The karyotype of a patient with Turner syndrome shows:
   A. 44 autosomes and XO.
   B. 43 autosomes and XYY.
   C. 44 autosomes and XXY.
   D. 44 autosomes and XYY.

7. Hypothetically an autosomal-dominant trait would be clinically present in:
   A. 25% of the offspring of an affected parent.
   B. 50% of the offspring of an affected parent.
   C. 75% of the offspring of an affected parent.
   D. Only in males, never in female offspring.

8. Patients with an X-linked hereditary condition:
   A. Are always men.
   B. Have cells with many Barr bodies.
   C. Are always women.
   D. Are generally affected more severely if they are men.

9. The major concern for a dental hygienist when treating a patient with cyclic neutropenia should be:
   A. The number of circulating neutrophils.
   B. Viral infections.
   C. Chipping away of enamel.
   D. Exfoliating teeth because of short roots.

10. A 9-year-old boy exhibits markedly swollen red and bleeding gingiva. In addition, he has tooth mobility, and the intraoral radiographs show marked alveolar bone atrophy with vertical periodontal pockets. Which of the following will be found in this child if he were to have the Papillon-Lefèvre syndrome?
    A. Diminished sweating
    B. Lack of anterior vestibular sulcus
    C. Blue sclerae
    D. Palmar and plantar hyperkeratosis

11. In all inherited varieties of gingival fibromatosis, the gingival enlargement is characterized by a marked:
    A. Collagenization of the connective tissue.
    B. Hyperplasia of the covering epithelium.
    C. Chronic inflammatory cellular infiltrate.
    D. Alveolar bone hypertrophy.

12. A 14-year-old boy is seen in consultation because of bilateral mandibular swelling. Radiographs show a bilateral multilocular lesion in the ascending mandibular rami. The mother of this patient has similar findings. The most likely diagnosis is:
    A. Ellis–van Creveld syndrome.
    B. Nevoid basal cell carcinoma syndrome.
    C. Cleidocranial dysplasia.
    D. Cherubism.

13. A 19-year-old woman is diagnosed with cleidocranial dysplasia. She has absent clavicles and a mushroom-shaped skull. Which of the following conditions is she also most likely to have?
    A. Taurodontism
    B. Pegged lateral incisors
    C. Supernumerary teeth
    D. Large pulp chambers

14. Which of the following is the most serious component of Gardner syndrome?
    A. Mandibular osteomas
    B. Multiple odontomas
    C. Intestinal polyposis
    D. Teeth hypercementosis

15. Two characteristic clinical components of mandibulofacial dysostosis are:
    A. Lack of clavicles and delayed teeth eruption.
    B. Hypoplastic mandible and deafness.
    C. Hypodontia and dysplastic nails.
    D. Cleft lip and fistulas of lower lip.

16. Odontogenic keratocysts are a clinical component of:
    A. Nevoid basal cell carcinoma syndrome.
    B. Neurofibromatosis of von Recklinghausen.
    C. MEN 2B syndrome.
    D. Cherubism.

17. Torus mandibularis and torus palatinus are similar in that both:
    A. Are inherited as an autosomal-dominant trait.
    B. Are more prevalent in females.
    C. Are inherited as an autosomal-recessive trait.
    D. Develop in childhood.

18. The cause of all forms of labial and palatal clefting is considered to be:
    A. Autosomal dominant.
    B. Autosomal recessive.
    C. Environmental.
    D. Multifactorial.

19. The major concern for a dental hygienist when treating a patient with Osler-Rendu–Parkes Weber syndrome should be:
    A. Severe infections.
    B. Spontaneous ulcerations.
    C. Gingival hemorrhage.
    D. Epithelial desquamation.

20. The most serious clinical manifestation of the MEN 2B syndrome is considered to be:
    A. Carcinoma of the thyroid gland.
    B. Carcinoma of the colon.
    C. Pheochromocytoma.
    D. Basal cell carcinomas.

21. Which of the following is true for von Recklinghausen disease?
    A. It is inherited as an autosomal-recessive trait.
    B. Patients have multiple neurofibromas.
    C. Patients have gingival fibromatosis.
    D. Patients experience a generalized whitening of the oral mucosa.

22. Teeth in snowcapped amelogenesis imperfecta have:
    A. A thin, brown enamel.
    B. Obliterated pulp chambers.
    C. Short, blunted roots.
    D. White hypocalcified enamel at the incisal and occlusal thirds.

23. In dentinogenesis imperfecta type II, teeth have:
    A. Roots that are short and thin.
    B. Dilacerated roots.
    C. Markedly brittle enamel.
    D. Hard, dense dentin.

24. The characteristic finding in permanent teeth affected with coronal dentin dysplasia is:
    A. Crowns with amber color.
    B. Thistle-shaped pulp chambers on radiographs.
    C. Markedly short roots.
    D. Large, square pulp chamber.

25. Patients with hypohidrotic ectodermal dysplasia characteristically have:
    A. Multiple tongue nodules.
    B. Hypodontia.
    C. Excessive amounts of hair.
    D. Blue sclerae.

26. Patients with hypophosphatasia characteristically have:
    A. Absence of root cementum.
    B. Obliterated pulp chambers.
    C. Increase in serum alkaline phosphatase levels.
    D. Marked gingival keratinization.

27. Taurodontic teeth:
    A. Are supernumerary.
    B. Have long roots.
    C. Are pyramidal in shape.
    D. Have thistle-shaped pulp chambers.

28. The order of the four stages of mitosis is:
    A. Prophase, telophase, metaphase, anaphase.
    B. Prophase, metaphase, anaphase, telophase.
    C. Metaphase, prophase, telophase, anaphase.
    D. Anaphase, metaphase, telophase, prophase.

CHAPTER 6 Synopsis

Condition/Disease	Cause	Age/Race/Sex	Location	Clinical Features
Trisomy 21	One extra chromosome No. 21	From birth	Systemic	Slanted eyes, gingivoperiodontitis, fissured tongue, hypodontia
Trisomy 13	One extra chromosome No. 13	From birth	Systemic	Bilateral CL/P, polydactyly microphthalmia
Turner Syndrome	One X chromosome missing	From birth, women	Systemic	Short, stature, webbing of neck, edema of hands
Klinefelter Syndrome	One extra X chromosome	From birth, men	Systemic	Tall stature, gynecomastia
Cat Cry Syndrome	Deletion 5p	From birth, M=F	Systemic	Catlike cry, severe mental retardation
Cyclic Neutropenia	AD gene ELA-2 19p13.3	From birth, M=F	Oral mucosa and periodontium	Gingivitis, periodontitis ulcers, hemorrhage
Papillon-Lefèvre Syndrome	AR, 11q14-21	From birth, M=F	Gingiva, periodontal ligament, palms and soles	Teeth mobility, pockets, palmoplantar hyperkeratosis
Focal Palmoplantar Gingival Hyperkeratosis	AD	From birth, M=F	Gingiva, palms, and soles	Keratosis of gingival, palms and soles
Laband Syndrome	AD	From birth, M=F	Gingiva	Marked gingival hyperplasia, abnormal nails, short fingers and toes
Gingival Fibromatosis, Hypertrichosis, Epilepsy, and Mental Retardation	AD	From birth, M=F	Gingiva, hair, central nervous system	Gingival hyperplasia, abundant body hair, epilepsy
Gingival Fibromatosis and Multiple Hyaline Fibromas	AD	From birth, M=F	Gingiva, nails mucosa, and skin	Gingival hyperplasia, hypertrophy of nails, multiple tumors
Cherubism	AD, 4p16	From birth, M=F	Mandible bilaterally	Bilateral enlargement of face
Ellis-van Creveld Syndrome (Chondroectodermal Dysplasia)	AR, 4p16	From birth, M=F	Gingival, teeth, alveolar ridge, hands	Absent upper vestibule, serrated lower alveolar ridge, polydactyly
Cleidocranial Dysplasia	AD, 6p21	From birth, M=F	Teeth, clavicles, skull	Supernumerary teeth absent clavicles, open fontanelles

AD, Autosomal dominant; *AR,* autosomal recessive.

Radiographic Features	Microscopic Features	Treatment	Diagnostic Process
None	None	Root planning, scaling	Karyotype shows trisomy 21
Extra fingers in hand	None	None	Karyotype shows trisomy 13
None	No Barr bodies in buccal smear	None	Karyotype shows absent X chromosome
Hypoplastic mandible	One Barr body, in buccal smear	None	Karyotype shows two X chromosomes
None	None	Dental care for mentally handicapped	Deletion of short arm of chromosome 5
Alveolar bone loss, pocket formation	Diminished neutrophils in peripheral blood	Root planing, scaling, antibiotics	Clinical and blood studies
Alveolar bone loss, severe periodontal disease	Profuse inflammatory infiltrate of soft dental tissues	Root planning, scaling, tooth fixation, retinoid for skin lesions	Clinical, genetic evaluation
None	Hyperorthokeratosis of affected areas	Maintain oral hygiene	Clinical and family history
Hypoplasia of terminal phalanges of fingers and toes	Profuse fibrosis and increase collagen of affect gingival	Maintain oral hygiene, surgical remodeling of gingival (recurrence)	Clinical and family history
None	Profuse fibrosis and increase collagen of affect gingiva	Maintain oral hygiene, surgical remodeling of gingival (recurrence)	Clinical and family history
None	Fibrosis of gingival, hyaline fibromas	Maintain oral hygiene, removal of fibromas	Clinical and family history
Multiple bilateral radiolucencies of mandibular ramus	Multinucleated giant cells in a loose connective tissue	Lesions fill in after puberty	Clinical, radiographs, and family history
Thinning of enamel	None	Reconstruction of upper vestibule, amputation of extra fingers	Clinical and family history
Multiple impacted teeth	Absent cellular cementum	Extractions orthodontia	Clinical, radiographs, and family history

Continued

CHAPTER 6 Synopsis (continued)

Condition/Disease	Cause	Age/Race/Sex	Location	Clinical Features
Gardner syndrome	AD, 5q21-22	From birth, M=F	Maxilla and mandible	Multiple osteomas, colon polyps, adenocarcinoma
Mandibulofacial Dysostosis	AD, 5q32-33.1	From birth, M=F	Mandible, teeth, ears	Hypoplastic mandible, malposed teeth, deafness
Nevoid Basal Cell Carcinoma Syndrome	AD, 9q22.3	From birth, M=F	Mandible, maxilla, skin	Multiple: odontogenic keratocysts and basal cell carcinoma
Hereditary Hemorrhagic Telangiectasia	AD, 9q3 and 12	Starts after teens	Mucous membranes and skin	Telangiectases, gingival bleeding
Multiple Mucosal Neuromas	AD, 10q-11.2	From birth, M=F	Oral mucosa, especially tongue	Multiple nodes on tongue tip, lips and cheek mucosa
Neurofibromatosis of von Recklinghausen	AD 17q11.2	From birth, M=F	Skin, oral mucosa, especially tongue	Multiple nodes on tongue and other mucosa
Peutz-Jeghers Syndrome	AD, 19p13.3	From birth, M=F	Skin, oral mucosa, small intestine	Pigmented macules in perioral skin and oral mucosa
White Sponge Nevus	AD, mutation mucosal keratin K4 or K13	At birth or develops at puberty	Buccal mucosa	Bilateral whitening of buccal mucosa
Amelogenesis Imperfecta Pitted Hypoplastic	AD	Visible when teeth erupt, M=F	All primary and permanent teeth	Random pinpoint pits on labial and lingual
Amelogenesis Imperfecta Hypocalcified Type	AD and AR	When teeth erupt, M=F	All primary and permanent teeth	Cheesy soft enamel, rapidly lost, anterior open bite
Amelogenesis Imperfecta Hypomaturation Type	AD, AR, and X-linked recessive	When teeth erupt, AD and AR, M=F; X-linked, more men	All primary and permanent teeth	Enamel softer than normal and chips easily
Amelogenesis Imperfecta Snow-Capped (Hypomaturation)	AD and X linked recessive	When teeth erupt, AD, M=F; X-linked, more men	All primary and permanent teeth	White discoloration surface enamel occlusal one third
Dentinogenesis Imperfecta	AD gene 4q13-21	When teeth erupt	All primary and permanent teeth	Bulbous crowns, opalescent brown bluish crown
Radicular Dentin Dysplasia	AD	When teeth erupt	All primary and permanent teeth	Normal crowns in size and color

AD, Autosomal dominant; *AR,* autosomal recessive.

Radiographic Features	Microscopic Features	Treatment	Diagnostic Process
Odontomas and osteomas in jaws	Review osteoma and colonic cancer	Surgery of: polyps and/or carcinoma, odontomas, osteomas	Clinical, radiographs, and family history
Obtuse mandibular angle, small condyle	None	Plastic surgery, orthodontia maintain oral hygiene	Clinical, radiographs, and family history
Multiple radiolucencies of the jaws bifid rib	Review odontogenic keratocyst (Chapter 5) and basal carcinoma (Chapter 7)	Surgical removal of cysts and basal cell carcinomas	Clinical, radiographs, and family history Microscopic
None	Capillary dilations	Care must be taken during scaling because of marked bleeding tendency	Clinical and family history
None	Review neurofibroma and thyroid carcinoma	Preventive thyroidectomy and excision of oral neurofibromas	Clinical and family history, microscopic
Spine anomalies	Review neurofibroma and neurofibrosarcoma,	Surgical removal of neurofibromas	Clinical and family history, microscopic
Intestinal polyps	Melanin apposition in skin and oral mucosas	Removal of intestinal polyps if needed	Clinical and family history
None	Thick layer of orthokeratin and clear cells	Maintain oral hygiene	Clinical and family history, microscopic
Enamel thinner than normal	Abnormal enamel matrix thinner than normal	Aesthetic dentistry operative procedures	Clinical and family history
Enamel has "moth-eaten" appearance	Enamel of normal thickness, poorly calcified	Jacket crowns, metal crowns, aesthetic dentistry	Clinical and family history
Enamel has same radiolucency as dentin	Large amounts of enamel matrix	Jacket crowns, metal crowns, aesthetic dentistry	Clinical and family history
None	Not Available	Aesthetic dentistry if the patient wants it	Clinical and family history
Short pointed roots, absent pulp chambers	Abnormal globular dentin, trapped odontoblasts	Aesthetic dentistry crowns operative procedures	Clinical and family history
Short pointed roots, absent pulp chambers	Abnormal tubular dentin and osteodentin	Prosthesis if teeth are lost	Radiographs and family history

Continued

CHAPTER 6 Synopsis (continued)

Condition/Disease	Cause	Age/Race/Sex	Location	Clinical Features
Coronal Dentin Dysplasia	AD gene 4q13-21	When teeth erupt	All primary teeth	Primary teeth amber in color, permanent normal
Hypohidrotic Ectodermal Dysplasia	X-linked recessive and AR Xq12-q13.1 AR 2q11-13	From birth, X-linked all males; AR, M=F	Skin, sweat, hair, both dentitions	Few teeth are formed, little sweat fear hairs
Hypophosphatasia	AR 1p36.1-34	From birth, M=F	Bones, teeth	Premature loss of primary anterior teeth
Hypophosphatemic Vitamin E– Resistant Rickets	X-linked dominant	From birth, more males	Bones, teeth	Multiple periapical radiolucencies (cyst, granuloma)

AD, Autosomal dominant; *AR,* autosomal recessive.

Radiographic Features	Microscopic Features	Treatment	Diagnostic Process
Primary absent pulp chambers, permanent molars "bow tie" pulp, uniradicular teeth, "thistle-shaped" pulp	Abnormal dentin in primary teeth, permanent teeth with pulp stones	Regular dental and dental hygiene care	Clinical, radiographs, and family history
Almost no teeth present	Reduced and abnormal sweat pores	Dental implants and/or dental prosthesis	Clinical, radiographs, and family history
Large pulp chambers	Absence of root cementum	Space retainers or dental prosthesis	Clinical, radiographs, and family history
Large pulp chambers, large pulp horns	Abnormal globular dentin, large cracks in dentin	Endodontics and regular dental hygiene care	Clinical, radiographs, and family history

Chapter 7 Neoplasia

Anne Cale Jones, Paul D. Freedman, Joan A. Phelan

OBJECTIVES

After studying this chapter, the student will be able to:

1. Define each of the words in the vocabulary list for this chapter.
2. Explain the difference between a benign tumor and a malignant tumor.
3. Define leukoplakia and erythroplakia.
4. Describe the clinical and histologic features of the calcifying odontogenic cyst and compare and contrast this lesion to the ameloblastoma.
5. Define the following neoplasms, describe the clinical features of each, and explain how they are treated: papilloma, squamous cell carcinoma, verrucous carcinoma, basal cell carcinoma, pleomorphic adenoma, monomorphic adenoma, adenoid cystic carcinoma, mucoepidermoid carcinoma, ameloblastoma, calcifying epithelial odontogenic tumor, adenomatoid odontogenic tumor (AOT), odontogenic myxoma, central cementifying and ossifying fibromas, benign cementoblastoma, ameloblastic fibroma, ameloblastic fibro-odontoma, odontoma, peripheral ossifying fibroma, lipoma, neurofibroma and schwannoma, granular cell tumor, congenital epulis, rhabdomyosarcoma, hemangioma, lymphangioma, Kaposi sarcoma, melanocytic nevi, malignant melanoma, torus, exostosis, osteoma, osteosarcoma, chondrosarcoma, leukemia, lymphoma, multiple myeloma, and metastatic jaw tumors.

VOCABULARY

Anaplastic **(an'ĕplas'tik)** Characterized by a loss of differentiation of cells and their orientation to one another; a characteristic of malignant tumors.

Benign **(be-nīn')** A condition that, if untreated or with symptomatic therapy, will not become life threatening.

Benign tumor **(be-nīn' too'mor)** A tumor that is not malignant **and** favorable for treatment and recovery.

Carcinoma **(kar"si-no'mah)** Malignant tumor of epithelium.

Central **(sen'tral)** Occurring within bone.

Dysplasia **(dis-pla'ze-ah)** Disordered growth; alteration in size, shape, and organization of adult cells.

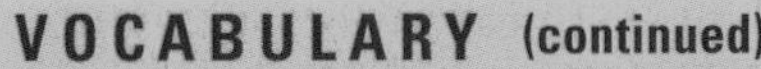

Encapsulated **(en-kap'su-lt-ed)** Surrounded by a capsule of fibrous connective tissue.

Enucleation **(ē-nū'klē-ā'shŭn)** Surgical removal without cutting into the lesion

Excision **(eksizh'ən)** Surgical removal

Hyperchromatic **(hi"per-kro-mat'āik)** Staining more intensely than normal.

Hyperplasia **(hi"per-pla'zĕ-ah)** Abnormal increase in the number of cells in an organ or tissue.

Immunoglobulin **(im'yĕnō-glăb'yĕlin)** A protein, also called an antibody, synthesized by plasma cells in response to a specific antigen.

In situ **(in sĭtoo)** Confined to the site of origin without invasion of neighboring tissues.

Invasion **(in-va'zhun)** Infiltration and active destruction of surrounding tissues.

Leukoplakia **(loo-kō-plā'kē-ah)** Clinical term used to identify a white, plaquelike lesion of the oral mucosa that cannot be wiped off or diagnosed as any other disease.

Malignant **(mah-lig'nant)** Resistant to treatment; able to metastasize and kill the host; describing cancer.

Malignant tumor **(mah-lig'nant too'mor)** Cancer; a tumor that is resistant to treatment and may cause death; a tumor that has the potential for uncontrolled growth and dissemination or recurrence, or both.

Metastasis **(mă-tas'tah-sis)** (plural, metastases [mĕ-tas'tah-sēz]) Transport of neoplastic cells to parts of the body remote from the primary tumor and the establishment of new tumors at those sites.

Metastatic tumor **(met"ah-stat'ik too'mor)** Tumor formed by cells that have been transported from the primary tumor to sites not connected with the original tumor.

Mitotic figure **(mi-tot'ik fig'ur)** (mitosis [mi-to'sis]) Dividing cells caught in the process of mitosis.

Neoplasia **(ne"o-pla'ze-ah)** New growth; the formation of tumors by the uncontrolled proliferation of cells.

Neoplastic **(nē"ō-plas'tik)** Pertaining to the formation of tumors by the uncontrolled proliferation of cells.

Neoplasm **(ne'o-plazm)** Tumor; a new growth of tissue in which growth is uncontrolled and progressive.

Nevus **(ne'vus)** (plural, nevi [ne'vi]) Circumscribed malformation of the skin or oral mucosa presumed to be of hereditary origin; also, a benign tumor of melanocytes (nevus cells).

Odontogenic **(o-don"to-jen'ik)** Tooth forming.

Oncology **(ong-kol'o-je)** Study of tumors or neoplasms.

Pedunculated **(pidungk'yēlā'tid)** Attached by a stalk.

Peripheral **(pĕ-rif'er-al)** Occurring outside of bone.

Pleomorphic **(ple"o-mor'fik)** Occurring in various forms.

Primary tumor **(pri'mer-e too'mor)** Original tumor; the source of metastasis.

Sarcoma **(sar-ko'mah)** Malignant tumor of connective tissue.

Sessile **(ses'il)** Attached by a base.

Tumor **(too'mor)** Neoplasm; also, a swelling or enlargement.

Undifferentiated **(un-difĕr-en'shē-āt'ed)** Absence of normal differentiation; anaplasia; a characteristic of some malignant tumors.

DESCRIPTION OF NEOPLASIA

Neoplasia means new growth. It is a process in which cells exhibit uncontrolled proliferation. A **neoplasm** is a mass of such cells. Although the word **tumor** means swelling, it is commonly used as a synonym for neoplasm. The study of tumors is called **oncology.** *Onco* in Greek means swelling or mass.

For neoplasia to occur, an irreversible change must take place in the cells, and this change must be passed on to new cells, resulting in uncontrolled cell multiplication. In most cases the initial stimulus that triggers the process of cell change is not known. Regulatory processes maintain the size of normal tissues. The regulatory processes that maintain the size of normal tissues do not function correctly in a neoplasm; therefore it exhibits unlimited and unregulated growth.

Like **hyperplasia,** which is described in Chapter 2, neoplasia is an abnormal process. With hyperplasia, normal cells proliferate in a normal arrangement in response to tissue damage, and the proliferation stops when the stimulus is removed. Although the size of the tissue may be greater than normal, the growth of the tissue is still under control. Reactive lesions such as the irritation fibroma, denture-related hyperplasia (epulis fissuratum), and the pyogenic granuloma described in Chapter 2 are examples of hyperplasia. In contrast, neoplasia is a completely abnormal process; the cells are abnormal, and the proliferation of these cells is uncontrolled and unlimited.

CAUSES OF NEOPLASIA

Many agents—principally chemicals, viruses, and radiation—have been shown to cause **neoplastic** transformation of cells in the laboratory. Hundreds of chemicals have been shown to cause cancer in animals. In addition, certain chemicals, viruses, and radiation have been shown to cause certain cancers in humans. Neoplastic transformation may also occur spontaneously secondary to a genetic mutation. Viruses that cause tumors are called **oncogenic viruses.** Radiation from sunlight, x-rays, nuclear fission, or other sources is well established as a cancer-producing agent in humans.

CLASSIFICATION OF TUMORS

Tumors are divided into two categories: **benign** and **malignant.** A **benign tumor** or neoplasm remains localized. It may be **encapsulated,** which means that it is walled off by surrounding fibrous connective tissue. Sometimes a benign tumor can invade adjacent structures, but it does not have the ability to spread to distant sites. In contrast, a **malignant tumor** both invades and destroys surrounding tissue and has the ability to spread throughout the body. **Cancer** is synonymous with malignancy.

Benign tumors almost always resemble normal cells, whereas malignant tumors vary in their histologic appearance. Malignant tumors composed of neoplastic cells that resemble normal cells are called *well-differentiated tumors.* Malignant tumors may also be poorly differentiated. The cells of these tumors have only some of the characteristics of the tissue from which they were derived. Still others may be **undifferentiated** or **anaplastic** and do not resemble at all the tissue from which they were derived. Malignant tumors are often composed of cells that vary in size and shape **(pleomorphic)** (Figure 7-1). The nuclei of these cells are darker than those of normal cells **(hyperchromatic)** and exhibit an increased nuclear cytoplasmic ratio (see Figure 7-1). Normal and abnormal **mitotic figures** are seen in the nucleus of the neoplastic cells (see Figure 7-1, *A*). Abnormal mitotic figures are those that are not dividing normally; therefore the shape of the dividing nucleus does not follow the shape of a normal mitotic figure. Table 7-1 compares benign and malignant tumors.

NAMES OF TUMORS

The prefix of the name of a tumor is determined by the tissue or cell of origin. The suffix *oma* is used to indicate a tumor. For example, a benign tumor of fat is called a **lipoma,** and a benign tumor of bone is called an **osteoma.** Malignant tumors are named in a similar fashion. Malignant tumors of epithelium are called **carcinomas,** and malignant tumors of connective tissue are called **sarcomas.** The prefix of the name of a malignant tumor is also determined by the tissue or cell of origin. Therefore a malignant tumor of squamous epithelium is called a **squamous cell carcinoma** or an **epidermoid carcinoma**, and a malignant tumor of bone is called an **osteosarcoma** (osteogenic sarcoma). Carcinomas are about 10 times more common than sarcomas. Table 7-2 lists tumors according to their tissue or cell of origin.

TREATMENT OF TUMORS

Benign tumors generally are treated by surgical **excision,** which can be accomplished through wide local excision or **enucleation.** Malignant tumors are treated by surgery, chemotherapy, or radiation therapy; a combination is often used.

Because many different types of tissues are present in the oral cavity, many different types of tumors can arise in this location. These neoplasms can be either benign or malignant. In this chapter the neoplasms are classified according

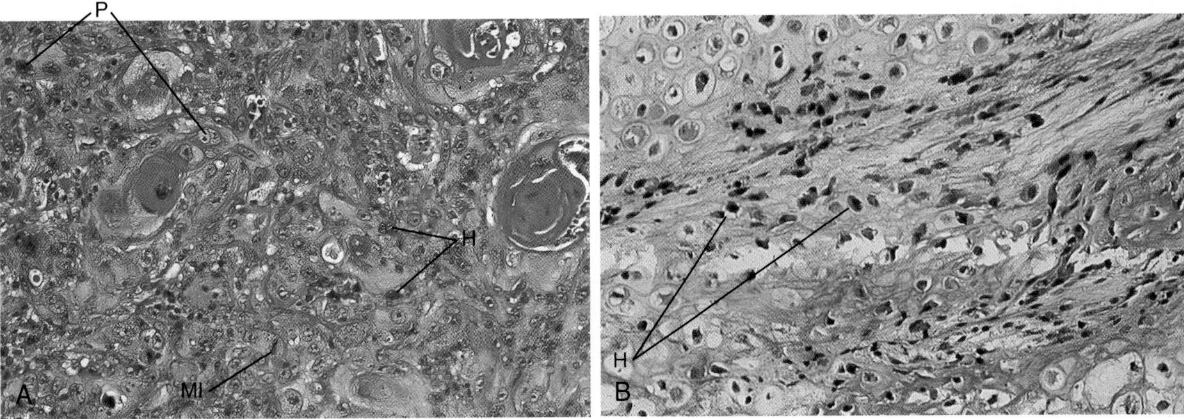

FIGURE 7-1 ■ Photomicrographs of malignant tumors show pleomorphic *(P)* and hyperchromatic *(H)* nuclei and mitotic figures *(MI)*. **A,** Squamous cell carcinoma. **B,** Osteosarcoma.

Table 7-1

Comparison of Benign and Malignant Tumors

Benign	Malignant
Usually well differentiated	Well differentiated to anaplastic
Usually slow growth	Slow-to-rapid growth
Mitotic figures are rare	Mitotic figures may be numerous
Usually encapsulated	Invasive and unencapsulated
No metastasis	Metastasis likely

to their tissue of origin. Benign tumors are described first, followed by their malignant counterparts.

EPITHELIAL TUMORS

Three different types of **epithelial tumors** occur in the oral cavity: (1) tumors derived from squamous epithelium, (2) tumors derived from salivary gland epithelium, and (3) tumors derived from **odontogenic** epithelium. A few of the lesions included in this section are not true tumors. The reasons for their inclusion are explained in their descriptions.

TUMORS OF SQUAMOUS EPITHELIUM

PAPILLOMA

The **papilloma** is a benign tumor of squamous epithelium that presents as a small, exophytic, **pedunculated** or **sessile** growth. These tumors are composed of numerous papillary projections that may be either white or the color of normal mucosa (Figure 7-2). They are often described as cauliflower-like in appearance. Most cases arise on the soft palate or tongue. A papilloma may occur at any age, and an equal sex predilection is noted. Microscopic examination demonstrates numerous fingerlike or papillary projections composed of normal stratified squamous epithelium surfaced by a thickened layer of keratin. A central core of fibrous connective tissue supports each papillary projection. The color of the lesion depends on the amount of surface keratin; the more keratin, the whiter the lesion appears clinically.

Other oral lesions that may resemble a papilloma clinically are a verruca vulgaris (common wart) and condyloma acuminatum (venereal wart). These two lesions are caused by human papillomaviruses and are described in Chapter 4. They are differentiated from the papilloma by microscopic examination. Special staining procedures can be used to identify viral particles within these lesions.

The papilloma is treated by surgical excision, which must include the base of the growth. With adequate excision, the papilloma usually does not recur.

PREMALIGNANT LESIONS

Leukoplakia

In any discussion of premalignant lesions of the oral mucosa, it is important to define the term **leukoplakia.** Leukoplakia is a clinical term and does not refer to a specific histologic appearance. It is defined as a white plaquelike lesion of the oral mucosa that cannot be rubbed off and cannot be diagnosed as a specific disease (Figure 7-3).

Leukoplakia is sometimes referred to as *idiopathic leukoplakia* to emphasize that the specific cause of the lesion is not known. The white lesion illustrated in Figure 7-4 is more accurately called **tobacco pouch keratosis** rather than a leukoplakia because the direct cause of the lesion is known.

The microscopic appearance of leukoplakia varies; therefore a biopsy is essential to establish a definitive diagnosis. Most leukoplakias are the result of hyperkeratosis

Table 7-2

Names of Tumors

Tissue of Origin	Benign Tumor	Malignant Tumor
Epithelium		
Squamous cells	Papilloma	Squamous cell or epidermoid carcinoma
Basal cells		Basal cell carcinoma
Glands or ducts	Adenoma	Adenocarcinoma
Neuroectoderm		
Melanocytes	Nevus	Melanoma
Connective Tissue		
Fibrous	Fibroma	Fibrosarcoma
Cartilage	Chondroma	Chondrosarcoma
Bone	Osteoma	Osteosarcoma
Fat	Lipoma	Liposarcoma
Endothelium		
Blood vessels	Hemangioma	Angiosarcoma
Lymphatic vessels	Lymphangioma	Lymphangiosarcoma
Muscle		
Smooth muscle	Leiomyoma	Leiomyosarcoma
Striated muscle	Rhabdomyoma	Rhabdomyosarcoma

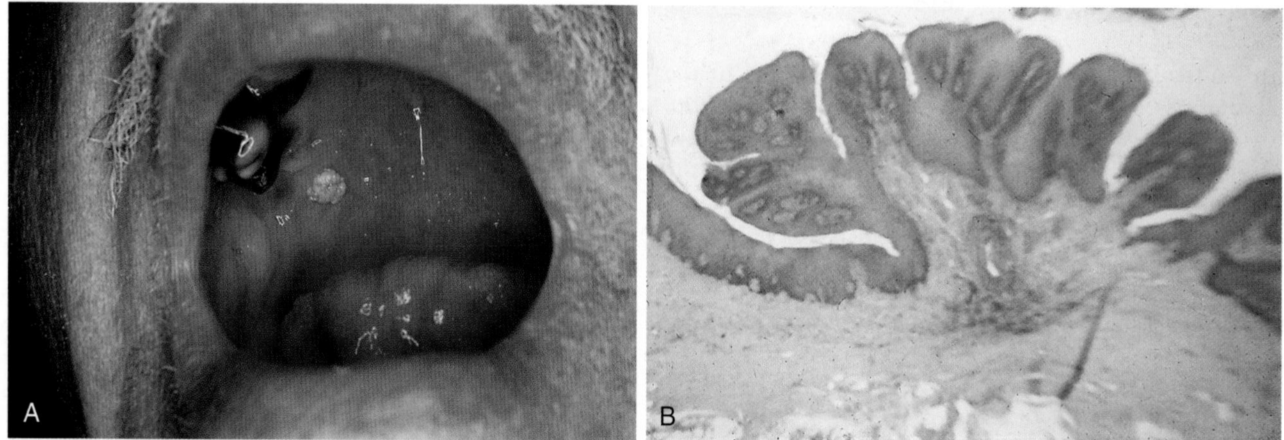

FIGURE 7-2 ■ **A,** Clinical appearance of a papilloma of the oral mucosa shows a cauliflower-like appearance and rough surface resulting from fingerlike projections. **B,** Microscopic appearance of a papilloma shows fingerlike projections surfaced by squamous epithelium and supported by thin cores of fibrous connective tissue.

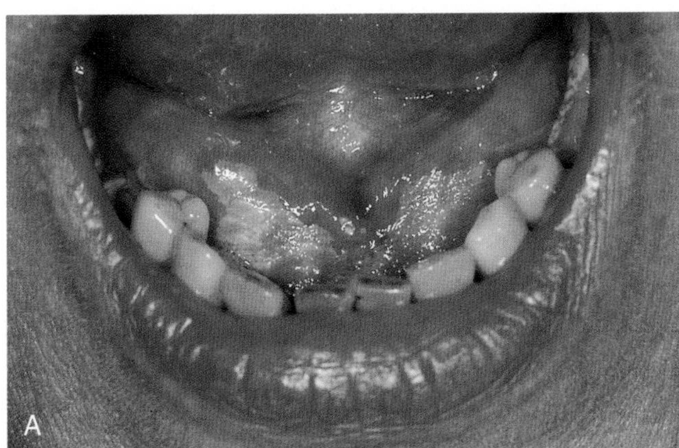

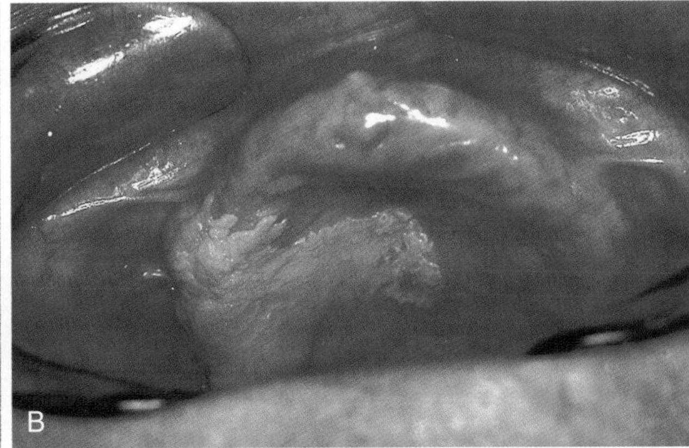

FIGURE 7-3 ■ Clinical appearance of leukoplakia. **A,** Floor of the mouth. **B,** Maxillary alveolar mucosa and palate. The cause of these lesions could not be identified.

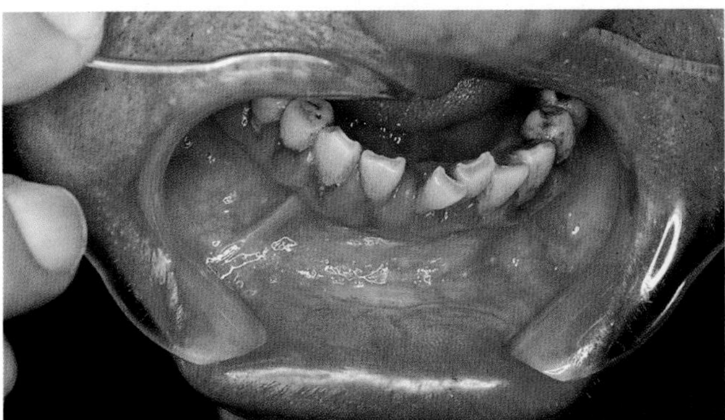

FIGURE 7-4 ■ Clinical appearance of a white lesion that was associated with tobacco chewing (tobacco pouch keratosis). This lesion developed on the lower labial mucosa at the site where the tobacco was held.

(thickening of the keratin layer) or a combination of epithelial hyperplasia (thickening of the prickle cell or spinous layer) and hyperkeratosis. When examined microscopically, a leukoplakia may also show epithelial **dysplasia**, a premalignant condition, or even squamous cell carcinoma, a malignant tumor of squamous epithelium. Depending on the study, approximately 5% to 25% of leukoplakias examined microscopically demonstrated epithelial dysplasia. Studies have also revealed that leukoplakia found on the floor of the mouth, ventrolateral tongue, and lip is more likely to represent epithelial dysplasia or squamous cell carcinoma than leukoplakia occurring in other areas of the oral cavity.

When a white lesion is identified in the oral cavity, the first goal is to identify the cause. Any associated irritation should be removed. If the lesion does not resolve, a biopsy and histologic examination of the tissue must be performed. Any white lesion that is diagnosed as epithelial dysplasia or that cannot be diagnosed as a specific disease should be removed completely. When leukoplakia is found on the floor of the mouth, ventrolateral tongue, or lip, the lesion should be removed regardless of the histologic appearance since there is an increased risk of squamous cell carcinoma developing in these areas.

The treatment of leukoplakia depends on the histologic diagnosis. The treatment of epithelial dysplasia and squamous cell carcinoma is discussed in the sections that follow.

Erythroplakia

Erythroplakia is a clinical term used to describe an oral mucosal lesion that appears as a smooth red patch or a granular red and velvety patch. A lesion that shows a mixture of red and white areas is generally called **speckled leukoplakia** rather than erythroplakia. Most cases of erythroplakia occur in the floor of the mouth, tongue, and soft palate. Erythroplakia is much less common than leukoplakia. In one study 60 cases of leukoplakia were seen for every one case of erythroplakia. When examined microscopically, 90% of cases of erythroplakia demonstrate epithelial dysplasia or squamous cell carcinoma. Because of these microscopic findings, erythroplakia is considered a more serious clinical finding than leukoplakia (a biopsy must be performed to establish a definitive diagnosis).

Treatment of erythroplakia depends on the histologic diagnosis.

Epithelial Dysplasia

Epithelial dysplasia is a histologic diagnosis that indicates disordered growth. It is considered a premalignant condition. Lesions that microscopically exhibit epithelial dysplasia frequently precede squamous cell carcinoma. Unlike squamous cell carcinoma, the cellular changes in epithelial dysplasia may revert to normal if the stimulus such as tobacco smoking is removed. Epithelial dysplasia may present clinically as an erythematous lesion (erythroplakia), a white lesion (leukoplakia), or a mixed erythematous and white lesion (speckled leukoplakia). Lesions often arise in the floor of the mouth or tongue. The term *dysplasia* may also be used to describe lesions that occur in tissues other than epithelium.

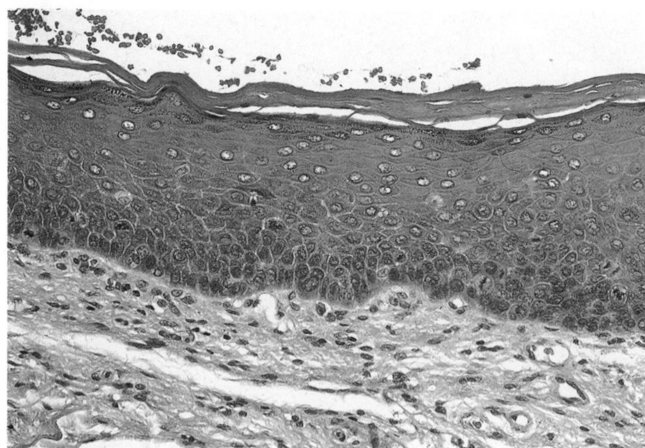

FIGURE 7-5 ■ Microscopic appearance of epithelial dysplasia. Loss of the normal stratification of the epithelium, hyperplasia of the basal cells, and enlarged and hyperchromatic nuclei are seen.

Dysplasia in other tissues (such as bone) is not considered a premalignant process. Microscopic examination of epithelial dysplasia demonstrates abnormal maturation of epithelial cells with disorganization of the epithelial layers; hyperplasia of the basal cells; and epithelial cells with enlarged and hyperchromatic nuclei, increased nuclear cytoplasmic ratios, abnormal keratinization, and increased numbers of normal and abnormal mitotic figures (Figure 7-5). Microscopically epithelial dysplasia differs from squamous cell carcinoma in that there is no **invasion** of the abnormal epithelial cells through the basement membrane into the underlying tissue. Severe dysplasia involving the full thickness of the epithelium is called carcinoma **in situ.**

All dysplastic lesions should be excised surgically. Close long-term follow-up examinations are indicated because of the potential for recurrence.

SQUAMOUS CELL CARCINOMA

Squamous cell carcinoma, or epidermoid carcinoma, is a malignant tumor of squamous epithelium. It is the most common primary malignancy of the oral cavity and, like other malignant tumors, can infiltrate adjacent tissues and metastasize to distant sites. Squamous cell carcinoma usually metastasizes to lymph nodes of the neck and then to more distant sites such as the lungs and liver. Clinically squamous cell carcinoma usually presents as an exophytic ulcerative mass (Figure 7-6), but early tumors may be erythematous and plaquelike (erythroplakia), white and plaquelike (leukoplakia), or a mixture of erythematous and white areas (speckled leukoplakia). Squamous cell carcinoma can infiltrate and destroy bone (see Figure 7-6, *D*).

The essential microscopic feature of a squamous cell carcinoma is the invasion of tumor cells through the epithelial basement membrane into the underlying connective tissue (Figure 7-7, *A*). Invasive sheets and nests of neoplastic squamous cells characterize this tumor. Although squamous cell carcinoma is a malignant tumor, it exhibits features that allow the cells to be recognized as squamous epithelial cells. In well-differentiated tumors these features are easily recognized; however, they may not be easily seen in a poorly differentiated squamous cell carcinoma. Because keratin is a product of squamous epithelium, well-differentiated tumors show keratin formation. In addition to normal surface keratin, the keratin may be seen in individual cells within the tumor and as structures called **keratin pearls** (Figure 7-7, B). The neoplastic cells are not normal cells. They contain large hyperchromatic nuclei and numerous mitotic figures. Some of the mitotic figures appear normal, whereas others are bizarre (see Figure 7-7, *B*).

Squamous cell carcinomas may occur anywhere in the oral cavity, but most tumors arise on the floor of the mouth, ventrolateral tongue, soft palate, tonsillar pillar, and retromolar areas. The clinical appearance of squamous cell carcinoma occurring in several different locations is seen in Figure 7-6.

Squamous cell carcinomas may occur on the vermilion border of the lips and skin of the face (Figure 7-8). In this location they are associated with sun exposure (actinic cheilitis and actinic keratosis) and tend to be more common in individuals with fair skin. The prognosis for squamous cell carcinoma of the lips and skin is much better than that for squamous cell carcinoma of the oral mucosa. Sun exposure causes recognizable changes of the vermilion border of the lips. The color changes from dark and uniform to mottled grayish-pink. The interface of the vermilion border and the skin becomes blurred, and linear fissures are seen at right angles to the line of the interface. Histologically damage from sun exposure is seen as changes that range from degeneration of the collagen under the epithelium to a condition called **solar or actinic cheilitis,** in which mild-to-severe epithelial dysplasia occurs. Fair-skinned individuals should be advised either to avoid the sun or to use a sun block.

The majority of squamous cell carcinomas occur in patients over 40 years of age. In the past men have outnumbered women; however, in the last 30 years there has been an increased incidence of squamous cell carcinoma in women. This is most likely a result of the increased number of women who smoke and the fact that women outnumber men in older age-groups.

Risk Factors

Several risk factors have been associated with the development of squamous cell carcinoma. The most significant is tobacco—including cigar, pipe, and cigarette smoking; snuff dipping; and tobacco chewing. Alcohol consumption appears to add to the risk of oral squamous cell carcinoma, especially in individuals who also use tobacco products. There is no

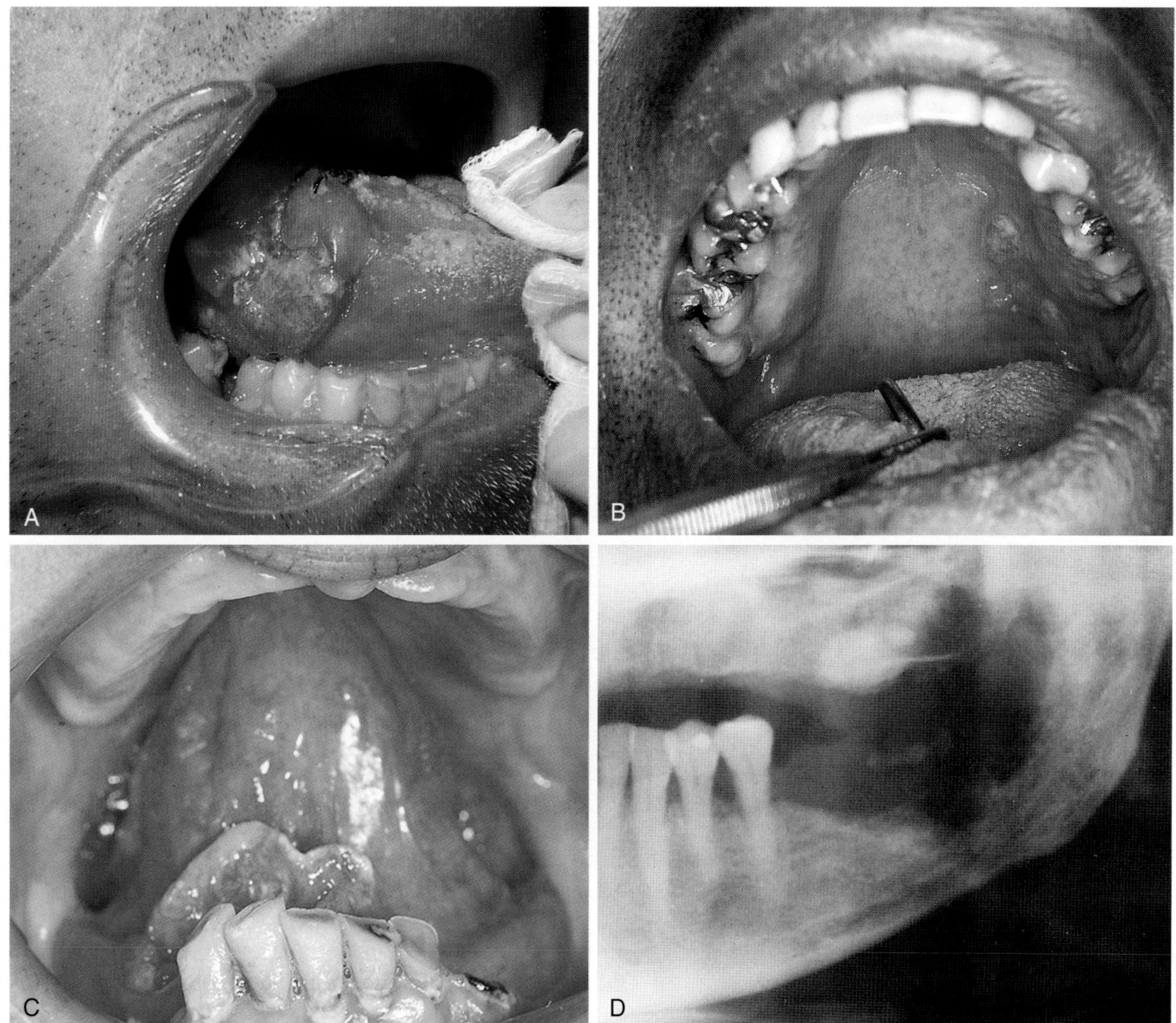

FIGURE 7-6 ■ **A,** Clinical appearance of a squamous cell carcinoma of the posterolateral tongue shows an exophytic, ulcerated mass. **B,** Clinical appearance of a squamous cell carcinoma on the left side of the soft palate and fauces. **C,** Clinical appearance of a squamous cell carcinoma on the floor of the mouth. **D,** Left side of a panoramic radiograph shows destruction of the mandible by a squamous cell carcinoma. (**C** courtesy Dr. Edward V. Zegarelli.)

evidence that chronic irritation is an initiating factor in the development of oral cancer.

Treatment and Prognosis

Squamous cell carcinoma generally is treated by surgical excision. Radiation therapy or chemotherapy may be used in combination with surgery. Occasionally radiation therapy is used alone. The prognosis of squamous cell carcinoma is related to the size and location of the tumor and the presence or absence of metastases. The smaller the tumor at the time of treatment, the better the prognosis. For oral squamous cell carcinoma, determining the size of the tumor and the presence or absence of cervical lymph node involvement and distant **metastasis** is important in predicting the patient's prognosis. These are assessed using a system called the **TNM staging system;** the higher the stage, the worse the prognosis (Box 7-1 and Table 7-3). Metastasis to cervical lymph nodes is associated with a much poorer prognosis, as is the presence of distant metastasis. Therefore it is important to identify asymptomatic areas of leukoplakia and erythroplakia while they are small and remove all potentially premalignant lesions.

Patients who have undergone radiation therapy for malignant tumors of the head and neck often experience severe xerostomia (dry mouth) as a result of radiation damage to the salivary gland tissue. These patients require preventive

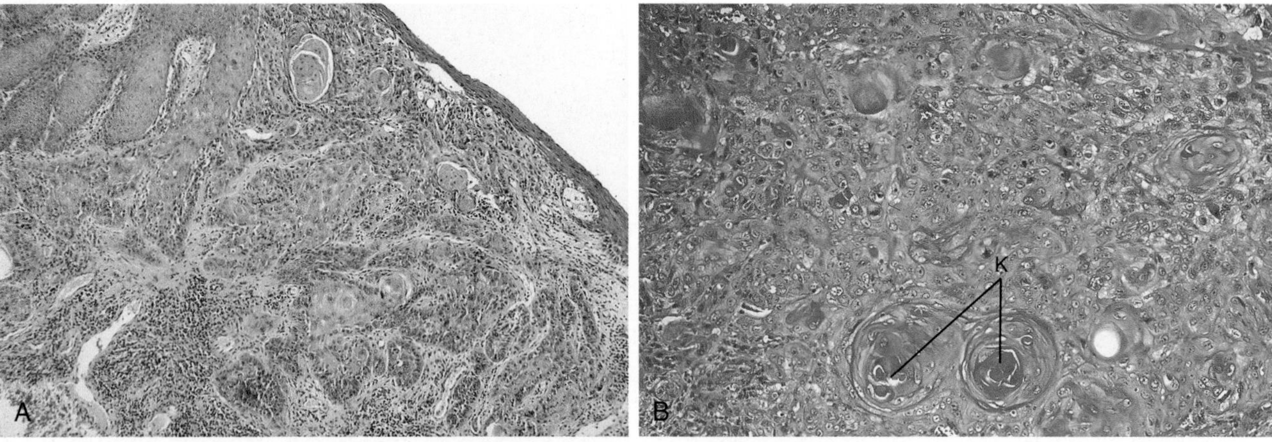

FIGURE 7-7 ■ **A,** Microscopic appearance (low power) of a squamous cell carcinoma shows infiltration of the tumor into the connective tissue. **B,** High-power photomicrograph shows abnormal keratinization *(K).*

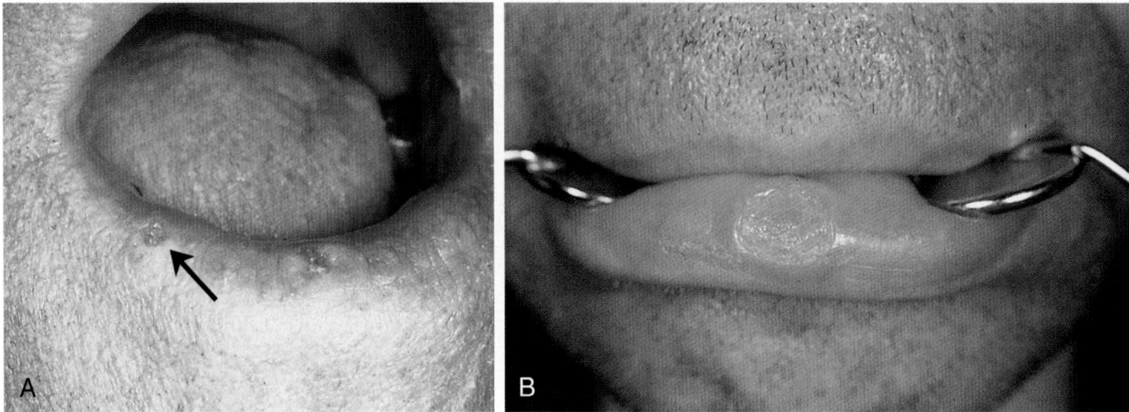

FIGURE 7-8 ■ Clinical appearance of squamous cell carcinoma of the lower lip *(arrow).* The reader should also note actinic (solar) cheilitis in **A**. (Courtesy Dr. Edward V. Zegarelli.)

Box 7-1

TNM Staging System for Oral Squamous Cell Carcinoma

T: Tumor

T_1: Tumor less than 2 cm in diameter
T_2: Tumor 2-4 cm in diameter
T_3: Tumor greater than 4 cm in diameter
T_4: Tumor invades adjacent structures

N: Node

N_0: No palpable nodes
N_1: Ipsilateral (same side as primary tumor) palpable nodes (same side as tumor)
N_2: Contralateral (opposite side from primary tumor) or bilateral nodes
N_3: Fixed palpable nodes

M: Metastasis

M_0: No distant metastasis
M1: Clinical or radiographic evidence of metastasis

Adapted from Sobin LH, Wittekind C, editors: *International union against cancer TNM classification of malignant tumours,* ... ·w York, 2002, Wiley-Liss.

dental care consisting of nutritional counseling, topical fluoride application, and meticulous home care. Oral manifestations of therapy for oral cancer is included in Chapter 9.

VERRUCOUS CARCINOMA

Verrucous carcinoma is a specific type of squamous cell carcinoma that is separated from other squamous cell carcinomas because it has a much better prognosis. Clinically it appears as a slow-growing exophytic tumor with a pebbly white and red surface (Figure 7-9). Most cases occur in men over 55 years of age and involve the vestibule and buccal mucosa. Verrucous carcinoma occurs most often in individuals who use smokeless tobacco products. Microscopic examination demonstrates a tumor composed of numerous papillary epithelial proliferations. The spaces between these papillary projections are filled with keratin. The epithelium is well differentiated, does not contain atypical cells, and exhibits broad-based rete pegs that penetrate deeply into the connective tissue. The epithelial basement membrane is intact, and the tumor does not show invasion of tumor cells through the basement membrane, as is seen in squamous cell carcinoma.

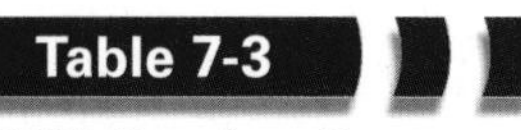

TNM Staging System

	Tumor	Node	Metastasis
Stage I	T_1	N_0	M_0
Stage II	T_2	N_0	M_0
Stage III	T_3	N_0	M_0
	T_1	N_1	M_0
	T_2	N_1	M_0
	T_3	N_1	M_0
Stage IV	T_1	N_2	M_0
	T_2	N_2	M_0
	T_3	N_2	M_0
	T_1	N_3	M_0
	T_2	N_3	M_0
	T_3	N_3	M_0
	T_4	N_0	M_0
	Any patients with M_1		

Adapted from Sobin LH, Wittekind C, editors: *International union against cancer TNM classification of malignant tumours,* ed 6, New York, 2002, Wiley-Liss.

Verrucous carcinoma is treated by surgical excision. Although it is a carcinoma, it usually does not metastasize; therefore the prognosis is better for verrucous carcinoma than for squamous cell carcinoma. If it is not treated, it can cause extensive local damage. Close long-term follow-up is necessary for patients with this condition.

BASAL CELL CARCINOMA

Basal cell carcinoma is a malignant skin tumor associated with excessive sun exposure. This particular neoplasm does not occur in the oral cavity. Basal cell carcinoma frequently arises on the skin of the face and appears as a nonhealing ulcer with characteristic rolled borders (Figure 7-10). Most cases arise in white adults, and no sex predilection is seen.

A basal cell carcinoma is composed of a proliferation of basal cells derived from the surface stratified squamous epithelium. Microscopic examination demonstrates nests and islands of basal epithelial cells in the underlying connective tissue. In most cases the tumor cells are well differentiated.

Basal cell carcinoma is a locally invasive tumor that can become quite large and disfiguring if it is not removed. Surgical excision is the treatment of choice, and radiation therapy may be used to treat large lesions. Only rarely does a basal cell carcinoma metastasize. As a general rule, a patient should be referred to an oral and maxillofacial surgeon or dermatologist to have a biopsy performed on any nonhealing ulcer of the skin or lips that has been present for more than 10 days.

SALIVARY GLAND TUMORS

Benign and malignant tumors may arise in either the major or the minor salivary glands. Tumors may occur within the parotid, submandibular, or sublingual glands; or they may involve any of the minor salivary glands located throughout the oral cavity. Intraorally minor salivary gland tumors are located most commonly at the junction of the hard and soft palates. They can also occur on the labial and buccal mucosa, the retromolar area, the floor of the mouth, and rarely the tongue (Figure 7-11). Tumors of minor salivary gland origin are much more common in the upper lip than in the lower lip.

Because the origin of these tumors is glandular epithelium, benign tumors of salivary gland origin are called **adenomas.** Although some malignant salivary gland tumors are called **adenocarcinomas,** most have more specific names such as adenoid cystic carcinoma and mucoepidermoid carcinoma. All salivary gland tumors are diagnosed on the basis of their microscopic appearance. A biopsy and microscopic examination of the tissue are required to establish a specific diagnosis.

PLEOMORPHIC ADENOMA (BENIGN MIXED TUMOR)

The **pleomorphic adenoma** is a benign salivary gland tumor. It is the most common salivary gland neoplasm and accounts for about 90% of all benign salivary gland tumors. Microscopic examination reveals an encapsulated tumor composed of tissue that appears to be a mixture of both epithelium and connective tissue (Figure 7-12). For this reason the tumor is often called the **benign mixed tumor.** The connective tissue–like part can vary from loose and dense fibrous connective tissue to cartilage. The tissue that looks like connective tissue is derived from a salivary gland cell called a **myoepithelial cell.**

The most common extraoral location for the pleomorphic adenoma is the parotid gland. The most common intraoral site is the palate. However, these tumors can occur wherever salivary gland tissue is present. Clinically the pleomorphic adenoma appears as a slowly enlarging, nonulcerated, painless, dome-shaped mass (see Figure 7-11, *A* and *C*). The surface can be ulcerated if traumatized. Its size can range from a few to several centimeters. Most pleomorphic adenomas occur in individuals over 40 years of age, and a female predilection has been noted. Pleomorphic adenomas have also been reported in children.

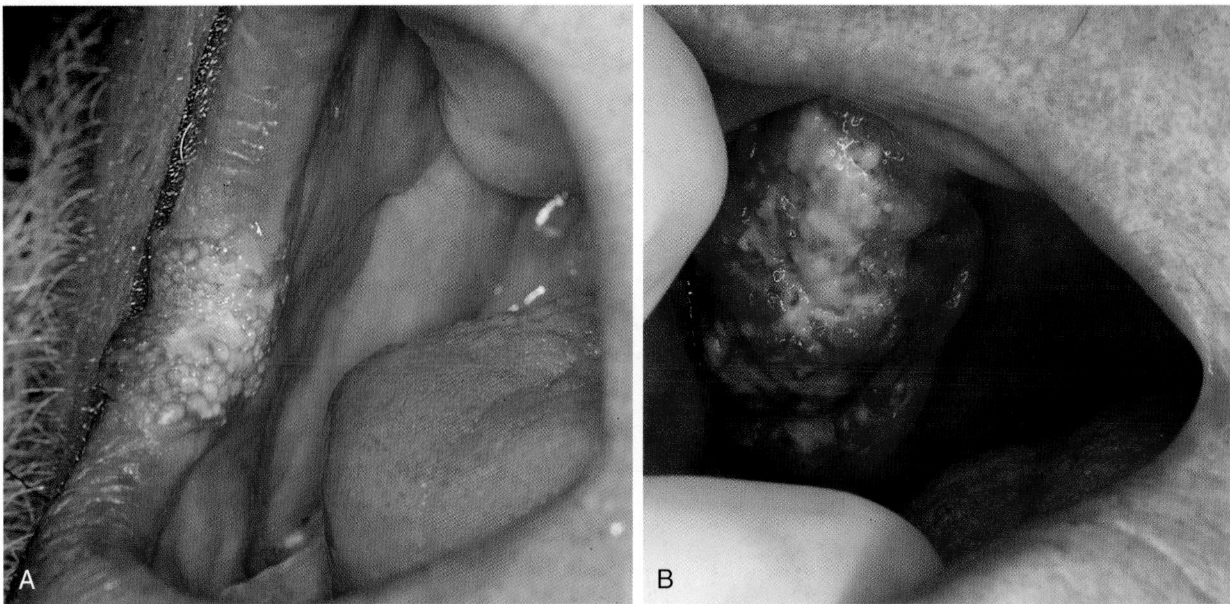

FIGURE 7-9 ■ **A,** Clinical appearance of a verrucous carcinoma occurring on the commissure and anterior buccal mucosa. **B,** Maxillary alveolar ridge.

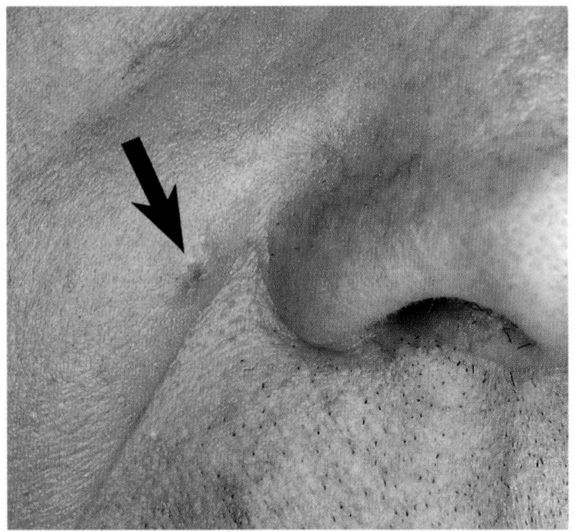

FIGURE 7-10 ■ Clinical appearance of a basal cell carcinoma *(arrow)* illustrating the characteristic "rolled" borders.

The pleomorphic adenoma is treated by surgical excision. The extent of the surgery depends on the location of the tumor. Clinicians treat parotid gland tumors by removing the part of the parotid gland containing the tumor (partial parotidectomy), whereas minor salivary gland tumors are treated by more conservative surgical excision. The pleomorphic adenoma grows by extension of projections of tumor into the surrounding tissue. Therefore some tumors are difficult to remove completely. Recurrence rates vary and are related to the adequacy of the initial surgical removal. Pleomorphic adenomas have been known to undergo malignant transformation; this occurrence is known as a **carcinoma arising in a pleomorphic adenoma.**

MONOMORPHIC ADENOMA

The **monomorphic adenoma** is a benign encapsulated salivary gland tumor that occurs less frequently than the pleomorphic adenoma. It is composed of a uniform pattern of epithelial cells (Figure 7-13). These tumors do not have the connective tissue–like component seen in a pleomorphic adenoma. They occur most commonly in adult women, with a predilection for the upper lip and buccal mucosa. Several specific types of monomorphic adenoma based on their histologic patterns have been identified. The **papillary cystadenoma lymphomatosum** is a unique type of monomorphic adenoma. It is also called *Warthin's tumor.* Microscopic examination of this particular variant demonstrates an encapsulated tumor composed of two types of tissue: epithelial and lymphoid (Figure 7-14). The epithelial component is neoplastic. It lines papillary projections that protrude from cystic structures. Sheets of lymphocytes surround the cystic structures. In some cases the lymphoid component demonstrates germinal center formation. Warthin's tumor presents as a painless, soft, and compressible or fluctuant mass, usually located in the parotid gland. Intraoral examples are very rare. This tumor often develops bilaterally and occurs predominantly in adult men.

All monomorphic adenomas are treated by surgical excision. Recurrence is rare.

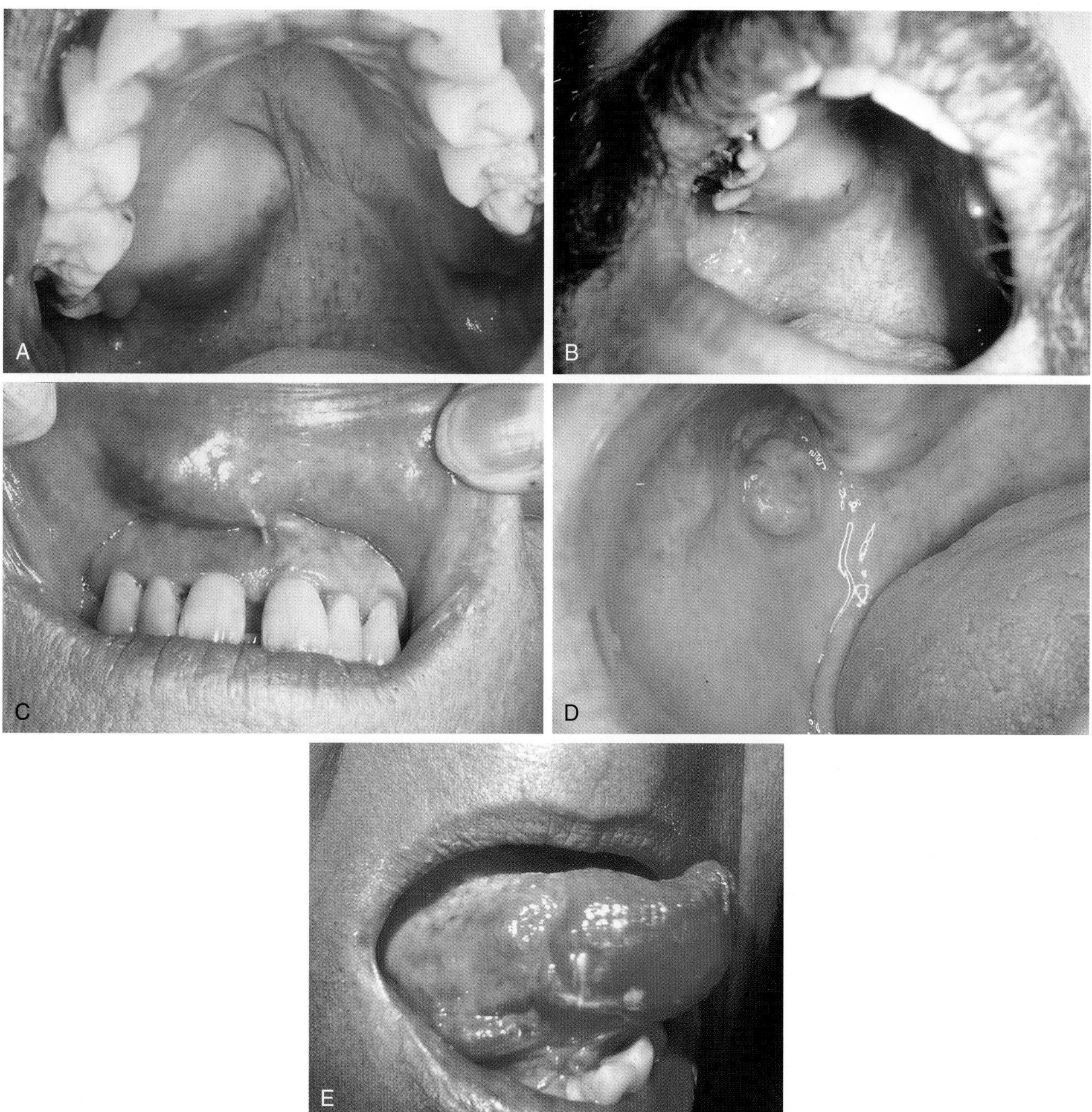

FIGURE 7-11 ■ **A,** Benign salivary gland tumor of the palate (pleomorphic adenoma). **B,** Malignant salivary gland tumor of the palate (adenoid cystic carcinoma). Biopsy site should be noted. **C,** Benign salivary gland tumor of the upper lip (pleomorphic adenoma). **D,** Malignant salivary gland tumor of the buccal mucosa (mucoepidermoid carcinoma). **E,** Malignant salivary gland tumor of the tongue (adenoid cystic carcinoma).

ADENOID CYSTIC CARCINOMA (CYLINDROMA)

The **adenoid cystic carcinoma** (see Figure 7-11, *E*) is a malignant tumor of salivary gland origin that can originate from either major or minor salivary gland tissue. It is unencapsulated and infiltrates surrounding tissue. This tumor is composed of small, deeply staining, uniform epithelial cells arranged in perforated round-to-oval islands. The microscopic appearance of adenoid cystic carcinoma has been likened to that of Swiss cheese (Figure 7-15). These round and oval islands represent cylinders of tumor; therefore this tumor has also been called a **cylindroma.** Although it is malignant, pleomorphic cells and mitotic figures are rarely seen. Malignancy is recognized on the basis of the unique microscopic features. The adenoid cystic carcinoma is a slow-growing malignant tumor.

The most common extraoral site for an adenoid cystic carcinoma is the parotid gland. The most common intraoral site is the palate. Most tumors appear as slowly growing masses that can exhibit surface ulceration (see Figure 7-11, *B* and E). Pain is often present because of the tendency of these tumors to surround nerves. Adenoid cystic carcinoma is more common in women than in men and is a tumor of adults; the majority of cases are diagnosed in the fifth and sixth decades of life.

The treatment of choice for adenoid cystic carcinoma is complete surgical excision. Radiation treatment has been attempted and has been shown to be of benefit in some cases. However, recurrence and persistent local invasion are common. Metastasis occurs late in the course of the disease. About 30% of patients experience cervical lymph node involvement. Distant metastases, most often involving the lungs, may occur after many years. In these cases the prognosis is poor.

MUCOEPIDERMOID CARCINOMA

Mucoepidermoid carcinoma is a malignant salivary gland tumor. It is an unencapsulated, infiltrating tumor composed of a combination of mucous cells interspersed with squamouslike epithelial cells called **epidermoid cells** (Figure 7-16).

Mucoepidermoid carcinomas involving the major glands occur most often in the parotid gland, whereas minor gland tumors are most common on the palate. They appear clinically as slowly enlarging masses (see Figure 7-11, *D*). Occasionally a mucoepidermoid carcinoma may arise **centrally** within bone (see Figure 7-16, *B*), usually in the mandibular premolar and molar region. In this location it appears as either a unilocular or a multilocular radiolucency (see Figure 7-16, *B*). A central mucoepidermoid carcinoma is derived from either salivary gland tissue trapped within bone or the transformed epithelial lining of a dentigerous cyst (a developmental odontogenic

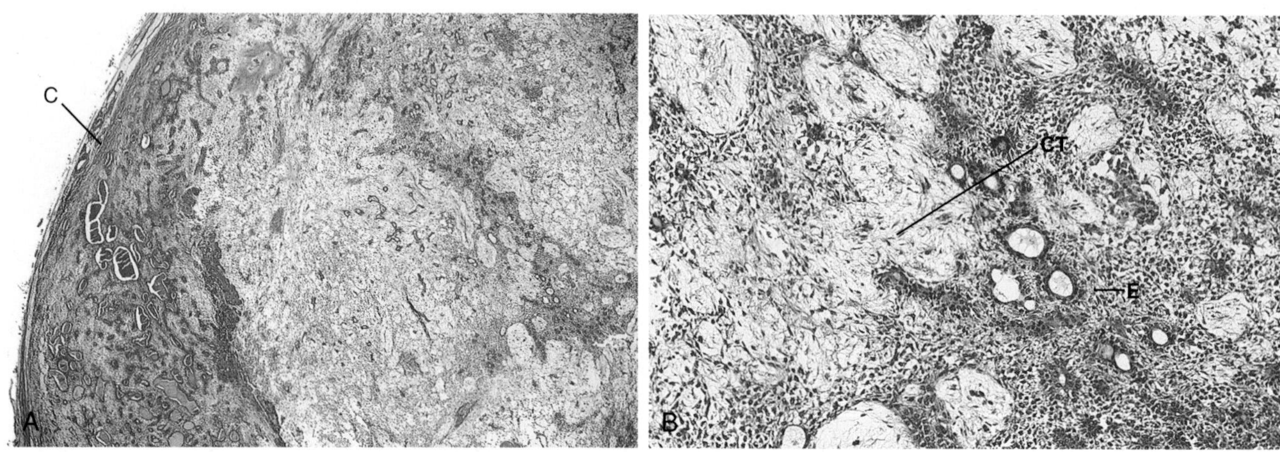

FIGURE 7-12 ■ Microscopic appearance of a pleomorphic adenoma. **A,** Low-power photomicrograph shows a capsule *(C).* **B,** High-power photomicrograph shows a mixture of epithelium *(E)* and connective tissue *(CT).*

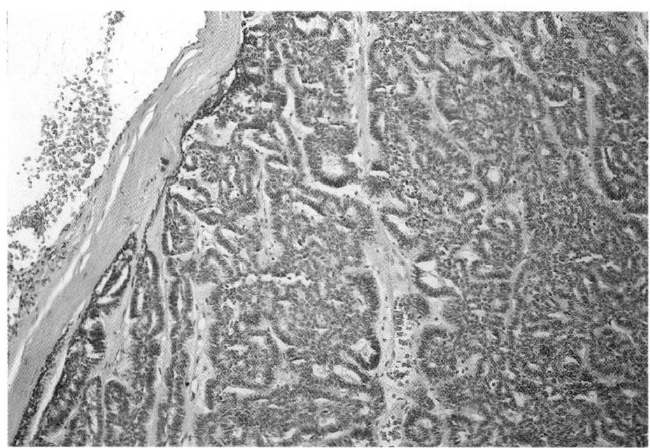

FIGURE 7-13 ■ Microscopic appearance (low power) of a monomorphic adenoma shows a capsule and a uniform pattern of epithelial cells.

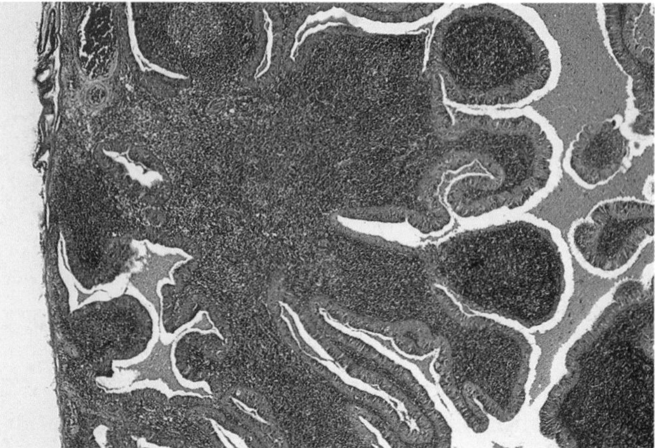

FIGURE 7-14 ■ Microscopic appearance of a papillary cystadenoma lymphomatosum (Warthin's tumor) shows spaces lined by epithelium and surrounded by lymphocytes.

cyst that forms around the crown of an unerupted or impacted tooth; see Chapter 5).

A mucoepidermoid carcinoma may occur over a wide age range. Although it usually occurs in adults after middle age, this tumor is the most common malignant salivary gland tumor in children. A female predilection is noted.

Treatment of the mucoepidermoid carcinoma consists of complete surgical excision, with close long-term follow-up for signs of recurrence and metastasis. The behavior of any one tumor is difficult to predict and is related to the histologic appearance of the tumor. Low-grade tumors have a 92% 5-year survival rate after initial treatment. For high-grade (more malignant) tumors, only 49% of patients survive 5 years after the initial treatment.

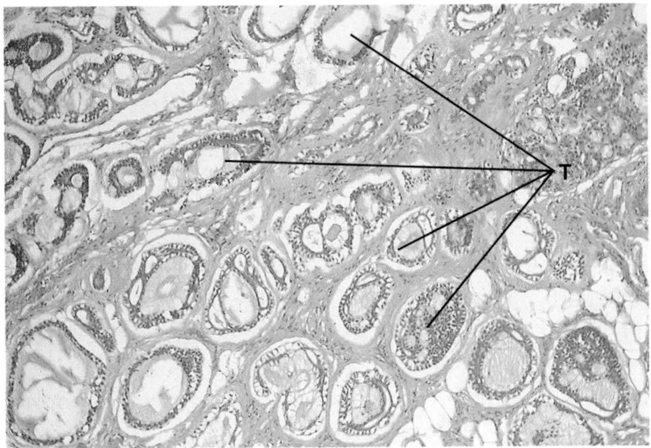

FIGURE 7-15 ■ Microscopic appearance of an adenoid cystic carcinoma shows perforated islands of uniform cells. Tumor *(T)* is seen infiltrating the adjacent adipose tissue.

OTHER MALIGNANT SALIVARY GLAND TUMORS

In addition to the adenoid cystic and the mucoepidermoid carcinomas, several other malignant salivary gland tumors exist, including polymorphous low-grade adenocarcinoma (lobular carcinoma), acinic cell adenocarcinoma, and other adenocarcinomas.

ODONTOGENIC TUMORS

Odontogenic tumors are derived from tooth-forming tissues. Tooth formation results from an interaction between odontogenic epithelium and odontogenic mesenchyme. Some odontogenic tumors are composed of epithelium only, some are composed of mesenchyme only, and others are composed of a mixture of both elements. Most odontogenic tumors are benign. Malignant odontogenic tumors occur but are rare. Table 7-4 presents a classification scheme for odontogenic tumors based on the derivation of the odontogenic tissue.

In addition to the odontogenic tumors described in this text, other uncommon odontogenic tumors such as the squamous odontogenic tumor and the central odontogenic fibroma exist. (See the references at the end of this chapter for more detailed information on these tumors.)

EPITHELIAL ODONTOGENIC TUMORS

Ameloblastoma

The **ameloblastoma** is a benign, slow-growing but locally aggressive epithelial odontogenic tumor that may arise in either the maxilla or the mandible. It is an unencapsulated

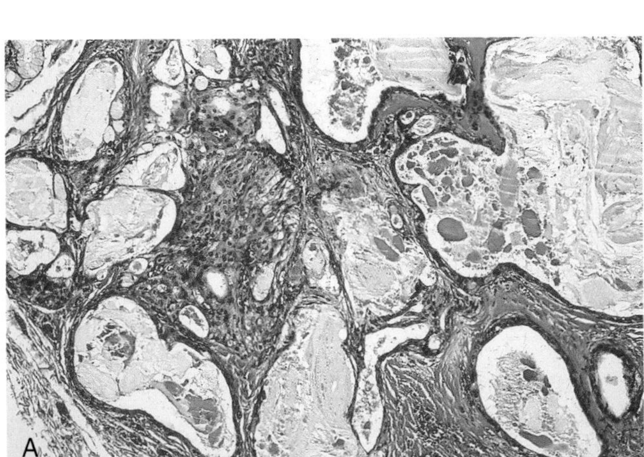

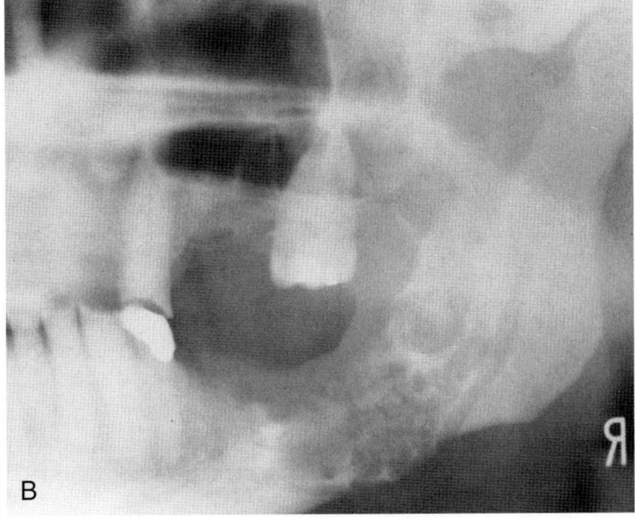

FIGURE 7-16 ■ **A,** Microscopic appearance (low power) of a mucoepidermoid carcinoma shows cystic structures, mucous cells, and epidermoid cells. **B,** Radiograph of a central mucoepidermoid carcinoma shows a multilocular radiolucency.

Table 7-4

Classification of Central Odontogenic Tumors

Epithelial Odontogenic Tumors	Mesenchymal Odontogenic Tumors	Mixed Odontogenic Tumors
Ameloblastoma	Odontogenic myxoma	Ameloblastic fibroma
Calcifying epithelial odontogenic tumor (CEOT)	Cementifying fibroma	Ameloblastic fibro-odontoma
Adenomatoid odontogenic tumor (AOT or OAT)	Ossifying fibroma Peripheral ossifying fibroma Benign cementoblastoma	Odontoma

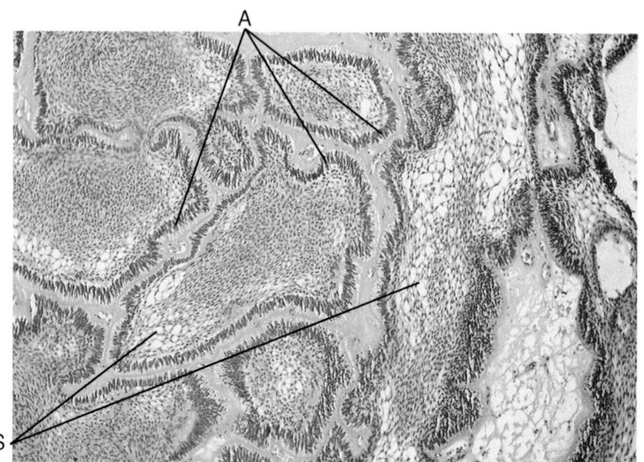

FIGURE 7-17 ■ Microscopic appearance (low-power) of a follicular ameloblastoma shows dental follicle-like islands composed of epithelial cells consisting of peripheral ameloblast-like cells *(A)* and stellate reticulum-like areas *(S)*.

tumor that infiltrates into surrounding tissue and can cause extensive destruction. When it occurs in the maxilla, death can result from direct extension into the brain and adjacent vital structures. An ameloblastoma is composed of ameloblast-like epithelial cells that surround areas resembling stellate reticulum. These cells are arranged in either dental follicle-like islands or interconnecting strands (Figure 7-17).

The classic radiographic appearance of an ameloblastoma is a multilocular soap bubble–like or honeycombed radiolucency (Figure 7-18). In smaller tumors the radiolucency may be unilocular. An ameloblastoma may arise anywhere in the jaws and can occur in association with a dentigerous cyst (Figure 7-19). However, 80% of ameloblastomas arise in the mandible, most often in the molar and ramus area. The molar area is also the most common location when they occur in the maxilla. The tumor may cause expansion of bone. The initial presentation is usually a slowly developing, asymptomatic swelling of the affected bone. The age range of individuals affected is broad, but most ameloblastomas occur in adults. No sex predilection is noted.

Ameloblastomas are treated by complete surgical removal. Recurrence is common. Occasionally these tumors occur in the gingiva and do not involve bone, in which case they are called **peripheral ameloblastomas.** These are also treated by surgical excision and differ from the central ameloblastomas in that they generally do not recur.

Calcifying Epithelial Odontogenic Tumor

The **calcifying epithelial odontogenic tumor,** also known as a *Pindborg tumor,* is a benign epithelial odontogenic tumor that occurs much less frequently than the ameloblastoma. It is a unique odontogenic tumor because the proliferating cells do not resemble odontogenic epithelium. The tumor is composed of islands and sheets of polyhedral (multisided) epithelial cells. Deposits similar to amyloid are seen in the tumor, and calcifications are seen within these deposits. The amyloid-like material is thought to represent a form of abnormal enamel protein (Figure 7-20, *A*). Radiographically the calcifying epithelial odontogenic tumor appears as a unilocular or multilocular radiolucency (Figure 7-20, *B*). Calcifications that form within the tumor appear as radiopacities within the radiolucency.

The majority of patients affected with this tumor are adults. However, the calcifying epithelial odontogenic tumor affects a broad age range that extends from young adults to elderly individuals. No sex predilection is noted. Reports of this tumor occurring in the mandible are twice as common as reports of it occurring in the maxilla. Although it can occur anywhere in the maxilla or mandible, the bicuspid and molar areas are the most common locations. Many neoplasms are associated with impacted teeth.

Treatment of the calcifying epithelial odontogenic tumor depends on the size and location of the tumor and involves complete surgical excision. Recurrence has been reported, but the recurrence rate is lower than that for an ameloblastoma.

Adenomatoid Odontogenic Tumor

The **adenomatoid odontogenic tumor** (AOT), also known as an **odontogenic adenomatoid tumor,** is an encapsulated, benign epithelial odontogenic tumor that has a distinctive age, sex, and site distribution. It also differs

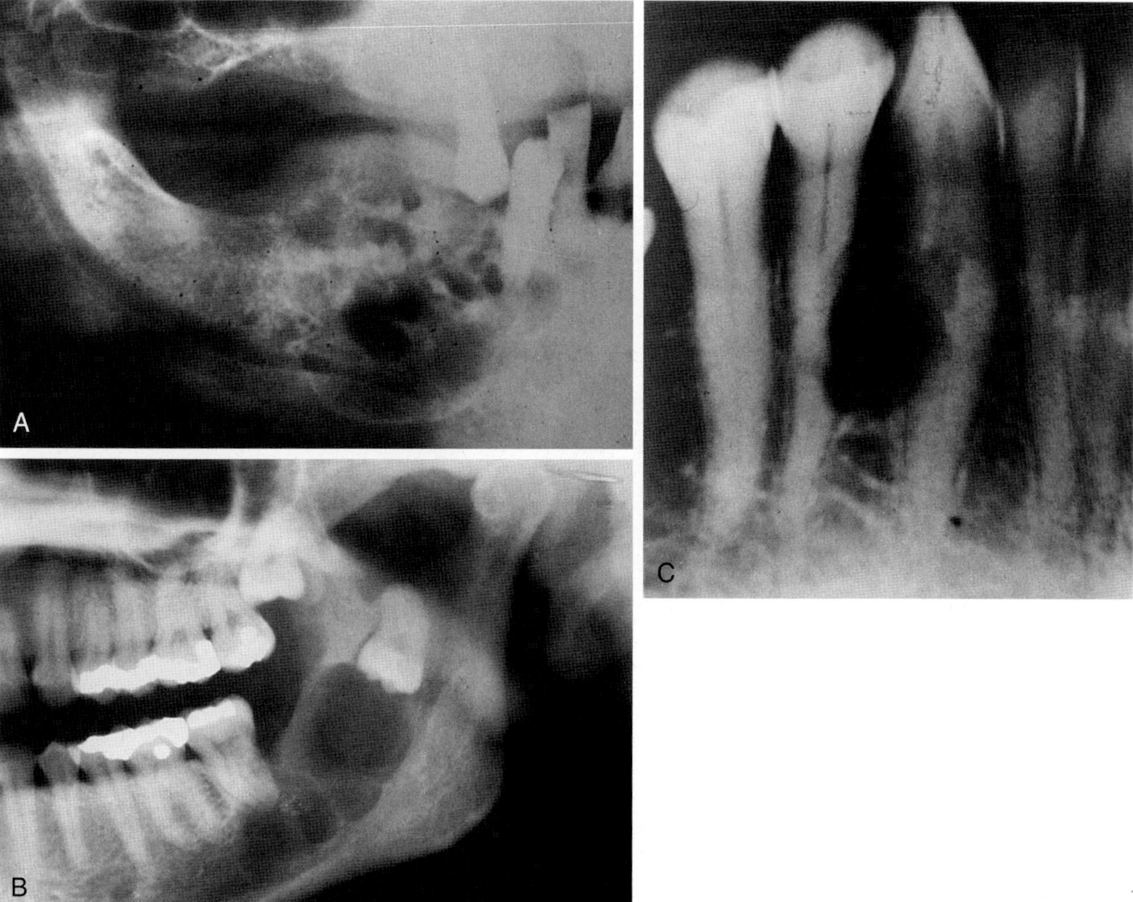

FIGURE 7-18 ■ **A,** Radiograph of an ameloblastoma shows multilocular radiolucency in the molar area of the mandible. **B,** Radiograph of an ameloblastoma shows a multilocular radiolucency in the molar area of the mandible. **C,** Radiograph of an ameloblastoma shows a small but multilocular radiolucency in the mandibular cuspid and bicuspid region.

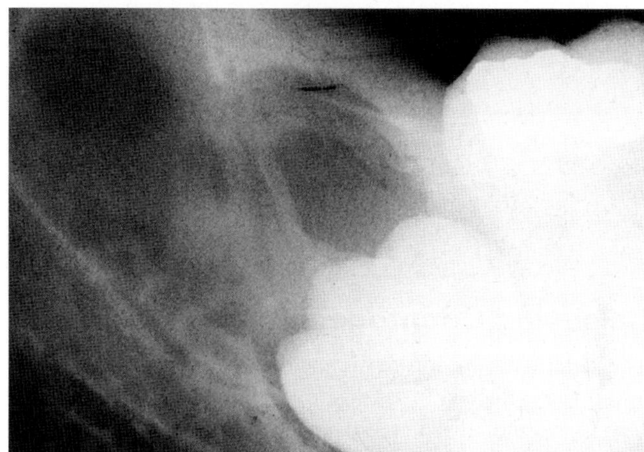

FIGURE 7-19 ■ Radiograph of an ameloblastoma that formed in association with an impacted tooth and dentigerous cyst.

from other epithelial odontogenic tumors in that it does not recur. Approximately 70% of AOTs occur in females under 20 years of age, and 70% involve the anterior part of the jaws. The maxilla is more commonly involved than the mandible. Many AOTs are associated with impacted teeth. Although a localized swelling may be present, most are asymptomatic and are discovered on routine radiographic examination.

Radiographically the AOT appears as a well-circumscribed radiolucency (Figure 7-21, *B*). Because of the frequent association with an impacted tooth, an adenomatoid odontogenic tumor often simulates a dentigerous cyst. However, unlike the dentigerous cyst (see Chapter 5), the adenomatoid odontogenic tumor extends beyond the cementoenamel junction and can involve 50% to 60% of the root. As calcifications form within the tumor, radiopaque areas of varying size are visible on radiographs. Histologic examination reveals a dense, fibrous connective tissue capsule surrounding ductlike structures, whorls, and large masses of cuboidal and spindle-shaped epithelial cells (Figure 7-21, *A*). The ductlike structures are

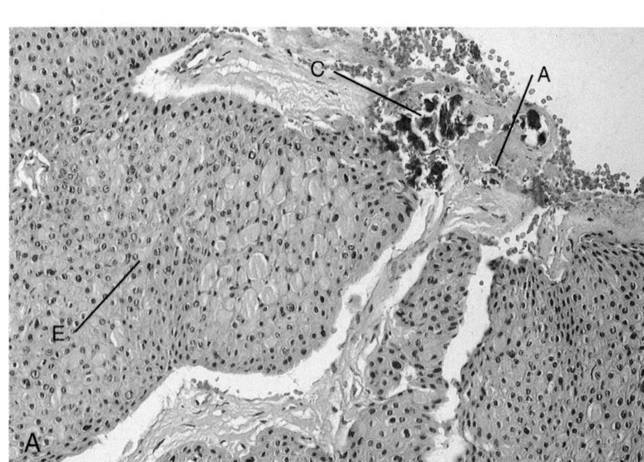

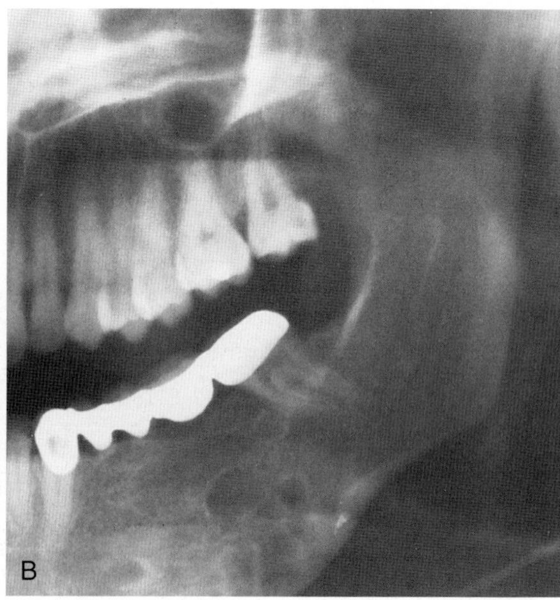

FIGURE 7-20 ■ Calcifying epithelial odontogenic tumor. **A,** Microscopic appearance (low power) of a calcifying epithelial odontogenic tumor shows sheets of epithelial cells *(E)*, amorphous material *(A)*, and calcifications *(C)*. **B,** Radiograph of a calcifying epithelial odontogenic tumor shows a multilocular radiolucency.

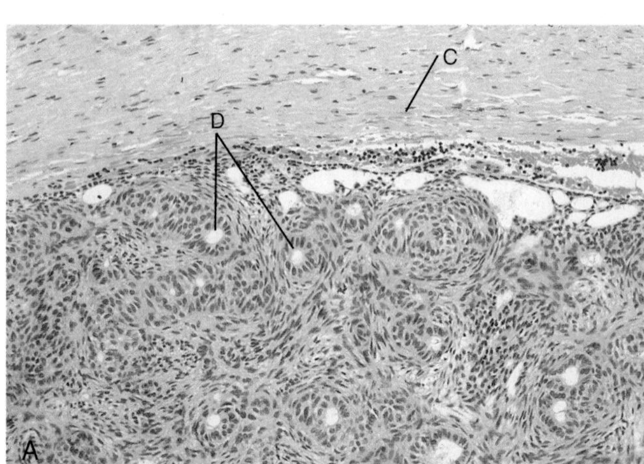

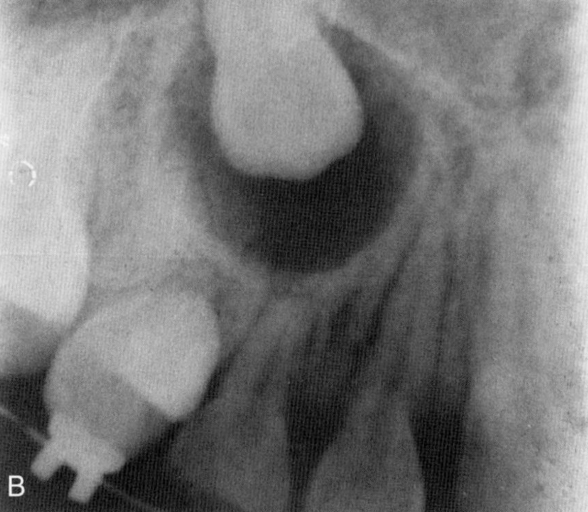

FIGURE 7-21 ■ Adenomatoid odontogenic tumor. **A,** Microscopic appearance of an adenomatoid odontogenic tumor shows the capsule *(C)*, epithelial cells, and ductlike structures *(D)*. **B,** Radiograph of an adenomatoid odontogenic tumor shows a unilocular radiolucency surrounding the crown of an unerupted maxillary cuspid.

one of the distinctive features of this tumor and are the reason for the name **adenomatoid,** or glandlike.

These structures are not ducts but actually ameloblast-like cells that resemble ducts because of their circular arrangement. Eosinophilic material is seen in the centers of these structures, and calcifications also form in this tumor.

The clinician should treat an adenomatoid odontogenic tumor conservatively by enucleation. The tumor is removed in its entirety since it is easily separated from the surrounding bone. Recurrence is rare.

Calcifying Odontogenic Cyst

The **calcifying odontogenic cyst** is a nonaggressive cystic lesion that affects a broad age range but is most commonly seen in individuals younger than 40 years of age. No sex predilection has been noted. A solid variant of the calcifying odontogenic cyst has been reported and has been suggested to represent a neoplasm rather than a cyst.

Histologic examination reveals a cystic structure lined by odontogenic epithelium with an associated and characteristic ghost cell keratinization (Figure 7-22, *A*). The epithelium

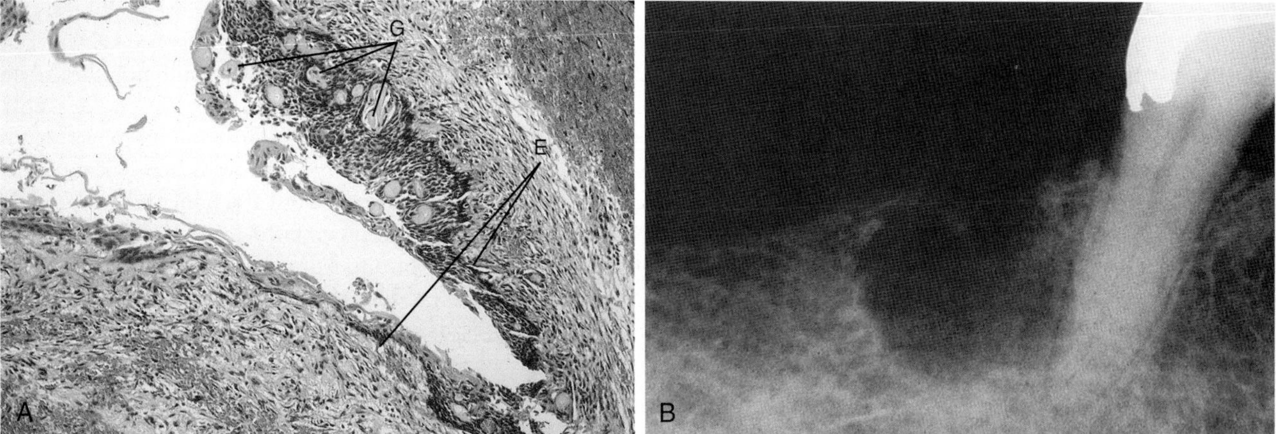

FIGURE 7-22 ■ Calcifying odontogenic cyst. **A,** Microscopic appearance of a calcifying odontogenic cyst shows a cystic structure lined by odontogenic epithelium *(E)* with associated ghost cells *(G).* **B,** Radiograph of a calcifying odontogenic cyst shows a unilocular radiolucency of the mandible.

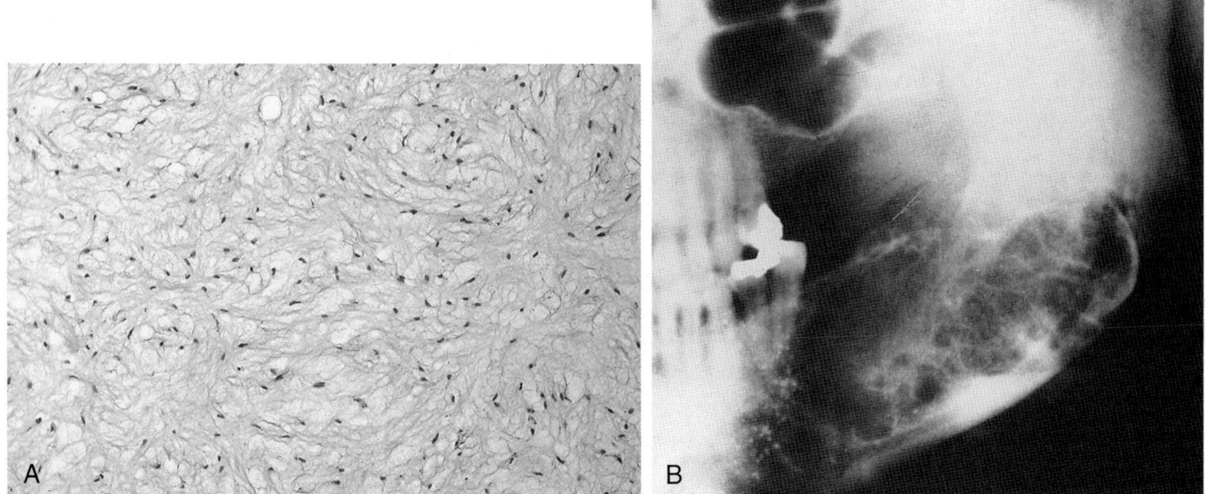

FIGURE 7-23 ■ **A,** Photomicrograph of an odontogenic myxoma shows background substance containing widely dispersed cells with long cytoplasmic processes. **B,** Radiograph of an odontogenic myxoma shows a multilocular, honeycombed radiolucency.

resembles that seen in an ameloblastoma, consisting of ameloblast-like cells and stellate reticulum-like areas. The ghost cells that are characteristic of this lesion exhibit a clear central area. They are thought to represent degenerating epithelial cells. The calcifying odontogenic cyst is usually a radiographically well-defined lesion that can present as either a unilocular or a multilocular radiolucency (Figure 7-22, *B*). Calcifications can occur and are seen as radiopaque areas.

The calcifying odontogenic cyst generally is treated by surgical enucleation. Although a few recurrences have been reported, it usually does not recur. The solid variant may exhibit more aggressive behavior and may be treated with a more extensive surgical procedure.

MESENCHYMAL ODONTOGENIC TUMORS

Odontogenic Myxoma

The **odontogenic myxoma** is a benign mesenchymal odontogenic tumor that occurs most often in young individuals between 10 and 29 years of age. No sex predilection is noted.

The odontogenic myxoma exhibits a multilocular, honeycombed radiolucency with poorly defined margins (Figure 7-23, *B*). The tumor may become quite large and cause tooth displacement. Although most cases occur in the posterior mandible, the odontogenic myxoma may arise anywhere in the maxilla or mandible. Histologic examination reveals a nonencapsulated infiltrating tumor composed of a pale-staining mucopolysaccharide ground substance that contains dispersed cells with long cytoplasmic processes (Figure 7-23, *A*). This tissue closely resembles tissue seen in the dental papilla, the mesenchymal component of tooth-forming tissue.

The odontogenic myxoma is treated by complete surgical excision. The extent of the surgery depends on the size of the tumor. The recurrence rate is approximately 25%, and most recurrences take place within 2 years following treatment.

Central Cementifying and Central Ossifying Fibromas

The **central cementifying fibroma** and **central ossifying fibroma** are benign well-circumscribed tumors classified as fibro-osseous lesions. They are considered variants of the same neoplasm since they are both composed of fibrous connective tissue and calcifications. In the central cementifying fibroma the calcifications are rounded and globular, resembling cementum (Figure 7-24, *A*), whereas in the central ossifying fibroma the calcifications more closely resemble bone trabeculae. Some tumors have a mixture of globular calcifications resembling cementum and bone trabeculae. These tumors are called central **cemento-ossifying fibromas.** This particular variant results from the potential of periodontal ligament cells to produce either cementum or bone.

The tumor usually occurs in adults in the third and fourth decades of life. Women are affected more often than men. Affected patients may be asymptomatic or demonstrate bone expansion or facial asymmetry. Radiographically the central cementifying and central ossifying fibroma are well-defined and demonstrate a radiolucent-to-radiopaque appearance, depending on the amount of calcified tissue

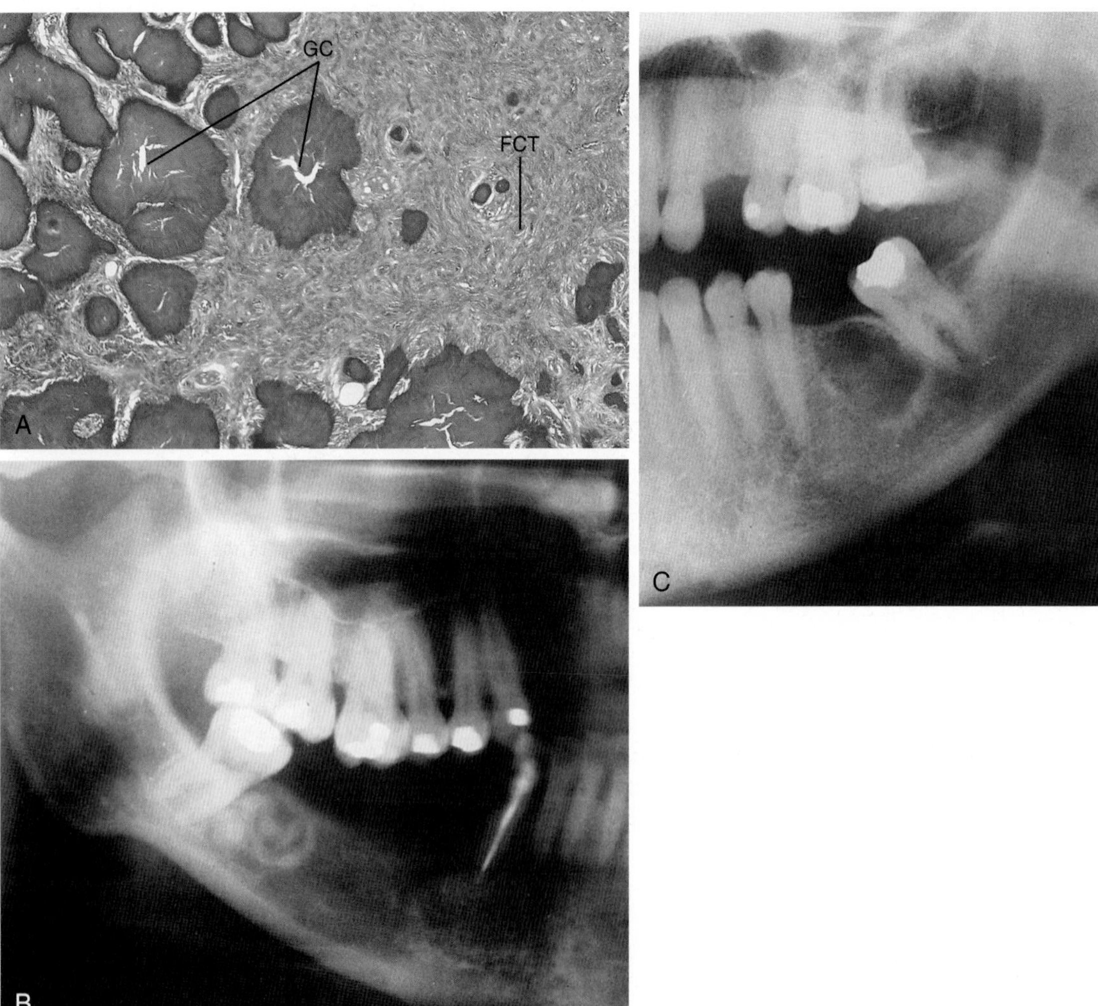

FIGURE 7-24 ■ **A,** Photomicrograph of a central cementifying fibroma shows rounded, globular calcifications *(GC)* and cellular fibrous connective tissue *(FCT).* **B,** Radiograph of a central cementifying fibroma shows a well-circumscribed radiolucent lesion. **C,** Radiograph of a central cementifying fibroma shows a radiolucent and radiopaque lesion.

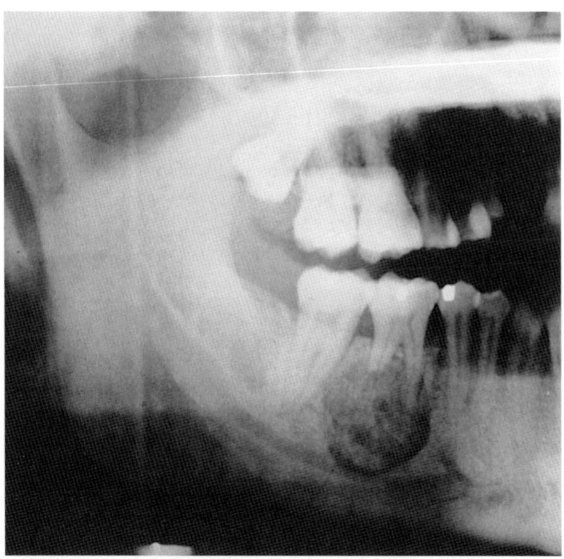

FIGURE 7-25 ■ Radiograph of a benign cementoblastoma shows a well-circumscribed radiopaque mass surrounded by a radiolucent halo and attached to the roots of a mandibular first molar.

present (Figure 7-24, *B* and *C*). The majority of cases occur in the mandible.

Other benign fibro-osseous lesions such as periapical cemento-osseous dysplasia and fibrous dysplasia (discussed in Chapter 8) may be histologically identical to the central cementifying and central ossifying fibroma. The radiographic appearance of each of these individual lesions is important in distinguishing them from one another.

The central cementifying and central ossifying fibromas are treated by surgical excision. Because these lesions are well delineated, they separate easily from the surrounding bone. Recurrence is rare.

Benign Cementoblastoma

The **benign cementoblastoma** is a cementum-producing lesion that is fused to the root or roots of a vital tooth. The tumor typically occurs in young adults. Unlike other odontogenic tumors, pain is a frequent symptom. The radiographic appearance is distinctive and consists of a well-defined radiopaque mass with a surrounding radiolucent halo (Figure 7-25). However, early in its development this lesion may be radiolucent and mimic inflammatory periapical disease The radiolucent halo represents the periodontal ligament. The neoplasm is usually seen in continuity with the root or roots of a mandibular molar or premolar tooth. Obliteration of the apex of the affected tooth is common. Occasional cases may cause localized bone expansion. Microscopic examination reveals a proliferation of cellular cementum fused to the root or roots of the affected tooth.

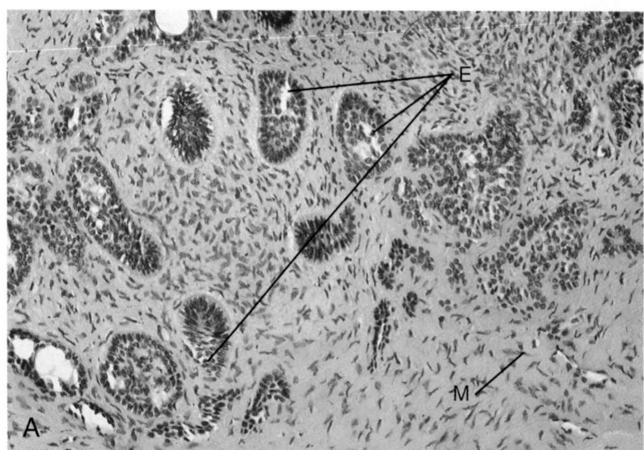

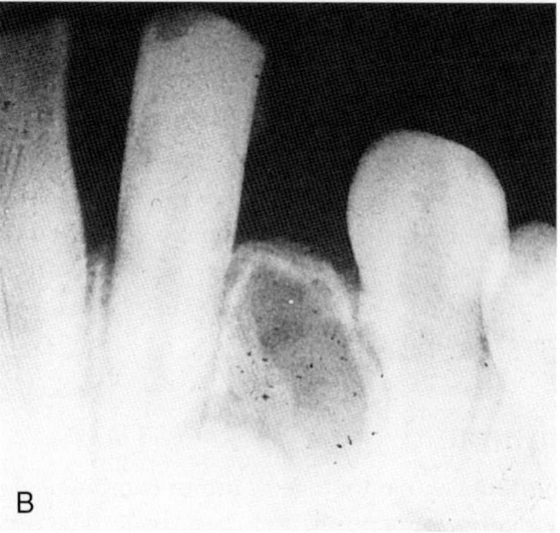

FIGURE 7-26 ■ **A,** Microscopic appearance of an ameloblastic fibroma shows a combination of odontogenic epithelium *(E)* and mesenchymal tissue *(M)*. **B,** Radiograph of an ameloblastic fibroma shows a poorly defined radiolucency.

Treatment of the benign cementoblastoma consists of enucleation of the tumor and removal of the involved tooth. It does not recur.

MIXED ODONTOGENIC TUMORS

Ameloblastic Fibroma

The **ameloblastic fibroma** is a benign, mixed odontogenic tumor that occurs in young children and adults. Most cases occur in individuals younger than 20 years of age. A male sex predilection is noted. The most common location is the mandibular bicuspid and molar region. Most patients are asymptomatic, but bone expansion or swelling may be noted. Radiographically the ameloblastic fibroma appears as either a well-defined or a poorly defined unilocular or multilocular radiolucency (Figure 7-26, *B*).

Histologic examination demonstrates a nonencapsulated odontogenic tumor composed of strands and small islands of ameloblast-like epithelial cells and tissue that resembles the dental papilla (Figure 7-26 *A*).

The ameloblastic fibroma is treated by surgical excision, and recurrence rate is low.

Ameloblastic Fibro-odontoma

The **ameloblastic fibro-odontoma** is a benign odontogenic tumor that has features of both an ameloblastic fibroma and an odontoma. Most cases occur in young adults, with an average age of 10 years. No sex predilection is noted. The ameloblastic fibro-odontoma typically arises in the posterior jaws and is often asymptomatic. However, some patients may experience swelling of the affected area.

Radiographic examination reveals a well-delineated radiolucent lesion that may be unilocular or multilocular. Calcifications of various size and shape are noted within the radiolucency. These calcifications represent tooth formation.

Microscopic examination demonstrates features similar to those described in the ameloblastic fibroma combined with structures that resemble teeth. Therefore various amounts of enamel, dentin, cementum, and pulp tissue are produced.

The ameloblastic fibro-odontoma is a well-circumscribed lesion that usually separates easily from the surrounding bone. It is treated by conservation surgical excision, and recurrence is unusual.

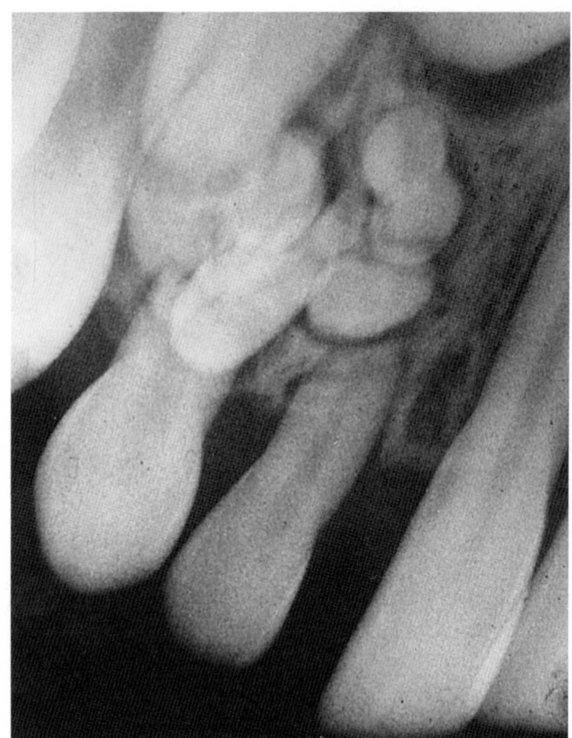

FIGURE 7-27 ■ Radiograph of a compound odontoma shows a collection of numerous, small, toothlike radiopacities surrounded by a radiolucent halo.

Odontoma

The **odontoma** is an odontogenic tumor composed of mature enamel, dentin, cementum, and pulp tissue. The odontoma is the most common of the odontogenic tumors. The two types of odontomas are compound and complex. A **compound odontoma** consists of a collection of numerous small teeth. Although compound odontomas may consist of many small teeth, they do not exhibit unlimited growth potential and therefore are more accurately developmental lesions than true tumors. A **complex odontoma** consists of a mass of enamel, dentin, cementum, and pulp that does not resemble a normal tooth.

Most odontomas are detected in adolescents and young adults. No sex predilection is noted. The compound odontoma is usually located in the anterior maxilla, and the complex odontoma most commonly occurs in the posterior mandible. The most common clinical manifestation of an odontoma is the failure of a permanent tooth to erupt. Most odontomas are small, but large lesions can cause swelling and displacement of erupted teeth. Odontomas can be associated with impacted or unerupted teeth and odontogenic cysts and tumors.

Radiographically compound odontomas appear as a cluster of numerous miniature teeth surrounded by a radiolucent halo (Figure 7-27). A complex odontoma appears as a radiopaque mass surrounded by a thin radiolucent halo (Figure 7-28).

Treatment of an odontoma consists of surgical excision. They generally do not recur.

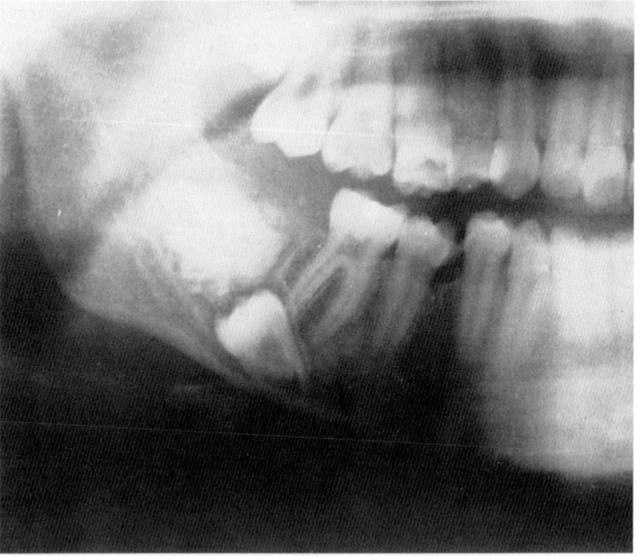

FIGURE 7-28 ■ Radiograph of a complex odontoma shows a radiopaque mass surrounded by a radiolucent halo.

PERIPHERAL ODONTOGENIC TUMORS

Peripheral Ossifying Fibroma

The peripheral ossifying fibroma is usually a well-demarcated sessile or pedunculated lesion that appears to originate from the gingival interdental papilla and is most likely derived from

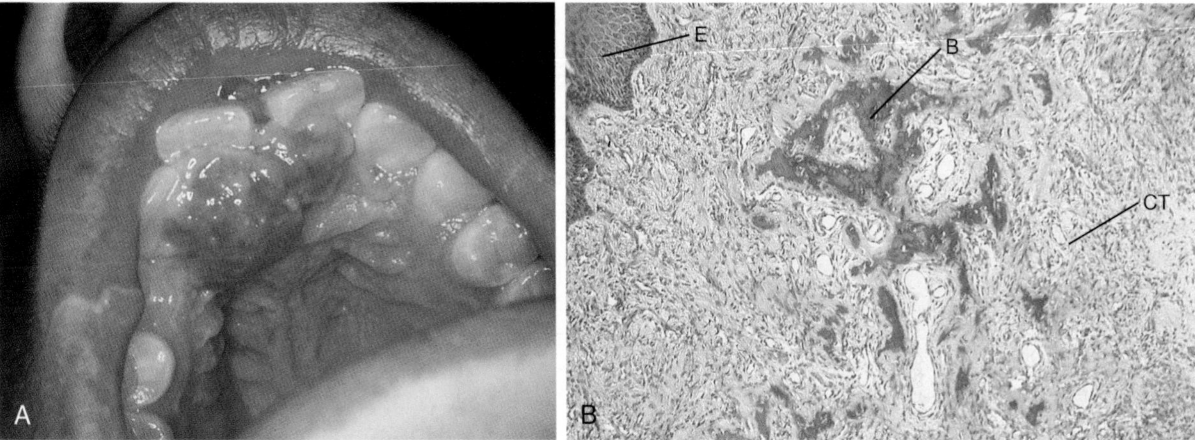

FIGURE 7-29 ■ **A,** Clinical appearance of a peripheral ossifying fibroma shows an exophytic lesion involving the palatal gingiva of the maxillary anterior teeth. **B,** Photomicrograph of a peripheral ossifying fibroma shows bonelike calcifications *(B)* in cellular fibrous connective tissue *(CT)*. A small amount of surface epithelium *(E)* is also visible.

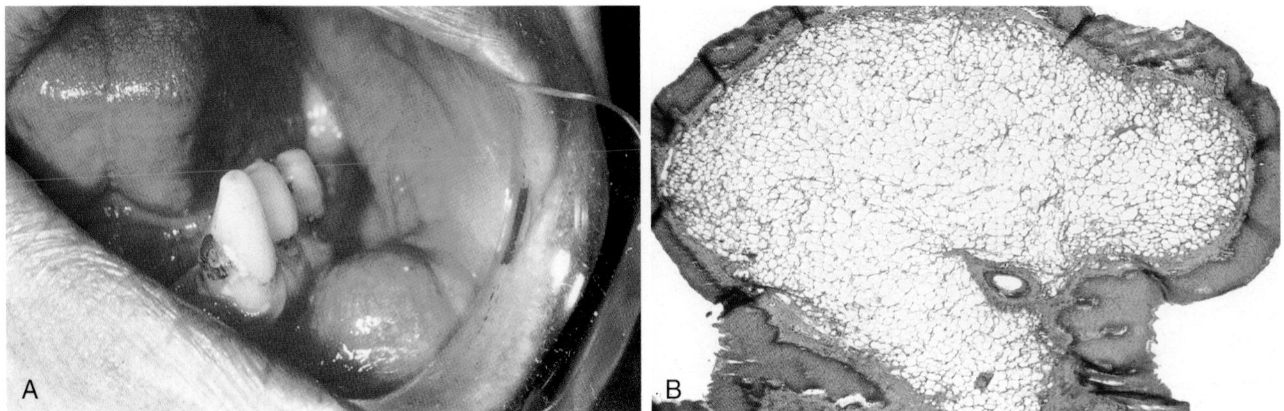

FIGURE 7-30 ■ **A,** Clinical appearance of a lipoma. **B,** Photomicrograph of a lipoma shows mature fat cells. (**A** courtesy Dr. Edward V. Zegarelli.)

cells of the periodontal ligament (Figure 7-29, *A*). It is more common in females than in males and often occurs in young individuals. It has been reported in children and adults.

It is composed of cellular fibrous connective tissue interspersed with scattered bone and cementum-like calcifications (Figure 7-29, *B*). Microscopically the peripheral ossifying fibroma is similar to the central cementifying fibroma and central ossifying fibroma.

Treatment of the peripheral ossifying fibroma consists of surgical excision with thorough scaling of the adjacent teeth to remove any irritants that can induce regrowth of the lesion. The recurrence rate for the peripheral ossifying fibroma is about 16%.

Other Peripheral Odontogenic Tumors

Several other odontogenic tumors have been reported to occur in the gingiva without underlying bone involvement. Although rare, these lesions are important to the dental hygienist because of their gingival location. The peripheral ameloblastoma (described earlier in this chapter) and the peripheral calcifying epithelial odontogenic tumor have been reported to occur in this location.

Treatment for the tumors described previously is surgical excision. After appropriate treatment recurrence is rare.

TUMORS OF SOFT TISSUE

Tumors of soft tissue include benign and malignant tumors of adipose tissue (fat), nerve, muscle, blood, and lymphatic vessels.

LIPOMA

The lipoma is a benign tumor of mature fat cells. Clinically it appears as a yellowish mass that is surfaced by a thin layer of epithelium (Figure 7-30, *A*). Because of this thin epithelium, a

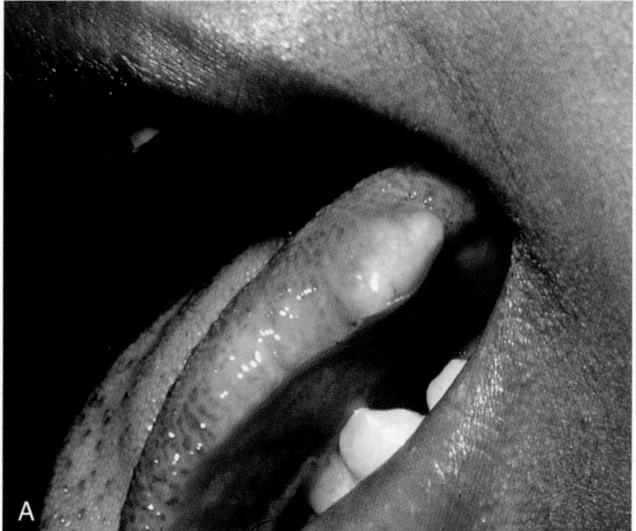

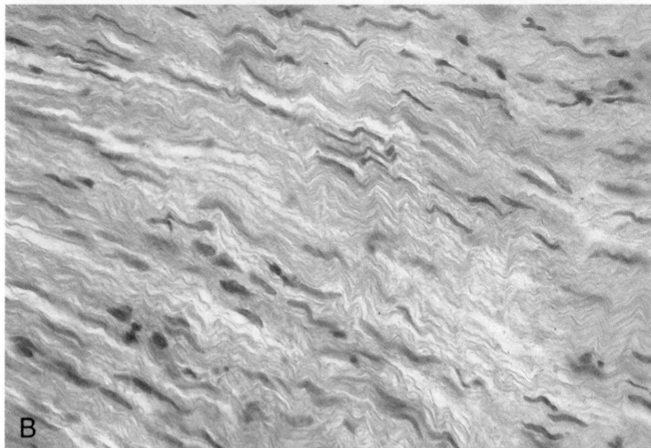

FIGURE 7-31 ■ **A,** Clinical appearance of a neurofibroma shows a nonulcerated mass on the lateral border of the tongue. **B,** Photomicrograph of a neurofibroma.

delicate pattern of blood vessels is usually seen on its surface. The majority of lipomas occur in individuals over 40 years of age, and no sex predilection is noted. The most common intraoral locations are the buccal mucosa and the vestibule. Microscopic examination reveals a well-delineated tumor composed of lobules of mature fat cells that are uniform in size and shape (Figure 7-30, *B*).

The lipoma is treated by surgical excision and generally does not recur.

TUMORS OF NERVE TISSUE

Neurofibroma and Schwannoma

The **neurofibroma** (Figure 7-31, *A*) and the **schwannoma** are benign tumors derived from nerve tissue. The schwannoma is also called a neurilemmoma. The schwannoma is derived from Schwann cells, and the neurofibroma is derived from Schwann cells and perineural fibroblasts. Both of these cells are components of the connective tissue surrounding a nerve. Although the neurofibroma and schwannoma are distinct tumors microscopically, they are quite similar in their clinical presentation and behavior and therefore are discussed together. The tongue is the most common intraoral location. Neurofibromas and schwannomas may occur at any age, and no sex predilection is noted. Microscopic examination of a neurofibroma reveals a fairly well-delineated but unencapsulated, proliferation of spindle-shaped Schwann cells and perineural fibroblasts (Figure 7-31, *B*). A schwannoma is composed of spindle-shaped Schwann cells arranged in palisaded whorls around a central pink zone. A connective tissue capsule surrounds the schwannoma.

A neurofibroma and a schwannoma are both treated by surgical excision. They generally do not recur. Malignant tumors of nerve tissue occur but are extremely rare.

Multiple neurofibromas occur in a genetically inherited disorder known as **neurofibromatosis of von Recklinghausen** or *von Recklinghausen's disease.* Patients with this syndrome have numerous neurofibromas on the skin and other sites in addition to other abnormalities. This syndrome is genetically inherited and is described in detail in Chapter 6.

Granular Cell Tumor

The **granular cell tumor** is a benign tumor composed of large cells with a granular cytoplasm. It most likely arises from a neural or primitive mesenchymal cell. The granular cell tumor most often occurs on the tongue, followed by the buccal mucosa. It appears as a painless, nonulcerated nodule (Figure 7-32, A). Most cases occur in adults, and a female sex predilection is noted. Microscopic examination reveals large oval-shaped cells with a granular cytoplasm. The granular cells are found in the connective tissue and between striated muscle fibers (Figure 7-32, *B*). The overlying surface epithelium may exhibit pseudoepitheliomatous hyperplasia, which is a benign proliferation of epithelium into the connective tissue (Figure 7-32, *C*).

This tumor is treated by surgical excision and does not recur.

Congenital Epulis

The **congenital epulis,** or congenital epulis of the newborn, is a benign neoplasm composed of cells that closely resemble those seen in the granular cell tumor. The neoplasm most likely arises from a primitive mesenchymal cell. This tumor is present at birth and appears as a sessile or pedunculated mass on the gingiva. It usually occurs on the anterior maxillary gingiva and almost always occurs in girls.

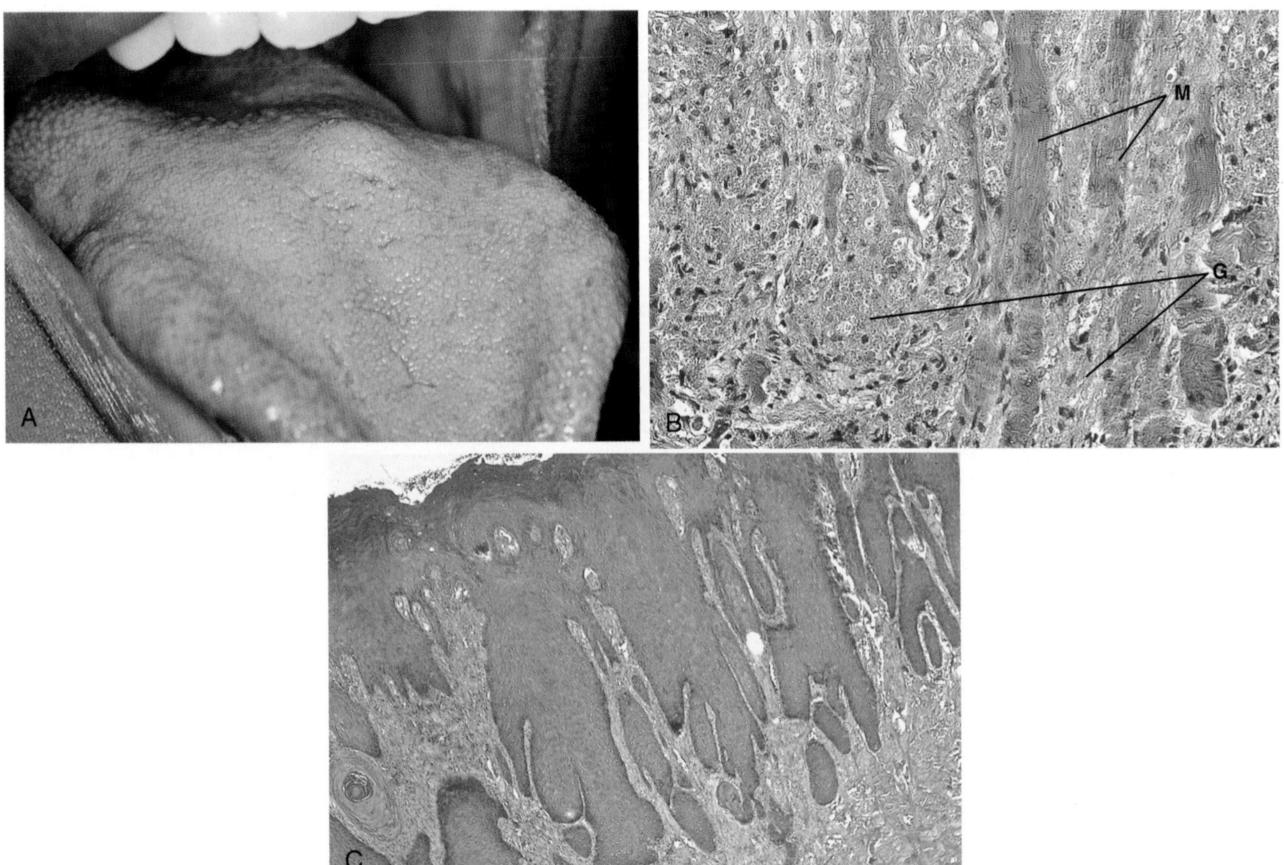

FIGURE 7-32 ■ **A,** Clinical appearance of a granular cell tumor of the tongue shows a nonulcerated mass. **B**, Photomicrograph of a granular cell tumor showing granular cell(s) *(G)* between striated muscle fiber(s) *(M).* **C**, Photomicroscope of a granular cell tumor showing overlying pseudoepitheliomatous hyperplasia. (**A** courtesy Dr. Sidney Eisig.)

The congenital epulis is treated by surgical excision and does not recur. Occasional examples have regressed without treatment.

TUMORS OF MUSCLE

Tumors of muscle are extremely uncommon in the oral cavity. The **rhabdomyoma,** a benign tumor of striated muscle, has been reported to occur on the tongue. The **leiomyoma,** a benign tumor of smooth muscle, may occur in association with blood vessels. These tumors are called **vascular leiomyomas** and occasionally occur in the oral cavity.

The **rhabdomyosarcoma,** a malignant tumor of striated muscle, is the most common malignant soft tissue tumor of the head and neck in children. It typically occurs in individuals under 10 years of age and has a male sex predilection. It is a rapidly growing, destructive tumor. The rhabdomyosarcoma is an aggressive malignant tumor that is best treated by a combination of multidrug chemotherapy, radiation therapy, and surgery. Despite treatment, the prognosis is poor.

VASCULAR TUMORS

Hemangioma

The **hemangioma** is a benign proliferation of capillaries (Figure 7-33, *A* and *B*). It is a common vascular lesion considered by many to represent a developmental lesion rather than a tumor because hemangiomas generally do not exhibit an unlimited growth potential. Some contain numerous small capillaries and are called **capillary hemangiomas.** Others contain larger blood vessels and are called **cavernous hemangiomas** (Figure 7-33, *C*).

Most are present at birth or arise shortly thereafter. More than half of the hemangiomas that occur in the body occur in the head and neck area. The tongue is the most common intraoral location. Involvement of the tongue often leads to marked enlargement (macroglossia). Hemangiomas are more common in girls than in boys. They also occur in adults as a

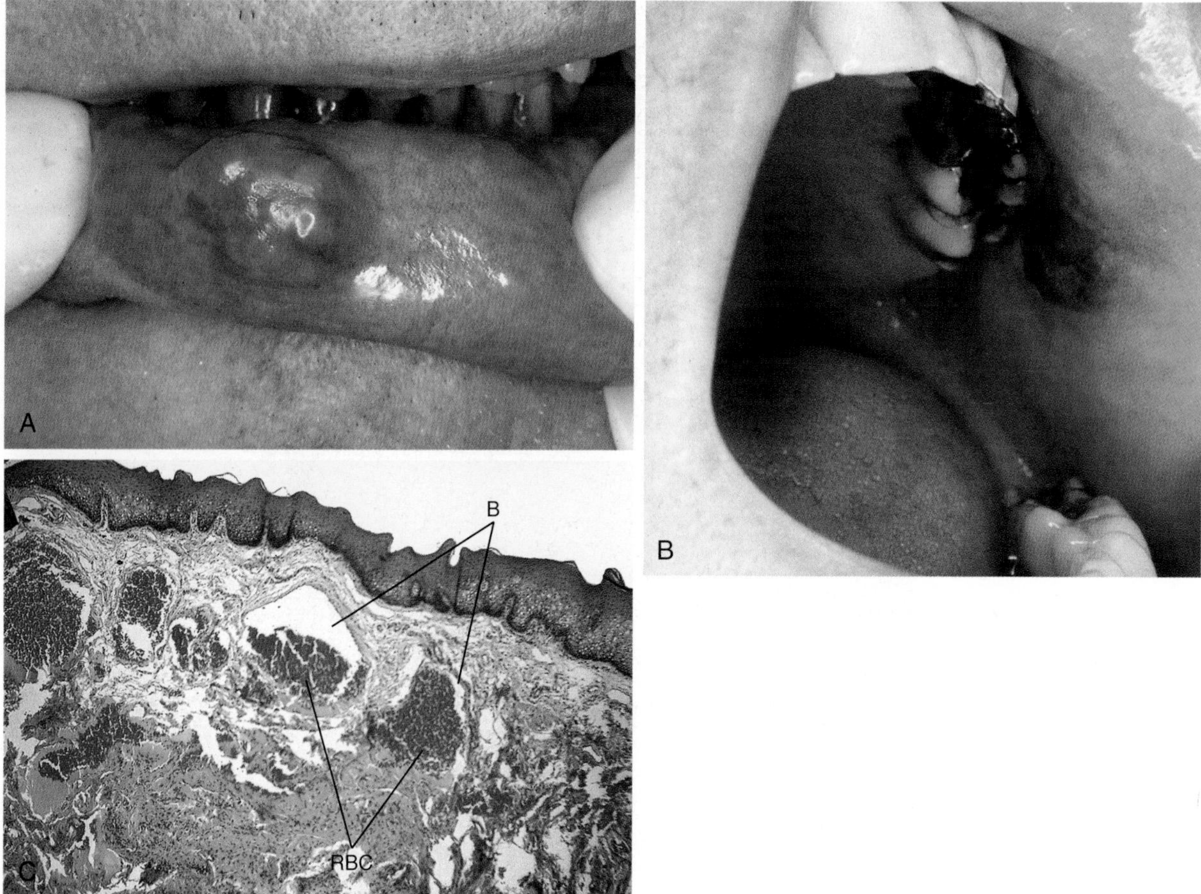

FIGURE 7-33 ■ Clinical appearance of a hemangioma of the lower lip **(A)** and of the buccal mucosa **(B)**. **C,** Microscopic appearance of a cavernous hemangioma showing large dilated blood vessels *(B)* filled with red blood cells *(RBC)*.

response to trauma and represent an abnormal proliferation of blood vessels during the healing process. They appear as variably sized, deep-red or blue lesions that frequently blanch when pressure is applied.

Many hemangiomas undergo spontaneous remission. Others can enlarge rapidly because of hemorrhage, thrombosis, or inflammation. Treatment is variable and includes surgery or the injection of a sclerosing solution into the lesion, which causes it to resolve.

Lymphangioma

The **lymphangioma** is a benign tumor of lymphatic vessels. It is less common than the hemangioma. Most lymphangiomas are present at birth, and half arise in the head and neck area. No sex predilection is noted. The most common intraoral location is the tongue, where the lymphangioma presents as an ill-defined mass with a pebbly surface. Involvement of the tongue may lead to macroglossia. A cystic lymphangioma in the neck is called a cystic hygroma. It is usually present at birth or develops shortly thereafter.

Lymphangiomas generally are treated by surgical excision and tend to recur.

Malignant Vascular Tumors

Malignant vascular tumors such as angiosarcoma may occur in the oral cavity but are rare. **Kaposi sarcoma** is a malignant vascular tumor and may arise in multiple sites, including the skin and oral mucosa. Classic Kaposi sarcoma occurs as multiple purplish tumors of the lower extremities in older men. The condition in these patients progresses slowly, usually resolves with low doses of radiation, and rarely causes death. With the advent of the human immunodeficiency virus (HIV) epidemic in the 1980s, Kaposi sarcoma has appeared in a much more aggressive form. In HIV-positive patients these lesions are often seen in the oral cavity, where they present as purple macules, plaques, or exophytic tumors. The hard palate and gingiva are the most common intraoral sites. Kaposi sarcoma associated with HIV infection is described in Chapter 4. It may also occur in patients with other forms of immunodeficiency, specifically patients who

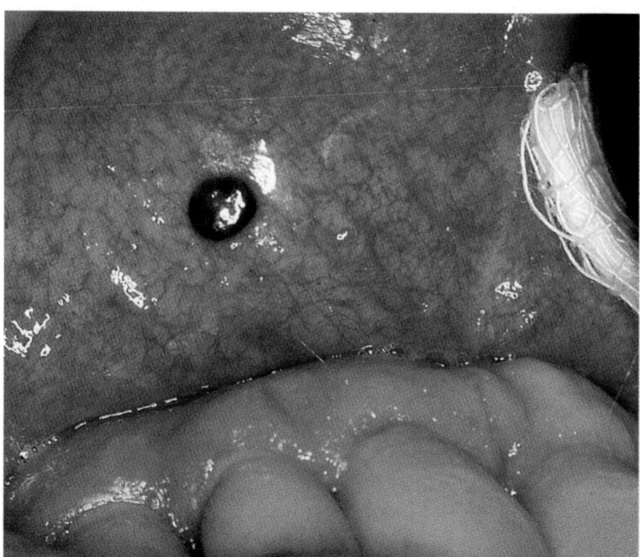

FIGURE 7-34 ■ Clinical appearance of a melanocytic nevus shows a well-defined pigmented lesion on the labial mucosa.

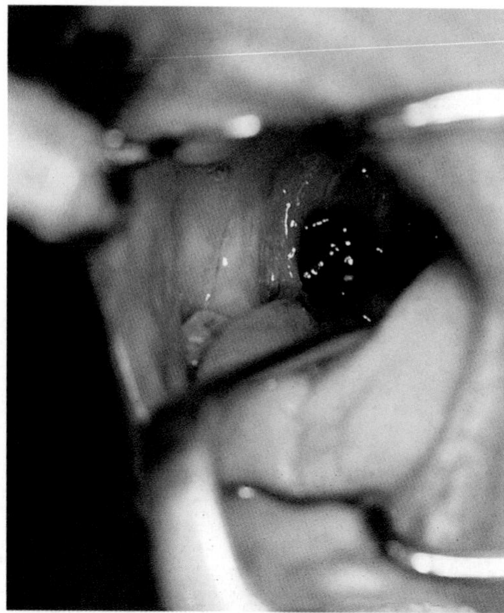

FIGURE 7-35 ■ Clinical appearance of a malignant melanoma shows a darkly pigmented lesion in the area of the fauces. (Courtesy Dr. Edward V. Zegarelli.)

have received immunosuppressive drug therapy as a result of organ transplantation.

Kaposi sarcoma is caused by a human herpesvirus (HHV) that is called both *human herpesvirus type 8* and *Kaposi sarcoma–associated herpesvirus.* Men are affected more often than women. Microscopic examination reveals a neoplasm composed of spindle-shaped cells mixed with slitlike spaces containing red blood cells.

Kaposi sarcoma is treated by surgical excision, radiation therapy, chemotherapy, or a combination of these therapies. In HIV-positive patients recurrence is common, and the disease may progress rapidly.

TUMORS OF MELANIN-PRODUCING CELLS

MELANOCYTIC NEVI

The word **nevus** (plural, nevi) has two meanings. Here the word is used to mean a benign tumor of melanocytes (melanin-producing cells), which are called **nevus cells.** Nevus also refers to a pigmented congenital lesion (a lesion present at birth). A hemangioma present at birth is an example of this second type of nevus.

Melanocytic nevi can arise on the skin or the oral mucosa. Intraoral tumors consist of tan-to-brown macules or papules that occur most often on the hard palate. The buccal mucosa is the second most common intraoral location (Figure 7-34). They occur twice as often in women as in men and are usually first identified in individuals between 20 and 50 years of age. Basal cell carcinomas are a component of the inherited nevoid basal cell carcinoma syndrome described in Chapter 6.

Most pigmented lesions that occur in the oral cavity are benign. Pigmented lesions that exhibit ulceration, an increase in size, or a change in color may be malignant.

A biopsy followed by microscopic examination is indicated for pigmented lesions of unknown cause, unknown duration, or recent onset. Surgical excision is the treatment of choice for intraoral melanocytic nevi. Recurrence is rare.

MALIGNANT MELANOMA

Malignant melanoma is a malignant tumor of melanocytes (Figure 7-35). Although the name malignant melanoma suggests that a benign counterpart exists, all melanomas are malignant. Most malignant melanomas arise on the skin as a result of prolonged exposure to sunlight. Primary malignant melanoma of the oral cavity is rare. However, malignant melanomas that arise on the skin may metastasize to the oral cavity.

Malignant melanoma usually presents as a rapidly enlarging blue-to-black mass. Malignant melanoma is a very aggressive tumor that exhibits an unpredictable behavior and early metastasis. The most common intraoral locations are the palate and maxillary gingiva. These neoplasms usually occur in adults older than 40 years of age.

Malignant melanomas are treated by surgical excision. Chemotherapy may be used in conjunction with surgery. The prognosis for oral malignant melanoma is poor.

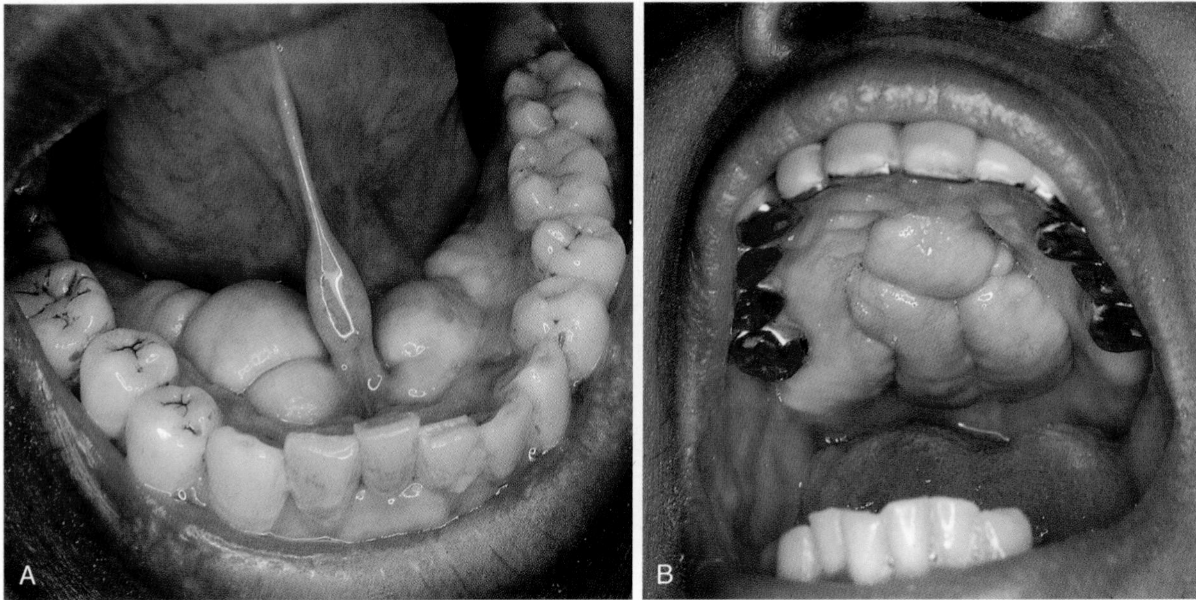

FIGURE 7-36 ■ **A,** Clinical appearance of bilateral lobulated mandibular tori. **B,** Clinical appearance of a lobulated torus palatinus.

TUMORS OF BONE AND CARTILAGE

TORUS

A **torus** (plural, tori) is a benign lesion composed of normal compact bone. Tori are located in the midline of the palate (**torus palatinus** or **palatal torus**) or the lingual aspect of the mandible in the area of the premolars (**torus mandibularis** or **mandibular torus**) (Figure 7-36, *A* and *B*). Tori are not true tumors. Because they have a hereditary basis, they are also discussed in Chapter 6. They are described in this chapter because of their resemblance to an osteoma. Tori occur in adults and are more common in women than in men. They present as an asymptomatic, bony hard, lobulated mass covered by epithelium with very little underlying fibrous connective tissue. Surface ulceration may occur if a torus is traumatized. Palatal or mandibular tori may result in radiopaque areas superimposed on tooth roots. The diagnosis is confirmed by the presence of a torus on clinical examination.

No treatment is necessary unless they interfere with the fabrication of a prosthetic appliance. If a prosthetic appliance needs to be constructed, a torus should be excised surgically.

EXOSTOSIS

An **exostosis** (plural, exostoses) is a small nodular excrescence of normal compact bone (Figure 7-37). Exostoses present as asymptomatic, bony hard nodules on the buccal aspect of the maxillary or mandibular alveolar ridges. Most cases occur in adults, and no sex predilection is noted. An increased incidence is noted in individuals who have a grinding or bruxing habit.

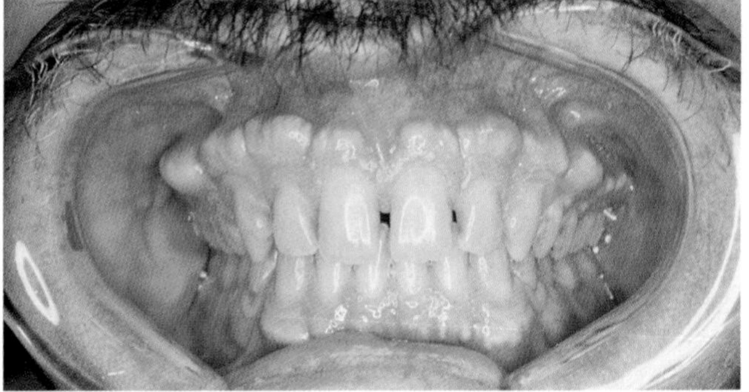

FIGURE 7-37 ■ Clinical appearance of exostoses on the labial and buccal aspect of the maxilla. Less prominent exostoses are noted on the labial and buccal aspect of the mandible.

No treatment is indicated unless they interfere with the fabrication of a prosthetic appliance. If a prosthetic appliance needs to be constructed, an exostosis should be excised surgically.

OSTEOMA

An osteoma is an asymptomatic benign tumor composed of normal compact bone. It is a slow-growing tumor that appears radiographically as either a sharply defined radiopaque mass within bone or a delineated mass attached to the outer surface of the bone (Figure 7-38). A large osteoma

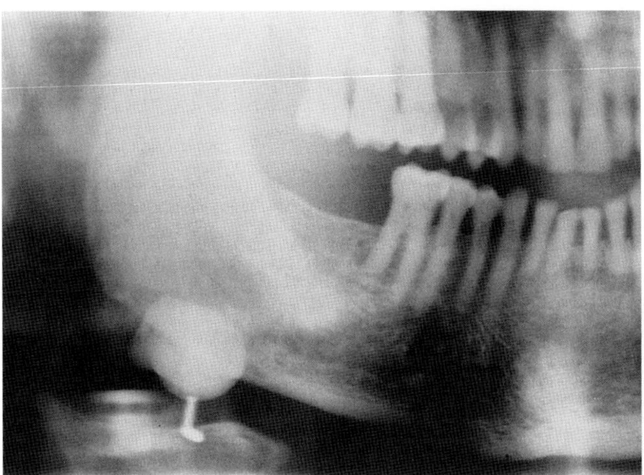

FIGURE 7-38 ■ Radiograph of an osteoma shows a radiopacity of the posterior mandible. (Courtesy Dr. Sidney Eisig.)

within bone may cause expansion of the involved bone. No sex predilection is noted. The most common location within the jaws is the posterior mandible. Osteomas are a component of Gardner syndrome that is transmitted genetically and described in Chapter 6.

Osteomas are treated by surgical excision and generally do not recur.

OSTEOSARCOMA

Osteosarcoma (osteogenic sarcoma) is a malignant tumor of bone-forming tissue. It is the most common primary malignant tumor of bone in patients under 40 years of age. Tumors that involve the long bones occur at an average age of 27 years, whereas the average age of occurrence for tumors that involve the jaws is about 37 years of age. These tumors occur in the mandible twice as frequently as in the maxilla and are more common in men than in women. Patients may experience a diffuse swelling or mass that is often painful (Figure 7-39, *A*). Some patients present initially with a toothache or exhibit tooth mobility. Paresthesia of the lip is common in tumors involving the mandible.

The radiographic appearance of an osteosarcoma varies from radiolucent to radiopaque (Figure 7-39, *B*). It is usually a destructive, poorly defined lesion and may or may not involve the adjacent soft tissue. Asymmetric widening of the periodontal ligament space and a sunburst pattern may be seen radiographically in some cases. Microscopic examination of this tumor shows pleomorphic and hyperchromatic cells and abnormal bone formation. Abnormal cartilage formation may also be present (Figure 7-39, *C*).

Currently osteosarcomas are treated with preoperative multiagent chemotherapy followed by surgery. Jaw tumors frequently recur after treatment. Only about 20% of patients with osteosarcoma of the jaws survive 5 years.

TUMORS OF CARTILAGE

Cartilaginous tumors of the jawbones are extremely rare and are more likely to be malignant than benign. A **chondroma** is a benign tumor of cartilage. A **chondrosarcoma** is a malignant tumor of cartilage (Figure 7-40). A chondrosarcoma may occur in either the maxilla or the mandible and is more common in men than in women. Most patients have enlargement of the affected bone.

Chondrosarcomas are treated by wide surgical excision. Radiation therapy and chemotherapy are not effective. The prognosis is poor. Only about 30% of patients with chondrosarcoma involving the jaws survive 5 years after the diagnosis.

TUMORS OF BLOOD-FORMING TISSUES

LEUKEMIA

Leukemia comprises a broad group of disorders characterized by an overproduction of atypical white blood cells. The atypical white blood cells proliferate in the bone marrow and then spill into the circulating blood and tissues. Several types of leukemia are classified according to the kind of cells that are proliferating: myelocytes, lymphocytes, or monocytes.

Leukemias are divided into two forms: acute and chronic. Acute leukemia is most common in children and young adults and is characterized by a proliferation of immature white blood cells (blasts). Chronic leukemia is characterized by an excess proliferation of mature white blood cells and most frequently occurs in middle-age adults. Leukemia occurs more often in men than in women.

Although oral involvement may occur in any type of leukemia, the monocytic variant most often exhibits oral lesions. A common oral manifestation of monocytic leukemia is diffuse gingival enlargement with persistent bleeding (Figure 7-41). (Leukemia is further described in Chapter 9.)

The treatment of leukemia consists of chemotherapy, radiation therapy, and corticosteroids. The prognosis depends on the type of leukemia and the extent of disease.

LYMPHOMA (NON-HODGKIN'S LYMPHOMA)

Lymphoma is a malignant tumor of lymphoid tissue. Numerous types of lymphoma exist, each of which is differentiated on the basis of microscopic findings. The characteristic clinical presentation is gradual enlargement of involved lymph nodes. Rarely a lymphoma may present as a primary lesion in the oral soft tissues or bone. However, most lymphomas involve either lymph nodes or aggregates of lymphoid tissue that are located in the digestive tract

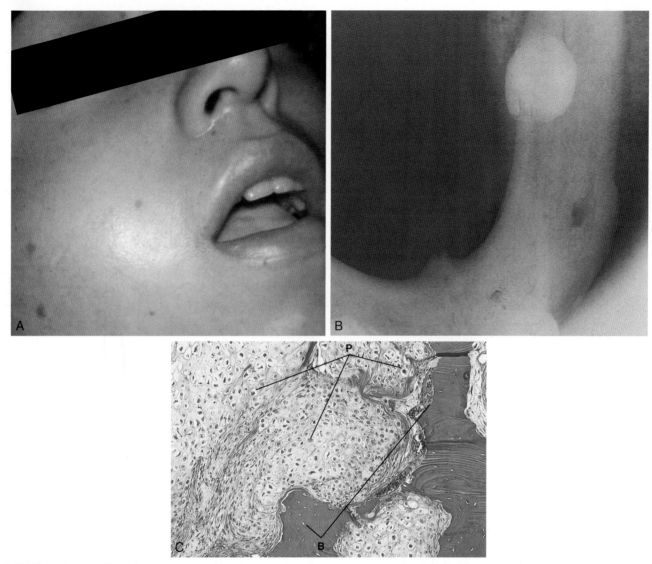

FIGURE 7-39 ■ **A,** Clinical appearance of an osteogenic sarcoma shows swelling. **B,** Radiograph of an osteogenic sarcoma in the left molar area shows a poorly defined radiopaque lesion. **C,** Microscopic appearance of an osteogenic sarcoma shows pleomorphic *(P)* and hyperchromatic cells and bone formation *(B).*

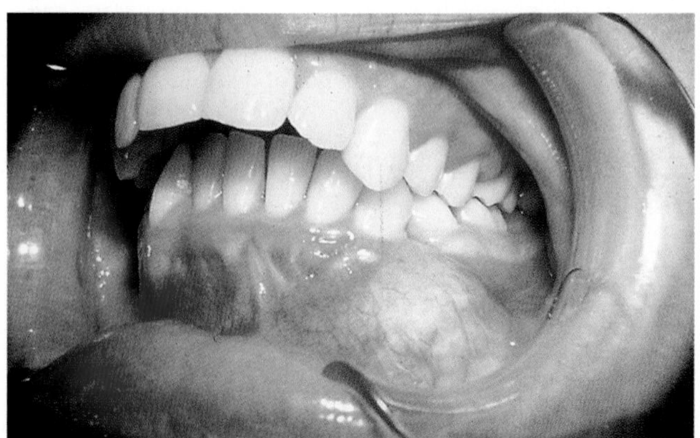

FIGURE 7-40 ■ Clinical appearance of a chondrosarcoma shows an exophytic mass in the anterior mandible.

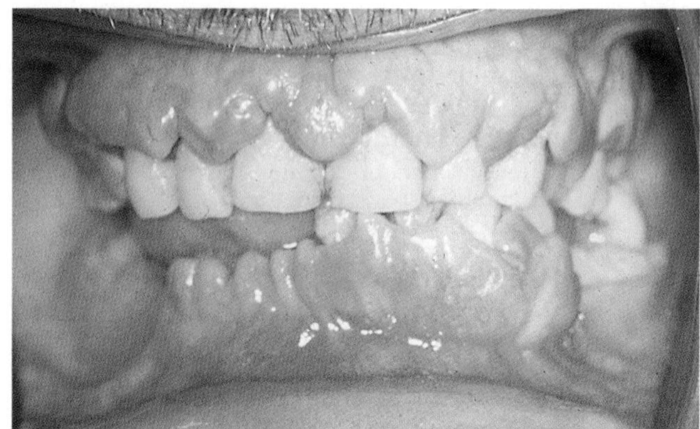

FIGURE 7-41 ■ Clinical appearance of a patient with leukemic infiltration of the gingiva resulting in diffuse enlargement. (Courtesy Dr. Edward V. Zegarelli.)

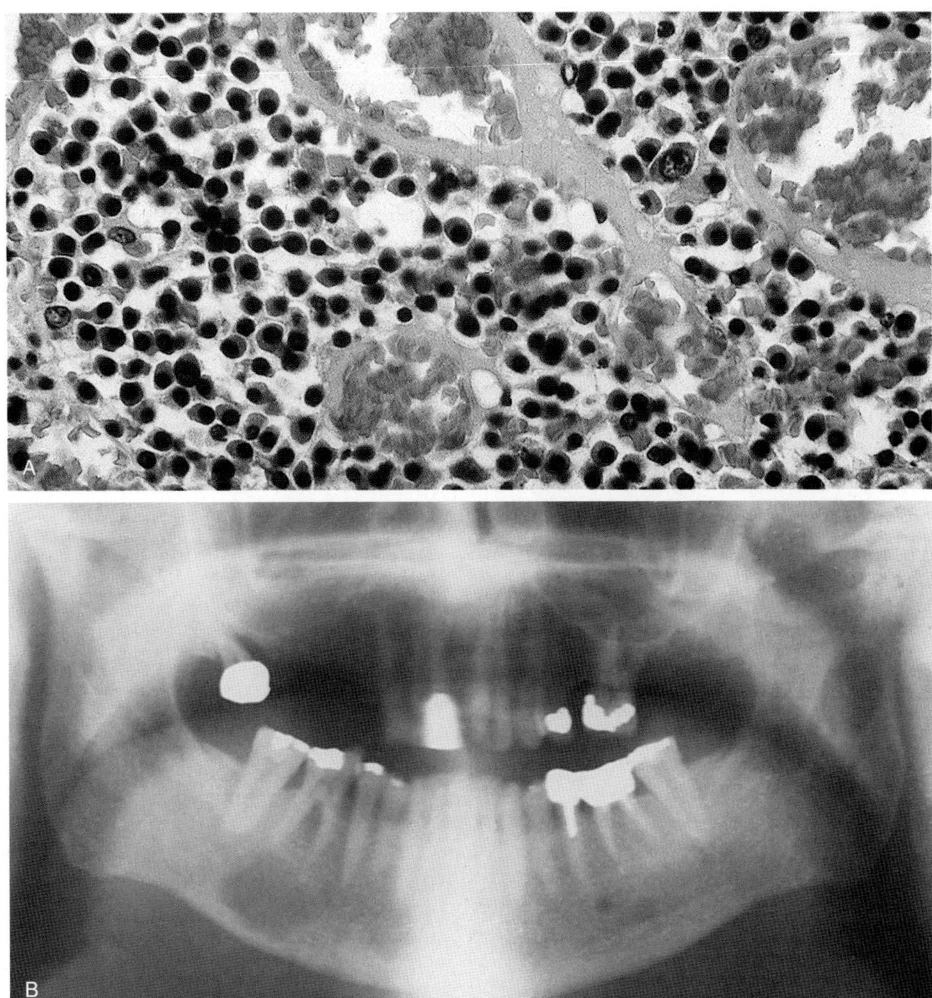

FIGURE 7-42 ■ Multiple myeloma. **A,** Microscopic appearance of multiple myeloma shows a proliferation of plasma cells. **B,** Radiograph shows multiple radiolucent lesions of the mandible in a patient with multiple myeloma.

from the oral cavity to the anus. In the oral cavity lymphoid tissue is located at the base of the tongue, soft palate, and pharynx (Waldeyer's ring). The most common location for intraoral lymphoma is the tonsillar area. Lymphomas usually occur in adults and are more common in men than in women.

Lymphoma is treated by radiotherapy, surgery, chemotherapy, or a combination of these therapies. The prognosis depends on the type of lymphoma and the extent of involvement.

MULTIPLE MYELOMA

Multiple myeloma is a systemic, malignant proliferation of plasma cells that causes destructive lesions in bone. The neoplastic plasma cells produce large amounts of **immunoglobulin.** Most patients are older than 40 years of age, and the disease occurs most commonly in the seventh decade of life. Men are affected more often than women. Patients usually experience bone pain and swelling. Pathologic fracture of an involved bone is common and typically occurs in bones weakened as a result of their destruction by the proliferation of neoplastic plasma cells (Figure 7-42, *A*).

Radiographically the involved bones show multiple radiolucent lesions. The disease can involve the skull, spine, ribs, pelvis, long bones, and jaws. The mandible is affected more often than the maxilla (Figure 7-42, *B*). Most patients have an elevation of a single type of immunoglobulin, which is detected by a process called immunoelectrophoresis. This elevation is called a **monoclonal spike.** Patients may have fragments of immunoglobulins in the urine. These fragments are called **Bence Jones proteins.**

The tumors are composed of sheets of well- to–poorly differentiated plasma cells.

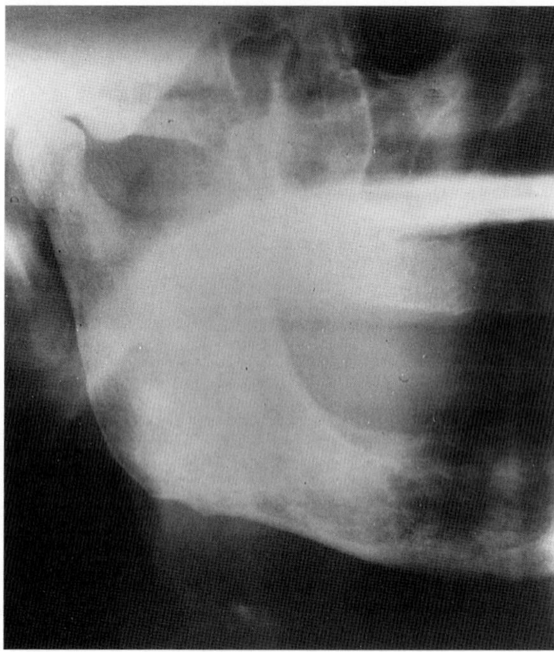

FIGURE 7-43 ■ Radiograph shows diffuse radiolucent and radiopaque changes resulting from metastatic carcinoma of the prostate gland.

A localized tumor of plasma cells in soft tissue is called an **extramedullary plasmacytoma.** Although these are rare tumors, they are more common in the head and neck region than anywhere else in the body. Many patients with extramedullary plasmacytoma will eventually develop multiple myeloma. Therefore patients with a single tumor of plasma cells must be evaluated to determine if the lesion is solitary or part of multiple myeloma.

Patients with multiple myeloma are treated with chemotherapy and radiation. The prognosis is poor. The most common cause of death is infection followed by renal failure. Only 18% of patients survive 5 years after the diagnosis.

METASTATIC TUMORS OF THE JAWS

Metastatic tumors of the jaws from primary sites elsewhere in the body are rare. Most of these tumors arise from the thyroid, breast, lungs, prostate gland, and kidneys. The most frequent intraoral site for metastatic tumors of the jaws is the mandible. Patients display various signs and symptoms, including pain, paresthesia or anesthesia of the lip, swelling, expansion of the affected bone, and loosening of the teeth in the involved area. Metastatic lesions usually appear several years after the primary lesion is discovered. Occasionally the oral metastatic tumor is the first manifestation of a **primary tumor** elsewhere. Most patients are adults, and men are affected more often than women.

The radiographic appearance of metastatic tumors varies (Figure 7-43). Lesions are usually poorly defined and radiolucent. The roots of the involved teeth may show a spiked appearance. Metastatic tumors from the breast, prostate gland, and lungs may form bone and therefore may show areas of radiopacity.

Histologically the metastatic tumor resembles the primary malignancy. Most metastatic tumors in the jaws are epithelial in origin, and most are adenocarcinomas.

Chemotherapy and radiation therapy are used to alleviate the discomfort of metastatic tumors in the jaws. The prognosis for patients with tumors that have metastasized to the jaws is poor.

Selected References

Books

Neville BW et al: *Oral and maxillofacial pathology,* ed 3, St Louis, 2009, Saunders.

Regezi JA, Sciubba JJ, Jordan RCK: *Oral pathology: clinical-pathologic correlations,* ed 5, St Louis, 2008, Saunders.

Kumar V, Cotran RS, Robbins SL: *Robbins basic pathology,* ed 8, Philadelphia, 2007, Saunders.

Journal Articles

Tumors of Squamous Epithelium

Abbey LM, Page DG, Sawyer DR: The clinical and histopathologic features of a series of 464 oral squamous cell papillomas, *Oral Surg Oral Med Oral Pathol* 49:419, 1980.

Damm DD et al: Leukoplakia of the maxillary vestibule—an association with Viadent? *Oral Surg Oral Med Oral Pathol Oral Radiol Endod* 87:61, 1999.

Fantasia JE, Damm DD: Oral Diagnosis: exophytic lesion of palatal mucosa: papilloma, *Gen Dent* 181:183, 2004.

Freitas MD et al: Clinicopathologic aspects of oral leukoplakia in smokers and nonsmokers, *Oral Surg Oral Med Oral Pathol Oral Radiol Endod* 102:199, 2006.

Kaugars GE et al: Actinic cheilitis: a review of 152 cases, *Oral Surg Oral Med Oral Pathol Oral Radiol Endod* 88:181, 1999.

Krutchkoff DF et al: Oral cancer: a survey of 566 cases from the University of Connecticut Oral Pathology Biopsy Service 1975-1986, *Oral Surg Oral Med Oral Pathol* 70:192, 1990.

Medina JE, Dichtel W, Luna MA: Verrucous-squamous carcinomas of the oral cavity: a clinicopathologic study of 104 cases, *Arch Otolaryngol* 110:437, 1984.

Padayachee A, Van Wyk CW: Human papillomavirus (HPV) in oral squamous cell papillomas, *J Oral Pathol* 16:353, 1987.

Shibuya H et al: Multiple primary cancer risk in patients with squamous cell carcinoma of the oral cavity, *Cancer* 60:3083, 1987.

Warnakulasuriya KAAS, Ralhan R: Clinical, pathological, cellular and molecular lesions caused by oral smokeless tobacco—a review, *J Oral Pathol Med* 36:63, 2007.

Leukoplakia and Erythroplakia

Shafer WG, Waldron CA: Erythroplakia of the oral cavity, *Cancer* 36:1021, 1975.

Silverman S Jr, Gorsky M, Lozada F: Oral leukoplakia and malignant transformation: a follow-up study of 257 patients, *Cancer* 53:563, 1984.

Waldron CA, Shafer WG: Leukoplakia revisited: a clinicopathologic study of 3256 oral leukoplakias, *Cancer* 36:1386, 1975.

Salivary Gland Tumors

Eveson JW, Cawson RA: Tumours of the minor (oropharyngeal) salivary glands: a demographic study of 336 cases, *J Oral Pathol* 14:500, 1985.

Pires FR et al: Intra-oral minor salivary gland tumors: a clinicopathological study of 546 cases, *Oral Oncol* 43:463, 2007.

Waldron CA, El-Mofty SK, Gnepp DR: Tumors of the intraoral minor salivary glands: a demographic and histologic study of 426 cases, *Oral Surg Oral Med Oral Pathol* 66:323, 1988.

Odontogenic Tumors

Ai-Ru L, Zhen L, Jian S: Calcifying epithelial odontogenic tumors: a clinicopathologic study of 9 cases, *J Oral Pathol* 11:399, 1982.

Buchner A, Ficarra G, Hansen LS: Peripheral odontogenic fibroma, *Oral Surg Oral Med Oral Pathol* 64:432, 1987.

Courtney RM, Kerr DA: The odontogenic adenomatoid tumor: a comprehensive study of 20 new cases, *Oral Surg Oral Med Oral Pathol* 39:424, 1975.

Daley TD, Wysocki GP: Peripheral odontogenic fibroma, *Oral Surg Oral Med Oral Pathol* 78:329, 1994.

Kaugars GE, Miller ME, Abbey LM: Odontomas, *Oral Surg Oral Med Oral Pathol* 67:172, 1989.

Shamaskin RG, Svirsky JA, Kaugars GE: Intraosseous and extraosseous calcifying odontogenic cyst (Gorlin cyst), *J Oral Maxillofac Surg* 47:562, 1989.

Ulmansky M et al: Benign cementoblastoma, *Oral Surg Oral Med Oral Pathol* 77:48, 1994.

Waldron CA, El-Mofty SK: A histopathologic study of 116 ameloblastomas with special reference to the desmoplastic variant, *Oral Surg Oral Med Oral Pathol* 63:441, 1987.

Lipoma

Furlong MA, Fanburg-Smith JC, Childers ELB: Lipoma of the oral and maxillofacial region: site and subclassification of 125 cases, *Oral Surg Oral Med Oral Pathol* 98:441, 2004.

Neurogenic Tumors

Cunha KS et al: Neurofibromatosis type I with periodontal manifestations: a case report and literature review, *Br Dent J* 196:457, 2004.

Vascular Tumors

Hernandez GA et al: Aneurysmal bone cyst versus hemangioma of the mandible, *Oral Surg Oral Med Oral Pathol* 76:790, 1993.

Tumors of Melanin-Producing Cells

Kaugars GE et al: Oral melanotic macules, *Oral Surg Oral Med Oral Pathol* 76:59, 1993.

Meleti M et al: Oral malignant melanoma: the Amsterdam experience, *J Oral Maxillofac Surg* 65:2181, 2007.

Tumors of Bone

Canadian Society of Otolaryngology—Head and Neck Surgery Oncology Study Group: Osteogenic sarcoma of the mandible and maxilla: a Canadian review (1980-2000), *J Otolaryngol* 33:139, 2004.

Forteza G, Colmenero A, Lopez-Barea F: Osteogenic sarcoma of the maxilla and mandible, *Oral Surg Oral Med Oral Pathol* 62:179, 1986.

Tumors of Blood-Forming Tissues

Lambertenghi-Deliliers G et al: Incidence of jaw lesions in 193 patients with multiple myeloma, *Oral Surg Oral Med Oral Pathol* 65:533, 1988.

Raubenheimer EJ, Dauth J, van Wilpe E: Multiple myeloma: a study of 10 cases, *J Oral Pathol* 16:383, 1987.

Metastatic Tumors

Hasimoto N et al: Pathological characteristics of metastatic carcinoma in the human mandible, *J Oral Pathol* 16:362, 1987.

REVIEW QUESTIONS

1. Which of the following are associated with the neoplastic transformation of cells?
   A. Chemicals
   B. Sunlight
   C. Viruses
   D. All of the above

2. Neoplasia involves:
   A. Abnormal proliferation of cells in response to tissue damage.
   B. Controlled proliferation of cells.
   C. Normal arrangement of proliferating cells.
   D. Irreversible change that results in an uncontrolled multiplication of cells.

3. Which of the following statements concerning leukoplakia is *true*?
   A. Most cases represent examples of epithelial dysplasia.
   B. Sites that are at high risk for epithelial dysplasia include the palate and gingiva.
   C. A biopsy should be performed to establish a diagnosis.
   D. Leukoplakia is less common than erythroplakia.

4. Which of the following is a characteristic of benign tumors?
   A. Numerous mitotic figures
   B. Pleomorphic cells
   C. Slow growth
   D. Metastasis likely

5. A small white exophytic lesion on the palate is a benign lesion composed of squamous epithelium. Papillary projections are arranged in a cauliflower-like appearance. It is most likely a:
   A. Papilloma.
   B. Fibroma.
   C. Neurofibroma.
   D. Granular cell tumor.

6. Which of the following is not a histologic characteristic of squamous cell carcinoma?
   A. Invasion of tumor cells into the connective tissue
   B. Pleomorphic epithelial cells
   C. Keratin pearls
   D. Cells with very small nuclei

7. Which of the following are the most common locations for intraoral squamous cell carcinoma?
   A. Upper labial mucosa, buccal mucosa, and hard palate
   B. Lower labial mucosa, maxillary gingiva, and buccal mucosa
   C. Floor of the mouth, ventrolateral tongue, and soft palate
   D. Anterior tongue, mandibular gingiva, and retromolar area

8. A patient with squamous cell carcinoma of the lateral tongue exhibits metastatic disease in the lungs. What clinical stage correlates with these findings?
   A. Stage I
   B. Stage II
   C. Stage III
   D. Stage IV

9. Which of the following represents the earliest clinical example of squamous cell carcinoma?
   A. Exophytic mass
   B. Erythematous plaque
   C. Nonhealing ulceration
   D. Destructive radiolucency

10. The most appropriate treatment for epithelial dysplasia is:
    A. Observation.
    B. Chemotherapy.
    C. Surgical excision.
    D. Repeat biopsy in 6 months.

11. Verrucous carcinoma is differentiated from squamous cell carcinoma because it:
    A. Does not occur in the oral cavity.
    B. Responds to chemotherapy.
    C. Has a better prognosis.
    D. Often metastasizes.

12. The most common intraoral location for salivary gland tumors is the:
    A. Lower lip.
    B. Buccal mucosa.
    C. Junction of the hard and soft palate.
    D. Anterior tongue.

13. Which of the following is an example of a malignant salivary gland tumor?
    A. Pleomorphic adenoma
    B. Warthin's tumor
    C. Monomorphic adenoma
    D. Adenoid cystic carcinoma

14. Which of the following statements concerning an ameloblastoma is *true*?
    A. It often occurs in young children.
    B. It is a radiopaque lesion.
    C. It often occurs in the mandibular molar and ramus area.
    D. It should be treated with radiation therapy.

15. The odontogenic tumor that characteristically appears as a well-circumscribed radiolucency located in the anterior maxilla of an adolescent girl is an:
    A. Ameloblastic fibroma.
    B. Ameloblastoma.
    C. Odontogenic myxoma.
    D. Adenomatoid odontogenic tumor.

16. Which odontogenic tumor most closely resembles the mesenchyme of the dental follicle?
    A. Benign cementoblastoma
    B. Odontogenic myxoma
    C. Complex odontoma
    D. Adenomatoid odontogenic tumor

17. A benign cementoblastoma may be recognized radiographically because:
    A. It is a well-circumscribed radiopaque lesion with a radiolucent halo attached to the root of a tooth.
    B. It has a radiolucent multilocular appearance.
    C. It is a radiolucent lesion surrounding the crown of an impacted tooth.
    D. It is an ill-defined radiolucent lesion containing scattered opacifications.

18. Which of the following lesions characteristically occurs on the alveolar mucosa?
    A. Congenital epulis
    B. Granular cell tumor
    C. Lymphangioma
    D. Lipoma

19. Human herpesvirus 8 is associated with:
    A. Lymphangioma.
    B. Rhabdomyosarcoma.
    C. Kaposi sarcoma.
    D. Schwannoma.

20. A compound odontoma differs from a complex odontoma in that a compound odontoma:
    A. Is composed of toothlike structures.
    B. Has unlimited growth potential.
    C. Is composed primarily of pulp tissue.
    D. Is located in the posterior mandible.

21. Peripheral odontogenic tumors are located on the:
    A. Tongue.
    B. Lower lip.
    C. Buccal mucosa.
    D. Gingiva.

22. A benign tumor of adipose tissue is called a:
    A. Lipoma.
    B. Schwannoma.
    C. Hemangioma.
    D. Lymphangioma.

23. The most common malignant soft tissue tumor of the head and neck in children is:
    A. Squamous cell carcinoma.
    B. Lymphoma.
    C. Rhabdomyosarcoma.
    D. Osteosarcoma.

24. Malignant melanoma of the oral cavity is rare; however, the most common intraoral location is the:
    A. Palate and maxillary gingiva.
    B. Tongue.
    C. Buccal mucosa.
    D. Retromolar area.

25. Which of the following neoplasms often occurs in the buccal mucosa or vestibule?
    A. Lipoma
    B. Congenital epulis
    C. Lymphangioma
    D. Melanocytic nevus

26. A malignant tumor of bone-forming tissue is called:
    A. Chondrosarcoma.
    B. Melanoma.
    C. Osteosarcoma.
    D. Rhabdomyosarcoma.

27. An overproduction of atypical white blood cells in the circulating blood is called:
    A. Lymphoma.
    B. Leukemia.
    C. Malignant melanoma.
    D. Multiple myeloma.

28. Which of the following is a malignant tumor of lymphocytes?
    A. Multiple myeloma
    B. Malignant melanoma
    C. Lymphoma
    D. Kaposi sarcoma

29. The cell involved in multiple myeloma is the:
    A. Lymphocyte.
    B. Histiocyte.
    C. Eosinophil.
    D. Plasma cell.

30. The most frequent intraoral site for metastatic tumors is the:
    A. Buccal mucosa.
    B. Mandible.
    C. Soft palate.
    D. Floor of the mouth.

31. Which of the following tumors is associated with von Recklinghausen's disease?
    A. Pleomorphic adenoma
    B. Lipoma
    C. Neurofibroma
    D. Fibroma

32. Which of the following is the most common odontogenic tumor?
    A. Odontoma
    B. Ameloblastoma
    C. Ameloblastic fibroma
    D. Odontogenic myxoma

33. Which of the following salivary gland tumors often occurs in adult men?
    A. Adenoid cystic carcinoma
    B. Monomorphic adenoma
    C. Papillary cystadenoma lymphomatosum
    D. Mucoepidermoid carcinoma

34. A benign tumor composed of a proliferation of capillaries is called a:
    A. Schwannoma.
    B. Hemangioma.
    C. Lipoma.
    D. Lymphangioma.

35. A white plaquelike lesion that cannot be rubbed off or diagnosed clinically as a specific disease is called:
    A. Speckled leukoplakia.
    B. Erythroplakia.
    C. Leukoplakia.
    D. Epithelial dysplasia.

36. All of the following are benign lesions that histologically contain bone or bonelike material except a(n):
    A. Torus.
    B. Odontoma.
    C. Exostosis.
    D. Central ossifying fibroma.

37. Which of the following malignant tumors may present as diffuse gingival enlargement with persistent bleeding?
    A. Multiple myeloma
    B. Leukemia
    C. Chondrosarcoma
    D. Osteosarcoma

38. Which of the following malignancies is characterized by a monoclonal spike on immunoelectrophoresis?
    A. Malignant melanoma
    B. Squamous cell carcinoma
    C. Multiple myeloma
    D. Leukemia

39. Which of the following malignant tumors has been reported to show a characteristic sunburst pattern on radiographic examination?
    A. Malignant melanoma
    B. Osteosarcoma
    C. Squamous cell carcinoma
    D. Rhabdomyosarcoma

40. All of the following neoplasms arise from squamous epithelium except a(n):
    A. Basal cell carcinoma.
    B. Verrucous carcinoma.
    C. Adenoid cystic carcinoma.
    D. Papilloma.

41. All of the following are true concerning solar cheilitis except one. Which one is the exception?
    A. Mottled grayish-pink discoloration of lower lip
    B. Distinct demarcation between vermilion border and skin
    C. More common in fair-skinned individuals
    D. Due to excessive exposure to sunlight

42. Which of the following has the best long-term prognosis?
    A. Verrucous carcinoma
    B. Squamous cell carcinoma
    C. Rhabdomyosarcoma
    D. Malignant melanoma

43. Which of the following does not arise in the oral cavity?
    A. Melanocytic nevus
    B. Malignant melanoma
    C. Basal cell carcinoma
    D. Verrucous carcinoma

44. Which of the following may undergo malignant transformation?
    A. Granular cell tumor
    B. Pleomorphic adenoma
    C. Monomorphic adenoma
    D. Hemangioma

45. Which of the following neoplasms occurs most often in males?
    A. Congenital epulis
    B. Mucoepidermoid carcinoma
    C. Pleomorphic adenoma
    D. Multiple myeloma

46. Pain is most often a clinical features of a(n):
    A. Schwannoma.
    B. Neurofibroma.
    C. Lipoma.
    D. Adenoid cystic carcinoma.

47. Central involvement of the jaws may occur with a:
   A. Granular cell tumor.
   B. Congenital epulis.
   C. Melanocytic nevus.
   D. Mucoepidermoid carcinoma.

48. Syndrome involvement may occur with a(n):
   A. Neurofibroma.
   B. Verrucous carcinoma.
   C. Pleomorphic adenoma.
   D. Ameloblastoma.

49. Which of the following neoplasms is least likely to occur in the jaws?
   A. Chondroma
   B. Osteoma
   C. Chondrosarcoma
   D. Osteosarcoma

50. Which of the following neoplasms has the worst long-term prognosis?
   A. Basal cell carcinoma
   B. Verrucous carcinoma
   C. Lymphangioma
   D. Metastatic tumor to the jaws

CHAPTER 7 Synopsis

Condition/Disease	Cause	Age/Race/Sex	Location	Clinical Features
Papilloma	Neoplastic	M=F	Soft palate, tongue	Exophytic fingerlike projections
Epithelial Dysplasia	Premalignant Smoking considered a risk factor	Age: adults	Floor of mouth, tongue	White erythematous or mixed white and erythematous mucosal lesion
Squamous Cell Carcinoma	Neoplastic	Age: over 40 M>F	Most common sites: floor of mouth, tongue, lips	Exophytic mass, ulcerated leukoplakia, erythroplakia
Verrucous Carcinoma	Neoplastic	Age: over 55 M>F	Most common sites: vestibule, buccal mucosa	Slow-growing exophytic mass papillary projections
Basal Cell Carcinoma	Neoplastic Associated with sun exposure	Age: over 40 M=F Whites	Skin of face	Nonhealing ulcer rolled borders
Pleomorphic Adenoma	Neoplastic	Age: over 40 F>M	Parotid gland Most common intraoral site; palate	Nonulcerated, dome-shaped
Monomorphic Adenoma	Neoplastic	Adults F>M	Most common oral sites: upper lip and buccal mucosa	Smooth-surfaced mass
Adenoid Cystic Carcinoma	Neoplastic	Adults F>M	Parotid gland Most common oral site: palate	Mass, often painful Surface may be ulcerated
Mucoepidermoid Carcinoma	Neoplastic	F>M	Parotid gland Most common oral site: palate Some are central in mandible	Asymptomatic swelling or mass
Ameloblastoma	Neoplastic	Adults M=F	Intraosseous Peripheral tumors also occur Mandible>maxilla Posterior>anterior	Slow growing, Expansion of bone

N/A, Not applicable.
*Not covered in text.

Radiographic Features	Microscopic Features	Treatment	Diagnostic Process
N/A	Papillary projections surfaced by stratified squamous epithelium covering connective tissue cores	Surgical extraction	Microscopic
N/A	Abnormal maturation of epithelial cells Hyperplasia of basal cells, disorganization of epithelial layers, increased nuclear/cytoplasmic ratios, cells with enlarged and hyperchromatic nuclei Abnormal keratinization Increased numbers of normal and abnormal mitotic figures No invasion of abnormal cells into underlying tissue	Surgical extraction	Microscopic
N/A	Invasion of tumor cells through basement membrane into underlying connective tissue Pleomorphic epithelial cells, normal and abnormal miotic figures	Surgical excision Radiation therapy Chemotherapy	Microscopic
N/A	Papillary epithelial projections Well-differentiated epithelium with normal-appearing epithelial cells Broad-based rete pegs with intact basement membrane	Surgical excision	Microscopic
N/A	Proliferation of basal epithelial cells Broad rete pegs penetrate deeply into the connective tissue	Surgical excision Radiation therapy	Microscopic
N/A	Encapsulated tumor Mixture of epithelium and tissue that resembles varying forms of connective tissue	Surgical excision	Microscopic
N/A	Encapsulated epithelial tumor with a uniform pattern of epithelial cells	Surgical excision	Microscopic
N/A	Unencapsulated, infiltrating tumor composed of small, deeply staining, uniform epithelial cells arranged in perforated round-to-oval islands	Surgical excision Radiation therapy	Microscopic
When intraosseous, unilocular or multilocular Radiolucency	Unencapsulated Infiltrating tumor composed of a combination of mucous cells and squamouslike epithelial cells	Surgical excision	Microscopic
Unilocular or multilocular radiolucency	Unencapsulated, infiltrating tumor composed of ameloblast-like epithelial cells surrounding areas resembling stellate reticulum	Surgical excision	Microscopic

Continued

CHAPTER 7 Synopsis (continued)

Condition/Disease	Cause	Age/Race/Sex	Location	Clinical Features
Calcifying Epithelial Odontogenic Tumor	Neoplastic	Adults M=F	Posterior mandible	Asymptomatic, slow-growing expansion of bone
Adenomatoid Odontogenic Tumor	Neoplastic	Age: over 20 F>M	70% involve anterior maxilla and mandible Maxilla>mandible	Asymptomatic swelling
Calcifying Odontogenic Cyst	Cyst with neoplastic variant	Age: over 40 M=F	Maxilla and mandible	Asymptomatic Swelling Root resorption
Odontogenic Myxoma	Neoplastic	Age: 10-29 M=F	Mandible>maxilla	Asymptomatic expansion of bone
Central Cementifying and Ossifying Fibromas	Neoplastic	Age: adults F>M	Mandible (90%)	Asymptomatic expansion, facial asymmetry
Benign Cementoblastoma	Neoplastic	Age: younger than 25 M=F	Most occur associated with a mandible molar	Localized expansion, pain, vital teeth
Ameloblastic Fibroma	Neoplastic	Age: younger than 20 M>F	Posterior mandible	Asymptomatic Swelling
Ameloblastic Fibro-odontoma	Neoplastic	Age: younger than 10	Posterior Maxilla and mandible	Asymptomatic Swelling
Odontoma	Neoplastic	Age: children and young adults M=F	Most common locations: anterior maxilla, posterior mandible	Lack of eruption Swelling
Peripheral Ossifying Fibroma	Probably reactive	Age: children and young adults F>M	Gingiva	Nodular, sessile, or pedunculated mass

N/A, Not applicable.
*Not covered in text.

Radiographic Features	Microscopic Features	Treatment	Diagnostic Process
Unilocular or multilocular radiolucency with scattered calcifications	Unencapsulated, infiltrating tumor composed of islands and sheets of polyhedral epithelial cells Calcifications and eosinophilic deposits in tumor	Surgical excision	Microscopic
Well-defined radiolucency associated with an impacted tooth Radiopacities within the radiolucency	Encapsulated tumor composed of ductlike epithelial structures, masses of cubodial and spindle-shaped epithelial cells with eosinophilic material and calcifications	Surgical enucleation	Microscopic
Unilocular or multilocular Radiolucency Radiopacities within the radiolucency	Cyst lined by odontogenic epithelium with associated ghost cell keratinization Ameloblast-like cells and stellate reticulum-like areas	Enucleation	Microscopic
Multilocular, honeycombed radiolucency	Unencapsulated, infiltrating tumor composed of pale-staining substance containing widely dispersed cells with small nuclei	Surgical excision	Radiographic
Wide-defined unilocular lesion, varying degrees of opacities	Well-circumscribed tumor composed of fibrous connective tissue and rounded globular calcifications, bone trabeculae, or both	Surgical excision	Radiographic Microscopic
Well-defined radiopaque mass in continuity with root or roots of the affected tooth	*	Enucleation of the tumor Removal of the associated tooth	Radiographic Microscopic
Well-defined unilocular or multilocular radiolucency	Nonencapsulated tumor composed of both strands and small islands of odontogenic epithelium and tissue that resembles the dental papilla	Surgical excision	Microscopic
Well-defined radiolucency with associated calcifications Calcifications may resemble teeth	Strands and small islands of odontogenic epithelium and tissue that resembles the dental papilla combined with tooth structures	Surgical excision	Microscopic
Compound: cluster of miniature teeth Complex: radiopaque mass	Mature enamel, dentin, cementum, and pulp Compound: from multiple small teeth Complex: form irregular mass	Surgical excision	Radiographic Microscopic
N/A	Exophytic lesion composed of connective tissue interpreted with scattered bone or cementum-like calcifications	Surgical excision Scale teeth	Microscopic Clinical

Continued

CHAPTER 7 Synopsis (continued)

Condition/Disease	Cause	Age/Race/Sex	Location	Clinical Features
Lipoma	Neoplastic	Age: most over 40 M=F	Most common intraoral locations: buccal mucosa, vestibule	Yellowish mass with delicate pattern of blood vessels on the surface
Neurofibroma/ Schwannoma	Neoplastic	Age: any M=F	Most common intraoral location: tongue	Asymptomatic nodule
Granular Cell Tumor	Neoplastic	Age: 30-50 F>M	Most common locations: tongue, buccal mucosa	Asymptomatic nodule
Congenital Epulis	Neoplastic	Present at birth (congenital) F>M	Anterior maxillary gingiva	Sessile or pedunculated mass
Rhabdomyosarcoma	Neoplastic	Age: frequently younger than 10 M>F	Head and neck	Rapidly growing destructive tumor
Hemangioma	Congenital/ developmental Adults/response to trauma	Age: adults Congenital F>M	Most common oral site: tongue	Deep red–to-blue mass Blanches with pressure
Lymphangioma	Neoplastic/ developmental	Congenital M=F	Most common oral site: tongue	Ill-defined mass with a pebbly surface
Kaposi Sarcoma	Neoplastic human herpesvirus 8	M>F	Most common oral sites: hard palate and gingiva	Purple macules, plaques, or exophytic tumors
Melanocytic Nevi	Developmental	Age: 20-50 F>M	Most common oral sites: hard palate and buccal mucosa	Tan/brown macules or papules
Malignant Melanoma	Neoplastic	Age: over 40	Most common oral sites: hard palate and maxillary	Rapidly enlarging blue and black mass
Torus	Genetic	Age: adults F>M	Midline of hard palate Lingual aspect of mandible	Asymptomatic, bony hard, lobulated mass

N/A, Not applicable.
*Not covered in text.

Radiographic Features	Microscopic Features	Treatment	Diagnostic Process
N/A	Well-delineated tumor composed of lobules of mature, uniform fat cells	Surgical excision	Microscopic
N/A	Neurofibroma: well-delineated, diffuse proliferation of spindle-shaped cells Schwannoma: encapsulated proliferation of Schwann cells arranged in palisaded whorls around central pink zones	Surgical excision	Microscopic
N/A	Unencapsulated tumor composed of large cells with a granular cytoplasm Overlying epithelium exhibits pseudoepitheliomatous hyperplasia	Surgical excision	Microscopic
N/A	Unencapsulated tumor composed of large cells with granular cytoplasm (similar to cell in granular cell tumor)	Surgical excision	Microscopic
N/A	*	Surgical excision Multiagent chemotherapy Radiation therapy	Microscopic
N/A	Vascular lesion composed of numerous small capillaries or larger blood vessels	Injection of sclerosing solution Spontaneous remission	Clinical Microscopic
N/A	Lesion composed of lymphatic vessels	Surgical excision	Clinical Microscopic
N/A	Unencapsulated tumor composed of spindle-shaped cells mixed with slitlike spaces containing red blood cells	Surgical excision Radiation therapy Chemotherapy	Microscopic Clinical
N/A	Benign tumor composed of nevus cells	Surgical excision	Clinical Microscopic
N/A	Malignant tumor	Surgical excision	Microscopic
Radiopaque mass superimposed on tooth roots	Benign, compact bone	None unless necessary for fabrication of prosthetic appliance	Clinical

Continued

CHAPTER 7 Synopsis (continued)

Condition/Disease	Cause	Age/Race/Sex	Location	Clinical Features
Exostosis	Possibly reactive	Age: adults M=F	Buccal aspect of maxillary and mandibular ridges	Asymptomatic, bony hard nodules
Osteoma	Neoplastic	M=F	Intraosseous	Asymptomatic
Osteosarcoma	Neoplastic	Most common primary malignant tumor of bone in patients younger than 40 M>F	Mandible 2 × maxilla	Painful, diffuse swelling or mass Expansion of involved bone
Chondrosarcoma	Neoplastic	M>F	Maxilla and mandible	Enlargement of involved bone
Leukemia	Neoplastic	M>F	Gingiva	Diffuse gingival enlargement with persistent bleeding
Lymphoma	Neoplastic	Adults M>F	Most common oral site: tonsillar area	Enlargement of involved tissue
Multiple Myeloma	Neoplastic	Adults M>F	Mandible>maxilla	Bone pain, swelling
Metastatic Tumors	Neoplastic	Adults M>F	Mandible>maxilla	Pain Paresthesia Swelling Expansion of bone

N/A, Not applicable.
*Not covered in text.

Radiographic Features	Microscopic Features	Treatment	Diagnostic Process
Occasionally seen radiopacity	Benign, compact bone	None unless necessary for fabrication of prosthetic appliance	Clinical
Sharply defined radiopaque mass	Benign, compact bone	None unless necessary for fabrication of prosthetic appliance	Microscopic
Destructive, poorly defined radiolucency to radiopacity Asymmetric widening of the periodontal ligament space Sunburst pattern	Malignant tumor of bone*	Surgical excision Multiagent chemotherapy	Microscopic
*	Malignant tumor of cartilage*	Wide surgical excision	Microscopic
N/A	Atypical white blood cells in circulating blood and tissues	Chemotherapy Radiation therapy Corticosteroids	Laboratory Microscopic
N/A	Malignant tumor of lymphoid tissue	Radiation therapy Chemotherapy	Laboratory Microscopic
Multiple radiolucent lesions	Malignant proliferation of plasma cells	Chemotherapy	Laboratory Microscopic
Variable Usually poorly defined and radiolucent Tooth roots may show spiked appearances Some may show area of radiopacity	Resemble primary malignancy	Chemotherapy Radiation	Microscopic

Nonneoplastic Diseases of Bone

Anne Cale Jones, Joan A. Phelan, Olga A.C. Ibsen

OBJECTIVES

After studying this chapter, the student will be able to:

1. Define benign fibro-osseous lesions.
2. Define dysplasia as it relates to bone diseases and differentiate the term from epithelial dysplasia.
3. List the benign fibro-osseous lesions that occur in the jawbones.
4. Describe the clinical, radiographic, and microscopic features of periapical cemento-osseous dysplasia, focal cemento-osseous dysplasia, and florid cemento-osseous dysplasia.
5. Compare and contrast periapical cemento-osseous dysplasia, focal cemento-osseous dysplasia, and florid cemento-osseous dysplasia.
6. Compare and contrast monostotic fibrous dysplasia with polyostotic fibrous dysplasia.
7. Compare and contrast the radiographic appearance, histologic appearance, and treatment of fibrous dysplasia of the jaws with those of ossifying fibroma of the jaws.
8. Compare and contrast the three types of polyostotic fibrous dysplasia.
9. Describe the histologic appearance of Paget disease of bone and describe its clinical and radiographic appearance when the maxilla or mandible is involved.
10. Describe the clinical, radiographic and microscopic features of the central giant cell granuloma.
11. Describe the cause of osteomalacia and rickets.

VOCABULARY

Benign fibro-osseous lesion (be-nīn′ fi″bro-os′e-ĕs le′zhĕn) Benign lesion of bone characterized histologically by cellular fibrous connective tissue admixed with irregularly shaped bone trabeculae or cementoid material.

Dysplasia (dis-pla′ze-ah) Disordered growth.

Nonneoplastic diseases of bone that affect the maxilla and mandible fall into multiple categories. Inherited diseases that affect bone are discussed in Chapter 6, and benign and malignant neoplasms of bone, including central and peripheral cementifying and ossifying fibromas, are discussed in Chapter 7. Central and peripheral giant cell granulomas are included in Chapter 2, and aneurysmal bone cyst is included in Chapter 5. The purpose of this chapter is to delineate several other nonneoplastic diseases of bone that are important for a dental hygienist to understand but are not covered elsewhere in this text. These include three forms of cemento-osseous dysplasia: (1) periapical, (2) focal, and (3) florid. In addition, the dental hygienist should also be familiar with the various types of fibrous dysplasia and the clinical and radiographic features of Paget disease and osteomalacia.

The term **dysplasia** as used in this chapter in the context of the cemento-osseous dysplasias and fibrous dysplasia refers to the disordered production of cementum and bone. This term in this context should not be confused with dysplasia as used in the context of epithelial dysplasia. Epithelial dysplasia connotes a premalignant condition affecting squamous epithelium.

BENIGN FIBRO-OSSEOUS LESIONS

Benign fibro-osseous lesions that affect the maxilla and mandible include central and peripheral cementifying and ossifying fibromas (see Chapter 7), periapical cemento-osseous dysplasia, focal cemento-osseous dysplasia, florid cemento-osseous dysplasia, and fibrous dysplasia (Box 8-1).

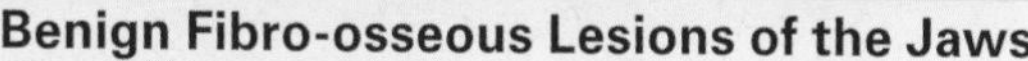

Box 8-1

Benign Fibro-osseous Lesions of the Jaws

- Fibrous dysplasia
  - Monostotic type
  - Polyostotic types
    - Jaffe type
    - Albright syndrome
  - Craniofacial type
- Central ossifying fibroma
- Cementifying fibroma
- Peripheral ossifying fibroma
- Periapical cemento-osseous dysplasia (cementoma)
- Florid cemento-osseous dysplasia

PERIAPICAL CEMENTO-OSSEOUS DYSPLASIA

Periapical cemento-osseous dysplasia is a relatively common disease of unknown cause that affects periapical bone (Figure 8-1, *A* and *B*). The term **cementoma** is often used for this disease. However, because the disease does not represent a neoplasm, this term is inappropriate and should be avoided.

The lesion is asymptomatic and is discovered on routine radiographic examination. It occurs most commonly in the anterior mandible of patients older than 30 years of age. It is more common in women than men. Many studies have shown a predilection for this disease in black women. Early lesions are well circumscribed and radiolucent and may mimic periapical disease. Teeth in the affected area are vital unless they are coincidentally carious or have been traumatized. With time the lesions become increasingly calcified; therefore older lesions are radiolucent with central opacifications.

The diagnosis of periapical cemento-osseous dysplasia is usually established on the basis of observation of its characteristic clinical and radiographic features. A biopsy may be necessary in cases in which the characteristic radiographic features are not evident. Histologic examination reveals a fibro-osseous lesion. Like other fibro-osseous lesions, periapical cemento-osseous dysplasia is composed of a combination of fibrous tissue and calcifications. The calcifications in this lesion may resemble bone, cementum, or both. Early lesions consist mainly of fibrous tissue, whereas older lesions contain fibrous connective tissue interspersed with numerous calcifications (Figure 8-1, *C*). If a patient demonstrates radiographic changes characteristic of an early lesion, close follow-up examinations may be necessary to ensure that a correct diagnosis was established. Once the condition is recognized, no treatment is necessary. The lesion remains asymptomatic and localized.

FOCAL CEMENTO-OSSEOUS DYSPLASIA

Focal cemento-osseous dysplasia is an asymptomatic fibro-osseous lesion that shares similar histologic features with periapical cemento-osseous dysplasia and florid cemento-osseous dysplasia. However, it differs from these two lesions in that it has unique clinical and radiographic features.

Focal cemento-osseous dysplasia usually occurs in women between 30 and 50 years of age; and, unlike periapical and florid cemento-osseous dysplasia, it is reported to be more common in white than black individuals. It typically arises in the posterior mandible and appears as an isolated, well-delineated radiolucent-to-radiopaque lesion that is less than 1.5 cm in size.

Biopsy and histologic examination usually are necessary to establish a diagnosis of focal cemento-osseous dysplasia. A characteristic surgical feature of focal cemento-osseous dysplasia is that it is composed of numerous gritty pieces of soft and hard tissue. This finding is distinctly different from the characteristic surgical features of a central cementifying or ossifying fibroma. These latter tumors present as a circular mass of hard tissue that separates easily from the adjacent normal bone. The gritty tissue removed from focal cemento-osseous dysplasia represents fibrous connective tissue interspersed with bone trabeculae and cementum-like material.

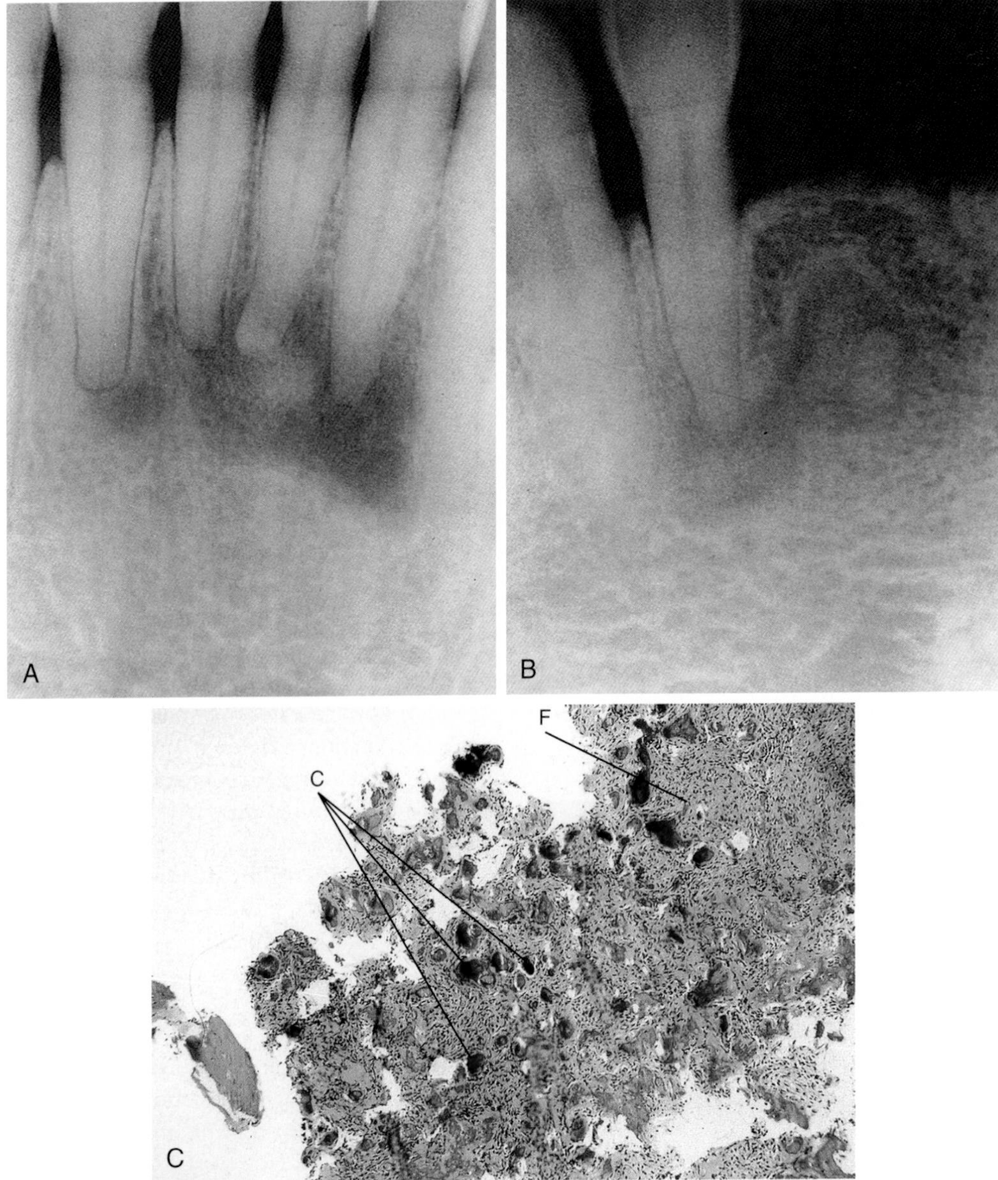

FIGURE 8-1 ■ **A** and **B,** Radiographs of periapical cemento-osseous dysplasia. **C,** Microscopic appearance of periapical cemento-osseous dysplasia shows a combination of cellular fibrous connective tissue *(F)* and calcified tissue *(C).*

Once a definitive diagnosis has been established, no further treatment is necessary. The prognosis for focal cemento-osseous dysplasia is excellent. Occasionally this lesion has progressed to florid cemento-osseous dysplasia.

FLORID CEMENTO-OSSEOUS DYSPLASIA

Florid cemento-osseous dysplasia is another fibro-osseous lesion characterized by disordered cementum and bone development. This lesion characteristically involves multiple quadrants in the maxilla and mandible.

Florid cemento-osseous dysplasia occurs most often in black women older than 40 years of age. The cause of this disease is unknown. Radiographically it differs from periapical cemento-osseous dysplasia in that it typically affects more than one quadrant of the maxilla and mandible, often in the posterior areas. Occasionally an early radiolucent phase similar to that seen in periapical cemento-osseous dysplasia may be identified. However, the majority of cases are composed of masses of irregular opacification. (Figure 8-2).

Florid cemento-osseous dysplasia is often diagnosed on the basis of its characteristic clinical presentation and radiographic appearance. Because of these findings, treatment is often unnecessary. However, in an edentulous patient the sclerotic masses may perforate the mucosa, resulting in a communication between the oral environment and

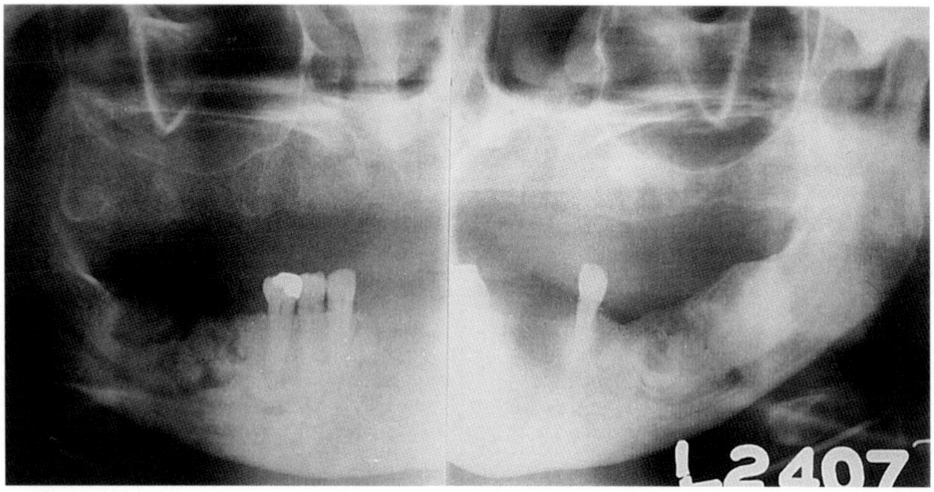

FIGURE 8-2 ■ Florid cemento-osseous dysplasia. Pantomographic radiograph shows irregular radiopaque masses in both the left and right mandible.

the underlying bone. This complication may lead to the development of an osteomyelitis, necessitating antibiotic therapy and surgical intervention.

FIBROUS DYSPLASIA

Fibrous dysplasia is a disease that is characterized by the replacement of bone with abnormal fibrous connective tissue interspersed with varying amounts of calcification. Although the cause is unknown, several theories have been proposed. One of the most widely accepted theories is that the unusual fibrous proliferation is the result of abnormal mesenchymal cell function. Several types of fibrous dysplasia exist; each type shares similar microscopic features, but the clinical presentation and associated systemic signs and symptoms differ. Histologically fibrous dysplasia is classified as a benign fibro-osseous lesion. It is composed of vascularized, cellular fibrous connective tissue interspersed with irregular trabeculae of bone emerging from the connective tissue.

Types of Fibrous Dysplasia

Monostotic FIbrous Dysplasia

Monostotic fibrous dysplasia, the most common type of fibrous dysplasia, is characterized by involvement of a single bone. The mandible and maxilla are commonly affected, and the maxilla is more frequently involved than the mandible. Other bones may be affected, including the ribs, femur, and tibia. Monostotic fibrous dysplasia is most commonly diagnosed in children and young adults; no sex predilection is seen. Clinical examination reveals a painless swelling or bulging of the buccal plate of the maxilla or mandible. The expanding nature of the lesion may lead to malocclusion, tipping, or displacement of adjacent teeth. However, the teeth are rarely mobile.

Polyostotic Fibrous Dysplasia

Polyostotic fibrous dysplasia is characterized by involvement of more than one bone. It typically occurs in children, and a definite female gender predilection is seen. The skull, clavicles, and long bones are often affected; and most cases are asymptomatic. When the long bones are involved, they may exhibit bowing and an associated dull aching pain. Patients with polyostotic fibrous dysplasia often demonstrate skin lesions. These lesions appear as light-brown macules called **café au lait spots.** Several forms of polyostotic fibrous dysplasia exist. Craniofacial fibrous dysplasia is the term used for polyostotic fibrous dysplasia that involves the maxilla with extension into the sinuses and adjacent zygoma, sphenoid, and occipital bones. Another form of polyostotic fibrous dysplasia is called the Jaffe type (or Jaffe-Lichtenstein type). It involves multiple bones along with associated café au lait macules on the skin. The most severe form of polyostotic fibrous dysplasia is called Albright syndrome (or McCune-Albright syndrome). This condition is characterized by endocrine abnormalities, including precocious puberty in females, and stunting or deformity of skeletal growth in both sexes as a result of early epiphyseal plate closure. Precocious puberty is exhibited by menses, pubic hair, and breast development in children as young as 2 years of age. Other complications of Albright syndrome include diabetes mellitus and hyperthyroidism. Café au lait skin macules may occur in this form of polyostotic fibrous dysplasia.

Clinical examination reveals a painless enlargement of the affected bone or bones. Jaw involvement typically appears as a painless, progressive, unilateral enlargement of the maxilla or mandible. When fibrous dysplasia involves the maxilla, the disease usually extends into the maxillary sinuses. Involvement of the jaws may occur in any type of fibrous dysplasia. The classic radiographic appearance of fibrous dysplasia is a diffuse radiopacity that is described as "looking like

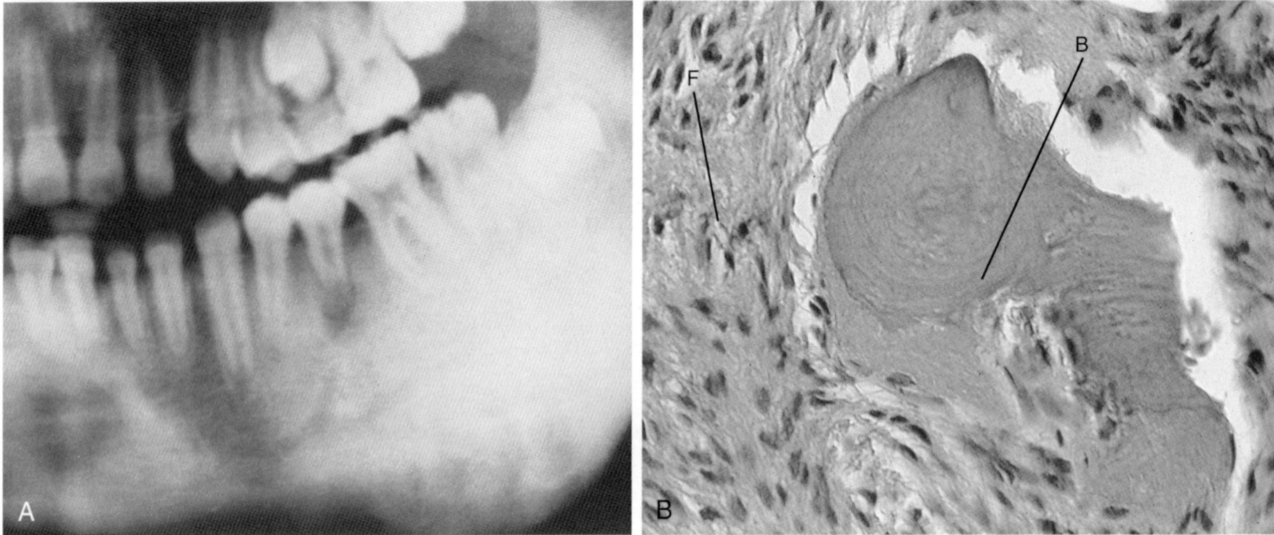

FIGURE 8-3 ■ Fibrous dysplasia. **A,** Radiograph of fibrous dysplasia demonstrating indistinct borders that blend into the adjacent normal bone. **B,** Microscopic appearance (high power) of fibrous dysplasia shows cellular fibrous connective tissue *(F)* and irregular trabeculae of bone *(B)*. (**A** courtesy Drs. Paul Freedman and Stanley Kerpel.)

ground glass" (Figure 8-3, *A*). The abnormal bone blends into the adjacent normal bone, making it difficult to determine the periphery of the lesion. A unilocular or multilocular radiolucency, a patchy radiolucency with central opacifications, and a dense radiopacity have also been observed in fibrous dysplasia. The radiolucent or radiopaque appearance of fibrous dysplasia depends on the degree of calcification present in the lesion. Lesions that are primarily radiolucent contain an abundance of fibrous connective tissue with few calcifications, whereas more radiopaque lesions are composed predominantly of calcified tissue and a scant amount of fibrous connective tissue.

The diagnosis of fibrous dysplasia is established by correlating the microscopic findings along with the characteristic clinical features and radiographic appearance. Histologic examination reveals a benign fibro-osseous lesion (Figure 8-3, *B*). The microscopic appearance is characterized by cellular fibrous connective tissue interspersed with irregularly shaped bone trabeculae. Fibrous dysplasia of the maxilla or mandible is distinguished from a central cementifying or ossifying fibroma on the basis of review of the radiographic findings. In fibrous dysplasia the radiographic changes blend into the surrounding normal bone. In a central cementifying or ossifying fibroma, a tumor that can demonstrate microscopic features similar to fibrous dysplasia, the radiographic findings consist of a well-delineated lesion that is easily delineated from the surrounding normal bone. Likewise other fibro-osseous lesions such as periapical cemento-osseous dysplasia and florid cemento-osseous dysplasia can be distinguished from fibrous dysplasia on the basis of an examination of their distinct clinical and radiographic features. Fibrous dysplasia is treated surgically by recontouring the affected bone for cosmetic reasons. No treatment exists for severe and progressive polyostotic fibrous dysplasia. Radiation treatment of fibrous dysplasia is contraindicated because it has been associated with malignant transformation.

PAGET DISEASE OF BONE

Paget disease of bone, also called *osteitis deformans* and *leontiasis ossea*, is a chronic metabolic bone disease. It is characterized by resorption, osteoblastic repair, and remineralization of the involved bone. The cause is unknown. Several theories have been proposed, and a viral cause is suspected. The disease occurs most commonly in men over the age of 50. It typically involves the pelvis and spinal column. When found in the jawbones, the maxilla is more commonly affected than the mandible.

The clinical manifestations of Paget disease depend on the bone involved. Enlargement of the affected bone is common, and the patient often complains of pain. When the maxilla or mandible is involved, spacing between the teeth increases as the bone enlarges (Figure 8-4, *A*). Edentulous patients may complain that their dentures no longer fit. When other bones of the skull are involved, clinical manifestations include severe headache, dizziness, and deafness. These symptoms occur because the enlarging bone impinges on cranial nerves as they exit the skull. The classic radiographic appearance is a patchy radiolucency and radiopacity that has been referred to as a *cotton-wool appearance* (Figure 8-4, *B*). However, this only occurs in the later stages of Paget disease. In earlier stages the radiographic appearance is not as unique. Hypercementosis, loss of the lamina dura, and obliteration of the periodontal ligament may also occur.

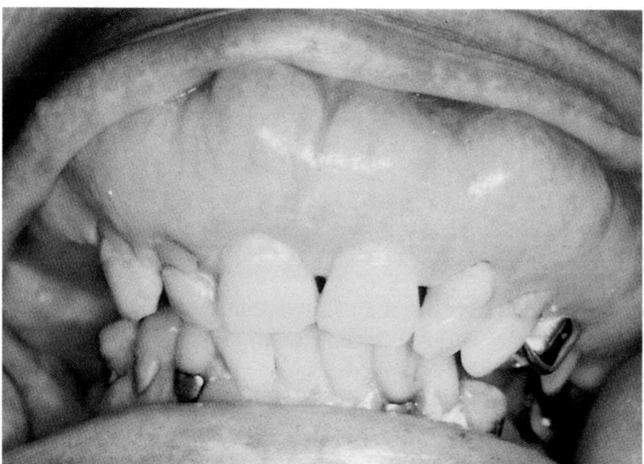

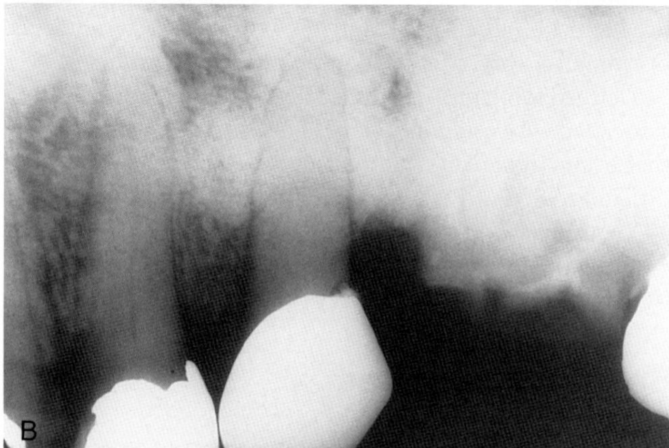

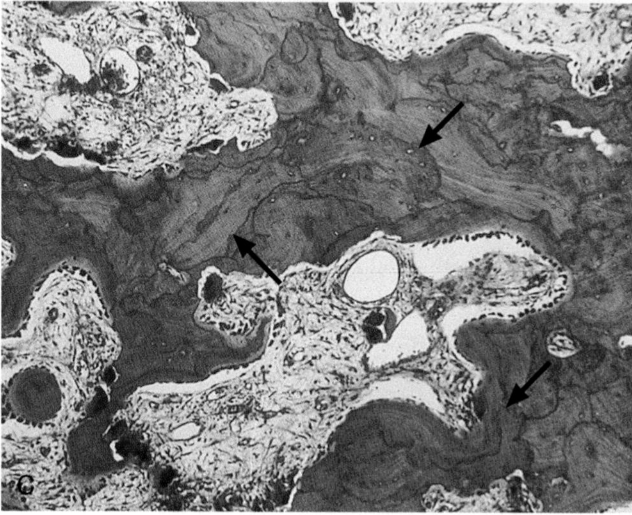

FIGURE 8-4 ■ Paget disease. **A,** Enlargement of the maxilla with spaces between the teeth. **B,** Radiograph demonstrating irregular opacification that is also referred to as a *cotton-wool appearance.* In areas, the lamina dura is obliterated. **C,** Microscopic appearance of Paget disease shows bone trabeculae surfaced by numerous osteoclasts and osteoblasts. The prominent reversal lines *(arrows)* seen here characterize the mosaic bone pattern of bone.

Laboratory evaluation is important in establishing the diagnosis of Paget disease. The serum alkaline phosphatase level is significantly elevated in active disease. Two different measurements are used to evaluate the serum alkaline phosphatase level. In Bodansky units the normal serum alkaline phosphatase value is 1.5 to 5.0. In Paget disease the serum alkaline phosphatase value can be as high as 250 Bodansky units. Another measurement used for evaluating the serum alkaline phosphatase level is the King-Armstrong unit (KAU). Normal values are 5 to 10 KAU. In patients with Paget disease KAU values may be as high as 200. Histologic examination reveals bone trabeculae surfaced by numerous osteoclasts and osteoblasts (Figure 8-4, *C*). The involved bone demonstrates prominent reversal lines that result from the resorption and deposition of bone; this pattern has been described as **mosaic bone.** The connective tissue between the bone trabeculae is so well vascularized that the overlying skin may feel warm when touched. Treatment of Paget disease is experimental. The disease is slowly progressive. Complications include fracture of the involved bone and development of malignant tumors, particularly osteosarcoma. Heart disease is a rare complication of Paget disease.

CENTRAL GIANT CELL GRANULOMA (CENTRAL GIANT CELL LESION)

The giant cell granuloma is a non-neoplastic lesion of unclear pathogenesis. It has also been called a giant cell reparative granuloma; however, evidence that this lesion represents a reparative response is lacking. The giant cell granuloma is composed of well vascularized connective tissue containing many multinucleated giant cells. Red blood cells and chronic inflammatory cells are also seen in this lesion. The giant cell granuloma occurs in both peripheral (gingival or alveolar mucosa) and central (located within the bone of the maxilla or mandible) locations. The peripheral giant cell granuloma is described in Chapter 2.

The central giant cell granuloma occurs within the bone of the maxilla or mandible, primarily in children and young adults. Studies have reported its occurrence more commonly in females than in males. These lesions are common in the anterior segments of the maxilla and mandible and are uncommon in the ramus of the mandible. Patients with central giant cell granulomas may complain of discomfort from the lesions, but pain is not a common feature. Most central giant cell granulomas are discovered on routine radiographs. The lesion is slow growing and destructive and produces a radiolucency in the bone. The borders of the radiolucency may be either sclerotic or ill defined, and they may be unilocular or multilocular (Figure 8-5). Divergence of the roots of teeth adjacent to the lesion is a common feature of central giant cell granuloma. Lesions are treated by surgical removal and occasionally recur.

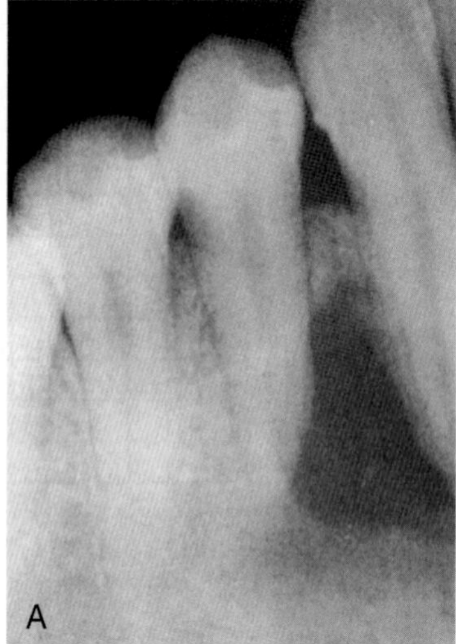

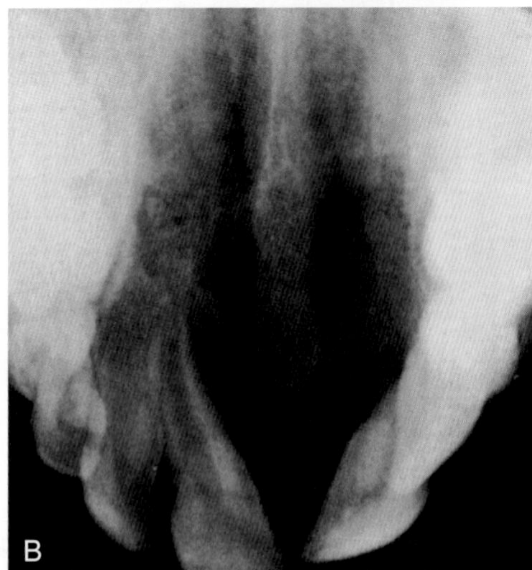

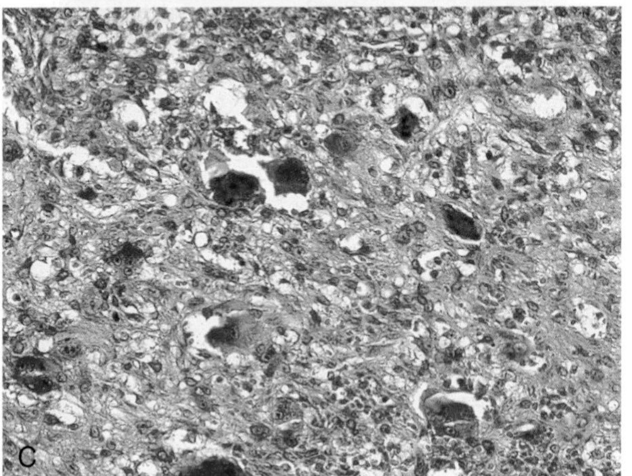

FIGURE 8-5 ■ Radiographs of central giant cell granulomas showing multilocular radiolucencies in the mandible **(A)** and maxilla **(B)**. **C,** Microscopic appearance of a central giant cell granuloma showing the same features as a peripheral giant cell granuloma except for the absence of surface mucosa.

A lesion of bone identical to the central giant cell granuloma (often called **brown tumor**) occurs in patients with hyperparathyroidism (discussed in Chapter 9). They are not surgically removed because they resolve when the underlying disease is successfully treated.

OSTEOMALACIA

Osteomalacia is a disease of bone that develops over a long period of time as the result of calcium deficiency. When this disease occurs in young children, it is usually caused by a nutritional deficiency of vitamin D, and the associated disease is termed *rickets.* An inherited form of vitamin D deficiency called **hypophosphatemic vitamin D–resistant rickets** is included in Chapter 6. In adults the disease may be related to various problems such as a malabsorption syndrome, drugs, liver and kidney disease, and the chronic use of antacids. Osteomalacia may also be induced by certain tumors.

Delayed tooth eruption and periodontal disease have been associated with osteomalacia. Changes in bone trabeculation that occur in patients with osteomalacia may be subtle and difficult to detect. Pathologic fractures may also occur.

Treatment is based on identification of the cause of the vitamin D deficiency and includes nutritional supplementation with vitamin D and dietary calcium.

Selected References

Books

Neville BW et al: *Oral and maxillofacial pathology,* ed 3, St. Louis, 2009, Saunders.

Regezi JA, Sciubba JJ, Jordan RCK: *Oral pathology: clinical-pathologic correlations,* ed 5, St Louis, 2008, Saunders.

Journal Articles

Bessho K et al: Monostotic fibrous dysplasia with involvement of the mandibular canal, *Oral Surg Oral Med Oral Pathol* 68:396, 1989.

Collins MT: Spectrum and natural history of fibrous dysplasia of bone, *J Bone Miner Res* 21 Suppl 2:99, 2006.

Hadjipavlou AG, Gaitanis IN, Kontakis GM: Paget disease of the bone and its management, *J Bone Joint Surg* 84:160, 2002.

MacDonald-Jankowski DS: Fibro-osseous lesions of the face and jaws, *Clin Radiol* 59:11, 2004.

Regezi JA: Odontogenic cysts, odontogenic tumors, fibro-osseous, and giant cell lesions of the jaws, *Mod Pathol* 15:331, 2002.

Singer SR et al: Florid cemento-osseous dysplasia and chronic diffuse osteomyelitis: report of a simultaneous presentation and review of the literature, *J Am Dent Assoc* 136:927, 2005.

Siris ES: Paget disease of bone, *J Bone Miner Res* 13:1061, 1998.

Summerlin Don-John, Tomich CE: Focal cemento-osseous dysplasia: a clinicopathologic study of 221 cases, *Oral Surg Oral Med Oral Pathol* 78:611, 1994.

Whyte MP: Clinical practice: Paget disease of bone, *New Engl J Med* 355:593, 2006.

Zacharin M: The spectrum of McCune Albright syndrome, *Pediatr Endocrinol Rev* 4(suppl):412, 2007.

REVIEW QUESTIONS

1. A 48-year-old black woman has multiple asymptomatic, radiopaque masses in the mandible and maxilla. No expansion of bone is noted. The most likely diagnosis is:
   A. Central cementifying fibromas.
   B. Periapical cemento-osseous dysplasia.
   C. Florid cemento-osseous dysplasia.
   D. Focal cemento-osseous dysplasia.

2. All of the following are examples of benign fibro-osseous lesions *except:*
   A. Fibrous dysplasia.
   B. Periapical cemento-osseous dysplasia.
   C. Central ossifying fibroma.
   D. Odontoma.

3. Which of the following is characterized by precocious puberty in females?
   A. Monostotic fibrous dysplasia
   B. Albright syndrome
   C. Jaffe-Lichtenstein type of fibrous dysplasia
   D. Periapical cemento-osseous dysplasia

4. Periapical cemento-osseous dysplasia is characteristically located in the:
   A. Posterior mandible.
   B. Posterior maxilla.
   C. Anterior maxilla.
   D. Anterior mandible.

5. Periapical cemento-osseous dysplasia is also known as a(n):
   A. Odontoma.
   B. Cementoblastoma.
   C. Cementifying fibroma.
   D. Cementoma.

6. Which of the following diseases are associated with café au lait spots?
   A. Polyostotic fibrous dysplasia
   B. Paget disease
   C. Monostotic fibrous dysplasia
   D. Focal cemento-osseous dysplasia

7. What is the name of the type of fibrous dysplasia that involves the maxilla and adjacent bones?
   A. Facial
   B. Jaffe
   C. Craniofacial
   D. Monostotic

8. Bone resorption, osteoblastic repair, loss of the lamina dura, hypercementosis, and cotton-wool radiopacities are characteristics of:
   A. Albright syndrome.
   B. Letterer-Siwe disease.
   C. Paget disease.
   D. Fibrous dysplasia.

9. The most characteristic radiographic appearance of fibrous dysplasia is described as a:
   A. Cotton-wool appearance.
   B. Ground glass appearance.
   C. Well-circumscribed radiopacity.
   D. Well-circumscribed radiolucency.

10. All of the following are histologic features seen in Paget disease except one. Which one is the exception?
    A. Osteoblasts and osteoclasts
    B. Bone with prominent irregular dark lines
    C. Well-vascularized fibrous connective tissue
    D. Pleomorphic nuclei and atypical mitotic figures

11. Which of the following is diagnosed on the basis of a characteristic radiographic appearance?
    A. Paget disease
    B. Osteomalacia
    C. Florid cemento-osseous dysplasia
    D. Focal cemento-osseous dysplasia

12. In patients with fibrous dysplasia, which of the following is the only recommended treatment modality?
    A. Surgery
    B. Radiation therapy
    C. Chemotherapy
    D. Antibiotics

13. Which of the following is helpful in the diagnosis of Paget disease?
    A. Serum alkaline phosphatase
    B. Serum vitamin D
    C. Serum calcium
    D. Urinalysis

14. Osteomalacia is usually caused by a deficiency of:
    A. Vitamin B_{12}.
    B. Vitamin A.
    C. Alkaline phosphatase.
    D. Calcium.

15. Osteomalacia in children is called:
    A. Rickets.
    B. Fibrous dysplasia.
    C. Osteogenesis imperfecta.
    D. Albright syndrome.

16. Which of the following diseases may be associated with malignant transformation into an osteosarcoma?
    A. Paget disease
    B. Periapical cemento-osseous dysplasia
    C. Focal cemento-osseous dysplasia
    D. Florid cemento-osseous dysplasia

17. Which of the following diseases demonstrates multiple fragments of gritty material when it is removed from the jaws?
    A. Periapical cemento-osseous dysplasia
    B. Focal cemento-osseous dysplasia
    C. Florid cemento-osseous dysplasia
    D. Central cemento-ossifying fibroma

CHAPTER 8 Synopsis

Condition/ Disease	Cause	Age/Race/Sex	Location	Clinical Features
Periapical	Reactive	Age: >30 F>M Race: more common in black	Anterior mandible	Asymptomatic Vital teeth
Focal Cemento-osseous Dysplasia	Reactive	Age: 30-50 F>M Race: more common in white	Posterior mandible	Asymptomatic
Florid Cemento-osseous Dysplasia	Reactive	Age > 40 F > M Race: more common in black	Multiple areas Maxilla and mandible	Asymptomatic
Fibrous Dysplasia	Cause unknown	Children and young adults M = F	Monostotic Maxilla > mandible Ribs, femur, tibia Craniofacial Maxilla and adjacent bones Jaffe type: More than one bone Albright syndrome: Many bones involved	All types: enlargement of involved bones Maxilla/mandible involved Malocclusion, tipping or displacement of teeth Jaffe type and Albright syndrome: Café au lait macules on the skin Extensive, progressive bone involvement Café au lait macules on the skin Endocrine abnormalities
Paget Disease of Bone	Chronic metabolic bone disease Cause unknown	Age: older than 50 M>F	Typically pelvis and spinal column When affecting the jaws: Maxilla > mandible	Enlargement of the involved bone, patient may complain of pain in affected bone With involvement of maxilla or mandible, spacing between teeth; when edentulous, dentures no longer fit
Central Giant Cell Granuloma	Unknown	Children/Young adults	Within bone of maxilla and Mandible Usually anterior Segments	Usually asymptomatic
Osteomalacia	Long-term deficiency of calcium Children: nutritional deficiency of vitamin D Adults: malabsorption syndromes, drugs, liver disease, kidney disease, chronic use of antacids	Children: rickets Adults: osteomalacia	Generalized bone disease	Children: delayed tooth eruption Pathologic fractures Periodontal disease

*Not covered in text.

18. Leontiasis ossea or osteitis deformans are two other names for:
    A. Rickets.
    B. Osteomalacia.
    C. Fibrous dysplasia.
    D. Paget disease.

19. The central giant cell granuloma:
    A. May occur on the tongue.
    B. May present as a multilocular radiolucency.
    C. Occurs primarily in men older than 60 years of age.
    D. Is histologically the same as a periapical granuloma.

Radiographic Features	Microscopic Features	Treatment	Diagnostic Process
Well-defined radiolucency to radiopacity at area of tooth apex	Fibrous connective tissue and calcification	None	Radiographic
Well-defined radiolucency to radiopacity	Fibrous connective tissue with round globular calcifications and bone trabeculae	None	Radiographic Microscopic if diagnosis not certain
Multiple areas Radiolucency to radiopacity	Fibrous connective tissue with dense sclerotic masses of bone, cementum, or both	None unless complicated by osteomyelitis	Radiographic
Diffuse "ground-glass"–appearing radiolucency Abnormal bone blends into normal bone Unilocular and multilocular radiolucencies have been described	Benign fibro-osseous lesion	Surgical recontouring of affected bone for cosmetic reasons	Radiographic Microscopic
Patchy radiolucency/radiopacity (*cotton-wool* appearance) Hypercementosis and loss of lamina aura also described	Mosaic bone: reversal lines in bone with osteoblasts and osteoclasts lining the trabeculae Well-vascularized fibrous tissue	Experimental	Radiographic Laboratory Elevated alkaline phosphate
Unilocular to multilocular radiolucency Divergence of tooth roots is a common feature	Many multinucleated giant cells in well-vascularized connective tissue	Surgical excision	Microscopic
Subtle changes in bone trabeculation	*	Children: vitamin D and dietary calcium Adults: dependent on cause	*

Oral Manifestations of Systemic Diseases

Olga A.C. Ibsen, Joan A. Phelan, Anthony T. Vernillo

OBJECTIVES

After studying this chapter, the student will be able to:

1. Define each of the words in the vocabulary list for this chapter.
2. Describe the difference between gigantism and acromegaly and list the physical characteristics of each.
3. State the oral manifestations of hyperthyroidism.
4. Describe the difference between primary and secondary hyperparathyroidism.
5. List the oral and systemic manifestations that occur in the uncontrolled diabetic state.
6. List the major clinical characteristics of type 1 and type 2 diabetes.
7. Define Addison disease and describe the changes that occur on the skin and oral mucosa in a patient with Addison disease.
8. Compare and contrast the cause, laboratory findings, and oral manifestations of each of the following: iron deficiency anemia, pernicious anemia, folic acid deficiency, and vitamin B deficiency.
9. Compare and contrast the definitions and oral manifestations of thalassemia major and sickle cell anemia.
10. Define celiac sprue.
11. Describe the difference between primary and secondary aplastic anemia.
12. Describe the oral manifestations of polycythemia.
13. Explain why platelets may be deficient in polycythemia vera.
14. Describe the most characteristic oral manifestations of agranulocytosis.
15. Describe and contrast acute and chronic leukemia.
16. State the purpose of each of the following laboratory tests: platelet count, bleeding time, prothrombin time, partial thromboplastin time, and international normalized ratio.
17. List two causes of thrombocytopenic purpura.
18. Describe the oral manifestations of thrombocytopenia and nonthrombocytopenic purpura.

OBJECTIVES (continued)

19. Define hemophilia and describe its oral manifestations and treatment.
20. Describe the difference between primary and secondary immunodeficiency.
21. Describe the oral problems that would be expected to occur in a patient with radiation-induced xerostomia.
22. List two drugs that are associated with gingival enlargement.

VOCABULARY

Agranulocytosis **(ah-gran″u-lo-si-to′sis)** Marked decrease in the number of granulocytes, particularly neutrophils.

Anemia **(ah-ne′me-ah)** Reduction of the number of red blood cells, quantity of hemoglobin, or volume of packed red blood cells to less than normal.

Aplasia **(ā-pla′zhe-ah)** (adjective, aplastic) Lack of development.

Arthralgia **(ar-thral′-jĭ-ah)** Severe pain in a joint.

Atherosclerosis The process by which lipid accumulates within the walls of large and medium-sized arteries. It leads to reduced blood flow to and death of vital organs.

Autoimmunity **(aw″to-ĭ-mu′nĭ-te)** Immune-mediated destruction of the body's own cells and tissues; immunity against self.

Catabolism **(kah-tab′ah-lizm)** Component of metabolism that involves the breakdown of tissues.

Coagulation **(ko-ag″u-la′shun)** Formation of a clot.

Ecchymosis **(ek″ĭ-mo′sis)** Small, flat, hemorrhagic patch larger than a petechia on the skin or mucous membrane.

Fibrin **(fi′brin)** Insoluble protein that is essential to the clotting of blood.

Hematocrit **(he-mat′ah-krit)** Volume percentage of red blood cells in whole blood.

Hemolysis **(he-mol′ĭ-sis)** Release of hemoglobin from red blood cells by destruction of the cells.

Hemostasis **(he″mo-sta′sis)** Stoppage or cessation of bleeding.

Hepatomegaly **(hep″ah-to-meg′ah-le)** Enlargement of the liver.

Hormone **(hor′mōn)** Secreted molecules produced in the body that have a specific regulatory action on target cells that are distant from their sites of synthesis; an endocrine hormone is frequently carried by the blood from its site of release to its target.

Hypercalcemia **(hi″per-kal-se′me-ah)** Excess calcium in the blood.

Hyperglycemia **(hi″per-gli-se′me-ah)** Excess glucose in the blood.

Hypochromic **(hi″po-kro′mik)** Stained less intensely than normal.

Hypophosphatemia **(hi″po-fos″fah-te′me-ah)** Deficiency of phosphates in the blood.

Insulin **(in′sū-lin)** Hormone produced in the pancreas by the beta cells in the islets of Langerhans; insulin regulates glucose metabolism and is the major fuel-regulating hormone.

Insulin shock Profound hypoglycemia, or low blood sugar, that necessitates emergency intervention.

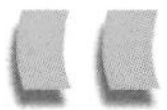

VOCABULARY (continued)

Ketoacidosis (ke"to-ah"sĭ-do'sis) Accumulation of acid in the body resulting from the accumulation of ketone bodies.

Microcyte (mi'kro-sĭt) Red blood cell that is smaller than normal.

Myalgia (mi-al'-jĕ-ah) Muscle pain.

Neutropenia (nu"tro-pe'ne-ah) Decreased number of neutrophils in the blood.

Osteoporosis (os"te-o-po-ro'sis) Abnormal rarefaction of bone.

Parathormone (par"ah-thor'mōn) Parathyroid hormone.

Petechia (pe-te'ke-ah) Minute red spot on the skin or mucous membrane caused by escape of a small amount of blood.

Platelet (plāt'let) Disc-shaped structure, also called a thrombocyte, found in the blood; it plays an important role in blood coagulation.

Polycythemia (pol"e-si-the'me-ah) Increase in the total red blood cell mass in the blood.

Polydipsia (pol"i-dip'se-a) Chronic excessive thirst and intake of fluid.

Purpura (pur'pu-rah) Blood disorders characterized by purplish or brownish-red discolorations caused by bleeding into the skin or tissues.

Receptor (re-sep'ter) Cell surface protein to which a specific hormone can bind; such binding leads to biochemical events.

Splenomegaly (sple"no-meg'ah-le) Enlargement of the spleen.

Thrombocyte (throm'bo-sīt) Platelet.

Thrombocytopenia (throm"bo-si"to-pe'ne-ah) Decrease in the number of platelets in circulating blood.

Many diseases that affect the body as a whole are associated with alterations of the oral mucosa, maxilla, and mandible. Systemic diseases can cause mucosal changes such as ulceration or mucosal bleeding. Generalized immunodeficiency can lead to the development of opportunistic diseases such as infection and neoplasia. Bone disease can affect the maxilla and mandible, and systemic disease can cause dental and periodontal changes. Drugs prescribed for a systemic disease can affect the oral tissues.

Local factors are frequently involved in manifestations of systemic disease in the oral mucosa. In some systemic diseases the mucosa is more easily injured; therefore mild irritation and chronic inflammation can cause lesions that would not occur without the presence of the systemic disease.

This chapter includes systemic diseases that have oral manifestations. Some overlapping occurs among the diseases included in this chapter and those included in other chapters. Some of the diseases discussed in this chapter could have been included appropriately in other chapters. Included here are endocrine disorders, disorders of red and white blood cells, disorders of **platelets** and other bleeding and clotting disorders, and immunodeficiency disorders. Oral changes can be similar for several different systemic diseases, and similar oral lesions can occur without the presence of systemic disease. Because of this, many oral lesions described in this chapter are also described elsewhere in this text.

ENDOCRINE DISORDERS

The endocrine system consists of a group of integrated glands and cells that secrete **hormones**. The secretion of hormones by these glands is controlled by feedback mechanisms in which the amount of hormone circulating in blood triggers factors that control production. Diseases of this system can result from (1) conditions in which too much or too little hormone is produced, and (2) from either dysfunction of the glands themselves or a problem in the mechanism that controls hormone production. Some of the endocrine gland diseases in which oral changes occur are included here.

HYPERPITUITARISM

Hyperpituitarism is excess hormone production by the anterior pituitary gland. It is caused most often by a benign tumor (**pituitary adenoma**) that produces growth hormone.

If the increase in growth hormone production occurs during development before the closure of the long bones, **gigantism** results. **Acromegaly** results when the hypersecretion occurs in adult life.

Clinical Features and Oral Manifestations

Gigantism includes excessive growth of the overall skeleton. Affected individuals can be more than 8 feet tall and weigh several hundred pounds; and as adults they experience headaches, chronic fatigue, and muscle and joint pain.

Acromegaly affects both men and women and most commonly occurs in the fourth decade of life. The onset is slow and insidious. Patients experience poor vision, sensitivity to light, enlargement of the hands and feet, and an increase in rib size. The facial changes include enlargement of the maxilla and mandible, frontal bossing (an enlargement of the bones of the forehead), and enlargement of the nasal bones. An enlargement of the maxillary sinus also occurs, which causes a characteristically deep voice. The enlargement of the maxilla and mandible results in separation of teeth and malocclusion. Mucosal changes such as thickened lips and macroglossia (enlarged tongue) have also been described in patients with acromegaly (Figure 9-1).

Diagnosis and Treatment

The diagnosis of hyperpituitarism involves measurement of growth hormone, and treatment often involves pituitary gland surgery.

HYPERTHYROIDISM

Hyperthyroidism, also called **thyrotoxicosis,** is characterized by excessive production of thyroid hormone. It is much more common in women than in men. Hyperthyroidism has several different causes. The most common cause is a condition called *Graves disease.* The exact cause of Graves disease is not clear, but it appears to result from an autoimmune disorder in which a substance that abnormally stimulates the thyroid gland is produced. Other causes of hyperthyroidism include hyperplasia of the gland, benign and malignant tumors of the thyroid, pituitary gland disease, and metastatic tumors.

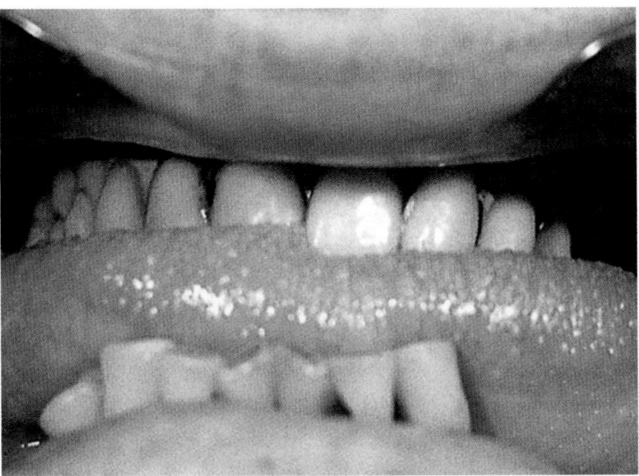

FIGURE 9-1 ■ Enlarged tongue (macroglossia) in a patient with acromegaly.

Clinical Features

The clinical features of hyperthyroidism include goiter, rosy complexion, erythema of the palms, excessive sweating, fine hair, and softened nails. Exophthalmos (protrusion of the eyeballs) may be seen. Anxiety, weakness, restlessness, and cardiac problems may be associated with the disorder.

Oral Manifestations

Hyperthyroidism in children may lead to premature exfoliation of deciduous teeth and premature eruption of permanent teeth. In adults **osteoporosis** may occur, which may affect alveolar bone. Dental caries and periodontal disease appear to develop and progress more rapidly in these patients than in other patients. Burning discomfort of the tongue has also been reported.

Treatment

Treatment of hyperthyroidism may include surgery, medications to suppress thyroid activity, or the administration of radioactive iodine. The treatment of hyperthyroidism is the most common cause of hypothyroidism. Clinical mismanagement of hyperthyroidism may lead to hypothyroidism and is thus described as iatrogenic or clinician-caused disease.

HYPOTHYROIDISM

Hypothyroidism is characterized by decreased output of thyroid hormone. When hypothyroidism is present during infancy and childhood, it is known as **cretinism.** In older children and adults the condition is known as **myxedema.** Causes include developmental disturbances, autoimmune disease, iodine deficiency, drugs, and pituitary disease. In infants facial and oral changes include thickened lips, enlarged tongue, and delayed eruption of teeth. Adults with hypothyroidism may have an enlarged tongue.

HYPERPARATHYROIDISM

Hyperparathyroidism results from excessive secretion of parathyroid hormone (**parathormone**) (PTH), which is secreted by the parathyroid glands. The four parathyroid glands are located near the thyroid gland. PTH plays an important role in calcium and phosphorus metabolism.

Elevated blood levels of calcium (**hypercalcemia**), low levels of blood phosphorus (**hypophosphatemia**), and abnormal bone metabolism characterize hyperparathyroidism.

Hyperparathyroidism may be the result of hyperplasia of the parathyroid glands, a benign tumor of one or more of the parathyroid glands (parathyroid adenoma), or (less commonly) a malignant parathyroid tumor. The disease is found in middle-age adults and is far more common in women than in men.

Calcium is obtained mainly from dairy products and plays an important role in the contraction of all types of muscle. PTH maintains normal blood levels of calcium through its effects on the kidney, gastrointestinal tract, and bone. It increases the uptake of dietary calcium from the gastrointestinal tract and is able to move calcium from bone to circulating blood when necessary. The hormone appears to be able to remove calcium from bone through the action of osteoclasts.

Hyperparathyroidism that results from an abnormality of the parathyroid glands is called *primary hyperparathyroidism*. Secondary hyperparathyroidism occurs when calcium is abnormally excreted by the kidneys and the parathyroid glands increase their production of PTH to maintain adequate blood levels of calcium. The most common cause of secondary hyperparathyroidism is kidney failure. Problems with absorption of nutrients and fat-soluble vitamins such as vitamin D through the gut or small intestine are also an important cause of hyperparathyroidism.

Clinical Features

The clinical manifestations of hyperparathyroidism are varied. Patients with mild cases can be asymptomatic. Joint pain or stiffness may be present. The disease can affect the kidneys, skeletal system, and gastrointestinal system. In severe disease lethargy and coma can occur.

Oral Manifestations

The oral manifestations of hyperparathyroidism include changes in the bone of the mandible and maxilla. The chief oral manifestation is the appearance of well-defined unilocular or multilocular radiolucencies (Figure 9-2, *A*). Microscopically these lesions appear indistinguishable from central giant cell granulomas (described in Chapter 2) (Figure 9-2, *B*). There have also been reports of a few cases of peripheral giant cell granulomas associated with hyperparathyroidism. Other radiographic changes that occur in hyperparathyroidism include a generalized mottled appearance of the bone and partial loss of the lamina dura. Loosening of teeth can also occur.

Diagnosis and Treatment

The diagnosis of hyperparathyroidism involves the measurement of PTH blood levels and can also include serum calcium and phosphorus measurements. Treatment is directed at correcting the cause of the increased production of the hormone. Causes of increased production of hormone can include tumors, renal disease, and vitamin D deficiency. Bone lesions resolve when the hyperparathyroidism is treated successfully.

DIABETES MELLITUS

Diabetes mellitus is a chronic disorder of carbohydrate (glucose) metabolism and is characterized by abnormally high blood glucose levels (**hyperglycemia**), which result from a lack of the hormone **insulin**, defective insulin that does not work effectively to lower blood glucose levels, or increased insulin resistance because of obesity. Diabetes is appropriately considered a syndrome because it has several components, including both acute and chronic complications. This

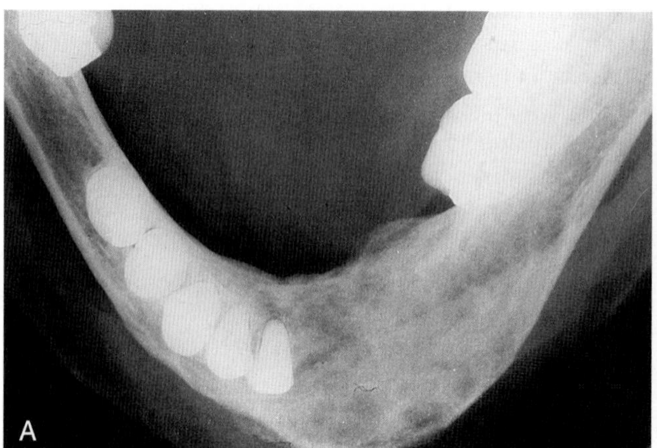

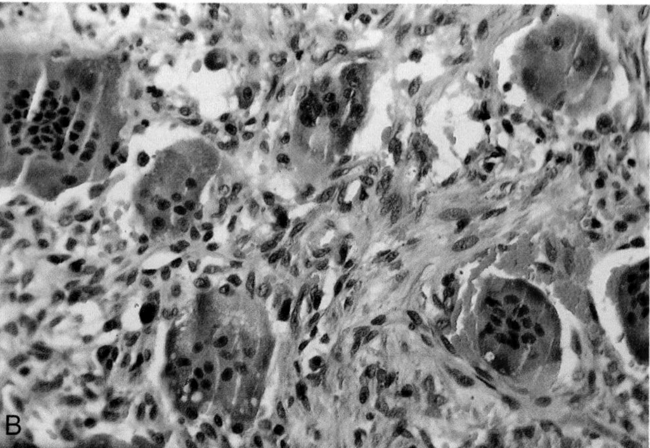

FIGURE 9-2 ■ **A,** Radiograph of a mandibular lesion in a patient with hyperparathyroidism. **B,** Microscopic appearance of a jaw lesion occurring in a patient with hyperparathyroidism. The histologic appearance is identical to that of a central giant cell granuloma. (**A** courtesy Drs. Paul Freedman and Stanley Kerpel.)

disorder of carbohydrate metabolism also leads to disorders of protein and fat metabolism. Normally glucose signals the beta cells of the pancreas to make insulin. This hormone is then secreted directly into the bloodstream to facilitate the uptake of glucose into fat and skeletal muscle cells. In the presence of insulin, fat and skeletal muscle cells can use glucose as an energy source. When insulin is lacking, these cells are starved of energy. Without insulin to meet the body's demand for carbohydrate, tissues are broken down (**catabolism**), and weight loss occurs, as well as severe hyperglycemia that can lead to diabetic coma. Furthermore, the production of ketone acid from the breakdown of fatty tissue is a life-threatening condition and is a common metabolic disturbance in type 1 (insulin-dependent) diabetes. These ketone acids (acetone) can lower the pH of the blood (**ketoacidosis**), an acute condition that can lead to coma and death. White blood cell function is affected in patients with diabetes mellitus. Phagocytic activity of macrophages is reduced; chemotaxis of neutrophils is delayed; and lymphocyte function (T lymphocytes) is also adversely affected. These changes increase a patient's susceptibility to infection. In addition, collagen production is abnormal, thus affecting the healing process. With chronic hyperglycemia, collagen and other proteins become tagged with carbohydrate. These resulting advanced glycation end products (AGEs) impair healing and may also play a contributory role in the progression of atherosclerosis. Atherosclerosis leads to death of heart muscle (myocardial infarction or heart attack), stroke, and kidney failure.

The precise cause of diabetes mellitus is unknown. Genetic and environmental factors have been implicated in its onset. Sixteen million Americans have been diagnosed with diabetes mellitus. It is estimated that an additional seven million Americans have undiagnosed diabetes and therefore are at risk for life-threatening complications of untreated diabetes.

Types of Diabetes

Insulin-Dependent Diabetes Mellitus

Two major types of diabetes have been recognized and classified. The first type **(type 1 diabetes)** is called **insulin-dependent diabetes mellitus (IDDM). Autoimmunity** appears to play a key role in the development of type 1 diabetes, leading to the destruction of the insulin-producing beta cells of the pancreas and ultimately profound insulin deficiency. Only 3% of all diabetic patients have this type of diabetes. Type 1 diabetes can occur at any age, but its time of onset is usually at a peak age of 20 years. The onset is abrupt and can have the three Ps (or the complications of these signs): (1) **polydipsia** (excessive thirst and intake of fluid), (2) **polyuria** (excessive urination), and (3) **polyphagia** (excessive appetite). Patients usually have a thin body build.

Complications can occur in 90% of individuals with type 1 diabetes within 20 years of diagnosis. Difficulty in controlling blood glucose levels is a major problem for patients with IDDM. In recent years it has become increasingly evident that long-term rigorous control of blood glucose levels is important in minimizing the extent of chronic complications in patients with IDDM. Damage to the small blood vessels (microvascular disease) in diabetes leads to complications with organ systems; these include particularly the eye, kidney, and nerves. Atherosclerosis of medium-size blood vessels (macrovascular disease) in diabetes affects, for example, the coronary and cerebral arteries. The former supply blood to the heart, whereas the latter bring blood to the brain. Macrovascular disease is best minimized, however, with good control of serum cholesterol and blood pressure. Thus, a diabetic must control not only blood sugar but also serum cholesterol and blood pressure to reduce the likelihood of vascular complications. Rigorous control of glucose is more likely achieved with multiple subcutaneous injections of insulin throughout the day to simulate physiologic conditions rather than with a single daily injection. Multiple insulin injections, proper diet, exercise, and frequent determinations of blood glucose levels at home constitute the current approach to the management of the patient with type 1 diabetes. In some cases oral hypoglycemic medications (typically used in type 2 diabetes) are added as part of the medical management of patients with type 1 diabetes. These drugs may enhance the action of injected insulin. However, multiple insulin injections can more readily lead to low blood sugar **(hypoglycemia)**; severe hypoglycemia (**insulin shock**) constitutes a medical emergency. The disease is controlled by replacement of the hormone insulin; however, insulin injections are not a cure for diabetes. All patients with IDDM remain dependent on insulin for their entire lives. Studies are now in progress to assess the efficacy of nasal preparations of insulin; to monitor the transplantation of insulin-producing beta cells to control blood glucose in humans; and to determine if stem cell infusions into animals will reverse diabetes. If these approaches are successful, some patients may be spared from life-time injections.

An increasing number of patients with type 1 diabetes are now entering insulin pump therapy. The patient must still monitor blood sugar levels by testing several times a day. The insulin pump is external and approximately the size of a pager; it delivers insulin through plastic tubing placed under the skin. The patient programs the pump to deliver small amounts of rapid-acting insulin on the hour over a 24-hour period according to the patient's metabolic needs. Thus the pump can maintain even more rigorous, predictable control of blood sugar levels than multiple insulin injections. Insulin dosage with the pump is also lower than with multiple insulin injections, making life-threatening hypoglycemia less frequent. Very recent advances in technology now include replaceable blood glucose sensors in the pump. These sensors monitor blood glucose levels and have an alarm to tell the patient when glucose levels are too low or too high. However, the blood glucose sensors do not tell the pump how much insulin to automatically deliver to the patient. The patient must still deliver the insulin from the pump because the pump still lacks "a brain." Frequent blood sugar testing is still necessary. With further advances in pump technology, the sensor may tell the pump if the blood sugar is too high and then the pump might automatically deliver the right amount of insulin to match the blood sugar for that patient. Such improvements in pump design would then "close the loop," and possibly represent the technological equivalent of a cure for diabetes. The patient with diabetes who uses insulin pump therapy should carry a backup supply of syringes in case the pump fails to deliver insulin; such failure can lead to the rapid development of ketoacidosis, resulting in signs and symptoms of nausea, abdominal cramps, disorientation, and fatigue.

Noninsulin-Dependent Diabetes Mellitus

The second type **(type 2 diabetes)** is **noninsulin-dependent diabetes mellitus (NIDDM).** Increased insulin resistance, rather than profound insulin deficiency, is characteristic of type 2 diabetes. Approximately 95% of all diabetic patients have type 2 diabetes. The onset of this type of diabetes is gradual and usually occurs in patients who are 35 to 40 years of age or older. When the metabolic rate starts to slow down with age, on comes the contributing factor of weight gain. However, there is now an epidemic of type 2 diabetes among children in major U.S. cities, particularly in minority neighborhoods; this epidemic has significant social, cultural, and ethical dimensions. Poor, high-crime neighborhoods in the inner cities restrict control of free space; people are less likely to get out and exercise; this may contribute to obesity. Hence, where you live may be an even more important determinant in developing type 2 diabetes than a person's genetic make-up. Fast-food companies also target their advertisements to the minority neighborhoods where less expensive but high-caloric food is a strong inducement—this is an ethically objectionable practice because it causes harm. Children are thus likely to succumb to pressures from other children and eat high caloric foods. Studies have shown that second- and third-generation individuals whose parents were born in countries with a low diabetes rate ultimately approximate the diabetes rate in the United States. The Western diet is "obesogenic." The urban minority populations tragically bear the brunt of diabetes in the United States and suffer from its myriad life-threatening complications. Dentists and dental hygienists can play a major role in educating their patients about diabetes and oral health and, in doing so, advance public health.

Obesity is a common finding in many people with type 2 diabetes, and therefore, this form of diabetes may be preventable. Obesity probably decreases the number of **receptors** for insulin binding in sensitive tissues such as fat and muscle, thereby leading to the development of the diabetic state. Hormones from fatty tissue (adipokines) may also contribute to insulin resistance. Complications are less common in this type of diabetes than in type 1 diabetes. However, the onset of type 2 diabetes among children is of extreme concern because life-threatening and debilitating complications may occur in young adulthood at the active peak of life. Some patients achieve control of blood glucose levels with diet and weight reduction alone, whereas others require oral hypoglycemic agents. These medications also lower blood glucose levels but, unlike insulin, are not given by injection. However, some patients with type 2 diabetes require insulin injections to obtain control of blood glucose levels. In April 2005 the Food and Drug Administration approved Byetta, an injectable product for the treatment of type 2 diabetes; it was made available to pharmacies in June 2005. Byetta is not insulin. It is delivered subcutaneously (like insulin) at a fixed dose before the morning and evening meals. Byetta lowers blood sugar and has the potential to help restore the response of the body's insulin-producing cells. Hypoglycemia is also less frequent than with insulin administration and occurs when patients are taking only a specific type of oral medication. This relatively new drug represents a significant advance in the management of type 2 diabetes for patients who cannot control their blood sugar by past conventional therapy.

Clinical Features

The vascular system is the most severely affected system in diabetes, leading to a myriad number of devastating systemic complications. Accelerated atherosclerosis (thickening of the blood vessel wall from fibrofatty plaques), is a common complication of diabetes leading to impaired circulation of blood and impaired transport of oxygen and nutrients to tissues. Heart attack caused by atherosclerosis of the coronary arteries is the most common cause of death among patients with diabetes. This blood vessel disease also increases the risk of ulceration and gangrene of the feet, high blood pressure, kidney failure, and stroke. Gangrene of the lower extremities is about 100 times more common in patients with diabetes than in the general population. Blood vessel changes in the eye (diabetic retinopathy, microvascular, or small artery disease) can lead to hemorrhage, which can result in blindness. The nervous system can also be affected in diabetes. This is partly the result of vascular damage and results in a variety of neurological complaints such as numbness or tingling in the fingers and toes. A patient with frost-bite, for example, may have little or no feeling in the fingers or toes. In such instances, the frost-bite may lead to death of tissue, necessitating amputation of fingers or toes. Decreased resistance to infection is seen, particularly in uncontrolled diabetes. Skin infections, especially furuncles (boils), urinary tract infections, and tuberculosis are common.

A skin disorder called **acanthosis nigrans** has been reported to be associated with type 2 diabetes mellitus and has been suggested to be a useful clinical indicator in screening for type 2 diabetes. Obesity in children and adults appears to increase the risk of development of this skin condition.

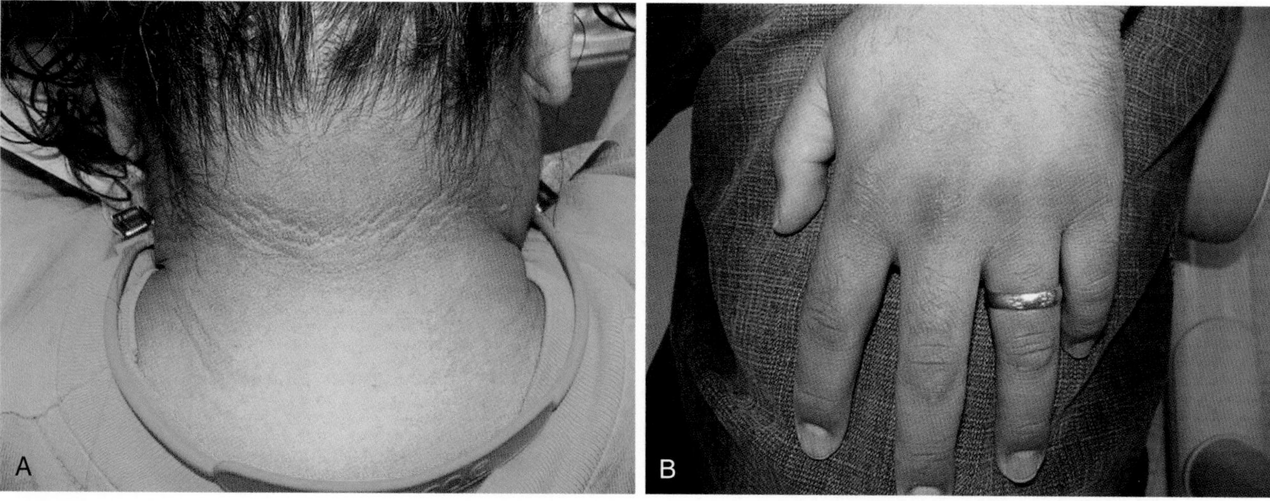

FIGURE 9-3 ■ **A,** Acanthosis nigricans affecting the back of the neck. **B,** Acanthosis nigricans affecting the hand. (Courtesy Lang Crawford.)

Acanthosis nigricans is characterized by hyperpigmented, velvety-textured plaques that appear symmetrically distributed in folds and creases of the body. Acanthosis nigricans affecting the neck (Figure 9-3, *A*) and hands (Figure 9-3, *B*) may be identified by the dental hygienist during physical/clinical evaluation of a patient.

Oral Complications

The oral complications of diabetes are most severe when blood glucose levels are not controlled. In some patients control is difficult, even with careful monitoring of these levels and insulin injections. These patients are said to have **brittle diabetes** and may benefit from recent advances with insulin pump therapy.

Increased colonization of the oral mucosa by *Candida albicans* and an increased prevalence of oral candidiasis have been reported in patients with diabetes mellitus, as has mucormycosis, a rare fungal infection that affects the palate and maxillary sinuses. These infections generally are seen in poorly controlled or uncontrolled diabetes mellitus. (Both oral candidiasis and mucormycosis are described in Chapter 4.) The presence of such fungal infections is indicative of compromised innate and acquired immune responses that occur in diabetes mellitus.

Bilateral, asymptomatic parotid gland enlargement occurs in some patients; this results from either a deposition of fat or hypertrophy of the salivary gland tissue.

Xerostomia (dry mouth) is usually associated with uncontrolled diabetes mellitus. Dehydration of the oral tissues can result, increasing the risk of the development of oral candidiasis and dental caries, and may diminish taste sensation. Altered subgingival flora has been described in diabetes and may be the result of immunologic or salivary changes. Other significant oral findings include burning mouth syndrome, which may or may not be related to xerostomia. Burning mouth or tongue has been reported to occur in undiagnosed cases of type 2 diabetes. These may mostly resolve after medical diagnosis of the diabetes and subsequent treatment toward improving blood sugar control. Xerostomia can be a physically and psychologically debilitating condition.

Patients with diabetes mellitus have an accentuated response to plaque. The gingiva can be hyperplastic and erythematous, and acute and fulminating gingival abscesses can occur. Excessive periodontal bone loss, tooth mobility, and early tooth loss can also be associated with diabetes mellitus (Figure 9-4). Periodontal disease is considered to be a significant complication of diabetes. Slow wound healing and increased susceptibility to infection occur as a result of the immunologic changes and defective collagen production.

The patient with diabetes who is receiving good medical management and whose glucose levels are controlled can receive any indicated dental treatment. Early identification of oral infections is important. Infection aggravates diabetes because it often results in the loss of blood glucose control, thus creating a vicious cycle because susceptibility to infection is increased. Therefore elimination of infection is extremely important in patients with diabetes. Antibiotic medication, calculus and plaque removal, effective oral hygiene care, and adequate nutrition are especially important in the management of the patient with diabetes. One final point deserves mention here. People with well-controlled diabetes of either type can lead long, productive lives. However, diabetes control is not an "in-between." A patient either controls his or her diabetes, or does not—there is also no such thing as "mild" diabetes. Good control of diabetes represents a synthesis of effort between the physician, nurse, nutritionist, dentist, and dental hygienist. It is truly a team effort.

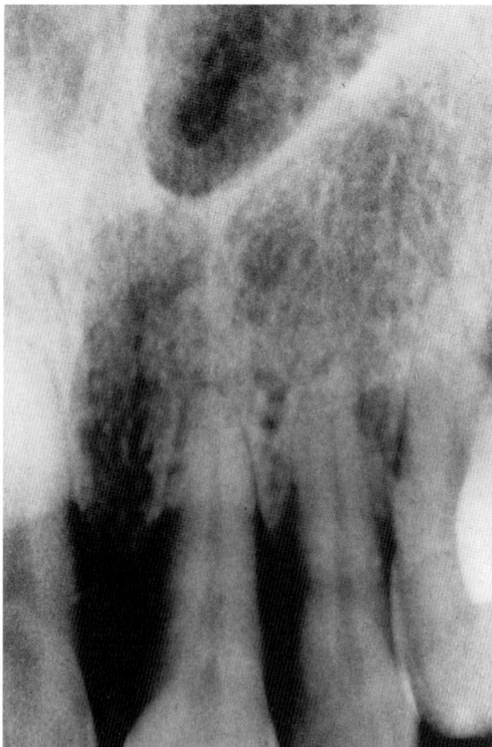

FIGURE 9-4 ■ Periapical radiograph of a patient with diabetes mellitus shows severe alveolar bone loss.

ADDISON DISEASE

Addison disease, also known as **primary adrenal cortical insufficiency**, is characterized by an insufficient production of adrenal steroids. A malignant tumor or tuberculosis may be responsible for destruction of the adrenal gland. However, in most cases the cause of the destruction of the adrenal cortex is unknown. In these patients the condition may be an autoimmune disease. Another known common cause is the spread of tuberculosis infection to the adrenal gland.

As a result of the decreased production of adrenal steroids, the pituitary gland increases its production of adrenocorticotropic hormone, which would normally increase the production of adrenal steroids. This hormone is similar to melanin-stimulating hormone and causes stimulation of melanocytes. Brown pigmentation (bronzing) of the skin occurs, and melanotic macules can develop on the oral mucosa. Treatment of Addison disease involves steroid replacement therapy.

BLOOD DISORDERS

The **complete blood count (CBC)** is important in the diagnosis of blood disorders. The CBC is a series of tests that examines the red blood cells, white blood cells, and platelets. It provides information about the number of each type of cell, the ratio of types of cells, and the appearance of the cells. The information included in a CBC and normal values are included in Box 9-1.

Box 9-1

Complete Blood Count Normal Adult Values

Red Blood Cells

Count: The total number of red blood cells (RBCs) mm^3 of whole blood
- Males: 4.6-6.2 × 10^6
- Females: 4.2-5.4 × 10^6

Hemoglobin: The amount of hemoglobin contained in 100 ml of whole blood
- Males: 13.5-18 g
- Females: 12-16 g

Hematocrit: The volume of packed RBCs in 100 ml of whole blood
- Males: 40%-54%
- Females: 38%-47%

Indices: Mean corpuscular (cell) volume: describes the average size of an individual RBC
- 80-96 mm^3

Mean corpuscular (cell) hemoglobin: indicates the amount of hemoglobin present in an RBC by weight
- 27-31 pg

Mean corpuscular (cell) hemoglobin concentration: indicates the proportion of each cell occupied by hemoglobin
- 32%-36%

White Blood Cells

Count: 4,000-11,000 mm^3

Differential count: The number of each type of white blood cell (WBC) expressed as a percentage of the total number of WBCs

Mature neutrophils (granulocytes)	50%-60%
Immature neutrophils (bands)	2%-4%
Lymphocytes	30%-40%
Monocytes	1%-9%
Basophils	0%-1%
Eosinophils	2%-3%

DISORDERS OF RED BLOOD CELLS AND HEMOGLOBIN

Anemia

Anemia is defined as a reduction in the oxygen-carrying capacity of the blood that in most cases is related to a decrease in the number of circulating red blood cells. There are many different types and causes of anemia.

Nutritional anemias occur when a substance necessary for the normal development of red blood cells is in scant supply in the bone marrow. The most common deficiencies are of iron, folic acid, or vitamin B_{12}. These deficiencies can occur when the intake of the nutrient is insufficient or when disorders of absorption prevent its uptake. Anemia can also occur when suppression of the bone marrow stem cells takes place, resulting in an inability of the bone marrow to produce red blood cells.

Oral manifestations are similar for all types of anemia and include skin and mucosal pallor, angular cheilitis, erythema and atrophy of the oral mucosa, and loss of filiform and fungiform papillae on the dorsum of the tongue. Circumvallate papillae and foliate papillae are not affected.

Iron Deficiency Anemia

Iron deficiency anemia occurs when an insufficient amount of iron is supplied to the bone marrow for red blood cell development. This type of anemia can occur as a result of a deficiency of iron intake, blood loss from heavy menstrual bleeding or chronic gastrointestinal bleeding, poor iron absorption, or an increased requirement for iron as in pregnancy or infancy.

The Plummer-Vinson syndrome can develop as a result of long-standing iron deficiency anemia. This syndrome includes dysphagia (difficulty swallowing), atrophy of the upper alimentary tract, and a predisposition to the development of oral cancer.

Clinical Features and Oral Manifestations

Iron deficiency anemia is most often asymptomatic. Nonspecific symptoms such as weakness and fatigue can occur. Oral mucosal signs in severe cases include angular cheilitis; pallor of the oral tissues; and an erythematous, smooth, painful tongue (Figure 9-5). The changes in the oral mucosa occur as a result of a lack of nutrients to the epithelium. The filiform papillae on the dorsum of the tongue disappear first because they have the highest metabolic requirements. Disappearance of the fungiform papillae can also occur in chronic and severe cases.

Diagnosis and Treatment

The diagnosis of iron deficiency anemia is made by laboratory tests, which show a low hemoglobin content of red blood cells and a reduced **hematocrit** value. Iron is needed for hemoglobin synthesis; therefore in iron deficiency anemia the red blood cells appear smaller than normal (microcytic) and lighter in color than normal (**hypochromic**). Increasing the intake of iron is the treatment for iron deficiency anemia; dietary supplements are usually used. The oral lesions resolve when the deficiency is corrected.

Pernicious Anemia

Pernicious anemia is a vitamin B_{12} deficiency that is caused by a deficiency of intrinsic factor, a substance secreted by the parietal cells of the stomach. Intrinsic factor is necessary for the absorption of vitamin B_{12}. Normally vitamin B_{12} is transported across the intestinal mucosa by intrinsic factor. An autoimmune mechanism is the most likely cause of pernicious anemia. Antibodies to components of gastric mucosa have been identified in patients with pernicious anemia. Other causes include surgical removal of the stomach (gastrectomy), gastric cancer, or gastritis. Vitamin B_{12} is needed for deoxyribonucleic acid (DNA) synthesis; when it is lacking, the development of rapidly dividing cells such as bone marrow cells and epithelial cells is affected.

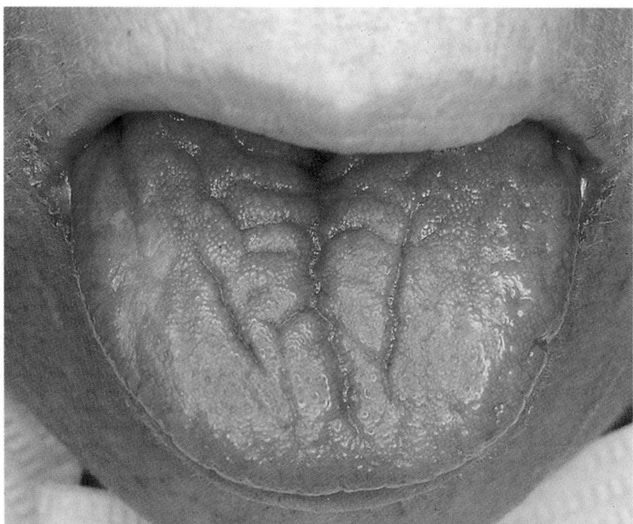

FIGURE 9-5 ■ Iron deficiency anemia. The tongue is devoid of filiform papillae. Angular cheilitis was also present in this patient.

Clinical Features and Oral Manifestations

The clinical signs of pernicious anemia are weakness, pallor, and fatigue on exertion. Other constitutional signs can include nausea, dizziness, diarrhea, abdominal pain, loss of appetite, and weight loss. Neurologic changes such as severe paresthesia may also occur in patients with pernicious anemia.

Oral manifestations of pernicious anemia include angular cheilitis; mucosal pallor; painful, atrophic and erythematous mucosa; mucosal ulceration; loss of papillae on the dorsum of the tongue; and burning and painful tongue (Figure 9-6).

Diagnosis and Treatment

The diagnosis of pernicious anemia is made by laboratory testing. The diagnostic features include low serum vitamin B_{12} levels and gastric achlorhydria (lack of hydrochloric acid). Pernicious anemia is a megaloblastic anemia. **Megaloblastic anemia** is characterized by red blood cells that are immature, abnormally large, and have nuclei (**megaloblasts**). Immature neutrophils and platelets are also seen in both the bone marrow and the circulating blood. The Schilling test, which detects an inability to absorb an oral dose of vitamin B_{12} (cyanocobalamin), is another method used to diagnose pernicious anemia. Treatment consists of injections of vitamin B_{12}.

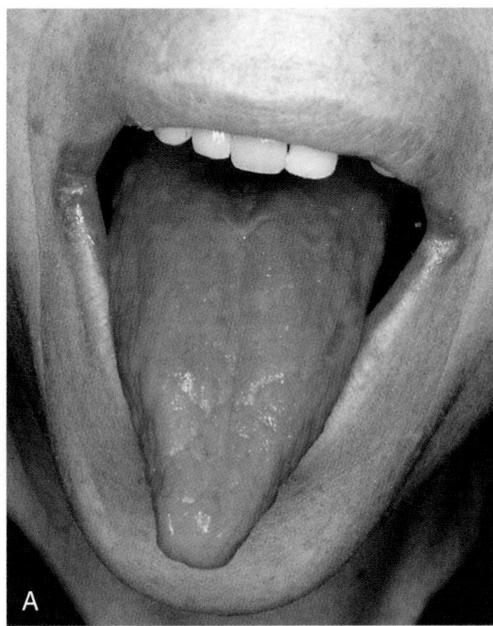
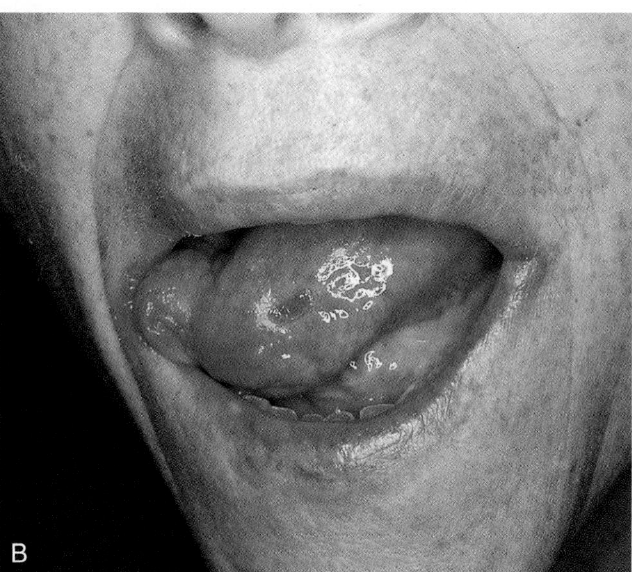

FIGURE 9-6 ■ Pernicious anemia. **A,** Angular cheilitis and depapillation of the tongue in a patient with pernicious anemia. **B,** The mucosa becomes atrophic in pernicious anemia and easily ulcerated. Note ulcer on left lateral aspect of tongue.

The oral mucosa improves in time, but the papillae on the dorsum of the tongue may not regenerate completely.

Folic Acid and Vitamin B_{12} Deficiency Anemia

Dietary deficiencies of **folic acid** and **vitamin B_{12}** can result in anemia and can occur in association with malnutrition and increased metabolic requirements. Malnutrition can occur in association with alcoholism, and pregnant women can experience a deficiency because of increased metabolic demands. Folic acid and vitamin B_{12} are essential for DNA synthesis.

Oral Manifestations

The oral manifestations are indistinguishable from those of pernicious anemia.

Diagnosis and Treatment

The diagnosis of these anemias is based on laboratory test results that include serum assays of folic acid and vitamin B_{12}. These are also megaloblastic anemias. Thus, as in pernicious anemia, the red blood cells are immature, abnormally large, and nucleated (megaloblasts). Treatment involves dietary supplements.

Thalassemia

Thalassemia, also called *Mediterranean* or **Cooley anemia,** is the name of a group of inherited disorders of hemoglobin synthesis. It has an autosomal inheritance pattern; no predilection for either sex is seen. The heterozygous form (see Chapter 6), in which only one gene at a locus is involved, is called **thalassemia minor** and can be asymptomatic or only mildly symptomatic. The homozygous form, in which the genes on both chromosomes are involved, is called **thalassemia major** and is associated with severe hemolytic anemia, which results from damage to the red blood cell membranes and destruction of the red blood cells.

Clinical Features and Oral Manifestations

The severe form of the disease begins early in life. The child has a yellowish skin pallor, fever, malaise, and weakness. An enlarged liver and spleen are common. The characteristic facies includes prominent cheekbones, depression of the bridge of the nose, an unusual prominence of the premaxilla, and protrusion or flaring of the maxillary anterior teeth. Intraoral radiographs show a peculiar trabecular pattern of the maxilla and mandible. There is a prominence of some trabeculae and a blurring and disappearance of others, resulting in a "salt and pepper" effect. Thinning of the lamina dura and circular radiolucencies in the alveolar bone have also been described.

Treatment

Treatment of thalassemia major is experimental. Blood transfusions and splenectomy have provided periods of remission. The prognosis is poor. However, these supportive therapies have extended life from early childhood to about 20 years of age.

Sickle Cell Anemia

Sickle cell anemia is an inherited disorder of the blood that is found predominantly in black individuals and those of Mediterranean origin. Persons who are heterozygous for the disease are generally asymptomatic. This is called **sickle cell trait.** Those who are homozygous are much more severely affected. The disease presents before age 30 years. Sickle cell anemia occurs as a result of an abnormal type of hemoglobin in red blood cells. Because of this abnormal hemoglobin, the cells develop a sickle shape in the presence of decreased oxygen; hence the name *sickle cell anemia.* Exercise, exertion, administration of a general anesthetic, pregnancy, or even sleep can trigger a sickling of the red blood cells. Because of the change in their shape, the red blood cells are no longer able to pass through small blood vessels and are destroyed more rapidly than normal.

Clinical Features and Oral Manifestations

The patient with sickle cell anemia experiences weakness, shortness of breath, fatigue, joint pain, and nausea. Oral manifestations are seen on dental radiographs (Figure 9-7). A loss of trabeculation takes place, with the appearance of large, irregular marrow spaces. This change is most prominent in the alveolar bone. Changes in the skull have been described as a hair-on-end pattern because the trabeculae radiate outward.

Diagnosis and Treatment

The sickle-shaped cells are seen on a blood smear (Figure 9-8). The number of red blood cells is usually low, as is the hemoglobin content. Management of sickle cell anemia is largely symptomatic and supportive and involves the administration of oxygen and intravenous and oral fluids. Sickle cell anemia can result in profound changes of the heart such as enlargement and lead to cardiac failure.

Celiac Sprue

Celiac sprue is a chronic disorder associated with sensitivity to dietary gluten, a protein found in wheat and wheat products. When gluten is ingested, there is injury to the intestinal mucosa. Malabsorption of other nutrients such as vitamin B_{12} and folic acid occurs because of mucosal injury. As a result, anemia and the oral and clinical signs associated with it develop.

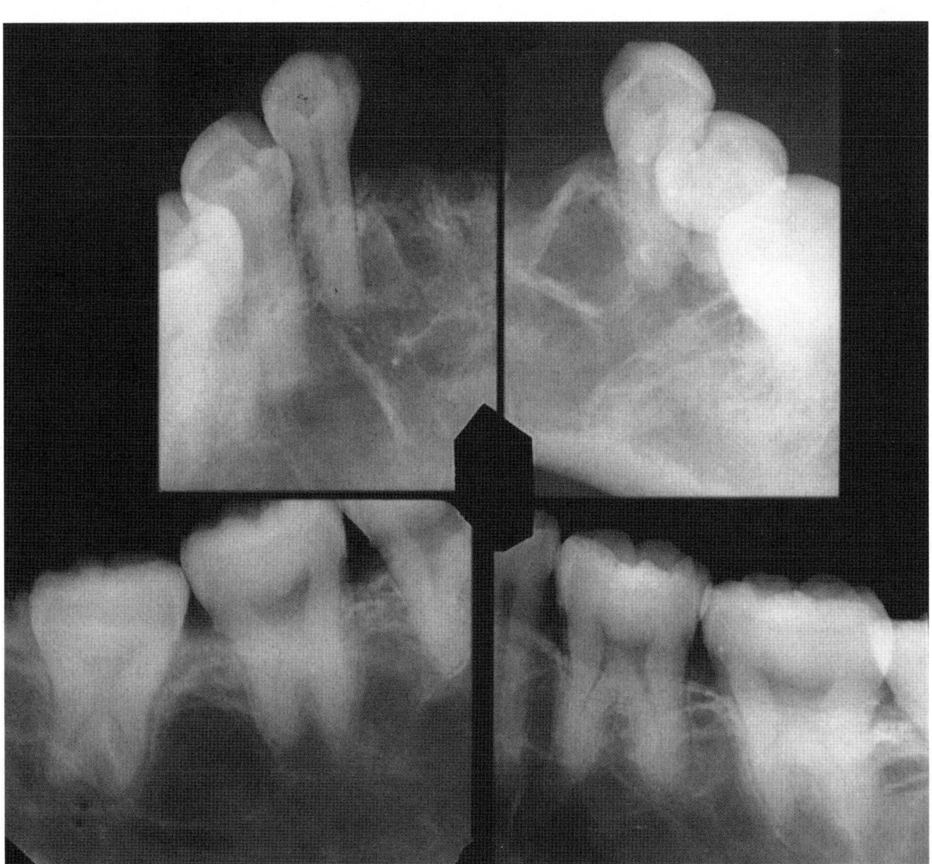

FIGURE 9-7 ■ Sickle cell anemia. Radiograph shows abnormal trabeculation. (Courtesy Dr. Edward V. Zegarelli.)

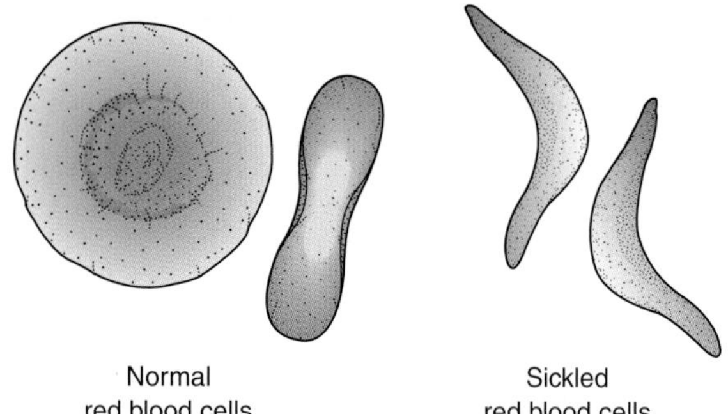

FIGURE 9-8 ■ Sickled red blood cells compared with normal red blood cells.

Clinical Features and Oral Manifestations

Systemic symptoms include diarrhea, nervousness, and paresthesia of the extremities. Oral manifestations include a painful burning tongue (glossitis), atrophy of the papillae of the tongue, and ulceration of the oral mucosa.

Diagnosis and Treatment

Patients should adhere to a gluten-free diet. Oral manifestations resolve when the systemic disease is under control.

Aplastic Anemia

In **aplastic anemia** patients experience a dramatic decrease in all the circulating blood cells (**pancytopenia**) because of a severe depression of bone marrow activity. All the blood cells are produced in the marrow (Figure 9-9). The cause of primary aplastic anemia is unknown. In secondary aplastic anemia the bone marrow failure is a result of a drug or chemical agent. Chemotherapy, radioactive isotopes, radium, and radiant energy have been associated with the development of aplastic anemia. Primary aplastic anemia occurs most frequently in young adults.

Oral Manifestations

These are related to the generalized decrease in white blood cells and platelets and include infection, spontaneous bleeding, **petechiae,** and purpuric spots (Figure 9-10).

Diagnosis and Treatment

In both forms of aplastic anemia a generalized decrease of circulating blood cells occurs. In addition to anemia, **leukopenia** (a decrease in white blood cells) and **thrombocytopenia** (a decrease in platelets) occur. White blood cells are essential in the defense against infection (see Chapters 3 and 4), and platelets are essential in the clotting of blood. Primary aplastic anemia is usually progressive and fatal. Treatment of secondary aplastic anemia involves removing the cause.

Polycythemia

Polycythemia is characterized by an increase in the number of circulating red blood cells. This increase can be either absolute or relative. Normal red blood cell production is carefully regulated and involves both the precursor cells in the bone marrow and the hormone erythropoietin, which is produced by the kidney.

Types of Polycythemia

The three forms of polycythemia are (1) polycythemia vera (primary polycythemia), (2) secondary polycythemia, and (3) relative polycythemia.

Polycythemia Vera (Primary Polycythemia). In polycythemia vera a neoplastic proliferation of bone marrow stem cells results in an abnormally high number of circulating red blood cells. The production of red blood cells is uncontrolled. The cause of this disorder is unknown. It is somewhat more common in men than in women, and the age of onset is usually between 40 and 60 years. It is generally seen in white individuals and is extremely rare in black individuals. The symptoms of polycythemia vera include headache, dizziness, and itching of the skin (pruritus). The increase in red blood cells leads to impaired blood flow, vascular stasis, and poor circulation. The formation of thrombi can cause a disruption of the blood supply to the brain, heart, or peripheral vessels. A decrease in platelets (thrombocytopenia) can occur because of the disruption of the marrow from which they are derived.

Secondary Polycythemia. In secondary polycythemia the increase in red blood cells is caused by a physiologic response to decreased oxygen. A decrease in oxygen in the blood triggers an increase in erythropoietin by the kidneys, which results in increased production of red blood cells. A number of factors can cause a decrease in oxygen, including pulmonary disease, heart disease, living at high altitudes, and an elevation in carbon monoxide. The increase in carbon monoxide has been associated with tobacco smoking.

Relative Polycythemia. This is caused by a decreased plasma volume and not an increase in red blood cells. In acute forms the cause is usually easily recognized. Causes of acute relative polycythemia include diuretic use, vomiting, diarrhea, or excessive sweating. A chronic form of relative polycythemia has been called stress polycythemia. Most patients with this type of polycythemia are middle-age white men who are under physiologic stress, mildly overweight, hypertensive, and heavy smokers. The risk of cerebrovascular accidents (stroke) and myocardial infarction (heart attack) is increased in these patients.

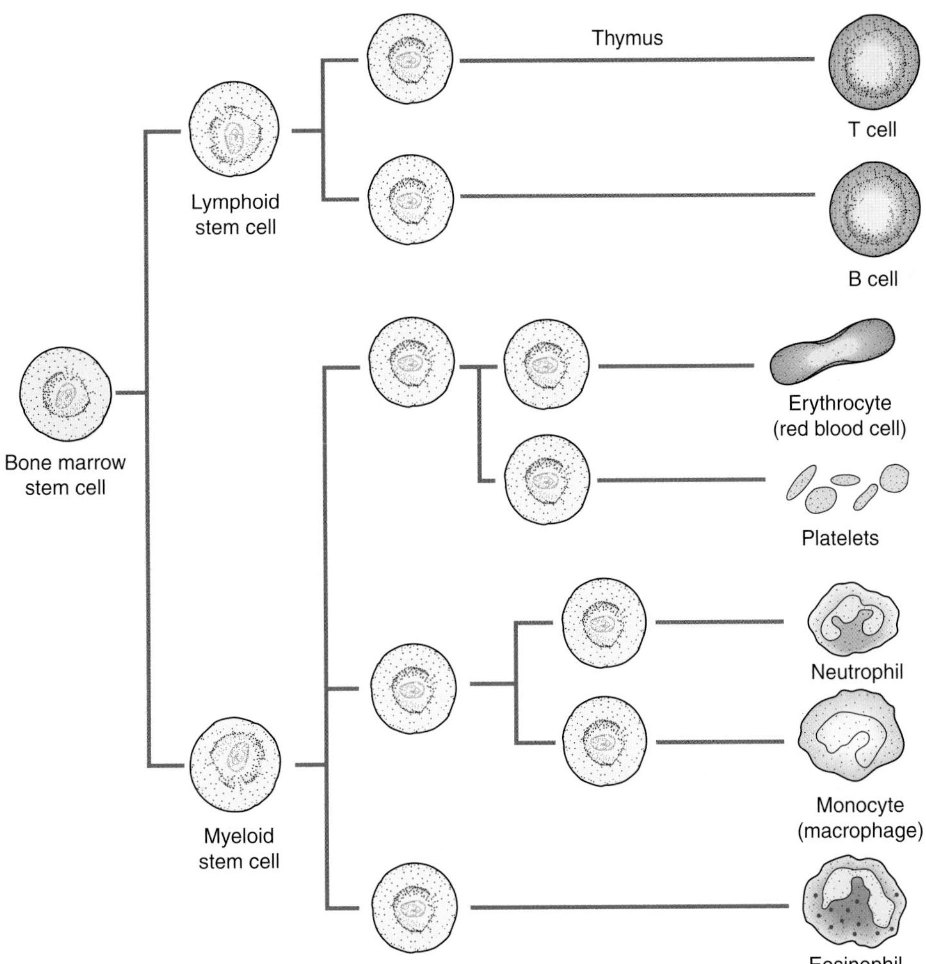

FIGURE 9-9 ■ Blood cells are derived from stem cells in the bone marrow.

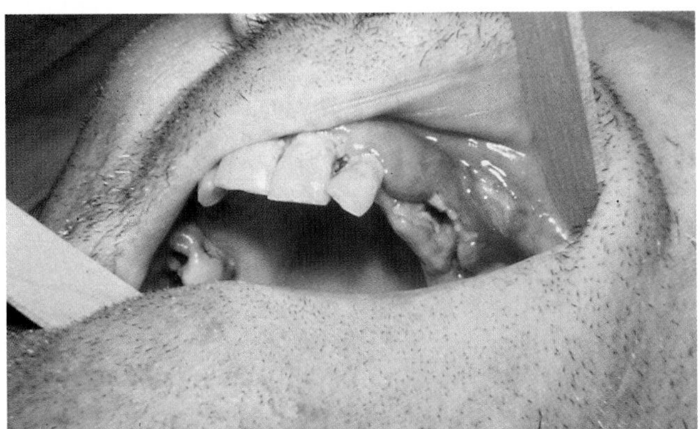

FIGURE 9-10 ■ Aplastic anemia. Severe oral infection occurred after extraction of teeth in this patient with aplastic anemia. (Courtesy Dr. Harry Lumerman.)

Oral Manifestations

The oral mucosa in patients with polycythemia may appear deep red to purple, and the gingiva may be edematous. The gingiva may bleed easily, and submucosal petechiae, **ecchymosis,** and hematoma formation can be present. There can be excessive bleeding after oral surgical procedures. Abnormalities of the oral mucosa result from an increase in circulating red blood cells, the impaired blood flow, and thrombocytopenia.

Diagnosis and Treatment

Diagnosis of the different forms of polycythemia involves laboratory testing and measurement of the hemoglobin content and the hematocrit. Treatment is related to the type of polycythemia and may include removal of causative factors, chemotherapy, and phlebotomy (bloodletting). Oral lesions generally do not require local treatment; however, patients tend to have increased bleeding after oral surgery.

DISORDERS OF WHITE BLOOD CELLS

Three groups of white blood cells are found in the circulation: granulocytes, lymphocytes, and monocytes. The three types of granulocytes are polymorphonuclear leukocytes (neutrophils), eosinophils, and basophils. The primary function of the neutrophils is to defend the body against foreign invaders such as bacteria, viruses, and fungi (described in Chapter 4). These cells are produced primarily in the bone marrow and are released into the circulating blood (see Figure 9-9). Their response to infection is known as the **inflammatory response** (see Chapter 2).

Agranulocytosis

In **agranulocytosis** a significant reduction in circulating neutrophils occurs (leukopenia), which has serious consequences. Any of the white blood cells can be involved, but leukopenia most commonly involves the neutrophils. A reduction in the number of circulating neutrophils is called **neutropenia.**

Agranulocytosis can result from either a problem in the development of neutrophils or a problem in accelerated destruction of neutrophils. Primary and secondary forms of agranulocytosis have been described. The cause of the primary form is unknown and may be an immunologic disorder. The secondary form of agranulocytosis is most commonly produced by drugs and other chemicals. Secondary agranulocytosis is most commonly seen in women.

Clinical Features and Oral Manifestations

Clinically patients experience a sudden onset of high fever, chills, jaundice **(icterus),** weakness, and sore throat. Orally the most characteristic feature is the presence of infection. Necrotizing ulcerations, excessive bleeding from the gingiva, and rapid destruction of the supporting tissue of the teeth have been described. Regional lymphadenopathy can accompany the oral problems.

Diagnosis and Treatment

The diagnosis is made by laboratory testing. The white blood cell count, which is normally 5000 to 10,000 cells/mm^3, is dramatically reduced to less than 1000 cells/mm^3. Treatment includes transfusions; antibiotics to control infection; and, in the secondary form, removal of the causative agent. Infections can become overwhelming and cause death. All surgical procedures, including dental hygiene procedures, are contraindicated.

Cyclic Neutropenia

Cyclic neutropenia is a form of agranulocytosis. A severe depression of granulocytes (neutrophils) occurs at periodic intervals. Cyclic neutropenia is described in detail in Chapter 6.

Leukemia

Leukemias are malignant neoplasms of the hematopoietic (blood-forming) stem cells. They are disorders that primarily originate in the bone marrow. The most dramatic feature of leukemias is the excessive number of abnormal white blood cells in the circulating blood. The pathogenesis is unknown. However, current investigations are focusing on oncogenic viruses (see Chapter 7). Many different types of leukemias exist. They are classified by the cell type involved and the maturity of the neoplastic cells (Box 9-2). Leukemias are described in this chapter with other abnormalities of blood. They also have been included in Chapter 7, together with other white blood cell neoplasms. Many different types of leukemias are known; this text gives only an overview of the two general categories, acute and chronic, with focus on the oral manifestations. The student is encouraged to use other texts for a more complete description of leukemias. Oral lesions are most common in acute leukemias but may also occur in chronic forms.

Box 9-2

Classification of Leukemias

Acute Leukemias
Acute lymphoblastic (lymphocytes) leukemia
Acute nonlymphoblastic leukemia (granulocytes, monocytes, erythrocytes)

Chronic Leukemias
Chronic lymphocytic leukemia
Chronic granulocytic (myeloid) leukemia

Acute leukemias

Acute leukemias are characterized by the presence of very immature cells (blast cells) and by a rapidly fatal course if not treated. They can involve immature lymphocytes (acute lymphoblastic leukemia) or immature granulocytes (acute myeloblastic leukemia). Acute lymphoblastic leukemia primarily affects children and young adults and has a good prognosis. Acute myeloblastic leukemia involves adolescents and young adults (age range 15 to 39 years), and the prognosis is not as good. The onset of acute leukemia is sudden and dramatic.

Clinical Features. Clinically patients experience weakness, fever, enlargement of lymph nodes, and bleeding. The lymph node enlargement can include cervical lymphadenopathy (enlargement of the lymph nodes in the neck) and is typically seen earlier in the course of disease, with the leukemias involving immature lymphocytes. A general loss of cells produced by the bone marrow occurs. The fatigue mainly results from anemia, the fever from infection, and the bleeding from a decrease in platelets (thrombocytopenia). In advanced disease enlargement of the spleen (**splenomegaly**) and liver (**hepatomegaly**) occurs when these organs are infiltrated by the leukemic cells.

Oral Manifestations. Oral manifestations can include gingival enlargement (which can be severe) caused by

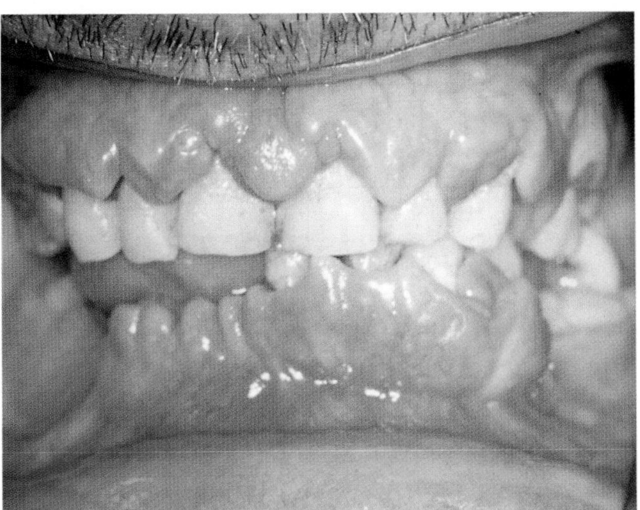

FIGURE 9-11 ■ Generalized gingival hyperplasia in a patient with leukemia. (Courtesy Dr. Edward V. Zegarelli.)

infiltration of leukemic cells (Figure 9-11) and oral infections (including acute necrotizing ulcerative gingivitis because white blood cells are not functioning). In addition, if a decrease in platelets occurs, bleeding gums, petechiae, and ecchymoses may be present. Toothache as the result of invasion of the pulp by leukemic cells has been reported.

Diagnosis And Treatment. In acute leukemia laboratory findings include an elevated white blood cell count with the presence of many immature cells, anemia, and a low platelet count. In young children with acute lymphocytic leukemia, the prognosis with treatment is very good. In adolescents and adults with acute myelocytic leukemia the prognosis is poor. Remissions occur with chemotherapy, and then relapses occur. Bone marrow transplantation is a treatment for this form of leukemia.

Chronic Leukemias

In addition, several different types of chronic leukemias exist. They are all characterized by a slow onset, and they all primarily affect adults. The disease can be present for months before a diagnosis is made, and occasionally the diagnosis is made during a routine physical examination based on laboratory testing. One of the forms of chronic leukemia, chronic myeloid leukemia, is associated with a distinctive chromosomal abnormality, the Philadelphia chromosome. Another form of chronic leukemia, chronic lymphocytic leukemia, is the most common form and accounts for about one quarter of the total cases of leukemia. It may be asymptomatic for a long time. About half the patients with this type of leukemia have abnormal karyotypes; however, the abnormality is different from the Philadelphia chromosome.

Clinical Features and Oral Manifestations. The clinical onset is slow. The symptoms are nonspecific and include easy fatigability, weakness, weight loss, and anorexia. Oral manifestations include pallor of the lips and gingiva, gingival enlargement, petechiae and ecchymosis, gingival bleeding, and atypical periodontal disease. Cervical lymphadenopathy may be an early manifestation of chronic leukemia.

Diagnosis and Treatment. The white blood cell count can increase to 500,000/mm^3, and most of the total cells can be leukemia cells. Remissions occur with chemotherapy; however, they are of short duration, and the long-term prognosis is poor. Bone marrow transplantation is used to treat both chronic and acute leukemia.

BLEEDING DISORDERS

Hemostasis

Patients with bleeding disorders can have one of a number of different defects.

Hemostasis (the cessation of bleeding) is a complex process that involves a number of events (Figure 9-12). When a blood vessel is damaged, marked constriction of the vessel (vasoconstriction) occurs in an attempt to stop the flow of blood. Platelets **(thrombocytes)** that are produced by the bone marrow and circulating in blood adhere to the damaged surface and aggregate to form a temporary clot. To stop the bleeding permanently, it is necessary for **fibrin** to be produced. Fibrin tightly binds the aggregating platelets to form a clot. A cascade of circulating plasma proteins that are made almost exclusively in the liver and called **clotting factors** or **coagulation factors** is necessary to convert the precursor fibrinogen to fibrin (Table 9-1; Figure 9-13).

Finally, anti-clotting mechanisms are activated to prevent the spread of more clots and to allow the clot to dissolve so that the damaged vessel can be repaired. This complexity is necessary to prevent inappropriate clotting. Successful hemostasis depends on the walls of the blood vessels, adequate numbers of functioning platelets, and adequate levels of properly functioning clotting factors.

Defects in hemostasis are caused by abnormalities of either platelets or coagulation factors. These defects can be diagnosed with a few laboratory tests (Table 9-2). Normal values may differ according to the specific test used and the individual laboratory.

Platelet Count

The **platelet count,** which is usually requested with a CBC, provides a quantitative or numeric evaluation of platelets. A normal platelet count should be 150,000 to 400,000/mm^3. A platelet count less than 100,000/mm^3 is considered thrombocytopenia. Spontaneous gingival bleeding can occur when a patient's platelet count is less than 20,000/mm^3. In addition, a physician can request specific clotting factor assays, which can also be performed in patients with suspected or known

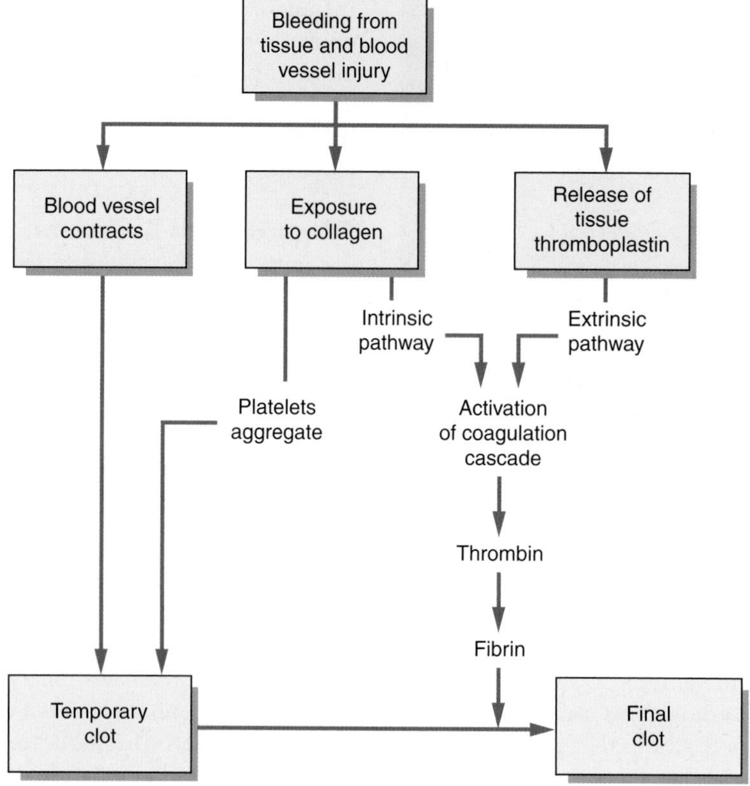

FIGURE 9-12 ■ Hemostasis.

Table 9-1

Factors Involved in Coagulation*

Factor Name	Name
I	Fibrinogen
II	Prothrombin
III	Tissue factor
IV	Calcium ions
V	Proaccelerin
VII	Proconvertin
VIII	Antihemophilic factor
IX	Plasma thromboplastin
X	Stuart factor
XI	Plasma thromboplastin antecedent
XII	Hageman factor
XIII	Fibrin-stabilizing factor

*Factors are numbered in the order in which they were discovered and not in the order in which they function. (No factor VI is included.)

clotting factor deficiencies. Nearly all bleeding disorders are caused by abnormalities of either platelets or clotting factors. Rarely bleeding disorders result from capillary fragility or weakness of the blood vessel walls.

Bleeding Time

The **bleeding time** provides an assessment of the adequacy of platelet function, not platelet number. The test measures how long it takes a standardized skin incision to stop bleeding by the formation of a temporary hemostatic plug or clot. The normal range of bleeding time depends on the way the test is performed but is usually between 1 and 6 minutes. The bleeding time is prolonged, or greater than 5 to 10 minutes, in patients with platelet abnormalities. Aspirin can also prolong the bleeding time but has no effect on the platelet count.

Prothrombin Time

The **prothrombin time (PT)** measures the patient's ability to form a clot. It is performed by measuring the time it takes for a clot to form when calcium and a tissue factor are added to the patient's plasma. A normal PT is usually between 11 and 16 seconds. The value is usually compared with a normal control, which is generated daily by the laboratory using standardized plasma. A prolonged or greater than normal PT can be associated with postoperative bleeding because

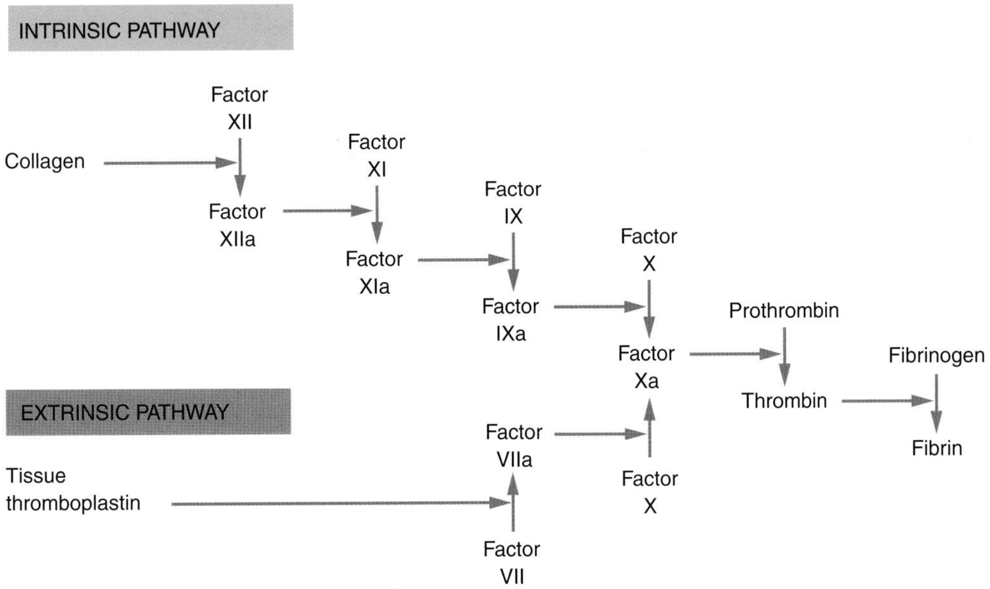

INTRINSIC PATHWAY
Collagen → Factor XII → Factor XIIa
Factor XIIa → Factor XI → Factor XIa
Factor XIa → Factor IX → Factor IXa
Factor IXa → Factor X → Factor Xa
Factor Xa → Prothrombin → Thrombin
Thrombin → Fibrinogen → Fibrin
EXTRINSIC PATHWAY
Tissue thromboplastin → Factor VII → Factor VIIa
Factor VIIa → Factor X → Factor Xa

FIGURE 9-13 ■ Coagulation cascade. Coagulation factors remain inactive until needed. As each coagulation factor becomes activated *(a)*, it is responsible for the activation of another factor until all have been activated and the final clot is formed. The two pathways by which this cascade is activated are the intrinsic and extrinsic pathways.

Table 9-2

Laboratory Tests for Hemostasis

Test	Normal Values
Platelet count (number of platelets)	150,000-400,000/mm^3
Bleeding time (platelet function)	1-6 minutes*
Prothrombin time (fibrin clot formation—extrinsic pathway)	11-16 seconds*
Partial thromboplastin time (fibrin clot formation—intrinsic pathway)	25-40 seconds*

*Normal values may differ according to the specific test used and the individual laboratory.

of abnormal clot formation. A prolonged PT is usually not associated with bleeding unless it is longer than 1.5 times the control. Most often physicians use PT to monitor anticoagulant therapy (as in coumarin or warfarin sodium) for preventing myocardial infarction. A more accurate determination of PT is the **international normalized ratio (INR)**, an expression of the ratio of PT to thromboplastin activity. The INR is more accurate because it is standardized from laboratory to laboratory. Values less than 3.0 are considered within normal range. Patients on anticoagulants such as warfarin may have INR values of 4 to 5.

Partial thromboplastin time

The **partial thromboplastin time (PTT)** also measures the effectiveness of clot formation. Two different pathways exist by which clot formation occurs. PT measures one of these, and PTT measures the other. The test is performed by measuring the time it takes for a clot to form after the addition of kaolin, a surface-activating factor, and cephalin, a substitute platelet factor, to the patient's plasma. A normal PTT is usually 25 to 40 seconds. Prolongation of the PTT to 45 to 50 seconds can be associated with mild bleeding problems. With further prolongation (more than 50 seconds) severe bleeding can occur. PTT is also used by physicians to monitor heparin therapy, which is commonly used for kidney hemodialysis in patients with renal failure.

Purpura

Purpura is a reddish-blue or purplish discoloration of the skin or mucosa that results from spontaneous extravasation of blood. It can be caused by a defect or deficiency in blood platelets or an increase in capillary fragility. A significant oral clinical finding is the oozing of blood at the gingival margins in several sites without the presence of gingivitis or inflammation. Petechiae, ecchymoses, and hemorrhagic blisters can also be present.

Thrombocytopenic Purpura

Thrombocytopenic purpura is a bleeding disorder that results from a severe reduction in circulating platelets. The normal platelet level is 150,000 to 400,000/mm^3 of blood.

Spontaneous bleeding occurs when platelet levels fall to less than 20,000/mm^3. When the cause is unknown, the condition is called **idiopathic thrombocytopenic purpura.** An autoimmune type of process has been identified for thrombocytopenia; therefore it is sometimes called *immune thrombocytopenia.* The condition can also be secondary to an existing disease or condition. **Secondary thrombocytopenic purpura** is often associated with drugs, including those used for cancer chemotherapy. The idiopathic or primary form is usually seen in young patients, with the greatest incidence occurring before the age of 10 years. No age predilection for the secondary type and no sex predilection for either type are seen.

Clinical and Oral Manifestations. Clinically spontaneous purpuric or hemorrhagic lesions of the skin develop that can vary in size and severity. In addition, these patients bruise easily, can have blood in the urine (hematuria), and have frequent nosebleeds (epistaxis). Oral manifestations include spontaneous gingival bleeding and clusters of petechiae or purpuric spots.

Diagnosis and Treatment. Laboratory tests show a significant decrease in platelets. Bleeding time can be prolonged to an hour or more, and the capillary fragility test result is positive. Treatment depends on the cause and includes transfusions, corticosteroids, and splenectomy. Any dental surgical procedure, including scaling, is contraindicated until laboratory test results confirm sufficient improvement in the patient's bleeding problem.

Nonthrombocytopenic Purpura

Nonthrombocytopenic purpuras are bleeding disorders that can result from either a defect in the capillary walls or disorders of platelet function. Vascular wall alterations occur in vitamin C deficiency and infections and can also result from chemicals and allergy. Many factors can cause disorders of platelet function, including drugs, allergy, and autoimmune disease. By far the most common reason for a prolonged bleeding time is the ingestion of drugs that affect platelet function. Ingestion of small doses of aspirin (0.3 to 1.5 g) produces an impairment of platelet function for 7 to 10 days. The nonsteroidal antiinflammatory drugs (e.g., ibuprofen, naproxen, indomethacin) can also adversely affect platelet function. Patients with kidney failure and those with leukemia can have impaired platelet function. **von Willebrand disease** is one of the most common inherited disorders of bleeding in humans. In most cases, it is transmitted as an autosomal-dominant disorder of platelet function. There are several autosomal-recessive variants that have been identified. Both men and women may be affected with this disorder.

Oral Manifestations. The oral manifestations in nonthrombocytopenic purpura are the same as those that occur in thrombocytopenic purpura and include spontaneous gingival bleeding, petechiae, ecchymoses, and hemorrhagic blisters.

Diagnosis and Treatment. The platelet count is normal in nonthrombocytopenic purpura. The bleeding time is prolonged. Treatment includes systemic corticosteroids, splenectomy, and permanent or temporary discontinuation of the causative agent.

Hemophilia

Hemophilia is a disorder of blood **coagulation** that results in severely prolonged clotting time. The problem results from a deficiency of one of the plasma proteins involved in the coagulation cascade that is necessary for the conversion of fibrinogen to fibrin (see Figure 9-12).

Types of Hemophilia

The two most common types of hemophilia are type A and type B. These types of hemophilia are inherited as X-linked recessive traits and therefore are transmitted through an unaffected carrier and occur in males and in homozygous females. The carrier mother may have a mildly prolonged coagulation time. (Inheritance patterns, including sex-linked inheritance, are described in Chapter 6.)

Type A hemophilia is the classic and most common type and is caused by a deficiency of the clotting factor called *plasma thromboplastinogen* or *factor VIII.* This deficiency is characterized by severe hemorrhage after even mild-to-moderate injury or surgery. Type B, or Christmas disease, is less common. The clotting defect is in **plasma thromboplastin** or **factor IX.**

Oral Manifestations

The oral manifestations of hemophilia are spontaneous gingival bleeding and ecchymoses. Patients have a risk of hemorrhage after oral surgery procedures and scaling.

Diagnosis and Treatment

The bleeding time and PT in hemophilia are normal, and the PTT is prolonged. Diagnosis involves identifying the missing factor, and treatment involves replacing it.

IMMUNODEFICIENCY

Immunity is described in Chapter 3. **Immunodeficiency** can involve the different parts of the immune system either alone or together. It can involve the cell-mediated (T-cell) response or the humoral (B-cell or antibody) response. Deficiencies in phagocytosis can also be considered deficiencies in immunity. Immunodeficiency diseases are divided into primary and secondary immunodeficiencies. Primary immunodeficiencies are those of genetic origin; secondary immunodeficiencies result from some other underlying disorder. The signs and symptoms that occur in a person with immunodeficiency depend on the degree of the deficiency and the type of immune response involved. The most common complication arising in persons with either primary or secondary immunodeficiency is infection. The type of infection is related to the type of immunodeficiency. Individuals with deficiency in humoral immunity are more likely to develop bacterial infections; those with deficiency in cell-mediated immunity are more likely to develop viral infections, fungal infections, and infections by intracellular bacteria such as tuberculosis. Autoimmune diseases and neoplasm may also be associated with certain immune deficiencies.

PRIMARY IMMUNODEFICIENCIES

Primary immunodeficiencies are immunodeficiencies of genetic origin and can involve B cells, T cells, or both. These primary immunodeficiencies have provided much information about the functions of the different immunologic responses and are extremely rare.

Three examples are included here. The first is **Bruton disease,** also called **X-linked congenital agammaglobulinemia** (lack of immunoglobulins), which is a disorder in which B cells do not mature. Plasma cells are deficient throughout the body; T cells are normal. Autoimmune diseases are common in these patients.

The second example is **DiGeorge syndrome,** which is also called **thymic hypoplasia**. It is a disorder in which the thymus is deficient or lacking; therefore T lymphocytes do not mature. Infants and children with this syndrome are extremely susceptible to fungal and viral infections and bacterial infections that require T- and B-cell cooperation. B lymphocytes and immunoglobulins are not affected.

The third example is **severe combined immunodeficiency.** Most infants with this type of immunodeficiency die within the first year of life and are vulnerable to all forms of viral, fungal, and bacterial infections.

SECONDARY IMMUNODEFICIENCIES

Secondary immunodeficiencies are those that occur as a result of an underlying disorder. They are much more common than the primary immunodeficiency disorders. Disorders that can have accompanying immunodeficiency include malnutrition, which can lead to inadequate synthesis of antibodies; viral infection; cancer; renal diseases in which antibodies are excreted abnormally; and Hodgkin's disease. They can also occur with the use of immunosuppressive drugs, including corticosteroids; drugs that are used, along with radiation, to suppress the immune system in organ and bone marrow transplantation and to treat autoimmune diseases; and drugs used for cancer chemotherapy. Table 9-3 lists some of the most common drugs that can cause immunodeficiency and the reasons they are generally used. Acquired immunodeficiency syndrome, which occurs as a result of infection with the human immunodeficiency virus (HIV), is an example of a secondary immunodeficiency. HIV infection is described in detail in Chapter 4. With the emergence of combination regimens of antiretroviral therapy, HIV infection is now a chronic illness amenable to treatment.

Table 9-3

Examples of Drugs That Can Cause Immunosuppression

Name	Use
Azathioprine	Prevention of rejection of renal transplants Treatment of rheumatoid arthritis
Cyclosporine	Prevention of rejection of renal transplants
Cyclophosphamide	Cancer chemotherapy
Methotrexate	Cancer chemotherapy
Prednisone	Treatment of autoimmune diseases (such as rheumatoid arthritis, pemphigus vulgaris, Behçet syndrome, lupus erythematosus)

ORAL MANIFESTATIONS OF THERAPY FOR ORAL CANCER

Oral cancer can be treated by surgery, radiation therapy, chemotherapy, or any combination of the three. Radiation therapy and chemotherapy can result in the development of several different oral manifestations.

RADIATION THERAPY

During **radiation therapy** the patient often experiences mucositis (Figure 9-14), which begins about the second week of therapy and subsides a few weeks after its completion. The mucositis is painful and appears as erythematous and ulcerated mucosa. Difficulty in eating, pain on swallowing, and loss of taste can occur as a result of the mucositis. If the radiation affects the major salivary glands, irreversible salivary gland destruction can occur, resulting in severe xerostomia. As a result, the mucosal tissues are easily irritated, and the patient is prone to the development of rampant caries (Figure 9-15) and oral candidiasis. Pilocarpine hydrochloride

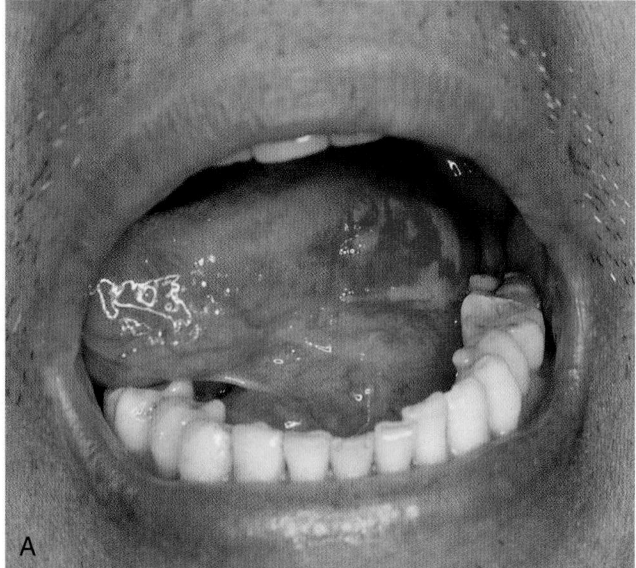

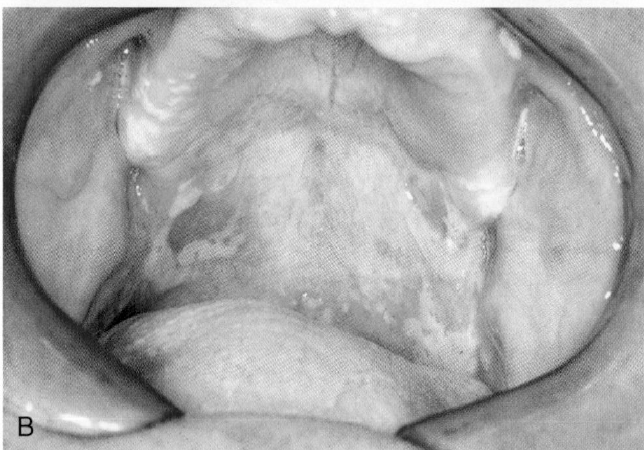

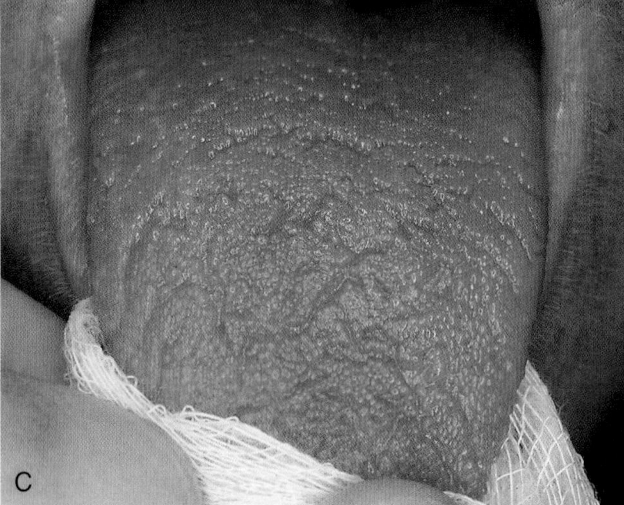

FIGURE 9-14 ■ **A** and **B,** Radiation mucositis. **C,** Postradiation xerostomia.

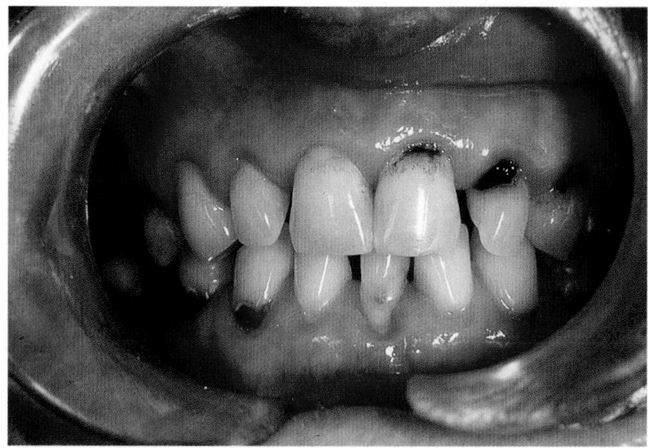

FIGURE 9-15 ■ Clinical appearance of radiation caries. (Courtesy Dr. Jonathan A. Ship.)

taken during the course of radiation treatment decreases the severity of radiation-induced xerostomia. A patient who has received radiation therapy for oral cancer is also at risk for the development of **osteoradionecrosis** (necrosis of bone from radiation therapy) because of the decreased blood supply to the bone after radiation therapy. Osteoradionecrosis develops in the mandible more frequently than in the maxilla, and the risk for its development does not decrease with time.

Patients for whom head and neck radiation is planned should have an oral evaluation before the initiation of radiation therapy. Potential sources of oral infection should be eliminated, and teeth for which the prognosis is questionable should be removed. The role of the dental hygienist in the management of patients receiving head and neck radiation treatment expected to result in xerostomia involves fluoride application both by the dental hygienist and the patient, patient education in oral hygiene care, and frequent follow-up appointments to ensure patient compliance.

Saliva substitutes can be used by the patient for symptomatic relief of xerostomia.

CHEMOTHERAPY

The complications of cancer **chemotherapy** are predictable and differ for the various types of chemotherapy used. Mucositis and oral ulceration are frequent complications because drugs used for cancer chemotherapy affect rapidly dividing cells and therefore the basal cells of the epithelium. The epithelium becomes atrophic and ulcerated with minor irritation. Cells of the bone marrow are also affected; therefore a decrease in all blood cells (red blood cells, white blood cells, and platelets) can result. The patient can experience anemia because of a decrease in red blood cells, is at increased risk for opportunistic infections (e.g., candidiasis) because of a decrease in white blood cells, and is at increased risk for bleeding problems because of a decrease in the number of platelets.

Before the initiation of cancer chemotherapy, the patient should receive an oral evaluation to identify and eliminate any source of oral infection that may exacerbate during the course of chemotherapy.

EFFECTS OF DRUGS ON THE ORAL CAVITY

Many drugs can cause changes in the oral tissues. Xerostomia can be caused by drugs used to control blood pressure. Antianxiety medications, antipsychotic medications, and antihistamines can also cause xerostomia (Figure 9-16). Drugs such as prednisone that suppress the immune system can increase the risk of candidiasis and other oral infections (Figure 9-17). Antibiotics can also increase the risk of candidiasis. Tetracycline taken when teeth are forming can cause tooth discoloration (Figure 9-18). Phenytoin (Dilantin) and nifedipine (Procardia) can cause gingival enlargement (Figure 9-19). Cyclosporine, an immunosuppressant drug used to prevent rejection of transplanted organs, can also cause gingival enlargement.

The complete medical history should include a listing of the medications taken by a patient and is useful in establishing the diagnosis of drug-induced oral lesions.

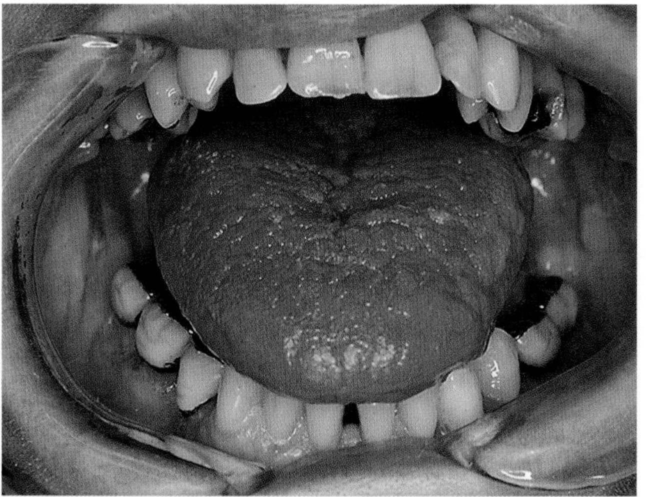

FIGURE 9-16 ■ Xerostomia caused by chlorpromazine (Thorazine) administration.

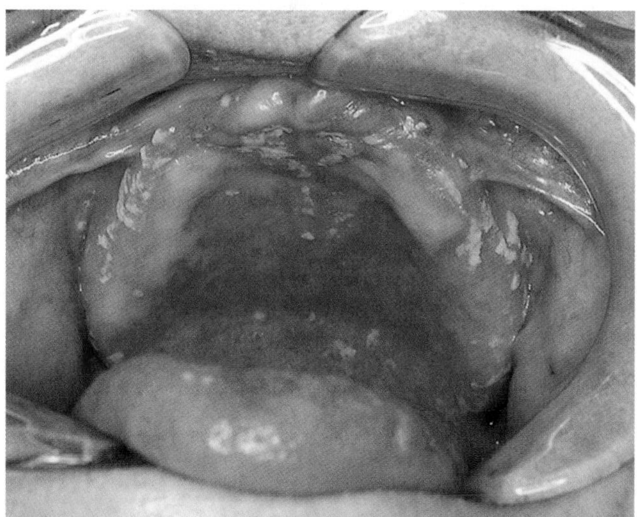

FIGURE 9-17 ■ Candidiasis in a patient taking prednisone for rheumatoid arthritis.

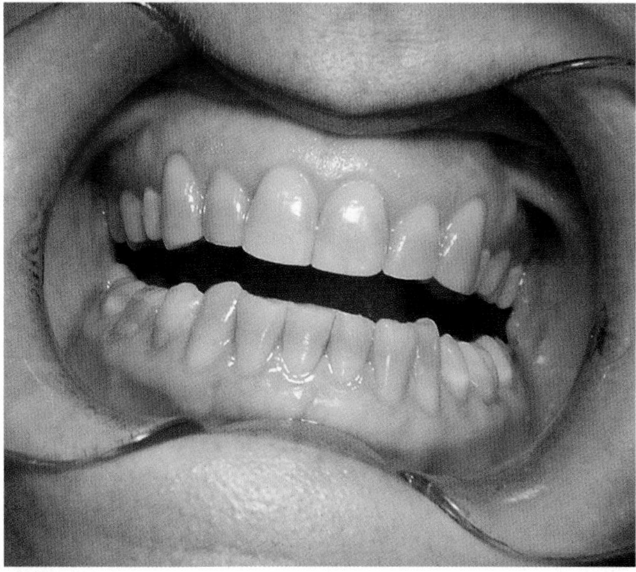

FIGURE 9-18 ■ Discoloration of teeth caused by tetracycline ingestion.

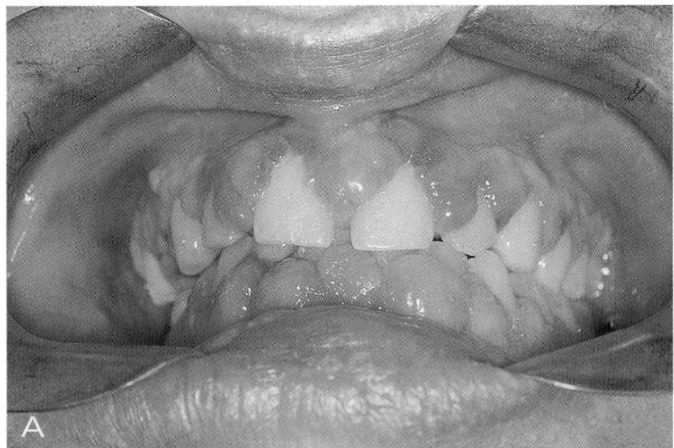

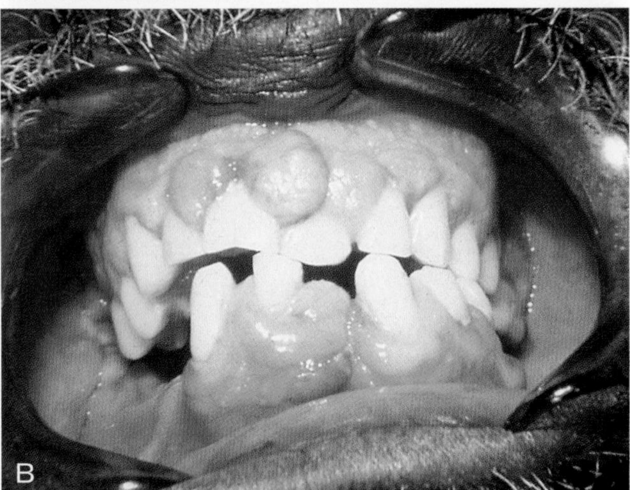

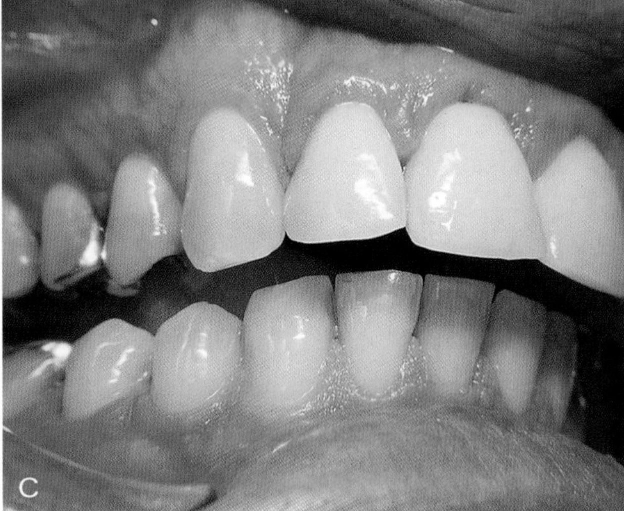

FIGURE 9-19 ■ Drug-induced gingival hyperplasia. **A,** Gingival enlargement caused by phenytoin (Dilantin). **B** and **C,** Gingival hyperplasia caused by nifedipine (Procardia). (**A** courtesy Dr. Edward V. Zegarelli; **B** and **C** courtesy Dr. Victor M. Sternberg.)

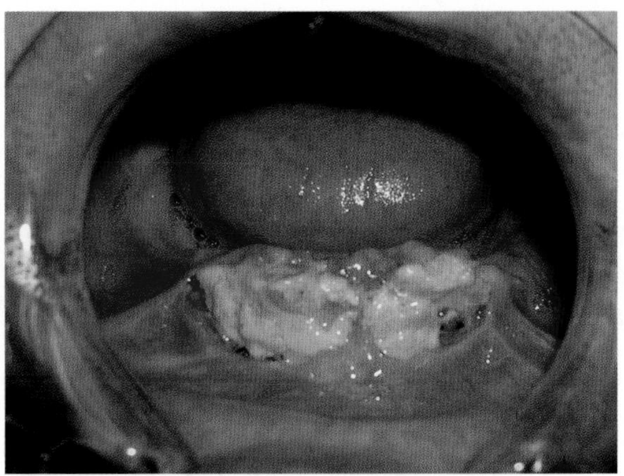

FIGURE 9-20 ■ Osteonecrosis associated with bisphosphonate therapy.

Recently, osteonecrosis of the maxilla and mandible associated with bisphosphonate therapy has been reported. (Figure 9-20). Intravenous bisphosphonate therapy has been used in patients with multiple myeloma and in patients with metastatic carcinoma of the breast and prostate to prevent tumor-associated bone destruction. The drug may also act against tumor cells. Bisphosphonate therapy is used experimentally in patients with Paget disease, and oral bisphosphonate therapy is used to treat osteoporosis. The American Academy of Oral and Maxillofacial Surgery has defined bisphosphonate-associated osteonecrosis (BON) as exposed, necrotic bone in the maxillofacial region that has persisted for more than 8 weeks in a patient with current or previous treatment with a bisphosphonate and no history of radiation therapy to the jaws. Intravenous bisphosphonate therapy is associated with a higher risk for the development of osteonecrosis of the jaws than oral bisphosphonate therapy. Local factors associated with this condition in patients on bisphosphonate medications include dentoalveolar surgery, history of inflammatory dental disease, and trauma to areas such as tori and exostoses where minimal soft tissue protects the bone. At present, there is no well-defined treatment for this condition. The medication remains in the bone for many years and therefore, discontinuation of the medication is not indicated to prevent or manage the condition.

Selected References

Books

Greenberg MS, Glick M, Ship JA: *Burket's oral medicine,* ed 11, Hamilton, 2008, BC Decker.

Little JW et al: *Dental management of the medically compromised patient,* ed 7, St Louis, 2008, Mosby.

Neville BW et al: *Oral and maxillofacial pathology,* ed 3, St Louis, 2009, Saunders.

Sciubba JJ, Regezi JA, Jordan RCK: *Oral pathology: clinical-pathologic correlations,* ed 5, Philadelphia, 2007, Saunders.

Vinay Kumar V, Abbas AK, Nelson F: *Robbins and Cotran pathologic basis of disease,* ed 7, Philadelphia, 2005, Saunders.

Wynn RL, Meiller TF, Crossley HL: *Drug information handbook for dentistry,* ed 14, Hudson, Ohio, 2008, Lexi-Comp.

Journal Articles

Avcu N et al: The relationship between gastric-oral *Helicobacter pylori* and oral hygiene in patients with vitamin B_{12}-deficiency anemia, *Oral Surg Oral Med Oral Pathol Oral Radiol Endod* 92:166, 2001.

Centers for Disease Control and Prevention: Iron deficiency—United States, 1999-2000, *MMWR Morb Mortal Wkly Rep* 51:89, 2002.

Chavez EM et al: A longitudinal analysis of salivary flow in control subjects and older adults with type 2 diabetes, *Oral Surg Oral Med Oral Pathol Oral Radiol Endod* 91:166, 2001.

Collin H et al: Oral symptoms and signs in elderly patients with type 2 diabetes mellitus, *Oral Surg Oral Med Oral Pathol Oral Radiol Endod* 90:299, 2000.

Fletcher PD, Scopp IV, Hersh RA: Oral manifestations of secondary hyperparathyroidism related to long-term hemodialysis therapy, *Oral Surg Oral Med Oral Pathol* 43:218, 1977.

Garg AK, Malo M: Manifestations and treatment of xerostomia and associated oral effects secondary to head and neck radiation therapy, *J Am Dent Assoc* 128:1128, 1997.

Guggenheimer J et al: Insulin-dependent diabetes mellitus and oral soft tissue pathologies. I. Prevalence and characteristics of non-candidal lesions, *Oral Surg Oral Med Oral Pathol Oral Radiol Endod* 89:564, 2000.

Guggenheimer J et al: Insulin-dependent diabetes mellitus and oral soft tissue pathologies. II. Prevalence and characteristics of *Candida* and candidal lesions, *Oral Surg Oral Med Oral Pathol Oral Radiol Endod* 89:570, 2000.

Hardin DS: Screening for type 2 diabetes in children with acanthosis nigricans, *Diabetes Educ* 32:547, 2006.

Hess LM et al: Factors associated with osteonecrosis of the jaw among bisphosphonate users, *Am J Med* 121:475, 2008.

Inokuchi T, Sano K, Kamingo M: Osteoradionecrosis of the sphenoid and temporal bones in a patient with maxillary sinus carcinoma: a case report, *Oral Surg Oral Med Oral Pathol* 70:278, 1990.

Khocht A, Schneider LC: Periodontal management of gingival overgrowth in the heart transplant patient: a case report, *J Periodontol* 68:1140, 1997.

Kong AS et al: Acanthosis nigricans and diabetes risk factors: prevalence in young persons seen in southwester US primary care practices, *Ann Fam Med* 5:202, 2007.

McDonough RJ, Nelson CL: Clinical implications of factor XII deficiency, *Oral Surg Oral Med Oral Pathol* 68:264, 1989.

Miranda J et al: Prevalence and risk of gingival enlargement in patients treated with nifedipine, *J Periodontol* 72:605, 2001.

Moore PA et al: Type 1 diabetes mellitus and oral health: assessment of periodontal disease, *J Periodontol* 70:409, 1999.

Moore PA et al: Type 1 diabetes mellitus and oral health: assessment of coronal and root caries, *Community Dent Oral Epidemiol* 29:183, 2001.

Moore PA et al: Type 1 diabetes mellitus, xerostomia and salivary flow rates, *Oral Surg Oral Med Oral Pathol Oral Radiol Endod* 92:281, 2001.

Ohishi M et al: Acute gingival necrosis caused by drug-induced agranulocytosis, *Oral Surg Oral Med Oral Pathol* 66:194, 1988.

Redding SW, Luce EB, Boren MW: Oral herpes simplex virus infection in patients receiving head and neck radiation, *Oral Surg Oral Med Oral Pathol* 69:578, 1990.

Ruggiero SL et al: Osteonecrosis of the Jaws and Bisphosphonate Therapy, *J Dent Res* 86:1013, 2007.

Sreebny LM, Valdini A, Yu A: Xerostomia. II. Relationship to nonoral symptoms, drugs and diseases, *Oral Surg Oral Med Oral Pathol* 68:419, 1989.

Vernillo AT: Diabetes mellitus: relevance to dental treatment, *Oral Surg Oral Med Oral Pathol Oral Radiol Endod* 91:263, 2001.

Vernillo AT: Dental considerations for the treatment of patients with diabetes mellitus, *J Am Dent Assoc* 134:24S, 2003.

Wahlin YB: Effects of chlorhexidine mouth rinse on oral health in patients with acute leukemia, *Oral Surg Oral Med Oral Pathol* 68:279, 1989.

Wu J, Fantasia JE, Kaplan R: Oral manifestations of acute myelomonocytic leukemia: a case report and review of the classification of leukemias, *J Periodontol* 73:664, 2002.

Newspaper Articles

Kleinfield NR: Diabetes and its awful toll quietly emerge as a crisis, *The New York Times,* January 9, 2006, pp A1, A18-A19.

Kleinfield NR: Living at an epicenter of diabetes: defiance and despair, *The New York Times,* January 10, 2006, pp A1, A20-A21.

Urbina I: In the treatment of diabetes, success often does not pay, *The New York Times,* January 11, 2006, pp A1, A22-A23.

Santora M: East meets west, adding pounds and peril, *The New York Times* January 12, 2006, pp A1, A22-A23.

REVIEW QUESTIONS

1. Hyperpituitarism results from an excessive production of growth hormone. Which of the following most often causes it?
   A. Pituitary adenoma
   B. Pituitary sarcoma
   C. Carcinoma in situ
   D. Ameloblastoma

2. Hyperthyroidism in children can lead to:
   A. Partial anodontia.
   B. Amelogenesis imperfecta.
   C. Ankylosis.
   D. Early exfoliation of the deciduous dentition and early eruption of the permanent teeth.

3. Hypercalcemia, hypophosphatemia, and abnormal bone metabolism are characteristic of which of the following conditions?
   A. Hyperthyroidism
   B. Hypothyroidism
   C. Hyperparathyroidism
   D. Hyperpituitarism

4. All of the following are chronic complications of diabetes mellitus *except:*
   A. Eye damage.
   B. Ketoacidosis.
   C. Atherosclerosis.
   D. Kidney failure.

5. Polydipsia, polyuria, and polyphagia are all characteristic of which of the following?
   A. Fibrous dysplasia
   B. Hyperthyroidism
   C. Type 1 diabetes mellitus
   D. Type 2 diabetes mellitus

6. Which of the following is not a feature of type 2 diabetes mellitus?
   A. Those with it have increased insulin resistance.
   B. It occurs at 40 years of age or older.
   C. Autoimmunity is the key to its development.
   D. Glucose control can be achieved without daily insulin injections in many cases.

7. Which of the following oral complications is not associated with diabetes mellitus?
   A. Candidiasis
   B. Xerostomia
   C. Excessive periodontal bone loss
   D. Purpura

8. Which one of the following is false concerning Addison disease?
   A. It is also known as primary adrenal cortical insufficiency.
   B. It is characterized by an insufficient production of adrenal steroids.
   C. It may be caused by a malignant tumor that destroys the adrenal gland.
   D. It is a condition in which the pituitary adenoma destroys the adrenal gland.

9. Which of the following statements is false regarding diabetes mellitus?
   A. Candidiasis may be indicative of compromised immunity in a patient with diabetes.
   B. Insulin pump therapy may lead to more predictable control of blood sugar.
   C. Hypoglycemic agents are more commonly used in the treatment of type 2 diabetes than in type 1 diabetes.
   D. Diabetes mellitus is not appropriately considered a syndrome.

10. Which of the following statements is false?
    A. Primary immunodeficiencies are less common than secondary immunodeficiencies.
    B. Persons with T-lymphocyte deficiencies are susceptible to viral and fungal infections.
    C. All primary immunodeficiencies are combined B-lymphocyte and T-lymphocyte deficiencies.
    D. Secondary immunodeficiency can result from corticosteroid medication.

11. Iron deficiency anemia can be caused by:
    A. Chronic blood loss.
    B. A deficiency of iron intake.
    C. An increased requirement for iron.
    D. All of the above

12. Thalassemia major is:
    A. Caused by a nutritional deficiency.
    B. The same as celiac sprue.
    C. An autoimmune condition.
    D. Associated with a severe hemolytic anemia.

13. Achlorhydria, failure to absorb vitamin B_{12}, and megaloblastic anemia are characteristic features of which of the following?
    A. Pernicious anemia
    B. Thalassemia
    C. Sickle cell anemia
    D. Thrombocytopenic purpura.

14. Which one of the following is not a characteristic of sickle cell anemia?
    A. It is an inherited blood disorder found predominantly in blacks.
    B. It occurs as a result of an abnormal type of hemoglobin and decreased oxygen in the red blood cells.
    C. The individual with sickle cell anemia can experience weakness, fatigue, and joint pain.
    D. Red blood cells are circular.

15. Which of the following is characterized by a decrease in platelets?
    A. Celiac sprue
    B. Thrombocytopenia
    C. Thalassemia
    D. Plummer-Vinson syndrome

16. Secondary aplastic anemia can be caused by:
    A. Chemotherapy.
    B. Dental radiographs.
    C. A genetic disorder.
    D. An autoimmune factor.

17. Which of the following is characterized by an abnormal increase in circulating red blood cells?
    A. Leukopenia
    B. Polydipsia
    C. Thrombocytopenia
    D. Polycythemia

18. Leukopenia most often involves which cell type?
    A. Eosinophils
    B. Neutrophils
    C. Basophils
    D. Erythrocytes

19. If a patient's white blood cell count is 1000/mm^3, the patient has:
    A. Leukopenia.
    B. Thrombocytopenia.
    C. Hemophilia.
    D. Cyclic neutropenia.

20. Excessive numbers of abnormal white blood cells are characteristic of:
    A. Agranulocytosis.
    B. Leukopenia.
    C. Cyclic neutropenia.
    D. Leukemia.

21. Normal bleeding time is usually between:
    A. 1 and 6 minutes.
    B. 2 and 3 minutes.
    C. 15 and 45 seconds.
    D. 10 and 15 minutes.

22. The normal prothrombin time is:
    A. 2 to 5 minutes.
    B. 11 to 16 seconds.
    C. 10 to 15 minutes.
    D. 1 to 6 seconds.

23. The international normalized ratio is:
    A. An expression of the ratio of prothrombin time to thromboplastin activity.
    B. More accurate than the prothrombin time because it is standardized from laboratory to laboratory.
    C. Used to determine the patient's ability to form a clot.
    D. All of the above

24. Symptoms of leukemia can be similar to those found in:
    A. Hepatitis.
    B. Amelogenesis imperfecta.
    C. Nonthrombocytopenic purpura.
    D. Mononucleosis.

25. Which of the following is not characteristic of primary hyperparathyroidism?
    A. Osteoclastic resorption
    B. Excessive production of parathyroid hormone
    C. Cotton-wool radiographic appearance
    D. Increased serum calcium

26. Osteonecrosis of the jaw is associated with:
    A. Antipsychotic medications
    B. Tetracycline
    C. Phenytoin
    D. Bisphophonates

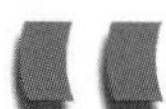

CHAPTER 9 Synopsis

Condition/Disease	Cause	Age/Race/Sex	Location
Hyperpituitarism	Excess growth hormone produced by the pituitary gland Most commonly caused by a pituitary adenoma	Children: gigantism Adults (most common fourth decade): acromegaly	Generalized bone involvement Affects only certain bones
Hyperthyroidism (Graves Disease)	Excessive production of thyroid hormone	Children and adults	Systemic disease
Hypothroidism	Decreased production of thyroid hormone	Children: cretinism	Systemic disease
Hyperparathyroidism	Excessive secretion of parathyroid hormone Primary: may be caused by hyperplasia or tumor of parathyroid glands Secondary causes include renal disease and vitamin D deficiency	Usually adults	Systemic disease

N/A, Not applicable.
*Not covered in text.

Clinical Features	Radiographic Features	Microscopic Features	Treatment	Diagnostic Process
Excessive growth of the skeleton overall Enlargement of the hands and feet Increase in rib size Enlargement of the mandible, maxilla, and maxillary sinus Separation of teeth with malocclusion Frontal bossing and enlargement of nasal bones	* *	N/A	May involve pituitary gland surgery	Laboratory
Rosy complexion, erythema of the palms, excessive sweating, fine hair and softened nails, exophthalmus Anxiety, weakness, restlessness, cardiac problems Children: premature exfoliation of deciduous and premature eruption of permanent teeth Adults: osteoporosis; dental caries and periodontal disease appear to progress rapidly	*	*	Suppression of thyroid activity May involve surgery, medication, radioactive iodine	Laboratory
Children: thickened lips, enlarged tongue, delayed eruption of teeth Adults: enlarged tongue	Delayed eruption pattern may be observed	*	*	*
Joint pain or stiffness, lethargy Loosening of teeth	Well-circumscribed bone lesions, changes in trabeculation, partial loss of lamina dura	Bone lesions-indistinguishable from central giant cell lesion	Dependent on cause	Laboratory

Continued

CHAPTER 9 Synopsis (continued)

Condition/Disease	Cause	Age/Race/Sex	Location
Diabetes Mellitus	Abnormally high blood glucose levels resulting from lack of the hormone insulin	Type I (IDDM) peak age of onset: 20 yrs Type 2: (NIDDM): 40 years or older	Systemic disease
Addison Disease	Insufficient production of adrenal steroids caused by: Autoimmune disease Malignant tumor of adrenal gland Tuberculosis Cause may be undetermined	*	Systemic disease
Pernicious Anemia	Deficiency of intrinsic factor (produced by parietal cells of the stomach) Autoimmune mechanism most likely	Usually adults	Systemic disease
Folic Acid and Vitamin B_{12} Deficiencies	Malnutrition Increased metabolic requirements		Systemic disease
Thalassemia **Thalassemia Major (Homozygous)** **Thalassemia Minor (Heterozygous)**	Inherited disorder (autosomal-dominant)	Begins in early childhood	Systemic disease Thalassemia major: severe symptoms Thalassemia minor: asymptomatic or mildly symptomatic

N/A, Not applicable.
*Not covered in text.

Clinical Features	Radiographic Features	Microscopic Features	Treatment	Diagnostic Process
Accelerated atherosclerosis resulting in impaired circulation of blood. Increased risk of ulceration, gangrene of the feet, high blood pressure, kidney failure, and stroke Acanthosis nigricans Eye damage and blindness Neurologic complaints Decreased resistance to infection, including oral candidiasis Slow wound healing Bilateral salivary gland enlargement Xerostomia (usually with uncontrolled diabetes) Accentuated response to dental plaque	Increased severity of periodontal bone loss	N/A	Control of blood glucose with insulin injections, oral hypoglycemic agents, and diet	Laboratory
Brown pigmentation of the skin and oral melanotic macules	N/A	Microcytic and hypochromic red blood cells	Increase in dietary iron intake	Laboratory
Weakness, fatigue, skin pallor, nausea, dizziness, diarrhea, abdominal pain, loss of appetite, weight loss Oral: angular cheilitis, pallor, painful, erythematous and depapillated tongue, mucosal ulceration	N/A	Abnormally large red blood cells (megaloblastic anemia)	Vitamin B_{12} by injection	Laboratory
Weakness, fatigue, skin pallor, nausea dizziness, diarrhea, abnormal pain, loss of appetite, weight loss Oral: angular cheilitis; pallor; painful, erythematous, and depapillated tongue; oral ulcers	N/A	Abnormally large red blood cells (megaloblastic)	Dietary supplements	Laboratory
Yellowish skin pallor, fever, malaise, weakness, enlarged liver and spleen Facies: prominent cheekbones, depression of the bridge of the nose, prominent premaxilla, protrusion or flaring of the maxillary anterior teeth	Atypical trabecular pattern ("salt and pepper effect") Thinning of the lamina dura Circular Radiolucencies in the alveolar bone also described	*	Experimental	Clinical Laboratory

Continued

CHAPTER 9 Synopsis (continued)

Condition/Disease	Cause	Age/Race/Sex	Location
Sickle Cell Anemia Sickle Cell Trait (Heterozygous)	Inherited disorder (autosomal-dominant pattern) Abnormal hemoglobin in red blood cells	Before age 30 Most in black individuals and those of Mediterranean origin Women > Men	Systemic disease
Celiac Sprue	Sensitivity to dietary gluten resulting in injury to the intestinal mucosa and subsequent anemia	N/A	Systemic disease
Aplastic Anemia	Decrease in all circulating blood cells because of a severe depression of bone marrow activity Primary: cause unknown Secondary: because of drug or chemical agent	Primary: young adults Secondary: any age	Systemic disease
Polycythemia	Abnormal increase in circulating red blood cells	Usually adults	Systemic disease
Polycythemia Vera (Primary polycythemia)	Neoplastic		
Secondary Polycythemia	Physiologic response to decreased oxygen		
Relative Polycythemia	Decreased plasma volume, not an increase in red blood cells		
Agranulocytosis	Marked reduction in circulating neutrophils (neutropenia) Primary: may be immunologic Secondary: drugs and other chemicals	N/A	Systemic disease
Cyclic Neutropenia	See Chapter 6		
Leukemia	Neoplastic Oncogenic viruses suggested	Children (acute lymphoblastic) Adolescents and young adults (acute myoblastic)	Systemic disease
		Adults (chronic leukemias)	Systemic disease

N/A, Not applicable.

*Not covered in text.

Clinical Features	Radiographic Features	Microscopic Features	Treatment	Diagnostic Process
Weakness, shortness of breath, fatigue, joint pain, nausea	Loss of trabeculation with large, irregular marrow spaces	Sickle-shaped red blood cells on blood smear	Symptomatic and supportive oxygen, intravenous and oral fluids	Laboratory
Same clinical features as anemias	N/A	*	Adherence to gluten-free diet	*
Infection, spontaneous bleeding, petechiae and purpuric spots	N//A	N/A	Primary: experimental, poor prognosis Secondary: removal of cause	Laboratory
Oral mucosa may appear deep red to purple Gingiva may be edematous and bleed easily	N/A	N/A	*	*
Petechiae, ecchymosis and hematoma formation can be present	N/A	N/A	*	*
Sudden onset of fever, chills, jaundice, weakness, and sore throat Oral infection with rapid periodontal destruction Gingival bleeding	N/A	N/A	Transfusions Antibiotics to control infection Removal of causative agent if identified	Laboratory
Weakness, fever, lymph node enlargement, bleeding, enlarged liver and spleen Gingival enlargement because of infiltration of leukemic cells, oral infections, spontaneous gingival bleeding, petechia, and ecchymoses	N/A	Enlarged gingival: infiltration of tissue by leukemic cells	Chemotherapy Bone marrow transplantation	Laboratory
Slow onset of symptoms Easy fatigability, weakness, weight loss, anorexia Pallor of the lips and gingiva, gingival enlargement, petechiae, ecchymosis, gingival bleeding, and atypical periodontal disease	N/A	Enlarged gingival-infiltration of tissue by leukemic cells	Chemotherapy Bone marrow transplantation	Laboratory

Continued

CHAPTER 9 Synopsis (continued)

Condition/Disease	Cause	Age/Race/Sex	Location
Thrombocytopenic Purpura	Severe reduction in circulating platelets		Systemic disease
Idiopathic Type (Primary Type)	Cause unknown	Primary and immune types	
Immune Type	Autoimmune disease	Usually children and young adults	
Secondary Type	Drugs: often chemotherapeutic agents	No age prediction for secondary type	
Hemophilia A and B	Inherited (X-linked)	Identified in childhood Affects boys	Systemic disease
Bisphosphonate-associated osteonecrosis	Bisphosphonate therapy for osteoporosis, multiple myeloma, metastatic carcinoma of the breast and prostate, and Paget disease	N/A	Maxilla and mandible

N/A, Not applicable.

*Not covered in text.

Clinical Features	Radiographic Features	Microscopic Features	Treatment	Diagnostic Process
Spontaneous hemorrhagic lesions of the skin and/or mucosa Gingival bleeding Frequent nose bleeds Blood in urine (hematuria)	N/A	N/A	Systemic corticosteroids, splenectomy Discontinuation of causative agent	Laboratory
Spontaneous bleeding, petechiae, ecchymoses Risk of hemorrhage after oral surgery and dental hygiene procedures	N/A	N/A	Replacement of missing clotting factors	Laboratory
Exposed bone persisting more than eight weeks in a patient taking bisphosphonate medication	*	*	*	Clinical Microscopic (rule out metastatic disease)

Diseases Affecting the Temporomandibular Joint

Kenneth E. Fleisher

OBJECTIVES

After studying this chapter, the student will be able to:

1. Label the following on a diagram of the temporomandibular joint: glenoid fossa of the temporal bone, articular disk, mandibular condyle, joint capsule, and superior belly of the lateral pterygoid muscle.
2. State the function of the muscles of mastication.
3. State three factors that have been implicated in the cause of temporomandibular disorders and three questions that would be appropriate to ask of a patient suspected of having a temporomandibular disorder.
4. List at least two symptoms that are suggestive of temporomandibular dysfunction.
5. State the function of radiographs in the evaluation of a patient with symptoms suggestive of temporomandibular dysfunction.
6. List five types of temporomandibular disorders.
7. List and describe the two main categories of treatment of temporomandibular disorders.
8. State the names of one benign and one malignant tumor that may affect the temporomandibular joint area.

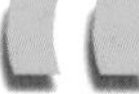

VOCABULARY

Arthrocentesis **(ahr"thro-sen-te'sis)** Surgical puncture of a joint followed by lavage of the joint space.

Arthrography **(ahr-throg'rah-fē)** Radiography of a joint after injection of opaque contrast material.

Arthroscopy **(ahr-thros'cah-pē)** Method for evaluating and manipulating a joint via the insertion of a camera and instruments.

Articulation **(ar-tik-ū-lā'shin)** Joint.

Auscultation **(aws-kul-tā'shin)** Listening to sounds within the body using a stethoscope.

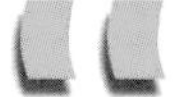

VOCABULARY (continued)

Crepitus (krep'i-tus) Dry, crackling sound.

Iatrogenic (i-at"ro-jen'ik) Induced inadvertently by a medical or dental care provider or by medical treatment or a diagnostic procedure.

Magnetic resonance imaging (MRI) Noninvasive diagnostic technique that uses radio waves to produce computerized images of internal body tissues.

Palpation (pal-pa'shĕn) Physical examination using pressure of the hand or fingers.

Sign (sīn) Objective evidence of disease that can be observed by a health care provider rather than by the patient.

Symptom (simp'tĕm) Subjective evidence of disease or a physical disorder that is observed by the patient.

Trismus (triz'mĕs) Inability to fully open the mouth.

Knowledge of the anatomy and function of the temporomandibular joint (TMJ) enables the dental hygienist to understand the diseases that affect the joint. Disorders of the TMJ include myofascial pain and dysfunction (MPD), internal derangements syndrome, osteoarthritis, and rheumatoid arthritis. Benign and malignant tumors can also affect the temporomandibular joint (Box 10-1).

ANATOMY OF THE TEMPOROMANDIBULAR JOINT

The TMJ is the **articulation** between the condyle of the mandible and the glenoid fossa of the temporal bone (Figure 10-1). It is a highly specialized joint that differs from other joints because of the fibrocartilage that covers the bony articulating surfaces, its ginglymoarthrodial (rotational and translational) movement, the fact that its function and overall health is dictated by jaw movement, and its dependence on the contralateral joint. An articular disk is interposed in the space between the temporal bone and the mandible. This disk divides the space into an upper (superior joint space) and a lower compartment (inferior joint space) (see Figure 10-1).

Box 10-1

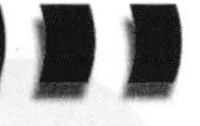

Commonly Used Abbreviations

MPD Myofascial pain and disfunction
TMD Temporomandibular disorder
TMJ Temporomandibular joint

Translational movements occur in the upper compartment, whereas the lower compartment functions primarily as the hinge or rotational component. The superior and inferior spaces contain **synovial fluid,** which is produced by the **synovial membrane** that lines the joint. The synovial fluid provides nourishment and lubrication of the avascular structures. The articular disk is attached to the lateral and medial aspects of the condyle, to the superior belly of the lateral pterygoid muscle, and to the joint capsule (see Figure 10-1). The disk and the bony surfaces are avascular (they do not contain blood vessels). The joint is further surrounded and protected by the fibrous connective tissue joint capsule.

Understanding the location and action of the **muscles of mastication** is important in the evaluation of disorders affecting the TMJ. **Palpation** of these muscles during a clinical evaluation is used to determine whether muscle spasm or dysfunctional muscle activity is occurring. The muscles of mastication comprise major muscles about the facial region that govern the movement of the mandible. They include the masseter, temporalis, medial pterygoid, lateral pterygoid, anterior digastric, and mylohyoid (suprahyoids) (Figures 10-2 to 10-4). The function of these muscles is to create the mandibular envelope of motion. Three of these muscles, the masseter, medial pterygoid, and temporalis, are elevator muscles that, when activated, close the mandible. The opening, or depressor, function is accomplished mainly by the lateral pterygoid muscle with some help from the anterior digastric muscle. Studies have shown that the two components of the lateral pterygoid muscle are active at different times in the functioning of the mandible (see Figure 10-4). The superior portion of the muscle seats the articular disk on the eminence of the articulating surface. The inferior belly is attached to the mandibular condyle and functions during mouth opening.

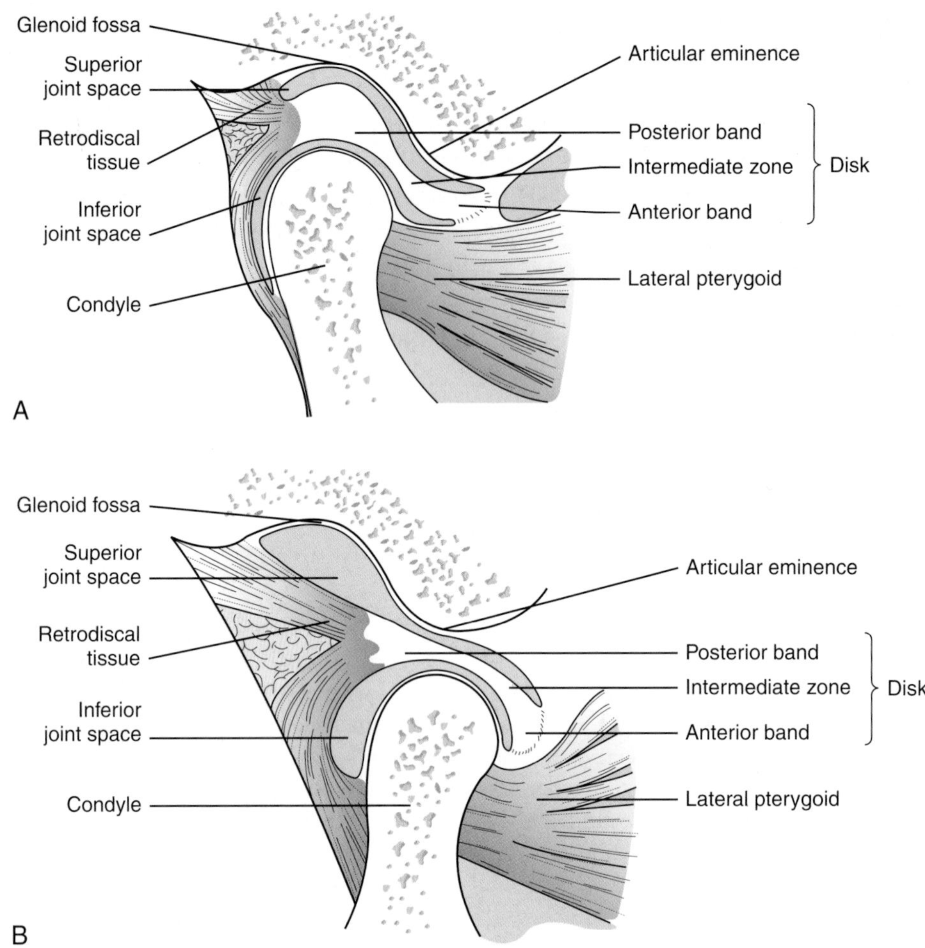

FIGURE 10-1 ■ Lateral views of the temporomandibular joint. **A,** Jaw closed. **B,** Jaw open. (From Kaplan AS, Assael LA: *Temporomandibular disorders,* Philadelphia, 1991, Saunders.)

NORMAL JOINT FUNCTION

The harmonious function of the TMJ depends on various factors. The anatomic relationship of the condyle-disk complex governs the smooth functioning of the mandible. This articulation, along with the muscles of mastication, provides the movement of the mandible. The muscles of mastication are the machinery that powers mandibular movement; the anatomic joint structures such as the condyle, articular eminence, and disk act as the gears or bearings of the jaw.

In **normal joint function** the jaw begins at a rest position of maximum occlusal contact. In this position the mandibular condyle rests within the glenoid fossa, with the articular disk situated between the condyle, roof of the glenoid fossa, and articular eminence (see Figure 10-1, *A* and *B*). The first phase of opening is characterized by rotational (hinge) movement of the condyle, followed by anterior translation (sliding movement) to approximately the anterior peak of the articular eminence. During translation the disk assumes a more posterior position in relation to the condyle. The inferior and superior joint spaces assume different configurations during each of these movements.

TEMPOROMANDIBULAR DISORDERS

Temporomandibular disorders (TMDs) are caused by abnormalities in the functioning of the TMJ or associated structures. They have been a clinical and diagnostic challenge in dentistry for many years. Hippocrates documented jaw dysfunction problems as early as the fifth century BC. However, it was not until 1934 that a syndrome of TMJ diseases was described. Dentists and oral and maxillofacial surgeons began to study the TMJ and related structures in an attempt to accurately describe the pathophysiology of disorders of this joint and establish the most effective treatment. Although up to 75% of the adult population has at least one **sign** and/or **symptom** of a temporomandibular disorder, most studies suggest that clinically significant TMD-related jaw pain, dysfunction, or both affects about 5% of the general population. Significantly

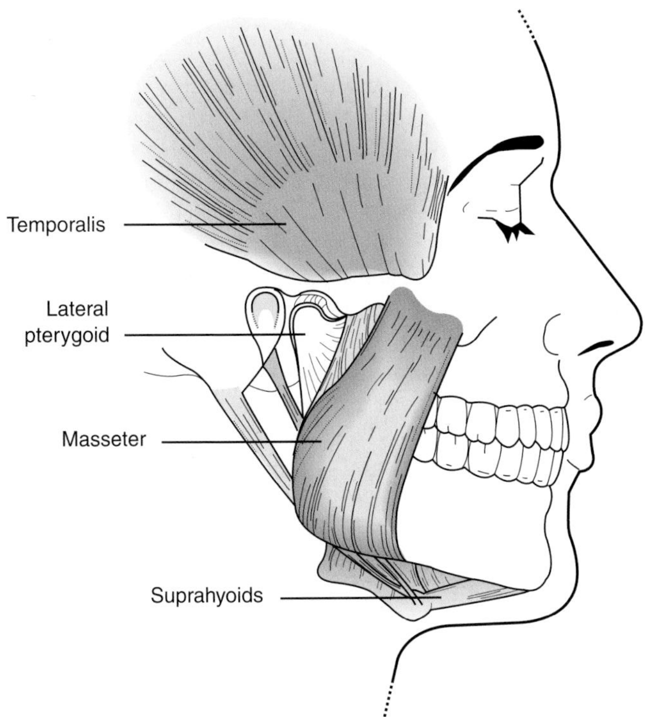

FIGURE 10-2 ■ Muscles of mastication: the temporalis, lateral pterygoid, masseter, and suprahyoid. (From Kaplan, AS, Assael LA: *Temporomandibular disorders,* Philadelphia, 1991, Saunders.)

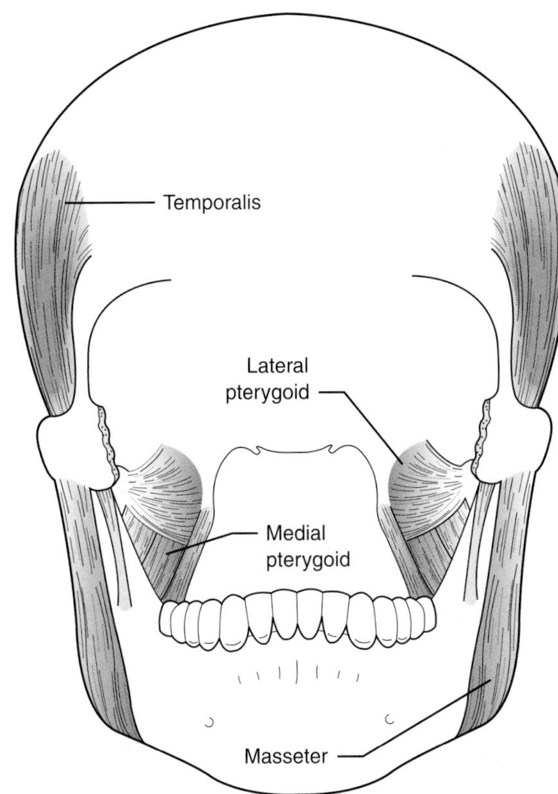

FIGURE 10-4 ■ Muscles of mastication. Illustrated are the four paired muscles of mastication: the masseter, temporalis, medial pterygoid, and lateral pterygoid. (From Kaplan AS, Assael LA: *Temporomandibular disorders,* Philadelphia, 1991, Saunders.)

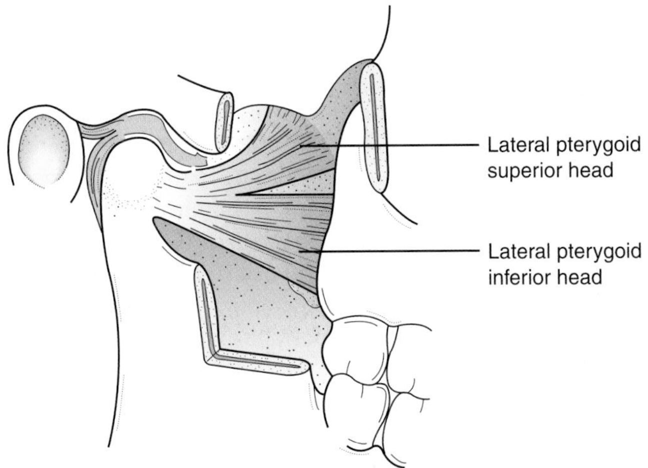

FIGURE 10-3 ■ Muscles of mastication. The two distinct heads of the lateral pterygoid muscle are illustrated. (From Kaplan AS, Assael LA: *Temporomandibular disorders,* Philadelphia, 1991, Saunders.)

more frequent and more severe TMD signs and symptoms are seen in women than men and in older adults.

PATHOPHYSIOLOGY OF TEMPOROMANDIBULAR JOINT DISORDERS

The cause of TMDs remains controversial, and many factors have been implicated. Trauma has been suggested as the most likely cause. Trauma affecting the TMJ is classified as *direct* (assault), *indirect* (whiplash injury), or secondary to *parafunctional habits* (clenching, bruxism). Other contributing factors include dentofacial deformities and psychosocial factors. Numerous studies continue to dispute the significance of occlusal relationships. TMJ abnormalities are also associated with a number of different systemic diseases. Rheumatoid arthritis and osteoarthritis are the most common and are described later in this chapter. TMJ disorders may also be the result of disorders in growth and development as seen in condylar hyperplasia or hypoplasia. **Iatrogenic** causes (resulting from the action of a health care provider) of TMDs include the indiscriminate use of corticosteroid injection into the joint.

PATIENT EVALUATION

Temporomandibular dysfunction can be caused by disorders of the muscles of mastication or internal derangements of the components of the joint. Evaluation involves a comprehensive history and a thorough clinical examination. An understanding of the procedures used in the evaluation of TMJ disorders is important to the dental hygienist. The dental hygienist does not generally perform a comprehensive examination of the TMJ area but may participate in diagnostic procedures related to the joint.

History

A history of aberrant growth, previous injuries, illnesses, musculoskeletal complaints, and possible emotional disturbances is an important consideration in the evaluation of patients with TMDs. The patient history specific to TMDs includes questions regarding the following:

- Joint symptoms (clicking, popping)
- Pain
- Problems with mastication
- Trismus
- Malocclusion
- Parafunctional habits (bruxing, clenching)
- Dental symptoms
- Extensive dental or orthodontic treatment
- History of surgical treatment of the jaws
- Progression of symptoms (sudden, gradual)
- Precipitating events (mastication, spontaneous, yawning)

Clicking and popping most commonly reflect disk displacement with reduction and occur in approximately 33% of asymptomatic patients. They are of little clinical consequence in the absence of pain or other symptoms relating to the TMJ because it is controversial as to whether these noises represent an adaptive response (i.e., normal variant) or an early symptom of progression to disk displacement without reduction. The incidence of orofacial pain among the adult population has been reported to be 26%; the differential diagnosis for evaluating patients with TMDs includes odontogenic pain (e.g., cracked tooth syndrome), headache, neuralgia (e.g., trigeminal neuralgia), fibromyalgia, otitis media, cervical spine pain, and tumor. Etiologies of **trismus** other than TMDs include odontogenic infection, oral surgery procedures, inferior alveolar nerve block, tumors, facial bone fractures, radiation therapy, and medications (e.g., phenothiazine)

Examination

A comprehensive examination of a patient related to TMJ disorders includes an examination of the joint, muscles of mastication, oral cavity, and cervical spine. Joint examination involves **auscultation** (using a stethoscope) and palpation. The clinician relates joint noises such as clicking, **crepitus** (crackling), or popping to the mandibular movement cycle. The muscles of mastication are palpated to determine tenderness. In addition to a thorough oral examination, the patient is asked to move the mandible in a normal rotation (hinge) and translatory (forward slide) cycle. Interincisal opening is measured, along with any obvious deviation of motion to the right or left side. The patient's ability to manipulate the mandible into right and left lateral excursions is noted. The patient is asked to protrude the mandible to determine whether any deviations or disk interferences exist within the joint. The patient's occlusion is evaluated to determine gross abnormalities and whether the occlusal abnormalities are related to the patient's temporomandibular problem. Finally, anesthetic injections (e.g., auriculotemporal nerve block, local infiltration) may be useful to distinguish between arthrogenous (joint related), myogenous (muscle related), and odontogenic (dental) pain.

Imaging

Radiographic studies may be helpful in determining the cause of the patient's pain or dysfunction. Several different types of radiographs and views are obtained to determine the shape of the condyle and whether evidence of degenerative joint disease exists (Figures 10-5 and 10-6). Radiographic evaluation of patients with TMDs typically includes panoramic or transcranial imaging. These radiographs are limited to identifying gross changes in bone. Several specialized diagnostic studies that are useful in the diagnosis of TMDs have become available over the past several years. Tomography may provide greater accuracy in assessing condylar position and range of mobility.

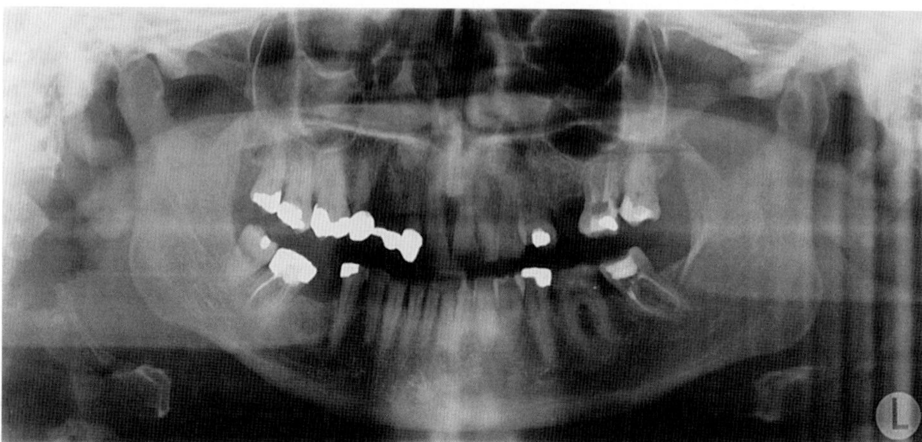

FIGURE 10-5 ■ Panoramic radiograph of a patient with temporomandibular dysfunction and normal anatomy of the mandibular condyles.

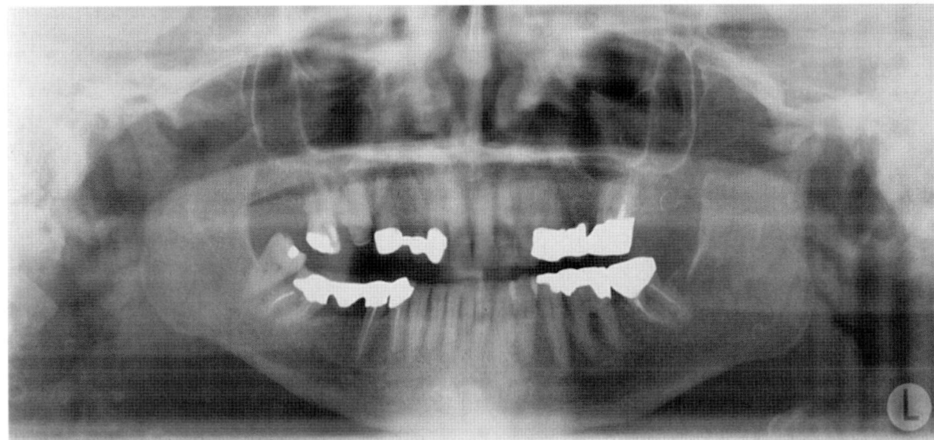

FIGURE 10-6 ■ Panoramic radiograph shows resorption of both the right and the left condyles. In this patient degenerative arthritis followed bilateral surgery of the temporomandibular joint. The left coronoid process was removed during surgery.

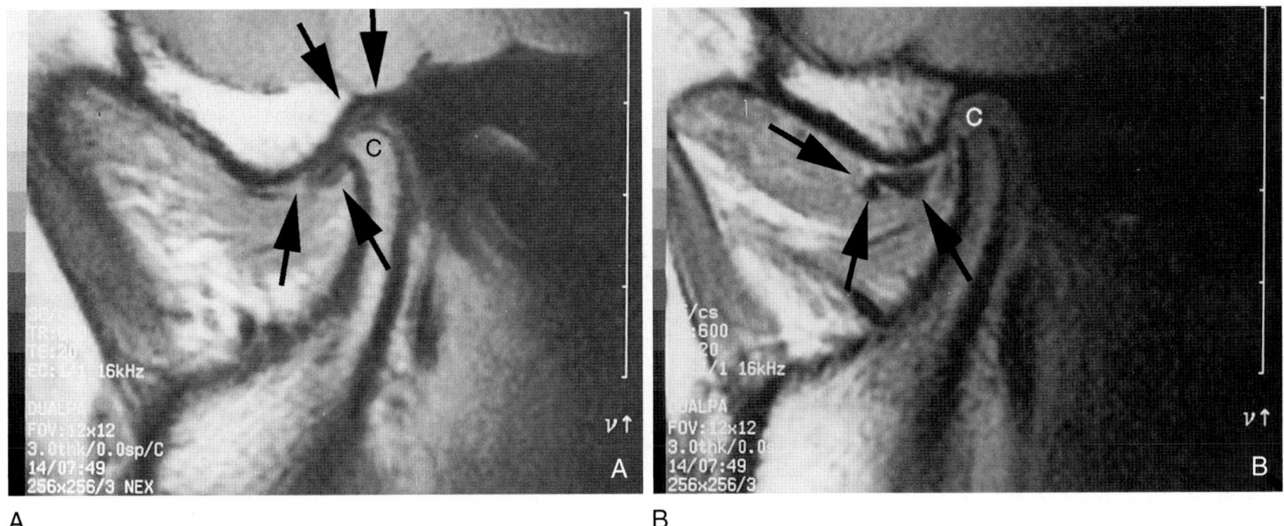

FIGURE 10-7 ■ **A,** Magnetic resonance imaging (MRI) scan of the right temporomandibular joint shows the normal position of the disk. *Arrows* point to the disk. **B,** MRI scan of the left temporomandibular joint in the same patient shows displacement of the disk. *C,* Condyle.

Computerized tomography is most accurate for identifying bone abnormalities; and **magnetic resonance imaging (MRI)** is mandatory for examining disk position, function, morphology, and the presence of joint effusions (inflammatory changes) (Figure 10-7). **Arthrography,** which utilizes a radiopaque contrast agent that is injected into the joint, may be useful when MRI is not tolerated and information regarding the position and morphology of the disk is required.

TYPES OF TEMPOROMANDIBULAR DISORDERS

Myofascial Pain and Dysfunction

MPD comprises at least 50% of all TMDs. It is characterized as dysfunctional muscle hyperactivity with regional pain, tenderness of the affected muscles, and variable amounts of reduced opening and complaints of malocclusion.

Internal Derangements

Internal derangements are divided into disk (meniscal) displacements, ankylosis, and hypermobility disorders.

Disk Displacement

Disk displacements are problems in which the disk (meniscus) is displaced. In some cases the disk is displaced anteriorly and returns to normal position on opening the mouth or movement away from the affected side (disk displacement with reduction). In another form of disk displacement the displaced disk acts as an obstacle to the sliding condyle. In this type of displacement patients complain of problems such as intermittent locking of the jaw; a sudden onset of limited mouth opening, usually associated with cessation of joint sounds; deflection of the mandible with a midline correction on opening; and restricted lateral excursive movements away from the affected side (disk displacement without reduction).

Ankylosis

Ankylosis of the TMJ is defined as immobility of the condyle because of fibrous or bony union between the articulating structures of the joint. Ankylosis can be classified by tissue type (fibrous, bony), location (intraarticular, extraarticular), and extent of fusion (complete, incomplete). Joint infection, usually after trauma, accounts for 50% of all TMJ ankylosis cases, but 30% result from trauma without infection. Fibrotic intraarticular ankylosis is the most common type seen in the TMJ. Trauma-induced hemorrhage (hemarthrosis) is a common cause of this type of ankylosis. Children are more prone to ankylosis because of greater osteogenic potential and less development of the joint meniscus.

Hypermobility Disorders

Hypermobility disorders include **dislocation** and **subluxation.** Dislocation occurs when one or both of the condyles translate anterior to the articular eminence, resulting in an open lock that the patient cannot reduce. Subluxation refers to hypermobility in which the patient is able to relocate the mandible back into the glenoid fossa.

Arthritis

Arthritis is defined as inflammation of a joint and is classified as either **osteoarthritis** or **rheumatoid arthritis**. Osteoarthritis, also referred to as degenerative joint disease, is the most common disease affecting the TMJ. It is characterized by degenerative changes of the articular cartilage with associated remodeling. Patients may have pain symptoms that are worse in the evening, as well as limited opening, muscle splinting, and crepitus of the TMJ. Rheumatoid arthritis is an inflammatory autoimmune disorder of the joints. Approximately 50% to 75% of patients with rheumatoid arthritis have involvement of the TMJ during the course of the disease. In rheumatoid arthritis patients may complain of pain that is worse in the morning, limited opening, occlusal changes, and preauricular edema and tenderness.

TREATMENT OF TEMPOROMANDIBULAR JOINT DISORDERS

Nonsurgical Treatment

Treatment goals for TMJ disorders involve improving function (range of motion) and reducing pain. Treatment typically begins with nonsurgical modalities. The first phase of nonsurgical treatment includes pharmacologic therapy, moist heat, physical therapy, soft mechanical diet, jaw stretching, and coordination exercises. This type of treatment is indicated for internal derangements, MPD, and the arthritides. Medications are used to control pain and inflammation. Muscle relaxants, botulism toxin, and antianxiety agents can be used to reduce muscle hypertonicity. Certain patients may also benefit from occlusal adjustment or orthodontic therapy to correct uneven tooth contacts or malocclusions respectively.

If a patient fails to improve or worsens after approximately 1 to 2 months of conservative nonsurgical management, the second phase, which involves the use of occlusal appliances, may be initiated. Depending on the type used, these function by relaxing muscles, protecting the dentition, stabilizing and protecting the joint, providing biofeedback by making patients aware of bruxing habits, or relieving the load on the disk to allow repair of damaged retrodiscal tissues. Recently botulism toxin (Botox) has been used to treat severe bruxism by providing muscle relaxation and thereby reducing inflammation of the masseter muscle and TMJ capsule.

Surgical Treatment

Patients with TMDs other than MPD may be considered for surgical treatment if they do not respond to nonsurgical therapy and continue to suffer from pain and functional impairment because of interferences in TMJ function. Various surgical techniques are used to treat TMDs. **Arthrocentesis** involves lavaging the joint through a needle. **Arthroscopy** allows direct visualization and manipulation of the joint. Condylotomy involves surgical repositioning of the condyle. **Open joint surgery** is used to perform disk repositioning, replacement or excision, and total joint reconstruction using a prosthetic device or autogenous graft.

Multidisciplinary Management

Additional considerations for patients with oral, facial, and head and neck pain may necessitate referral to other specialists such as a neurologist or otolaryngologist.

TUMORS OF THE TEMPOROMANDIBULAR JOINT

Tumors arising in the TMJ are rare. The most common benign tumors that arise in the condyle include the osteochondroma (Figure 10-8), osteoblastoma, chondroblastoma, and osteoma. Synovial chondromatosis is the most common benign neoplasm of the synovium and is characterized by the development of metaplastic, highly cellular cartilaginous foci in the synovial membrane that results in degenerative changes consistent with osteoarthritis; and by swelling, pain, and limitation of movement. Radiographic findings are variable and may include loose radiopaque bodies in the TMJ, degenerative changes of the articular surfaces, and variable widening or loss of joint space. Osteosarcoma (see Chapter 7) is one

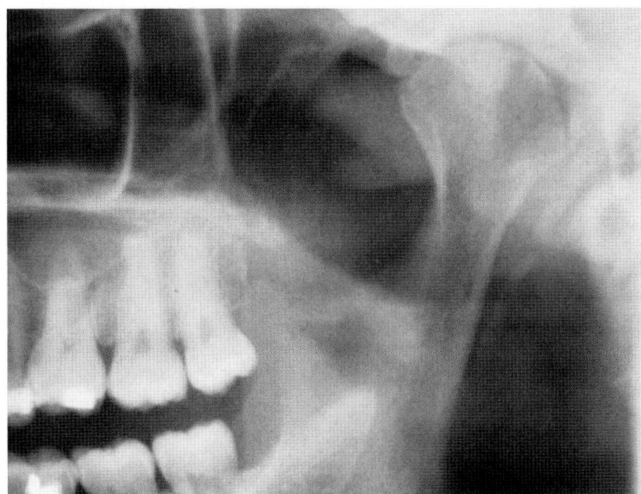

FIGURE 10-8 ■ Panoramic radiograph of an osteochondroma of the mandibular condyle. (Courtesy Dr. David L. Hirsch.)

of the most frequently occurring malignant bone tumors. Approximately 6% to 8% of all osteosarcomas occur in the jaws. Osteosarcoma of the TMJ has been reported.

Selected References

Books

Greenberg M, Glick M, Ship J: *Burket's oral medicine*, ed 11, Philadelphia, 2007, Lippincott.

Kaplan AS, Assael LA: *Temporomandibular disorders*, Philadelphia, 1991, Saunders.

Neville BW et al: *Oral and maxillofacial patholology*, ed 3, St Louis, 2009, Saunders.

Regezi JA, Sciubba JJ, Jordan RCK: *Oral pathology: clinical-pathologic correlations*, ed 5, St Louis, 2008, Saunders.

Journal Articles

Akerman S et al: Relationship between clinical and radiologic findings of the temporomandibular joint in rheumatoid arthritis, *Oral Surg Oral Med Oral Pathol* 66:639, 1988.

Carlsson GE: Epidemiology and treatment need for temporomandibular disorders, *J Orofac Pain* 13:232, 1999.

Clark GT, Kim YJ: A logical approach to the treatment of temporomandibular disorders, *Oral Maxillofac Surg Clin North Am* 7:149, 1995.

De Bont LGM, Kijkgraaf LC, Stegenga B: Epidemiology and natural progression of articular temporomandibular disorders, *Oral Surg Oral Med Oral Path Oral Radiol Endod* 83:72, 1997.

Dhanrajani PJ, Jonaidel O: Trismus: aetiology, differential diagnosis and treatment, *Dent Update* 29:88, 2002.

Dworkin SF et al: Epidemiology of signs and symptoms in temporomandibular disorders: clinical signs in cases and controls, *J Am Dent Assoc* 120:273, 1990.

Epstein JB, Caldwell J, Black G: The utility of panoramic imaging of the temporomandibular joint in patients with temporomandibular disorders, *Oral Surg Oral Med Oral Pathol Oral Radiol Endod* 92:236, 2001.

Kuttila M et al: TMD treatment need in relation to age, gender, stress, and diagnostic subgroup, *J Orofac Pain* 12:67, 1998.

Macfarlane TV et al: Oro-facial pain in the community: prevalence and associated impact, *Community Dent Oral Epidemiol* 30:52, 2002.

McNeill C et al: Temporomandibular disorders: diagnosis, management, education, and research, *J Am Dent Assoc* 120:253, 1990.

Nassif NJ, Al-Salleeh F, Al-Admawi M: The prevalence and treatment needs of symptoms and signs of temporomandibular disorders among young adult males, *J Oral Rehabil* 30:944, 2003.

Parker MW, Holmes EK, Terezhalmy GT: Personality characteristics of patients with temporomandibular disorders: diagnostic and therapeutic implications, *J Orofac Pain* 7:337, 1993.

Stohler CS: Muscle-related temporomandibular disorders, *J Orofac Pain* 13:273, 1999.

Takehana dos Santos D, Cavalcanti MGP: Osteosarcoma of the temporomandibular joint: report of 2 cases, *Oral Surg Oral Med Oral Pathol Oral Radiol Endod* 94:641, 2002.

Tan E, Janovic J: Treating severe bruxism with botulism toxin, *J Am Dent Assoc* 131:211, 2000.

Trieger N, Hoffman H, Rodriguez E: The effect of arthrocentesis of the temporomandibular joint in patients with rheumatoid arthritis, *J Oral Maxillofac Surg* 57:537, 1999.

REVIEW QUESTIONS

1. Disorders of the articulation between the mandible and maxilla are called:
   A. Synovial hyperplasias.
   B. Mandibulomaxillary dysfunction.
   C. Temporomandibular disorders.
   D. Mandibular dysfunction.

2. Using a stethoscope to listen to abnormal noises in the temporomandibular joint is called:
   A. Audiology.
   B. Auscultation.
   C. Arthrography.
   D. Crepitus.

3. Which of the following is the most important aspect of the management of temporomandibular diseases?
   A. Palpation of the muscles of mastication
   B. Using a nonsurgical approach
   C. Adjusting the occlusion
   D. Establishing an accurate diagnosis

4. Translational movements of the temporomandibular movements are:
   A. Hinge movements.
   B. Sliding movements.
   C. Rotational movements.
   D. Only used for diagnosis.

5. Which of the following is considered a parafunctional habit?
   A. Palpation
   B. Mastication
   C. Bruxing
   D. Trauma

6. Which of the following is a symptom of a temporomandibular disorder?
   A. Pain
   B. Malocclusion
   C. A history of surgical treatment of the jaws
   D. Occlusal adjustment

7. Which of the following comprises at least 50% of all temporomandibular disorders?
   A. Hypermobility
   B. Myofascial pain and dysfunction
   C. Internal disk derangements
   D. Osteoarthritis

8. Immobility of the temporomandibular joint because of fibrous or bony union between the articulating structures of the joint is called:
   A. Hypermobility.
   B. Ankylosis.
   C. Disk displacement.
   D. Osteoarthritis.

9. Which of the following is *not* a form of *surgical* treatment used for temporomandibular joint disorders?
   A. Arthrocentesis
   B. Condylotomy
   C. Joint reconstruction
   D. Occlusal appliance

10. Which of the following is the most common benign tumor of the synovium of the temporomandibular joint?
    A. Osteoblastoma
    B. Osteochondroma
    C. Chondroblastoma
    D. Synovial chondromatosis

Glossary

A

Abfraction A wedge-shaped lesion that typically occurs on the cervicofacial areas of teeth.

Abrasion The pathologic wearing away of tooth structure that results from repetitive mechanical habit.

Abscess A collection of pus that has accumulated in a cavity formed in the tissue.

Acantholysis Dissolution of the intercellular bridges of the prickle cell layer of the epithelium.

Acantholytic cells Cells detached from the epithelium that appear rounded. This process is caused by a loss of attachment between the epithelial cells. These cells are present with pemphigus vulgaris. Also known as *Tzanck cells.*

Acanthosis nigrans A skin condition characterized by hyperpigmented, velvety-textured plaques that appear symmetrically distributed in folds and creases of the body. It has been report to be associated with type 2 diabetes mellitus and has been used a clinical indicator when screening for it.

Acquired immune response A response by the body generated by the memory of past exposure to a foreign substance; this response is quicker when encountered a second time.

Acquired immunodeficiency syndrome A syndrome involving a defect in cell-mediated immunity that has a long incubation period, follows a protracted and debilitating course, manifests as opportunistic infections, and has a poor prognosis without treatment. It is caused by the retrovirus human immunodeficiency virus.

Acromegaly A condition caused by hyperfunction of the pituitary gland in adults.

Actinic cheilitis Degeneration of the tissue of the lips caused by sun exposure. Also called *solar cheilitis.*

Actinomycosis An infection caused by a filamentous bacterium called *Actinomyces israelii.* The most characteristic manifestation of the disease is the formation of abscesses that drain through fistulas.

Active immunity Immunity acquired naturally or artificially. It occurs naturally when a microorganism causes the disease. It occurs artificially when a person is injected with or ingests either altered pathogenic microorganisms or products of those microorganisms.

Acute Of short duration or of short and relatively severe course.

Acute inflammation The initial phase of inflammation that is of short duration, lasting only a few days.

Acute lymphonodular pharyngitis An infectious disease caused by the coxsackieviruses. It is characterized by fever, sore throat, and mild headache. Hyperplastic lymphoid tissue of the soft palate or tonsillar pillars appears as yellowish or dark pink nodules.

Acute necrotizing ulcerative gingivitis (ANUG) A painful erythematous gingivitis with necrosis of the interdental papillae. Also called necrotizing ulcerative gingivitis (NUG).

Acute osteomyelitis An acute inflammation of the bone and bone marrow. Acute osteomyelitis of the jaws is most commonly a result of the extension of a periapical abscess. Other potential causes include fracture of the bone, surgery, or bacteremia.

Addison disease A condition characterized by an insufficient production of adrenal steroids. Also known as *primary adrenal cortical insufficiency.*

Adenocarcinoma A nonspecific name for malignant tumors of gland origin.

Adenoid cystic carcinoma A slow-growing malignant tumor of salivary gland origin that can originate from either the major or minor salivary gland tissue. It is unencapsulated and infiltrates surrounding tissue.

Adenoma A benign tumor that originates from glandular epithelium.

Adenomatoid Glandlike.

Adenomatoid odontogenic tumor An encapsulated, benign epithelial odontogenic tumor that has a distinctive age, sex, and site distribution. Seventy percent occur in females under 20 years of age; 70% involve the anterior part of the jaws. May be associated with impacted teeth. Also known as an *odontogenic adenomatoid tumor.*

Agammaglobulinemia Lack of immunoglobulins.

Agranulocytosis A marked decrease in the number of granulocytes, particularly neutrophils.

Alleles Genes that are located at the same level or locus in the two chromosomes of a pair and that determine the same functions or characteristics.

Allergy A hypersensitive state acquired through exposure to a particular allergen. Reexposure to the same allergen elicits an exaggerated reaction.

Alveolar osteitis A postoperative complication of tooth extraction. After extraction the blood clot breaks down and is lost before healing occurs. The socket appears empty, and the bone surface is exposed. Also known as *dry socket*.

Amalgam tattoo A flat, bluish-gray lesion of the oral mucosa resulting from the introduction of amalgam particles into the tissue.

Ameloblastic fibroma A nonencapsulated, benign odontogenic tumor of mixed tissue origin that is composed of strands and small islands of ameloblast-like epithelial cells and mesenchymal cells that resemble the dental papilla. It occurs in young children and adults, and the most common location is the mandibular bicuspid and molar region. Most patients are asymptomatic, but bone expansion or swelling may be noted.

Ameloblastic fibro-odontoma A benign odontogenic tumor that has features of both an ameloblastic fibroma and an odontoma. It typically arises in the posterior jaws and is often asymptomatic.

Ameloblastoma A benign, slow-growing but locally aggressive epithelial odontogenic tumor that may arise in either the maxilla or the mandible. It is an unencapsulated tumor that infiltrates into surrounding tissue and can cause extensive destruction.

Amelogenesis imperfecta A broad group of conditions that affect the structural formation of enamel. The disease is divided into four main types: type I, hypoplastic; type II, hypocalcified; type III, hypomaturation; type IV, hypoplastic-hypomaturation.

Amenorrhea Abnormal temporary or permanent cessation of menstrual cycles.

Amino acid An organic compound containing the amino group NH_2. Amino acids are the main component of proteins.

Anaphylaxis A type of hypersensitivity or allergic reaction in which the exaggerated immunologic response results from the release of vasoactive substances such as histamine. The reaction occurs on reexposure to a foreign protein or other substance after sensitization.

Anaplastic A loss of differentiation of cells and their orientation to one another; a characteristic of malignant tumor tissue.

Anemia Reduction to less than normal of the number of red blood cells, quantity of hemoglobin, or volume of packed red blood cells in the blood.

Aneuploid Any extra number of chromosomes that do not represent an exact multiple of the total chromosome complement (e.g., trisomy [a pair with an identical extra chromosome] and monosomy [a missing chromosome from a pair]).

Aneurysmal bone cyst A pseudocyst that consists of blood-filled spaces surrounded by multinucleated giant cells and fibrous connective tissue. The radiolucent lesion typically bulges between the roots of teeth, creating a radiographic appearance termed *scalloping*.

Angioedema A lesion that appears as a diffuse swelling of tissue caused by increased permeability of deeper blood vessels. The skin covering the swelling appears normal.

Angular cheilitis Erythema or fissuring at the labial commissures. Angular cheilitis may be caused by factors such as nutritional deficiency; however, it most commonly results from *Candida* infection.

Ankyloglossia Extensive adhesion of the tongue to the floor of the mouth or the lingual aspect of the anterior portion of the mandible; caused by a short lingual frenum.

Ankylosed teeth Teeth in which bone has fused to cementum and dentin, preventing exfoliation of deciduous teeth and eruption of the underlying permanent tooth; ankylosed teeth typically appear submerged clinically.

Ankylosis Immobility of a joint because of fibrous or bony union between the articulating structures of the joint. Ankylosis can be classified by tissue type, location, and extent of fusion.

Anodontia Complete or almost complete congenital lack of teeth.

Anomaly Marked deviation from normal, especially as a result of congenital or hereditary defects.

Anorexia nervosa An eating disorder characterized by a distorted perception of body image, in addition to depression, intense fear of weight gain, and self-imposed starvation.

Antibody A protein molecule, also called an *immunoglobulin*, which is produced by plasma cells and reacts with a specific antigen.

Antibody titer The specific level of an antibody in the blood. It can be measured by laboratory tests.

Antigen Any substance that is able to induce a specific immune response.

Antigenic determinate The portion of an antibody that recognizes and binds to the antigen.

Antigens Foreign substances against which the immune system defends the body.

Aphthous ulcer Painful oral ulcer that frequently recurs in episodes. Also know as *canker sore* or *aphthous stomatitis.*

Aplasia Lack of development.

Aplastic anemia A type of anemia in which patients experience a dramatic decrease in all the circulating blood cells (pancytopenia) because of a severe depression of bone marrow activity. Can be primary (cause unknown) or secondary (caused by a drug or chemical agent).

Arthralgia Severe pain in a joint.

Arthritis Inflammation of a joint. It is classified as either osteoarthritis or rheumatoid arthritis.

Arthrocentesis Surgical puncture of a joint, usually for the withdrawal of fluid.

Arthrography Radiography of a joint after injection of an opaque contrast material.

Arthroscopy A method for evaluating and manipulating a joint by the insertion of a camera and instruments.

Articular disk A pad of fibrocartilage or dense fibrous tissue present in some synovial joints (e.g., the temporomandibular joint).

Articulation The location where bones are joined together.

Aspirin burn A type of chemical injury that occurs when a patient places an aspirin tablet directly on a tooth instead of swallowing it. The soft tissue becomes necrotic and appears white.

Atrophy The decrease in size and function of a cell, tissue, organ, or whole body.

Attrition The wearing away of tooth structure during mastication. Attrition occurs normally but may also be accelerated by teeth grinding against hard restorations.

Auscultation The act of listening to sounds within the body.

Autoantibody An antibody that reacts against an antigenic constituent of the person's own tissues.

Autoimmune disease A disease characterized by tissue injury caused by a humoral or cell-mediated immune response against constituents of the body's own tissues.

Autoimmunity Immune-mediated destruction of the body's own cells and tissues; immunity against self.

Autosomes (adjective, autosomal) The nonsex chromosomes that are identical for men and women.

B

B lymphocyte A lymphocyte, also called a *B cell,* which matures without passing through the thymus and later can develop into a plasma cell that produces antibodies.

Barr body Condensed chromatin of the inactivated X chromosome, which is found at the periphery of the nucleus of cells in women.

Basal cell carcinoma A malignant skin tumor associated with excessive sun exposure that appears as a nonhealing ulcer with characteristic rolled borders. It does not occur in the oral cavity.

Behçet syndrome A chronic, recurrent, autoimmune disease consisting primarily of oral ulcers, genital ulcers, and ocular inflammation. The oral ulcers that appear are similar to aphthous ulcers.

Bence Jones proteins Fragments of immunoglobulins found in the urine of patients with multiple myeloma.

Benign A condition that, if untreated or with treated with symptomatic therapy, will not become life threatening.

Benign cementoblastoma A cementum-producing tumor that is fused to the root or roots of a vital tooth. It typically occurs in young adults, and pain is a frequent symptom.

Benign fibro-osseous lesion A benign lesion of bone characterized histologically by cellular fibrous connective tissue mixed with irregularly shaped bone trabeculae or cementoid material.

Benign mixed tumor The most common of the benign salivary gland tumors. Also known as a *pleomorphic adenoma.*

Benign mucous membrane pemphigoid A chronic autoimmune disease that affects the oral mucosa, conjunctiva, genital mucosa, and skin. It is also known as *mucous membrane pemphigoid* and *cicatricial pemphigoid.*

Benign tumor A tumor that is not malignant; favorable for treatment and recovery.

Bleeding time A test that provides an assessment of the adequacy of platelet function. It measures how long it takes a standardized skin incision to stop bleeding by the formation of a temporary hemostatic plug or clot.

Brachydactyly Short fingers or toes or both.

Branchial arch One of a series of mesodermal bars located between the branchial clefts. During embryonic stages the arch contributes to the formation of the face, jaws, and neck.

Brittle diabetes A term used to describe diabetes in patients who have blood glucose levels that are unstable or are not well controlled.

Brush test A technique used to obtain information from oral mucosal epithelium. This technique uses a circular brush to obtain cells from the full thickness of the epithelium, including cells from the keratin layer through the basal layer.

Bruton disease A type of primary immunodeficiency in which B cells do not mature. Plasma cells are deficient throughout the body; T cells are normal. Also called *X-linked congenital agammaglobulinemia.*

Bruxism The grinding and clenching of the teeth together for nonfunctional purposes.

Bulimia An eating disorder characterized by food binges, usually of high caloric intake, followed by self-induced vomiting.

Bulla (adjective, bullous; plural, bullae) A circumscribed, elevated, fluid-filled lesion within or below the skin or mucous membranes that is larger than 5 mm in diameter and usually contains serous fluid.

Bullous lichen planus The type of lichen planus in which the epithelium separates from the connective tissue and erosions, bullae, or ulcers form.

C

Café au lait spots Light brown skin lesions.

Calcifying epithelial odontogenic tumor A benign epithelial odontogenic tumor in which the proliferating cells do not resemble odontogenic epithelium. The tumor is composed of islands and sheets of polyhedral (multisided) epithelial cells. It is also known as a *Pindborg tumor.*

Calcifying odontogenic cyst A nonaggressive cystic lesion lined by odontogenic epithelium with associated ghost cell keratinization.

Calcitonin A polypeptide secreted by the C cells of the thyroid gland.

Cancer Malignancy

Candidal leukoplakia A type of candidiasis that appears as a white lesion that does not wipe off the mucosa. An important diagnostic feature of this type of candidiasis is that it is treated with antifungal medication. Also called *chronic hyperplastic candidiasis* and *hypertrophic candidiasis.*

Candidiasis An overgrowth of the yeastlike fungus *Candida albicans.* It is the most common oral fungal infection. It can result from many different conditions, including antibiotic use, cancer, corticosteroid therapy, dentures, diabetes mellitus, and HIV infection. Also called *moniliasis* and *thrush.*

Capillary hemangioma A hemangioma that contains numerous small capillaries.

Carcinoma A malignant tumor of epithelial tissue origin.

Carrier In genetics a heterozygous individual who is clinically normal but who can transmit a recessive trait or characteristic; also, a person who is homozygous for an autosomal-dominant condition with low penetrance.

Catabolism Component of metabolism that involves the breakdown of molecules with the concomitant release of energy.

Cavernous hemangioma A hemangioma containing large blood vessels.

Celiac sprue A chronic disorder associated with a sensitivity to dietary gluten, a protein found in wheat and wheat products. When gluten is ingested, injury to the intestinal mucosa results.

Cell-mediated immunity Immunity in which the predominant role is played by T lymphocytes.

Cementogenesis The formation of cementum.

Cementoma An apical lesion associated with the apices of teeth. It may present as a mass of fibrous connective tissue, fibrous connective tissue with spicules of cementum, or calcified mass resembling cemetum and having few cellular elements.

Cemento-ossifying fibroma A tumor that has a mixture of globular calcifications resembling cementum and bone trabeculae that results from the potential of periodontal ligament cells to produce either cementum or bone.

Cementum Outermost layer of the root of the tooth.

Centimeter (cm) One hundredth of a meter. Equivalent to a little less than $\frac{1}{2}$ inch (0.393 of an inch).

Central cementifying fibroma A benign, well-circumscribed tumor classified as a fibro-osseous lesion. The calcifications are rounded and globular, resembling cementum. Affected patients may be asymptomatic or demonstrate bone expansion or facial asymmetry.

Central Occurring within the bone. In oral pathology a lesion occurring within the maxilla or mandible.

Central ossifying fibroma A benign, well-circumscribed tumor classified as a fibro-osseous lesion. The calcifications resemble bone trabeculae. Affected patients may be asymptomatic or demonstrate bone expansion or facial asymmetry.

Centromere The constricted portion of the chromosome that divides the short arms from the long arms.

Chancre Lesion of the primary stage of syphilis. It is highly infectious and forms at the site at which the spirochete enters the body.

Chemotaxis The directed movement of white blood cells to the area of injury by chemical mediators.

Chemotherapy Cancer treatment that uses chemical agents to modify or destroy cancer cells.

Cherubism A disorder beginning in childhood characterized by progressive bilateral facial swelling that can occur in either the maxilla or mandible, with involvement of the mandible being most common. The swollen jaws and raised eyes give a "chubby angel" appearance, and radiographs show multilocular radiolucent lesions.

Chiasmata The intercrossing of chromatids of the same or homologous chromosomes that takes place at metaphase of first meiosis for the purpose of genetic recombination.

Chickenpox A highly contagious disease caused by the varicella-zoster virus. It is characterized by vesicular and pustular eruptions of the skin and/or mucous membranes, along with systemic symptoms such as headache, fever, and malaise. It usually occurs in children.

Chondroma A benign tumor of cartilage.

Chondrosarcoma A malignant tumor of cartilage that can occur in either the maxilla or mandible.

Chromatid Either of the two vertical halves of a chromosome that are joined at the centromere.

Chromatin A general term used to refer to the material (DNA) that forms the chromosomes.

Chromosomes The small bodies in the nucleus of a cell that carry the chemical instructions for reproduction of the cell in addition to other cellular functions.

Chronic atrophic candidiasis The most common type of candidiasis affecting the oral mucosa. This type of candidiasis presents as erythematous mucosa, but the erythematous change is limited to mucosa that is covered by a full or partial denture. Also called *denture stomatitis.*

Chronic hyperplastic candidiasis A type of candidiasis that appears as a white lesion that does not wipe off the mucosa. An important diagnostic feature of this type of candidiasis is that it is treated with antifungal medication. Also called *candidal leukoplakia* and *hypertrophic candidiasis.*

Chronic hyperplastic pulpitis An excessive proliferation of chronically inflamed dental pulp tissue. Also called *pulp polyp.*

Chronic inflammation Inflammation that may last weeks, months, or indefinitely.

Chronic mucocutaneous candidiasis A severe form of candidiasis that usually occurs in patients who are severely immunocompromised. Oral involvement may appear as pseudomembranous, erythematous, or hyperplastic candidiasis. Angular cheilitis is common.

Chronic neutropenia A variety of neutropenia in which the intraoral manifestations are similar to those of cyclic neutropenia but are constant. Also known as *Kostmann syndrome*

Chronic osteomyelitis A long-standing inflammation of bone.

Chronic Persisting over a long time.

Chronic sclerosing osteomyelitis A condition that is characterized by an inflamed bone that has developed radiopacities.

Cicatricial pemphigoid A chronic autoimmune disease that affects the oral mucosa, conjunctiva, genital mucosa, and skin. It is also known as *mucous membrane pemphigoid* and *benign mucous membrane pemphigoid.*

Cleft lip Congenital anomaly of the face caused by the failure of fusion between the embryonic maxillary and medial nasal processes.

Cleft palate Congenital anomaly of the oral cavity caused by the failure of fusion between the embryonic palatal shelves.

Cleidocranial dysplasia A familial disease or congenital disorder characterized by retarded or failed formation of the clavicles; delayed closure of the sutures and fontanels of the skull; and delayed eruption of teeth, with formation of supernumerary teeth. Characterized by underdevelopment of the maxillae, agenesis or aplasia of the clavicle, abnormalities in other skeletal bones and muscles, and irregularities of the dentition.

Clotting factors A cascade of circulating plasma proteins (made almost exclusively in the liver) that are necessary to convert precursor fibrinogen to fibrin. Also called *coagulation factors.*

Coagulation factors A cascade of circulating plasma proteins (made almost exclusively in the liver) that are necessary to convert precursor fibrinogen to fibrin. Also called *clotting factors.*

Coagulation Formation of a clot.

Coalescence The process by which parts of a whole join together, or fuse, to make one.

Codominance The full expression in a heterozygote of both alleles of a pair of chromosomes, with neither influenced by the other. A good example is the AB blood group.

Codon The sequence of three bases in DNA that codes for one amino acid.

Cold sore The most common type of recurrent oral herpes simplex infection that occurs on the vermilion border of the lips. Also called *herpes labialis* or *fever blister*.

Coloboma A cleft generally seen on the iris or the eyelids.

Commissural lip pits Epithelium-lined blind tracts located at the corners of the mouth. This is a relatively common developmental anomaly.

Commissure The site of union of corresponding parts (e.g., the corners of the lips).

Complete blood count A series of tests that examines the red blood cells, white blood cells, and platelets.

Complex odontoma An odontogenic tumor that consists of a mass of enamel, dentin, cementum, and pulp, which does not resemble a normal tooth. It commonly occurs in the posterior mandible.

Compound odontoma An odontogenic tumor that consists of a collection of numerous small teeth. They do not exhibit unlimited growth potential and therefore are more accurately classified as developmental lesions rather than true tumors. They are usually located in the anterior maxilla.

Concrescence A condition in dentistry in which two adjacent teeth are united by cementum.

Condensing osteitis A change in bone near the apices of teeth; thought to be a reaction to low-grade infection.

Condyloma acuminatum A benign papillary lesion caused by human papillomavirus. Oral condylomas appear as papillary bulbous masses and can occur anywhere in the oral mucosa.

Congenital disorder A disorder that is present at birth. It can be either inherited or developmental.

Congenital epulis A benign neoplasm composed of cells that closely resemble those seen in the granular cell tumor. The neoplasm most likely arises from a primitive mesenchymal cell. This tumor is present at birth and appears as a sessile or pedunculated mass on the gingiva. Also known as *congenital epulis of the newborn*.

Congenital lip pit Congenital depression on the vermilion portion of the lower lip that may appear either unilaterally or bilaterally.

Congenital Present at and existing from the time of birth.

Congenital syphilis The type of syphilis that is transmitted from an infected mother to the fetus because the organism can cross the placenta and enter the fetal circulation.

Connective tissue disease Diseases in which the body's recognition mechanism breaks down and certain body cells are no longer tolerated. The immune system treats body cells as antigens. Also known as an autoimmune disease.

Consanguinity Blood relationship. In genetics the term is generally used to describe matings or marriages among close relatives.

Contact dermatitis Lesions resulting from the direct contact of an allergen with the skin.

Contact mucositis Lesions resulting from the direct contact of an allergen with the mucosa.

Corrugated Having a surface that appears wrinkled.

Coxsackieviruses A group of viruses named for the town in New York where it was first discovered. It causes several different infectious diseases. Three of these diseases have distinctive oral lesions: herpangina, hand-foot-and-mouth disease, and acute lymphonodular pharyngitis.

C-reactive protein (CRP) A protein produced in the liver that becomes elevated during episodes of acute inflammation or infection.

Crepitus A dry, crackling sound.

Cretinism The presence of hypothyroidism during infancy and childhood.

Crossing over The exchange of segments between chromatids of the same or homologous chromosomes that takes place at metaphase of first meiosis. Crossing over is the result of chiasmata.

Cyclic neutropenia A hereditary disease characterized by flulike symptoms and severe ulcerative gingivitis or gingivostomatitis. Cycles can occur every 3 to 4 weeks with painful, crater-like ulcers of variable size. Episodes can lead to severe periodontal disease, loss of alveolar bone, tooth mobility, and exfoliation of teeth.

Cylindroma Another name for adenoid cystic carcinoma; so-called because of its microscopic appearance, which shows round and oval islands that represent cylinders of tumor.

Cyst An abnormal pathologic sac or cavity that is lined with epithelium and enclosed in a connective tissue capsule.

Cyst of the palatine papilla A cyst found in the incisive papilla.

Cytokines Chemical mediators produced by the cells involved in the immune response.

D

Dark-field microscopy Examination of a microscopic specimen in which illumination causes the specimen to appear to glow against a dark background. Used to identify the syphilis spirochete.

Delayed hypersensitivity The type of hypersensitivity in which there is a latent period between the antigen introduction and the reaction. Cellular reactions are mediated by the T lymphocytes. It can be used to test for tuberculosis and is responsible for rejection of tissue grafts and transplanted organs.

Deletion In genetics the loss of part of a chromosome.

Dens evaginatus An accessory enamel cusp found on the occlusal tooth surface. This developmental anomaly occurs most often on the mandibular premolars.

Dens in dente "A tooth within a tooth"; a developmental anomaly that results when the enamel organ invaginates into the crown of a tooth before mineralization. Also called *dens invaginatus*.

Dens invaginatus "A tooth within a tooth"; a developmental anomaly that results when the enamel organ invaginates into the crown of a tooth before mineralization. Also called *dens in dente*.

Dental fluorosis A condition resulting from the ingestion of high concentrations of fluoride, causing the affected teeth to have a mottled discoloration of enamel.

Dental papilla The mesenchymal tissue within a tooth germ. After dentin is produced, the dental papilla is called the dental pulp.

Dentigerous cyst A cyst that forms around the crown of an unerupted or developing tooth. Also called a *follicular cyst*.

Dentin Body of the tooth. It surrounds the pulp and underlies the enamel on the crown and the cementum on the root of teeth.

Dentin dysplasia A genetic disturbance of the dentin characterized by early calcification of the pulp chambers and root canals and root resorption. It is subdivided into radicular dentin dysplasia and coronal dentin dysplasia.

Dentinogenesis imperfecta A disturbance of the dentin of genetic origin; characterized by early calcification of the pulp chambers and root canals, marked attrition, and an opalescent hue to the teeth. It may be hereditary and associated with osteogenesis imperfecta, or it may occur in isolation.

Dentinogenesis The formation of dentin.

Denture-induced fibrous hyperplasia A lesion caused by an ill-fitting denture. It is located in the vestibule adjacent to the denture border. It is composed of dense fibrous connective tissue surfaced by stratified squamous epithelium. Commonly called *epulis fissuratum* or *inflammatory hyperplasia*.

Denture stomatitis The most common type of candidiasis affecting the oral mucosa. This type of candidiasis presents as erythematous mucosa, but the erythematous change is limited to the mucosa covered by a full or partial denture. Also called *chronic atrophic candidiasis*.

Deoxyribonucleic acid (DNA) A substance composed of a double chain of polynucleotides; both chains coiled around a central axis form a double helix. DNA is the basic genetic code or template for polypeptide formation.

Dermoid cyst A developmental cyst that is often present at birth or noted in young children. It is uncommon in the head and neck but usually occurs in the anterior floor of the mouth. It is lined by orthokeratinized, stratified squamous epithelium surrounded by a connective tissue wall. The lumen is usually filled with keratin.

Desquamative gingivitis A clinical and descriptive term for gingival lesions that may be seen in lichen planus, pemphigus vulgaris, and mucous membrane pemphigoid. The gingival margin is ulcerated or eroded and shows loss of normal stippling.

Development The process by which an individual reaches maturity.

Developmental disorder A failure or disturbance that occurs during the process of prenatal development that can result in a lack, excess, or deformity of a body part. Also called *developmental anomaly*.

Diabetes mellitus A chronic disorder of carbohydrate (glucose) metabolism that is characterized by abnormally high blood glucose levels (hyperglycemia). This is caused by either a lack of the hormone insulin, defective insulin that does not work properly, or increased insulin resistance.

Differentiation The distinguishing of one thing from another.

Diffuse In the description of a lesion, the borders of the lesion are not well defined, and it is not possible to detect the exact parameters of the lesion.

DiGeorge syndrome A type of primary immunodeficiency in which the thymus is deficient or lacking; therefore T lymphocytes do not mature. Also called *thymic hypoplasia*.

Dilaceration An abnormal bend or curve in the root of a tooth.

Diploid Having two sets of chromosomes; the normal constitution of somatic cells.

Disk displacements Problems in which the disk of the temporomandibular joint (meniscus) is displaced.

Dislocation When one or both of the mandibular condyles translates anterior to the articular eminence, resulting in an open lock that the patient cannot reduce.

Disorder Derangement of function.

Distomolar A maxillary fourth molar; the second most common supernumerary tooth.

Dominant In genetics a trait or characteristic that is manifested when it is carried by only one of a pair of homologous chromosomes.

Double helix The coiled structure of double-stranded DNA in which strands linked by hydrogen bonds form a spiral configuration.

Down syndrome A type of abnormality in which three of chromosome 21 are found instead of two. This results in abnormal physical characteristics and mental impairment. Also called *trisomy 21*.

Dry socket A postoperative complication of tooth extraction. After extraction the blood clot breaks down and is lost before healing occurs. The socket appears empty, and the bone surface is exposed. Also known as *alveolar osteitis.*

Duplication A chromosome is larger than normal, the extra segment being copied from within the chromosome itself.

Dysplasia Disordered growth; alteration in size, shape, and organization of adult cells or structures.

E

Ecchymosis A small, flat, hemorrhagic patch larger than a petechia on the skin or mucous membrane.

Ectopic geographic tongue A term used to described the condition of geographic tongue when it is found on mucosal surfaces other than the tongue.

Ectopic lingual thyroid nodule A small mass of thyroid tissue located on the tongue, distant from the normal anatomic location of the thyroid gland. It is an uncommon developmental anomaly that results from the failure of the primitive thyroid tissue to migrate from its developmental location in the area of the foramen cecum on the posterior portion of the tongue to its normal position in the neck. Also called *lingual thyroid.*

Edema Excess plasma or exudate in the interstitial space of the tissues that causes swelling.

Ellis-Van Creveld syndrome A syndrome characterized by dwarfism, polydactyly, and possible retardation and congenital heart defects. Oral manifestations include fusion of the anterior portion of the maxillary gingiva to the upper lip from canine to canine. Most teeth have a conical shape and exhibit enamel hypoplasia.

Embedded teeth Teeth that do not erupt because of a lack of eruptive force.

Emigration The passage of white blood cells through the endothelium and wall of the microcirculation into the injured tissue.

Enamel Hard outer layer of the crown of the tooth.

Enamel hypocalcification A developmental anomaly that results in a disturbance of the maturation of the enamel matrix. It usually appears as a localized, chalky white spot on the middle third of smooth crowns, and the underlying enamel may be soft and susceptible to caries.

Enamel hypoplasia The incomplete or defective formation of enamel, resulting in the alteration of tooth form or color.

Enamel pearl A small, spheric enamel projection located on a root surface. Also called *enameloma.*

Enameloma A small, spheric enamel projection located on a root surface. Also called *enamel pearl.*

Encapsulated Surrounded by a capsule of fibrous connective tissue.

Endogenous Originating or produced within an organism or one of its parts.

Enucleation Surgical removal without cutting into the lesion; involves "scooping" out of a lesion along its peripheral borders.

Enzyme-linked immunosorbent assay A species-specific serologic laboratory procedure used to identify microorganisms infecting or inhabiting a tissue or organ system. Routinely used in HIV testing.

Eosinophilic granuloma of bone A solitary or chronic localized form of Langerhans cell disease. This form primarily affects older children and young adults. The skull and mandible are commonly involved with eosinophilic granuloma. The radiographic appearance varies, and the lesion may resemble periodontal disease or periapical inflammatory disease; or it may appear as a well-circumscribed radiolucency with or without a sclerotic border.

Epidemic parotitis A viral infection of the salivary glands caused by a paramyxovirus. The disease most commonly occurs in children and is characterized by painful swelling of the salivary glands, most commonly bilateral swelling of the parotid glands. Also called *mumps*.

Epidermal cyst A raised nodule in the skin of the face or neck. It is lined by keratinizing epithelium that resembles the epithelium of skin (epidermis). The cyst lumen is usually filled with keratin scales.

Epidermoid carcinoma A malignant tumor of squamous epithelium. It is the most common primary malignancy of the oral cavity and, like other malignant tumors, can infiltrate adjacent tissues and metastasize to distant sites. Also known as *squamous cell carcinoma*.

Epidermoid cells Squamouslike epithelial cells

Epilepsy A group of neurologic disorders characterized by recurrent episodes of convulsive seizures, sensory disturbances, abnormal behavior, and loss of consciousness.

Epistaxis Nosebleed.

Epithelial dysplasia A histologic diagnosis that indicates disordered growth. It is considered a premalignant condition.

Epithelial Pertaining to the epithelium.

Epithelial tumor A tumor that develops from epithelium. There are three types: (1) tumors derived from squamous epithelium, (2) tumors derived from salivary gland epithelium, and (3) tumors derived from odontogenic epithelium.

Epithelium The layer of cells that lines a body cavity.

Epstein-Barr virus A herpesvirus associated with several diseases that occur in the oral region, including infectious mononucleosis, nasopharyngeal carcinoma, Burkitt lymphoma, and hairy leukoplakia.

Erosion The loss of tooth structure resulting from chemical action.

Erosive lichen planus The type of lichen planus in which the epithelium separates from the connective tissue and erosions, bullae, or ulcers form.

Eruption cyst A cyst that forms in the soft tissue around the crown of an erupting tooth.

Erythema An abnormal redness of the skin or mucosa.

Erythema multiforme An acute, self-limited disease that affects the skin and mucous membranes. The cause is not clear, but some evidence exists that it is a hypersensitivity reaction.

Erythematous candidiasis A type of candidiasis characterized by an erythematous, often painful, mucosa. It may be localized to one area of the oral mucosa or be more generalized.

Erythroplakia A clinical term that is used to describe an oral mucosal lesion that appears as a smooth red patch or a granular red and velvety patch.

Euploid A cell or organism that has an integral multiple of the monoploid number of chromosomes.

Excision Surgical removal.

Exostosis (exostoses) A small nodular excrescence of normal compact bone. Exostoses present as asymptomatic, bony hard nodules on the buccal aspect of the maxillary or mandibular alveolar ridges.

Expressivity In genetics the degree of clinical manifestation of a trait or characteristic.

External tooth resorption Resorption of a tooth structure beginning at the outside of the tooth. It usually involves the root of the tooth but may involve the crown of an impacted tooth.

Extramedullary plasmacytoma A localized tumor of plasma cells located in soft tissue.

Extraosseous cyst A cyst that occurs in the soft tissue.

Exudate Inflammatory fluid formed as a reaction to injury of tissues and blood vessels.

F

Facial hemihypertrophy Localized enlargement affecting one side of the orofacial structures.

Facies The appearance of the face.

Factor IX A factor that is active in the formation of intrinsic blood thromboplastin. A deficiency results in Christmas disease (hemophilia B), which is caused by a decrease in the amount of thromboplastin formed. Also called *plasma thromboplastin*.

Familial Something that affects more members of a family than would be expected by chance.

Fever An elevation of body temperature to greater than the normal of 98.6° F (37° C).

Fever blister The most common type of recurrent oral herpes simplex infection that occurs on the vermilion border of the lips. Also called *cold sore* or *herpes labialis*.

Fibrin An insoluble protein that is essential to the clotting of blood.

Fibroma A broad-based, persistent exophytic lesion composed of dense, scarlike connective tissue containing few blood vessels. It occurs as a result of chronic trauma or an episode of trauma. It is also known as an *irritation fibroma* or *traumatic fibroma*.

Fibrous dysplasia A benign fibro-osseous lesion composed of vascularized, cellular fibrous connective tissue interspersed with irregular trabeculae of bone emerging from the connective tissue. It is characterized by the replacement of bone with abnormal fibrous connective tissue interspersed with varying amounts of calcification.

Fissure A cleft or groove, normal or otherwise, showing prominent depth.

Fissured Having surface clefting or grooves.

Fissured tongue Characterized by the dorsal surface of the tongue having deep fissures or grooves.

Fistula A drainage passage that bores through tissue, allowing drainage to the outside. It is formed at the expense of healthy, functioning tissue as the area that is lost becomes necrotic.

Fixed drug eruption Lesions that appear in the same site each time a drug is introduced.

Flare Redness of the skin or mucosa around an area of an irritant.

Florid cemento-osseous dysplasia A fibro-osseous lesion characterized by disordered cementum and bone development. It presents as a circular mass of hard tissue that easily separates from the adjacent normal bone. This lesion characteristically involves multiple quadrants in the maxilla and mandible.

Focal cemento-osseous dysplasia An asymptomatic fibro-osseous lesion typically arises in the posterior mandible. A characteristic feature is that it is composed of numerous gritty pieces of soft and hard tissue.

Focal epithelial hyperplasia A disease caused by a human papillomavirus (HPV) that is characterized by the presence of multiple whitish-to–pale pink nodules distributed throughout the oral mucosa. Also known as *Heck disease*.

Focal palmoplantar A syndrome characterized by areas of hyperkeratinization of the palms and soles and marked hyperkeratinization of the labial and lingual gingiva.

Folic acid A member of the vitamin B complex necessary for the normal production of red blood cells.

Follicular cyst A cyst that forms around the crown of an unerupted or developing tooth. Also called a *dentigerous cyst*.

Fordyce granules Clusters of ectopic sebaceous glands. They are most commonly seen on the lips and buccal mucosa. They are considered a variant of normal.

Frenectomy Surgical removal of a portion of the lingual frenum.

Frontal process Covering of the brain from which the forehead and other facial structures develops; located just above the stomodeum.

Fusion The union of two adjoining tooth germs.

G

Gamete Spermatozoon or ovum.

Gap 1 (G_1) phase The phase the cell enters after each cell division is completed and before the next division can occur.

Gap 2 (G_2) phase The phase that follows S phase that ends when mitotic division begins.

Gardner syndrome An inherited syndrome characterized by the presence of osteomas in various bones, especially in the frontal bones, mandible, and maxilla. Osteomas of the facial skeleton expand, obliterate the sinuses, and cause facial asymmetry. Intestinal polyps are also present, which become malignant after age 30. As known as *familial colorectal polyposis*.

Gemination "Twinning"; a single tooth germ attempts to divide, resulting in the incomplete formation of two teeth; the tooth usually has a single root and root canal.

Genes The hereditary units that are transmitted from one generation to another.

Genetic heterogeneity Having more than one inheritance pattern.

Geographic tongue A condition characterized by diffuse areas devoid of filiform papillae that develop on the dorsal and lateral borders of the tongue. These areas appear as erythematous patches that are surrounded by a white or yellow perimeter. The fungiform papillae are distinct within the erythematous patch.

Ghost cell Red blood cells that have lost their hemoglobin so that only the plasma membranes are observed in microscopic examinations of urine samples. The hemoglobin is destroyed by the presence of the urine.

Ghost teeth A developmental problem in which one or several teeth in the same quadrant radiographically exhibit a marked reduction in radiodensity and a characteristic ghostlike appearance. Very thin enamel and dentin are present. Also called *regional odontodysplasia*.

Giant cell granuloma A lesion that contains many multinucleated giant cells and well-vascularized connective tissue. It occurs only in the jaws.

Gigantism Excessive growth resulting in a stature larger than the range that is normal for age and race.

Gingival cyst A cyst appears as a small bulge or swelling of the attached gingiva or interdental papillae. It exhibits the same type of epithelial lining as the lateral periodontal cyst and is located in the soft tissue of the same area.

Gingival fibromatosis An enlargement of the gingiva that results from the marked collagenization of the fibrous connective tissue. It is a component of many different inherited syndromes.

Gingival fibromatosis with hypertrichosis An inherited syndrome characterized by gingival fibromatosis and excessive growth of hair (hypertrichosis), especially of the eyebrows, extremities, genitals, and sacral region.

Gingival fibromatosis with multiple hyaline fibromas An inherited syndrome characterized by gingival fibromatosis; hypertrophy of the nail beds; and multiple hyaline fibrous tumors developing on the nose, chin, head, back, fingers, thighs, and legs. Also known as the *Murray-Puretíc Drescher syndrome*.

Gingival hyperkeratosis A syndrome characterized by areas of hyperkeratinization of the palms and soles and marked hyperkeratinization of the labial and lingual gingiva.

Gingival hyperplasia Enlargement of gingiva.

Globular process A pair of bulges formed from the median nasal process that grow downward, forming a portion of the upper lip.

Globulomaxillary cyst A cyst found between the roots of the maxillary lateral incisor and cuspid. It is characterized by well-defined, pear-shaped radiolucency and is believed to be of odontogenic epithelial origin. When it is large enough, divergence of the roots of adjacent teeth can result.

Granular cell tumor A benign tumor composed of large cells with a granular cytoplasm. It likely arises from a neural or primitive mesenchymal cell. It most often occurs on the tongue or buccal mucosa. The tumor appears as a painless, nonulcerated nodule.

Granulation tissue The initial tissue formed in the connective tissue portion of the injury. It is immature tissue with many capillaries and fibroblasts.

Granuloma A tumorlike mass of inflammatory tissue consisting of a central collection of macrophages, often with multinucleated giant cells, surrounded by lymphocytes.

Granulomatous disease A disease characterized by the formation of granulomas.

Granulomatous inflammation A distinctive form of chronic inflammation characterized by the formation of granulomas.

Gumma A localized, noninfectious, destructive lesion that occurs during the tertiary stage of syphilis. The most common oral sites are the tongue and palate. The lesion appears as a firm mass that eventually becomes an ulcer.

H

Hairy leukoplakia An irregular, corrugated, white lesion that almost exclusively occurs on the lateral border of the tongue. Epstein-Barr virus has been identified in the epithelial cells of hairy leukoplakia and is considered to be the cause of the lesion.

Hairy tongue A condition in which the patient has an increased accumulation of keratin on the filiform papillae that results in either a light or dark "hairy" appearance.

Hand-foot-and-mouth disease An infectious disease caused by a coxsackievirus characterized by painful vesicles and ulcers that can occur anywhere in the mouth. Multiple macules or papules occur on the skin, typically on the feet, toes, hands, and fingers. Usually occurs in epidemics in children less than 5 years of age.

Hand-Schüller-Christian disease A chronic disseminated or multifocal form of Langerhans cell disease. This form occurs in children, usually less than 5 years of age. All changes are caused by localized collections of Langerhans cells. The triad includes single-to-multiple well-defined or "punched-out" radiolucent areas in the skull (may also occur in the jawbones), unilateral or bilateral exophthalmos, and diabetes insipidus that is caused by collections of macrophages in the sella turcica area, affecting the pituitary gland.

Haploid A cell with a single set of chromosomes. A gamete is haploid.

Hemangioma A benign proliferation of capillaries. It is a common vascular lesion considered by many to represent a developmental lesion rather than a tumor because it does not generally exhibit an unlimited growth potential.

Hematocrit The volume percentage of red blood cells in whole blood.

Hematoma A lesion that results from the accumulation of blood within tissue as a result of trauma.

Hemolysis The release of hemoglobin from red blood cells by destruction of the cells.

Hemophilia A disorder of blood coagulation that results in severely prolonged clotting time. The problem results from a deficiency of one of the plasma proteins involved in the coagulation cascade that is necessary for the conversion of fibrinogen to fibrin

Hemostasis The stoppage or cessation of bleeding.

Hepatomegaly Enlargement of the liver.

Hereditary hemorrhagic telangiectasia A syndrome characterized by multiple capillary dilations of the skin and mucous membranes. The skin of the face shows numerous pinpoint and spiderlike telangiectasias, especially on the lips, eyelids, and around the nose. Telangiectasias of the oral mucosa are prominent on the tip and anterior dorsum of the tongue; and the palate, gingiva, and buccal mucosa are often affected but to a lesser degree. Also known as *Osler-Rondu-Parks Weber syndrome.*

Herpangina An infectious disease caused by a coxsackievirus, characterized by vesicles on the soft palate, along with fever, malaise, sore throat, and difficulty swallowing (dysphagia). An erythematous pharyngitis is also present.

Herpes labialis The most common type of recurrent oral herpes simplex infection that occurs on the vermilion border of the lips. Also called a *cold sore* or *fever blister.*

Herpes simplex Infections caused by herpes virus types 1 and 2.

Herpes zoster A disease caused by the varicella-zoster virus that occurs in adults. It is characterized by a unilateral, painful eruption of vesicles along the distribution of a sensory nerve. Also called "*shingles.*"

Herpetic whitlow A painful infection of the fingers caused by the herpes simplex virus.

Herpetiform aphthous ulcer Tiny ulcers (1 to 2 mm) that resemble ulcers caused by the herpes simplex virus.

Hertwig's epithelial root sheath An epithelial structure that proliferates to shape the root of the tooth and induce the formation of the root dentin.

Heterozygote (adjective, heterozygous) Individual with two different genes at the allele loci.

Highly active antiviral therapy The combination of different types of antiretroviral (anti-HIV) drugs and drugs that prevent and treat opportunistic diseases that are used in the management of HIV infection.

Hives Multiple areas of well-demarcated swelling of the skin, usually accompanied by itching. The lesions are caused by localized areas of vascular permeability in the superficial connective tissue beneath the epithelium. Also know as *urticaria.*

hnRNA The fourth type of RNA. It is found within the nucleus and is the precursor of mRNA.

Homozygote (adjective, homozygous) An individual having identical genes at the allele loci.

Hormone A chemical substance produced in the body that has a specific regulatory effect on certain cells or a certain organ or organs.

Human immunodeficiency virus (HIV) A retrovirus that causes AIDS. It is transmitted through contact with an infected individual's blood, semen, cervical secretions, cerebrospinal fluid, or synovial fluid. It infects T-helper cells of the immune system and results in infection with a long incubation period averaging 10 years.

Human papillomavirus (HPV) A group of over 100 related viruses. HPVs are called *papillomaviruses* because some of the HPV types cause warts, or papillomas. The papillomaviruses are attracted to and are able to live only in squamous epithelial cells in the body.

Humoral immunity Immunity in which antibodies play the predominant role.

Hutchinson incisor Malformed incisor that results from the presence of congenital syphilis during tooth development. It is shaped like a screwdriver; broad cervically and narrow incisally, with a notched incisal edge.

Hypercalcemia An excess of calcium in the blood.

Hyperchromatic Staining more intensely than normal.

Hyperemia An excess of blood in a part of the body.

Hyperglycemia An excess of glucose in the blood.

Hypermobility An increase in the range of movement of a body part, especially a joint.

Hyperparathyroidism A condition that results from excessive secretion of parathyroid hormone (parathormone, or PTH), which is secreted by the parathyroid glands.

Hyperpituitarism Excess hormone production by the anterior pituitary gland.

Hyperplasia An abnormal increase in the number of normal cells in an organ or tissue.

Hypersensitivity A state of altered reactivity in which the body reacts to a foreign agent with an exaggerated immune response.

Hypertelorism Abnormally increased distance between two organs or parts. Orbital or ocular hypertelorism is abnormally increased distance between the orbits.

Hyperthermia Increased body temperature.

Hyperthyroidism A condition characterized by excessive production of thyroid hormone. Also called *thyrotoxicosis*.

Hypertrichosis The excessive growth of hair.

Hypertrophic candidiasis A type of candidiasis that appears as a white lesion that does not wipe off the mucosa. An important diagnostic feature of this type of candidiasis is that it is treated with antifungal medication. Also called chronic *hyperplastic candidiasis* and *candidal leukoplakia*.

Hypertrophy An enlargement of a tissue or organ caused by an increase in size but not in the number of cells.

Hypochromic Stained less intensely than normal.

Hypodontia Partial anodontia. The lack of one or more teeth.

Hypoglycemia Low blood sugar.

Hypohidrosis Abnormally diminished secretion of sweat.

Hypohidrotic ectodermal dysplasia The most severe form of ectodermal dysplasia. Its major characteristics are hypodontia, hypotrichosis, and hypohidrosis.

Hypophosphatasia A syndrome characterized by a decrease in serum alkaline phosphatase levels with increased urinary and plasma levels of phosphoethanolamine. This can cause total or partial aplasia of the cementum, an abnormal periodontal ligament in the primary teeth, and a decreased phosphatase level that has been linked to a premature loss of teeth.

Hypophosphatemia Deficiency of phosphates in the blood.

Hypophosphatemic vitamin D–resistant rickets A disorder characterized by low serum levels of phosphorus. This can be caused by low absorption of inorganic phosphate in the renal tubules, rickets, or osteomalacia. This condition demonstrates resistance to treatment with usual doses of vitamin D and a lack of other abnormalities.

Hypoplasia The incomplete development of an organ or tissue.

Hyposalivation Decreased salivary flow.

Hypothyroidism A condition characterized by decreased output of thyroid hormone.

Hypotrichosis Presence of less than the normal amount of hair.

I

Iatrogenic Induced inadvertently by a medical/dental care provider or by medical treatment or a diagnostic procedure.

Icterus A condition characterized by an abnormal accumulation of bilirubin (red bile pigment) in the blood and manifested by a yellowish discoloration of the skin, mucous membranes, and cornea. Also called *jaundice*.

Idiopathic thrombocytopenic purpura A condition in which spontaneous bleeding occurs for an unknown reason.

Idiopathic tooth resorption Resorption that can involve the crown of an impacted tooth or roots of teeth. The cause cannot be identified.

Immune complex A combination of antibody and antigen.

Immunity The ability for an organism to resist or not be susceptible to injury or infection.

Immunization A process by which resistance to an infectious disease is induced. It lowers the risk of a microorganism causing disease because it prepares the immune system to fight future attacks by the disease-causing microorganism.

Immunodeficiency A deficiency of the immune response caused by hypoactivity or decreased numbers of lymphoid cells.

Immunoglobulin A protein, also called an *antibody*, synthesized by plasma cells in response to a specific antigen.

Immunologic tolerance The recognition and nonresponsiveness of the immune system to the body's own cells and tissues.

Immunopathology The study of immune reactions involved in disease.

Impacted teeth Teeth that cannot erupt into the oral cavity because of a physical obstruction.

Impetigo A bacterial skin infection caused primarily by *Staphylococcus aureus* and occasionally by *Streptococcus pyogenes.* Impetigo most commonly involves lesions on the skin of the face or extremities.

In situ Confined to the site of origin without invasion of neighboring tissues.

Incubation period The period between the infection of an individual by a pathogen and the manifestation of the disease it causes.

Infectious mononucleosis An infectious disease caused by the Epstein-Barr virus. It is characterized by sore throat, fever, generalized lymphadenopathy, enlarged spleen, malaise, and fatigue. Palatal petechiae occur in infectious mononucleosis, usually appearing early in the course of the disease.

Inflammation A nonspecific response to injury that involves the microcirculation and its blood cells.

Inflammatory response The response of neutrophils to infection.

Inherited disorder A disorder caused by an abnormality in the genetic makeup (genes and chromosomes) of an individual that are transmitted from parent to offspring through the egg or sperm.

Injury An alteration in the environment that causes tissue damage.

Insulin A peptide hormone produced in the pancreas by the beta cells in the islets of Langerhans. Insulin regulates glucose metabolism and is the major fuel-regulating hormone.

Insulin shock Profound hypoglycemia, or low blood sugar, that necessitates emergency intervention.

Insulin-dependent diabetes mellitus The type of diabetes that usually includes patients being required to administer insulin to prevent ketosis. The onset is abrupt and may be characterized by polydipsia, polyuria, and polyphagia. Also called type 1 diabetes.

Internal derangement Disk (meniscal) displacements, ankylosis, and hypermobility disorders.

Internal tooth resorption Resorption usually involving a single tooth, often associated with an inflammatory response in the pulp. It can occur in any tooth.

International Normalized Ratio An expression of the ratio of prothrombin time to thromboplastin activity. It is a more accurate determination of prothrombin time (PT).

Intraoosseous cyst A cyst that occurs within the bone.

Intrinsic Naturally occurring within; essential.

Intrinsic staining Tooth discoloration that occurs as a result of the deposition of substances circulating systemically during tooth development.

Invaginate One portion of a structure infolds into another portion of a structure.

Invasion The infiltration and active destruction of surrounding tissues.

Inversion A portion of a chromosome arranged upside-down.

Iron deficiency anemia A condition that occurs when an insufficient amount of iron is supplied to the bone marrow for red blood cell development.

J

Jaundice A condition characterized by an abnormal accumulation of bilirubin (red bile pigment) in the blood and manifested by a yellowish discoloration of the skin, mucous membranes, and cornea. Also called *icterus*.

K

Kaposi sarcoma A malignant vascular tumor that may arise in multiple sites, including the skin and oral cavity. In HIV-positive patients these lesions are often seen on the hard palate and gingiva, where they present as purple macules, plaques, or exophytic tumors.

Karyotype A photomicrographic representation of a person's chromosomal constitution arranged according to the Denver classification.

Keloid Excessive skin scarring that appears raised and extends beyond its original boundaries.

Keratin pearl Rounded concentric masses of epithelial cells and keratin found in some squamous cell carcinomas.

Keratoconjunctivitis sicca The eye damage that occurs in Sjögren syndrome.

Ketoacidosis A metabolic acidosis resulting from the accumulation of ketone bodies. It is most commonly a consequence of untreated type I diabetes mellitus.

L

Laband syndrome An inherited syndrome characterized by gingival fibromatosis, dysplastic or absent nails, malformed nose and ears, hepatosplenomegaly, and hypoplasia of terminal phalanges of the fingers and toes.

Lack of penetrance The ability to carry a gene with a dominant effect without presenting any clinical manifestations.

Langerhans cell disease A disease formerly called histiocytosis X. Three entities traditionally grouped under the category of histiocytosis X are (1) Letterer-Siwe disease, (2) Hand-Schüller-Christian disease, and (3) solitary eosinophilic granuloma.

Lateral nasal processes The processes that form the sides of the nose.

Lateral palatine processes The processes that develop from the maxillary tissues laterally and grow to the midline to form the palate.

Lateral periodontal cyst A cyst named for its location. It is most often seen in the mandibular cuspid and premolar area and presents as an asymptomatic, a unilocular, or a multilocular radiolucent lesion located on the lateral aspect of a tooth root. A thin band of stratified squamous epithelium that exhibits focal epithelial thickenings lines the cyst.

LE cell A cell that is a characteristic of lupus erythematosus and other autoimmune diseases. It is a mature neutrophil that has phagocytized a spheric inclusion derived from another neutrophil.

Leiomyoma A benign tumor of smooth muscle that may occur in association with blood vessels.

Letterer-Siwe disease An acute disseminated form of Langerhans cell disease that usually affects children younger than 3 years of age. The disease resembles a lymphoma in that it generally has a rapidly fatal course that sometimes responds to chemotherapy.

Leukemia A form of cancer characterized by an overproduction of atypical white blood cells. Can be acute or chronic.

Leukocytosis A temporary increase in the number of white blood cells circulating in blood.

Leukoedema A condition characterized by generalized opalescence of the buccal mucosa.

Leukopenia A decrease in white blood cells.

Leukoplakia A clinical term used to identify a white, plaquelike lesion of the oral mucosa that cannot be wiped off and cannot be diagnosed as any other disease on a clinical basis.

Lichen planus A benign, chronic disease affecting the skin and oral mucosa. The lesions have a characteristic pattern of interconnecting lines called striae, resembling the pattern of the plant lichen as it grows on rocks and trees.

Linea alba A white raised line that forms commonly on the buccal mucosa at the occlusal plane and is usually considered a variant of normal.

Linear gingival erythema A type of gingival disease that develops in patients with HIV infection. It has three characteristic features: (1) spontaneous bleeding, (2) punctate or petechiae-like lesions on the attached gingiva and alveolar mucosa, and (3) a bandlike erythema of the gingiva that does not respond to therapy.

Lingual mandibular bone concavity Often referred to as a pseudocyst because it is not a pathologic cavity and is not lined with epithelium. It is characterized by a well-defined cystlike radiolucency in the posterior region of the mandible inferior to the mandibular canal that is caused by a lingual depression in the mandible, which contains normal salivary gland tissue. Also known as a *static bone cyst* or *Stafne bone cyst*.

Lingual thyroid nodule A small mass of thyroid tissue located on the tongue away from the normal anatomic location of the thyroid gland. It is an uncommon developmental anomaly that results from the failure of the primitive thyroid tissue to migrate from its developmental location in the area of the foramen cecum on the posterior portion of the tongue to its normal position in the neck. Also called *ectopic lingual thyroid nodule*.

Lingual varicosities Prominent lingual veins usually observed on the ventral and lateral surfaces of the tongue.

Lipoma A benign tumor of fat.

Lobule (adjective, lobulated) A segment or lobe that is part of a whole. Lobules sometimes appear fused together.

Local Confined to a limited part; not general or systemic.

Locus In genetics the position occupied by a gene on a chromosome.

Lymphadenopathy Any disease process that affects lymph nodes such that they become enlarged and palpable.

Lymphangioma A benign tumor of lymphatic vessels. The most common intraoral location is the tongue, where the lymphangioma presents as an ill-defined mass with a pebbly surface.

Lymphoepithelial cyst A cyst most commonly found in the major salivary glands. It is composed of a stratified squamous epithelial lining surrounded by a well-circumscribed component of lymphoid tissue. Also known as a *branchial cleft cyst* when located in the neck.

Lymphoid tissue Tissue composed of lymphocytes supported by a meshwork of connective tissue.

Lymphoma A malignant tumor of lymphoid tissue.

Lyon hypothesis The hypothesis postulated by Mary Lyon that states that during the early period of embryonic development the genetic activity of one of the X chromosomes in each cell of a female embryo is inactivated.

Lysosomal enzyme An enzyme found in the granular cytoplasm of a neutrophil. Lysosomal enzymes destroy substances after the cell has engulfed them.

M

Macrodontia Abnormally large teeth.

Macrophage A large, mononuclear phagocyte derived from monocytes. Macrophages become mobile when stimulated by inflammation and interact with lymphocytes in an immune response.

Macule An area that is usually distinguished by a color different from that of the surrounding tissue; it is flat and does not protrude above the surface of the normal tissue. A freckle is an example of a macule.

Magnetic resonance imaging A noninvasive diagnostic technique that uses radio waves to produce computerized images of internal body tissues.

Major aphthous ulcer An ulcer that is larger than 1 cm in diameter, is deeper, and lasts longer than a minor aphthous ulcer. The presence of multiple major aphthous ulcers is known as *Sutton disease* or *periadenitis mucosa necrotica recurrens.*

Major histocompatibility complex Unique cell surface molecules that help T cells to recognize antigen fragments.

Malaise A vague, indefinite feeling of discomfort, debilitation, or lack of health.

Malignant melanoma Malignant tumor of melanocytes that commonly arises on the skin as a result of prolonged exposure to sunlight.

Malignant Resistant to treatment; able to metastasize and kill the host; describing cancer.

Malignant tumor Cancer; a tumor that is resistant to treatment and may cause death; a tumor that has the potential for uncontrolled growth and dissemination or recurrence or both.

Mandibular processes The first branchial arch divides into two maxillary processes and the mandibular process (or mandibular arch). It forms the lower part of the cheeks, the mandible, and part of the tongue.

Mandibular tori Outgrowths of normal dense bone found on the lingual aspect of the mandible in the area of the premolars above the mylohyoid ridge.

Mandibulofacial dysostosis A syndrome characterized by developmental disturbance of the cranial bones and hypoplasia of the lower part of the face. The mandibular body is underdeveloped, and the eyes slant downward. The teeth are crowded and malposed. Also known as *Treacher-Collins syndrome.*

Margination A process during inflammation in which white blood cells tend to move to the blood vessel walls.

Maxillary exostoses Tori that generally develop on the buccal aspect of the maxillary alveolar ridge, usually in the molar and premolar area. They are generally symptomless.

Maxillary processes The first branchial arch divides into two maxillary processes and the mandibular process. The maxillary processes give rise to the upper part of the cheeks, the lateral portions of the upper lip, and part of the palate.

Measles A highly contagious disease causing systemic symptoms and a skin rash that results from a paramyxovirus. The disease most commonly occurs in childhood. Early in the disease, Koplik spots, which are small erythematous macules with white necrotic centers, may occur in the oral cavity.

Median mandibular cyst A rare cyst located in the midline of the mandible. It is characterized by a well-defined radiolucency that is seen below the apices of the mandibular incisors and is lined with squamous epithelium.

Median nasal process The process that forms the center and tip of the nose.

Median palatine cyst A cyst located in the midline of the hard palate. It is characterized by a well-defined unilocular radiolucency and is lined with stratified squamous epithelium that is surrounded by dense fibrous connective tissue.

Median rhomboid glossitis A flat or slightly raised oval or rectangular erythematous area in the midline of the dorsal surface of the tongue, beginning at the junction of the anterior and middle thirds and extending posterior to the circumvallate papillae. It is devoid of filiform papillae; therefore its texture is smooth. It may be associated with *Candida albicans.*

Megaloblastic anemia A type of anemia characterized by hyperplastic bone marrow changes and maturation arrest resulting from a dietary deficiency, impaired absorption, impaired storage and modification, or impaired use of one or more hematopoietic factors.

Megaloblasts Red blood cells that are immature, abnormally large, and have nuclei. Megaloblasts are seen in high numbers in the bone marrow in megaloblastic anemia.

Meiosis The two-step cellular division of the original germ cells, which reduces the chromosomes from 4nDNA to 1nDNA. The two steps are called *first meiosis* and *second meiosis.*

Melanin pigmentation Discoloration of the oral tissues produced by the deposition of melanin.

Melanin The pigment that gives color to the skin, eyes, hair, mucosa, and gingiva.

Melanocytes A pigment-producing cell in the skin, hair, and eye that determines their color. The pigment that melanocytes make is called *melanin*.

Mental retardation A disorder characterized by certain limitations in a person's mental functioning and in skills such as communicating, taking care of himself or herself, and social skills.

Metaphase The phase of cellular division in which the chromosomes are lined up evenly along the equatorial plate of the cell; during this time the chromosomes are most visible.

Metastasis (plural, metastases) The transport of neoplastic cells to parts of the body remote from the primary tumor and the establishment of new tumors in those sites.

Metastatic tumor A tumor formed by cells that have been transported from the primary tumor to a site not connected with the original tumor.

Meth mouth The extensive and rapid destruction of teeth due to methamphetamine abuse.

Methamphetamine A sympathomimetic amine related to amphetamine and ephedrine that enhances central nervous system stimulant activity. It is used to treat obesity, minimal brain dysfunction, and attention deficit hyperactivity disorder. It is also used illicitly as a recreational drug.

Microcirculation Small blood vessels, including arterioles, capillaries, and venules.

Microcyte A red blood cell that is smaller than normal.

Microdontia Abnormally small teeth.

Miliary tuberculosis The type of tuberculosis in which the bacteria is carried to widespread areas of the body and causes involvement of organs such as the kidneys and liver.

Millimeter (mm) One thousandth of a meter (a meter is equivalent to 39.3 inches). The periodontal probe is of great assistance in documenting the size or diameter of a lesion that can be measured in millimeters.

Minor aphthous ulcer The most commonly occurring type of ulcer. It appears as a discrete, round-to-oval ulcer that is up to 1 cm in diameter and exhibits a yellowish-white fibrin surface surrounded by a halo of erythema.

Mitochondria Cytoplasmic energy-producing organelles that have their own DNA in a circular chromosome.

Mitochondrial DNA Unique DNA that is inherited maternally.

Mitosis The way in which somatic cells divide so that the two daughter cells receive the same number of identical chromosomes.

Mitotic cycle The part of the life span of a somatic cell when cellular division is achieved by mitosis.

Mitotic figures The appearance of dividing cells caught in the process of mitosis.

Moniliasis An overgrowth of the yeastlike fungus *Candida albicans.* It is the most common oral fungal infection. It can result from many different conditions, including antibiotic use, cancer, corticosteroid therapy, dentures, diabetes mellitus, and HIV infection. Also called *candidiasis* and *thrush*.

Monoclonal spike An elevation of a single type of immunoglobulin detected by immunoelectrophoresis; seen in patients with multiple myeloma.

Monomorphic adenoma A benign encapsulated salivary gland tumor composed of a uniform pattern of epithelial cells. It occurs most commonly in adult females, with a predilection for the upper lip and buccal mucosa.

Monostotic fibrous dysplasia The most common type of fibrous dysplasia. It is characterized by involvement of a single bone. The mandible and maxilla are commonly affected; the maxilla is more frequently involved than the mandible.

Mosaic bone A pattern found in the involved bone of a patient with Paget disease of bone. It demonstrates prominent reversal lines that result from the resorption and deposition of bone.

mRNA The first type of RNA. It carries the message from the DNA to ribosomes, where proteins are produced.

Mucocele A lesion that forms when a salivary gland duct is severed and the mucous salivary gland secretion spills into the adjacent connective tissue.

Mucoepidermoid carcinoma An unencapsulated and infiltrating malignant salivary gland tumor composed of a combination of mucous cells interspersed with squamouslike epithelial cells. Major gland tumors occur most often in the parotid gland. Minor gland tumors occur most commonly on the palate.

Mucormycosis A rare fungal infection caused by an organism that is a common inhabitant of soil and is usually nonpathogenic. Infection occurs in diabetic and debilitated patients and often involves the nasal cavity, maxillary sinus, and hard palate; it can present as a proliferating or destructive mass in the maxilla. Also called *phycomycosis*.

Mucositis Mucosal inflammation.

Mucous cyst (mucous retention cyst) An epithelium-lined cystic structure that occurs in association with a salivary gland duct. Most are not true cysts but dilated salivary gland ducts that develop as a result of obstruction.

Mucous membrane pemphigoid A chronic autoimmune disease that affects the oral mucosa, conjunctiva, genital mucosa, and skin. It is also known as *cicatricial pemphigoid* and *benign mucous membrane pemphigoid.*

Mucous patches Oral lesions that appear in the secondary stage of syphilis. They are characterized by multiple, painless, grayish-white plaques covering ulcerated mucosa. They are very infectious.

Mulberry molar First molar with an irregularly shaped crown made up of multiple tiny globules of enamel instead of cusps, which imparts a berry-like appearance. Can be a manifestation of congenital syphilis.

Multifactorial conditions Conditions in which the phenotype results from a combination of genetic factors and environmental influences.

Multilocular A term used to describe a radiographic appearance of multiple rounded compartments or locules. These can appear "soap bubble like" or "honeycomb-like."

Multiple mucosal neuroma syndrome This syndrome is characterized by thick, large lips and possibly everted upper eyelids; affected patients are tall. Mucosal neuromas are prominent on the lips and anterior dorsal surface of the tongue. Also termed *multiple endocrine neoplasia syndrome (MEN syndrome).*

Multiple myeloma A systemic, malignant proliferation of plasma cells that causes destructive lesions in bone.

Mumps A viral infection of the salivary glands caused by a paramyxovirus. The disease most commonly occurs in children and is characterized by painful swelling of the salivary glands, most commonly bilateral swelling of the parotid glands. Also called *epidemic parotitis.*

Muscles of mastication The muscles that comprise the major muscles about the facial region that govern the movement of the mandible and chewing motions.

Mutation A permanent change in the arrangement of genetic material.

Myalgia Muscle pain.

Myoepithelial cell A specific type of salivary gland cell with contractile properties.

Myxedema The presence of hypothyroidism in older children and adults.

N

Nasolabial cyst A soft tissue cyst of the midlateral face with no alveolar bone involvement. It is lined with pseudostratified, ciliated columnar epithelium and multiple goblet cells. There is usually no associated radiographic change.

Nasopalatine canal cyst A cyst located within the nasopalatine canal or the incisive papilla. It arises from epithelial remnants of the embryonal nasopalatine ducts. Also know as an *incisive canal cyst.*

Natural killer cell (NK cell) A lymphocyte that is part of the body's initial innate immunity, which by unknown mechanisms is able to destroy cells recognized as foreign.

Natural passive immunity Antibodies from a mother pass through the placenta to the developing fetus. These antibodies protect a newborn infant from disease while the infant's own immune system matures.

Necrosis The pathologic death of one or more cells or a portion of tissue or organ, resulting from irreversible damage.

Necrotizing sialometaplasia A benign condition of the salivary gland characterized by moderately painful swelling and ulceration in the affected area. Most common on the hard palate.

Necrotizing stomatitis A condition characterized by extensive focal areas of bone loss along with the features of necrotizing ulcerative periodontitis.

Necrotizing ulcerative gingivitis (NUG) A painful erythematous gingivitis with necrosis of the interdental papillae. Also called *acute necrotizing ulcerative gingivitis* (ANUG).

Necrotizing ulcerative periodontitis A condition that resembles necrotizing ulcerative gingivitis in which patients experience pain, spontaneous gingival bleeding, interproximal necrosis, and interproximal cratering along with intense erythema and, most characteristically, extremely rapid bone loss.

Neoplasia New growth; the process of the formation of tumors by the uncontrolled proliferation of cells.

Neoplasm Tumor; a new growth of tissue in which the growth is uncontrolled and progressive.

Neoplastic Pertaining to the formation of tumors by the uncontrolled proliferation of cells.

Neurofibroma A benign tumor derived from Schwann cells and perineural fibroblasts, which are components of the connective tissue surrounding a nerve. The tongue is the most common intraoral location.

Neurofibromatosis of von Reckinghausen A syndrome characterized by multiple neurofibromas on the skin. Oral involvement is characterized by single or multiple tumors at any location in the oral mucosa. Café au lait skin pigmentation is common. Also called *von Recklinghausen disease*.

Neutropenia A diminished number of circulating neutrophils in the blood.

Neutrophil The first white blood cell to arrive at the site of injury and the primary cell involved in acute inflammation. The nucleus of this cell is multilobed. Also called a *polymorphonuclear leukocyte*.

Nevoid basal cell carcinoma syndrome A syndrome characterized by mild hypertelorism and mild prognathism, the appearance of basal cell carcinomas early in life, and multiple cysts of the jaws characterized histologically as odontogenic keratocysts. A variety of skeletal abnormalities may occur, including bifurcation of one or more ribs. Also known as *Gorlin syndrome*.

Nevus (plural, nevi) (1) A developmental tumor of melanocytes (melanin-producing cells). (2) A pigmented congenital lesion (a lesion present at birth).

Nevus cells Melanocytes (melanin-producing cells).

Nicotine stomatitis A benign lesion on the hard palate typically associated with pipe and cigar smoking. It may also occur with cigarette smoking.

Nikolsky sign Seen in some bullous diseases such as pemphigus vulgaris and bullous pemphigoid; the superficial epithelium separates easily from the basal layer on exertion of firm sliding manual pressure.

Nodule A palpable, solid lesion in soft tissue that is up to 1 cm in diameter and may be above, level with, or beneath the skin or mucosal surface.

Nondisjunction The result of chromosomes that were crossing over and did not separate; therefore, both migrate to the same cell.

Noninsulin dependent diabetes mellitus The type of diabetes that is characterized by increased insulin resistance. It includes patients who can maintain proper blood sugar levels without the administration of insulin. Obesity is common finding. Also called *type 2 diabetes*.

Nonodontogenic Not related to tooth development.

Nonthrombocytopenic purpuras Bleeding disorders that can result from either a defect in the capillary walls or disorders of platelet function.

Normal joint function The harmonious function of the temporomandibular joint and jaws.

Nucleotide A hydrolytic product of nucleic acid formed by a nitrogen-containing base, a five-carbon sugar (deoxyribose), and a phosphate.

O

Odontogenesis Tooth development.

Odontogenic adenomatoid tumor An encapsulated, benign epithelial odontogenic tumor that has a distinctive age, sex, and site distribution. Seventy percent occur in females under 20 years of age; 70% involve the anterior part of the jaws. May be associated with impacted teeth. Also known as an *adenomatoid odontogenic tumor*.

Odontogenic keratocyst An odontogenic developmental cyst with a unique histologic appearance. The lumen is lined by epithelium that is 8 to 10 cell layers thick and surfaced by parakeratin. The basal cell layer is palisaded and prominent; the interface between the epithelium and the connective tissue is flat. This cyst has a higher recurrence rate than many other odontogenic cysts.

Odontogenic myxoma A benign mesenchymal odontogenic tumor that occurs anywhere in the maxilla or mandible, with the mandible being more common. It may displace teeth and spread to other locations.

Odontogenic Arising from tooth-forming tissues.

Odontogenic tumor A tumor derived from tooth-forming tissues. Tooth formation results from an interaction between odontogenic epithelium and odontogenic mesenchyme. It is most often benign.

Odontoma An odontogenic tumor composed of mature enamel, dentin, cementum, and pulp tissue. The odontoma is the most common of the odontogenic tumors, and there are two types: compound and complex.

Olfactory pits Two pits that mark the future openings of the nose that develop on the surface of the frontal process.

Oligogenic inheritance Characteristics or traits that are inherited by the participation of several genes.

Oncology The study of tumors or neoplasms.

Oogenesis The process of formation of female germ cells (ova).

Open joint surgery Surgery used to perform disk repositioning, replacement or excision, and total joint reconstruction using a prosthetic device or autogenous graft.

Opportunistic infection A disease caused by a microorganism that does not ordinarily cause disease but becomes pathogenic under certain circumstances.

Opsonization The enhancement of phagocytosis.

Oral melanotic macule A flat, well-circumscribed brown lesion of unknown cause. They are usually small and may require biopsy and histologic examination for diagnosis.

Osteoarthritis This classification of arthritis is characterized by degenerative changes of the articular cartilage with associated remodeling. It is the most common disease affecting the temporomandibular joint. It is also referred to as *degenerative joint disease.*

Osteogenesis imperfecta A congenital disorder characterized by abnormally formed bones that fracture easily. Other abnormalities include blue sclerae (mild cases), bowing of the legs, curvature of the spine, deformity of the skull, and shortening of arms and legs (severe cases). The oral manifestation of this syndrome is a dentinogenesis imperfecta–like condition.

Osteoma Benign tumor of normal compact bone.

Osteomalacia A disease of bone that develops over a long period of time as the result of a deficiency of calcium. When this disease occurs in young children, it is usually caused by a nutritional deficiency of vitamin D, and the associated disease is termed *rickets.*

Osteoporosis A hereditary disease marked by abnormally porous bone lacking normal density.

Osteoradionecrosis Necrosis of bone from radiation therapy.

Osteosarcoma A malignant tumor of the bone-forming tissue. Also known as *osteogenic sarcoma.*

Ovum (plural, ova) The mature female germ cell.

P

Paget disease of bone A chronic metabolic bone disease characterized by resorption, osteoblastic repair, and remineralization of the involved bone. It typically involves the pelvis and spinal column. Also called *osteitis deformans* and *leontiasis ossea.*

Palatal papillomatosis A form of denture somatitis. Also called *papillary hyperplasia of the palate.*

Pallor Paleness of the skin or mucosal tissues.

Palpation The evaluation of a lesion by feeling it with the fingers to determine the texture of the area; the descriptive terms for palpation are *soft, firm, semifirm,* and *fluid filled;* these terms also describe the consistency of a lesion.

Pancytopenia A dramatic decrease in all the circulating blood cells.

Papillary cystadenoma lymphomatosum A unique type of monomorphic adenoma characterized by an encapsulated tumor composed of two types of tissue: epithelial and lymphoid. It presents as a painless, soft, compressible, or fluctuant mass, usually located in the parotid gland. It is also called a *Warthin tumor.*

Papillary Describing a small nipple-shaped projection or elevation usually found in clusters.

Papillary hyperplasia of the palate A form of denture somatitis. Also called *palatal papillomatosis.*

Papilloma A benign tumor of squamous epithelium that presents as a small, exophytic, pedunculated, or sessile growth. It is often described as cauliflower-like in appearance and occurs most often on the soft palate or tongue.

Papillon-Lefèvre syndrome An inherited disease characterized by marked destruction of the periodontal tissues of both dentitions with premature loss of teeth and hyperkeratosis of the palms of the hands and soles of the feet.

Papule A small circumscribed lesion usually less than 1 cm in diameter that protrudes above the surface of normal surrounding tissue.

Paramyxovirus A member of a family of viruses that include the organisms that cause influenza, mumps, and some respiratory infections.

Parathormone Parathyroid hormone.

Parenteral Administered by injection.

Paresthesia An abnormal alteration of touch sensation often perceived as prickling or tingling.

Partial thromboplastin time A test that measures the effectiveness of clot formation. It is performed by measuring the time it takes for a clot to form after the addition of kaolin, a surface-activating factor, and cephalin, a substitute platelet factor, to the patient's plasma.

Passive immunity The type of immunity in which antibodies produced by another person are used to protect an individual against infectious disease. This type of immunity can occur naturally or be acquired.

Pathogenic microorganism A microorganism that causes disease.

Pavementing Adherence of white blood cells to the walls of a blood vessel during inflammation.

Pedunculated Attached by a stemlike or stalklike base.

Pegged Resembling a small peg.

Pegged/absent maxillary lateral incisors A condition characterized by a lateral incisor that is small and peg shaped or congenitally lacking, either unilaterally or bilaterally. Both primary and secondary dentitions can be affected, but mostly the latter.

Pemphigus vulgaris A severe, progressive autoimmune disease that affects the skin and mucous membranes. It is characterized by intraepithelial blister formation that results from breakdown of the cellular adhesion between epithelial cells.

Penetrance The prevalence of individuals with a given genotype that manifest clinically the phenotype associated with that trait.

Periapical abscess An abscess composed of pus and surrounded by connective tissue containing neutrophils and lymphocytes. The abscess may develop directly from the inflammation in the pulp or in an area of previously existing chronic inflammation.

Periapical cemento-osseous dysplasia A relatively common disease of unknown cause that affects periapical bone. It is commonly seen in the anterior mandible.

Periapical granuloma A localized mass of chronically inflamed granulation tissue that forms at the opening of a pulp canal, generally at the apex of nonvital tooth root.

Periapical inflammation Inflammation at or around the root of a tooth.

Pericoronitis An inflammation of the mucosa around the crown of a partially erupted tooth. Usually the result of infection by bacteria that are part of the normal oral flora.

Peripheral Occurring outside of bone.

Peripheral ameloblastoma Ameloblastoma that occurs solely in the gingiva and not in the bone.

Peripheral giant cell granuloma A reactive lesion that occurs on the gingival or alveolar mucosa, typically anterior to the molars. It usually a result of local irritating factors.

Peripheral ossifying fibroma A well-demarcated sessile or pedunculated lesion that appears to originate from the gingival interdental papilla and is most likely derived from cells of the periodontal ligament

Pernicious anemia A vitamin B_{12} deficiency that is caused by a deficiency of intrinsic factor, a substance secreted by the parietal cells of the stomach.

Petechia A minute red spot on the skin or mucous membranes resulting from escape of a small amount of blood.

Peutz-Jeghers syndrome Syndrome characterized by multiple melanotic macular pigmentations of the skin and mucosa, which are associated with gastrointestinal polyposis.

Phagocytosis A process of ingestion and digestion by cells.

Pharyngitis Inflammatory condition of the tonsils and pharyngeal mucosa caused by many different organisms. Clinical features include sore throat, fever, tonsillar hyperplasia, and erythema of the oropharyngeal mucosa and tonsils.

Phenotype The physical and clinical visible characteristics of an individual. Genotype is the genetic composition. Phenotype is its observable appearance.

Pheochromocytoma A benign neoplasm that generally develops in ganglia around the adrenal glands. The tumor is often bilateral and is responsible for night sweats, high blood pressure, and episodes of severe diarrhea.

Philtrum The vertical groove in the midline of the upper lip.

Phycomycosis A rare fungal infection caused by an organism that is a common inhabitant of soil and is usually nonpathogenic. Infection occurs in diabetic and debilitated patients. It often involves the nasal cavity, maxillary sinus, and hard palate and can present as a proliferating or destructive mass in the maxilla. Also called *mucormycosis*.

Pituitary adenoma A benign tumor of the pituitary gland. Often causes hyperpituitarism.

Plasma cell A lymphoid or lymphocyte-like cell found in the bone marrow, connective tissue, and sometimes blood. It has the ability to produce immunoglobulins and is derived from B cells.

Plasma thromboplastin A factor that is active in the formation of intrinsic blood thromboplastin. A deficiency results in Christmas disease (hemophilia B), which is caused by a decrease in the amount of thromboplastin formed. Also called *factor IX*.

Platelet A disk-shaped structure, also called a *thrombocyte*, found in the blood, which plays an important role in blood coagulation.

Platelet count A quantitative or numeric evaluation of platelets.

Pleomorphic adenoma The most common of the benign salivary gland tumors. It is also called *benign mixed tumor*.

Pleomorphic Occurs in various forms.

Polycythemia An increase in the total red blood cell mass in the blood.

Polydactyly The presence of extra fingers or toes or both.

Polydipsia Chronic excessive thirst and intake of fluid. A possible sign of type 1 diabetes.

Polymorphonuclear leukocyte The most prevalent of the white blood cells containing a multilobed nucleus.

Polyostotic fibrous dysplasia A type of fibrous dysplasia characterized by involvement of more than one bone. The skull, clavicles, and long bones are commonly affected.

Polyphagia Excessive appetite. A possible sign of type 1 diabetes.

Polyploid Three (triploid) or four (tetraploid) complete sets of chromosomes. This has been occasionally described in humans and is incompatible with life.

Polyuria Excessive urination. A possible sign of type 1 diabetes.

Predilection A disposition in favor of something; preference.

Pregnancy tumor A pyogenic granuloma that may occur in pregnant women. They may be caused by changing hormonal levels and increased response to plaque.

Premaxilla The area of the palate that develops from the globular process. It forms the anterior part of the maxillae.

Primary adrenal cortical insufficiency A condition characterized by an insufficient production of adrenal steroids. Also known as *Addison disease.*

Primary dental lamina A band of ectoderm in each jaw on which proliferations of epithelial cells develop, which become the early enamel organs for each of the primary teeth.

Primary herpetic gingivostomatitis Oral disease caused by initial infection with the herpes simplex virus. It is characterized by painful, erythematous, and swollen gingiva and multiple tiny vesicles on the perioral skin, vermilion border of the lips, and oral mucosa. Patients also experience malaise and cervical lymphadenopathy.

Primary immunodeficiencies Immunodeficiencies of genetic origin that can involve B cells, T cells, or both. They provide information about the functions of the different immunologic responses and are extremely rare.

Primary Sjögren syndrome Lacrimal and salivary gland involvement without the presence of another autoimmune disease.

Primary tumor The original tumor; the source of metastasis.

Primordial cyst A cyst that develops in place of a tooth.

Proliferation The multiplication of cells.

Prothrombin time A test that measures the patient's ability to form a clot. It is performed by measuring the time it takes for a clot to form when calcium and a tissue factor are added to the patient's plasma.

Pruritis Itching.

Pseudocyst An abnormal cavity resembling a true cyst but that is not a pathologic cavity and is not lined with epithelium.

Pseudomembranous candidiasis A type of candidiasis in which a white curdlike material is present on the mucosal surface. When the material is wiped off, the underlying mucosa is erythematous.

Pulp polyp An excessive proliferation of chronically inflamed dental pulp tissue. Also called *chronic hyperplastic pulpitis.*

Purified protein derivative An antigen used to test if an individual has been exposed to and infected with *Mycobacterium tuberculosis.*

Purpura A group of disorders characterized by purplish or brownish-red discolorations caused by bleeding into the skin or tissues.

Purulent Containing or forming pus.

Pustule Variably sized circumscribed, pus-filled, elevated lesions.

Pyogenic granuloma A commonly occurring intraoral lesion that is characterized by a proliferation of connective tissue containing numerous blood vessels and inflammatory cells. It occurs in response to injury. The lesion does not produce pus and is not a true granuloma.

R

Radiation The process of emitting radiant energy in the form of waves or particles.

Radiation therapy The treatment of a disease or condition with a type of radiation.

Radicular cyst A cyst with a wall of fibrous connective tissue and a lining of stratified squamous epithelium that is attached to the root apex of a tooth with a dead pulp or a defective root canal filling.

Radiolucent The black or dark areas in a radiograph that result from the ability of radiant energy to pass through the structure. Less dense structures (e.g., the pulp) are radiolucent.

Radiopaque The white or clear appearance in a radiograph that results from the inability of radiant energy to pass through a structure. The more dense the structure (i.e., amalgam restorations), the whiter it appears in the radiograph.

Ranula A mucocele-like lesion that forms unilaterally on the floor of the mouth. It is associated with the sublingual and submandibular glands.

Raynaud phenomenon A disorder that affects the fingers and toes. Cold and emotional stress trigger a reaction, which is characterized by an initial pallor of the skin that results from vasoconstriction and reduced blood flow. The initial pallor is followed by cyanosis, which occurs because of the decreased blood flow.

Reactive connective tissue hyperplasia Proliferating exuberant granulation tissue and dense fibrous connective tissue resulting from overzealous repair.

Receptor A cell surface protein to which a specific hormone can bind; such binding leads to biochemical events.

Recessive In genetics a trait or characteristic manifested clinically with a double gene dose in autosomal chromosomes or with a single dose in males if the trait is X-linked.

Recurrent herpes simplex infection Herpes simplex virus that persists in a latent state, usually in the nerve tissue of the trigeminal ganglion, and causes localized recurrent infections. Recurrent infections are often produced by stimuli such as sunlight, menstruation, or stress.

Regeneration The process by which injured tissue is replaced with tissue identical to that present before the injury.

Regional odontodysplasia A developmental problem in which one or several teeth in the same quadrant radiographically exhibit a marked reduction in radiodensity and a characteristic ghostlike appearance. Very thin enamel and dentin are present. Also called *ghost teeth*.

Repair The restoration of damaged or diseased tissues.

Residual cyst A cyst that forms when a tooth is removed and all or part of a periapical cyst is left behind.

Reticular lichen planus The most common form of lichen planus. The lesions are composed of Wickham striae along with white, slightly raised plaque-like areas.

Retrocuspid papilla A sessile nodule on the gingival margin of the lingual aspect of the mandibular cuspids.

Rhabdomyoma A benign tumor of striated muscle that has been reported to occur on the tongue.

Rhabdomyosarcoma A malignant tumor of striated muscle that grows rapidly and is destructive. It is the most common malignant soft tissue tumor of the head and neck in children.

Rheumatic fever A childhood disease that follows a group A beta-hemolytic streptococcal infection, usually tonsillitis and pharyngitis. Characterized by an inflammatory reaction involving the heart, joints, and central nervous system.

Rheumatoid arthritis An inflammatory autoimmune disorder of the joints.

Rheumatoid factor An antibody against IgG found in serum and detectable on laboratory tests. It is associated with rheumatoid arthritis and other autoimmune diseases.

Ribonucleic acid (RNA) Single strands of polynucleotides found in all cells; different types of RNA have different functions in the production of proteins by the cell.

Ribosome The cytoplasmic organelles in which proteins are formed on the basis of the genetic code provided by an RNA template.

Root resorption Observed radiographically when the apex of the tooth appears shortened or blunted and irregularly shaped. It occurs as a response to stimuli, which can result from a cyst, tumor, or trauma.

rRNA The third type of RNA. It combines with several polypeptides to form ribosomes.

S

S phase The phase in which the replication of the DNA takes place.

Sarcoma A malignant tumor of connective tissue.

Scalloping around the roots The radiographic appearance of a radiolucent lesion that extends between the roots of multiple teeth, as seen in a traumatic bone cyst.

Scarlet fever Contagious childhood disease caused by group A beta-hemolytic *Streptococcus.* Characterized by a red rash, strawberry tongue, sore throat, fever, enlarged lymph nodes, and prostration.

Schwannoma A benign tumor derived from Schwann cells, a component of the connective tissue surrounding nerves. The tongue is the most common intraoral location.

Scoliosis Lateral curvature of the spine.

Scrofula Pertaining to tuberculosis, the enlargement of the submandibular and cervical lymph nodes. Also known as *tuberculous lymphadenitis*.

Secondary immunodeficiencies Immunodeficiencies that occur as a result of an underlying disorder. They are more common than the primary immunodeficiency disorders.

Secondary Sjögren syndrome The combination of another autoimmune disease with salivary and lacrimal gland involvement.

Secondary thrombocytopenic purpura The condition of thrombocytopenic purpura secondary to an existing disease or condition.

Serous A substance having a watery consistency; relating to serum.

Serum sickness A delayed allergic response after exposure to some antibiotics or antiserum. It is caused by an antibody reaction to an antigen in the donor serum. Symptoms include fever, painful swelling of the joints, renal disturbance or failure, edema around the eyes, carditis, and skin lesions.

Sessile Broad-based.

Severe combined immunodeficiency A genetic disorder in which both B cells and T cells of the immune system are crippled, leaving the patient extremely vulnerable to infectious diseases. Also known as *boy in the bubble syndrome*, made famous by a well-publicized case on television.

Shingles A disease caused by the varicella-zoster virus that occurs in adults. It is characterized by a unilateral, painful eruption of vesicles along the distribution of a sensory nerve. Also called *herpes zoster*.

Sialadenitis A painful swelling of a salivary gland that may be caused by obstruction or infection. It can be acute or chronic.

Sialolith A salivary gland stone.

Sicca syndrome A combination of dry mouth and dry eyes.

Sickle cell anemia An inherited disorder of the blood that is found predominantly in black individuals and those of Mediterranean origin. It occurs as a result of an abnormal type of hemoglobin in red blood cells that causes the cells to develop a sickle shape in the presence of decreased oxygen.

Sickle cell trait People who are heterozygous for sickle cell anemia.

Sign Objective evidence of disease that can be observed by a health care provider.

Simple bone cyst A pathologic cavity in bone that is not lined with epithelium. Also known as a *traumatic bone cyst*.

Single-gene inheritance Characteristics that are governed by the action of one gene.

Sjögren syndrome An autoimmune disease that affects the salivary and lacrimal glands, resulting in a decrease in saliva and tears.

Smoker's melanosis (smoking-associated melanosis) A type of melanosis in which the melanin pigmentation is associated with smoking and the intensity is related to the amount and duration of smoking.

Solar cheilitis Degeneration of the tissue of the lips caused by sun exposure. Also called *actinic cheilitis*.

Somatic cells All the cells of the human body with the exception of the primitive germ cells (oogonia and spermatogonia).

Speckled leukoplakia An oral mucosal lesion that shows a mixture of red and white areas.

Spermatogenesis The process of formation of spermatozoa (sperm).

Spermatozoon The mature masculine germ cell.

Spina bifida A defect in the spine caused by a lack of the vertebral arches through which the spinal cord protrudes.

Spina bifida occulta Similar to spina bifida, but with little or no protrusion of the spinal cord.

Splenomegaly Enlargement of the spleen.

Squamous cell carcinoma A malignant tumor of squamous epithelium. It is the most common primary malignancy of the oral cavity and, like other malignant tumors, can infiltrate adjacent tissues and metastasize to distant sites. Also know as *epidermoid carcinoma*.

Stafne bone cyst Often referred to as a pseudocyst because it is not a pathologic cavity and is not lined with epithelium. It is characterized by a well-defined cystlike radiolucency in the posterior region of the mandible inferior to the mandibular canal that is caused by a lingual depression in the mandible containing normal salivary gland tissue. Also known as a *lingual mandibular bone concavity* or *static bone cyst*.

Static bone cyst Often referred to as a pseudocyst because it is not a pathologic cavity and is not lined with epithelium. It is characterized by a well-defined cystlike radiolucency in the posterior region of the mandible inferior to the mandibular canal, which is caused by a lingual depression in the mandible, which surrounds normal salivary gland tissue. Also known as a *lingual mandibular bone concavity* or *Stafne bone cyst*.

Stevens-Johnson syndrome A severe form of erythema multiforme characterized by oral, ocular, and genital involvement.

Stomodeum The embryonic invagination that becomes the oral cavity.

Strawberry tongue Oral manifestation of scarlet fever in which the fungiform papillae are red and prominent, with the dorsal surface of tongue exhibiting either a white coating or erythema.

Striae Streaks or interconnecting lines that often result from rapidly developing tension in the skin.

Subclinical infection An infectious disease not detectable by the usual clinical signs.

Subluxation Hypermobility in which the patient is able to relocate the mandible back into the glenoid fossa.

Succedaneous Replacing or substituting for something else; often used when referring to the permanent teeth.

Supernumerary In excess of the normal or regular number, as in teeth or roots.

Supernumerary teeth Extra teeth found in the dental arches.

Symptom Subjective evidence of disease or a physical disorder that is observed by the patient.

Syndactyly Soft tissue or bone fusion or both of fingers and toes.

Syndrome A set of signs or symptoms or both occurring together.

Synovial fluid The transparent viscous fluid that is secreted by the synovial membrane and found in joint cavities.

Synovial membrane Tissue that forms a portion of the lining of some joints; (e.g., the temporomandibular joint).

Syphilis A disease caused by the spirochete *Treponema pallidum.* The organism is transmitted from one person to another by direct contact. It occurs in three stages: (1) primary, (2) secondary, and (3) tertiary.

Systemic lupus erythematosus An acute and chronic inflammatory autoimmune disease of unknown cause. It includes a wide spectrum of disease activity and signs and symptoms.

Systemic Pertaining to or affecting the body as a whole.

T

T lymphocyte A lymphocyte that passes through the thymus before migrating to tissues. The T lymphocyte, also called a T cell, is responsible for cell-mediated immunity and may modulate the humoral immune response.

Talon cusp An accessory cusp located in the area of the cingulum of a maxillary or mandibular permanent incisor.

Taurodontism A condition characterized by very large pyramid-shaped molars with large pulp chambers and short roots.

Tuberculous lymphadenitis Pertaining to tuberculosis, the enlargement of the submandibular and cervical lymph nodes. Also known as *scrofula.*

Temporomandibular disorders (TMDs) Abnormalities in the functioning of the temporomandibular joint or associated structures.

Thalassemia A group of inherited disorders of hemoglobin synthesis. Also called *Mediterranean* or *Cooley anemia.*

Thalassemia major The homozygous form of thalassemia in which genes on both chromosomes are involved.

Thalassemia minor The heterozygous form of thalassemia in which only one gene locus is involved.

Thrombocyte A platelet.

Thrombocytopenia Decrease in the number of platelets in circulating blood. It is sometimes called immune thrombocytopenia because an autoimmune type of process has been identified.

Thrombocytopenic purpura A bleeding disorder that results from a severe reduction in circulating platelets.

Thrush An overgrowth of the yeastlike fungus *Candida albicans.* It is the most common oral fungal infection. It can result from many different conditions, including antibiotic use, cancer, corticosteroid therapy, dentures, diabetes mellitus, and HIV infection. Also called *candidiasis* and *moniliasis.*

Thymic hypoplasia A type of primary immunodeficiency in which the thymus is deficient or lacking; therefore T lymphocytes do not mature. Also called *DiGeorge syndrome.*

Thymus A lymphoid organ that is situated in the chest. It reaches maximal development at about puberty and then undergoes gradual involution.

Thyroglossal tract (duct) cyst A cyst that forms along the same tract that the thyroid gland follows in development, from the area of the foramen cecum to its permanent location in the neck. Most occur below the hyoid bone. The epithelial lining varies from stratified squamous to ciliated columnar epithelium.

Thyrotoxicosis A condition characterized by excessive production of thyroid hormone. Also called *hyperthyroidism.*

TNM staging system A staging and classification system of malignant tumors. T: tumor size; N: lymph nodes involved; M: presence of metastasis. Created by the American Joint Committee on Cancer (AJCC).

Tobacco pouch keratosis A lesion caused by tobacco chewing, typically located in the mucobuccal fold.

Tonsillitis Inflammatory condition of the tonsils and pharyngeal mucosa caused by many different organisms. Clinical features include sore throat, fever, tonsillar hyperplasia, and erythema of the oropharyngeal mucosa and tonsils.

Torus (plural, tori) A benign lesion composed of normal compact bone.

Torus mandibularis An exophytic growth of bone occurring on the lingual aspect of the mandible in the area of the premolars. Also known as *mandibular tori.*

Torus palatinus An exophytic growth of bone occurring in the midline of the hard palate. Also known as *palatal torus.*

Translocation A portion of a chromosome attached to another chromosome.

Traumatic bone cyst A pathologic cavity in bone that is not lined with epithelium. Also known as a *simple bone cyst.*

Traumatic granuloma A hard, raised lesion resulting from persistent trauma.

Traumatic neuroma A lesion caused by injury to a peripheral nerve.

Traumatic ulcer An ulcer that occurs from some form or trauma such as biting the cheek, lip, or tongue; irritation from a denture; and injury from sharp edge of food.

Trismus Inability to open the mouth fully from one of many causes.

Trisomy 21 A type of abnormality in which three of chromosome 21 are found instead of two. This results in abnormal physical characteristics and mental impairment. Also called *Down syndrome.*

Trisomy A pair of chromosomes with an identical extra chromosome.

tRNA The second type of RNA. It transfers amino acids from the cytoplasm and matches them to the mRNA, positioning amino acids in the proper sequence to form polypeptides and proteins.

Tuberculosis An infectious chronic granulomatous disease usually caused by the organism *Mycobacterium tuberculosis.* The chief form of the disease is a primary infection of the lung.

Tumor A neoplasm; also a swelling or enlargement.

Turner tooth A permanent tooth showing enamel hypoplasia resulting from infection or trauma to the deciduous tooth.

Type 1 diabetes The type of diabetes that is characterized by profound insulin deficiency. It includes patients requiring the administration of insulin to prevent ketosis. The onset is abrupt and may be characterized by polydipsia, polyuria, and polyphagia. Also called *insulin-dependent diabetes mellitus.*

Type 2 diabetes The type of diabetes that is characterized by increased insulin resistance. It includes patients who can maintain proper blood sugar levels without the administration of insulin. Obesity is common finding. Also called *noninsulin dependent diabetes mellitus.*

Tzanck cells Detached rounded cells caused by a loss of attachment between the epithelial cells. Also known as *acantholytic cells.* These cells are present with pemphigus vulgaris.

U

Undifferentiated Absence of normal differentiation; anaplasia; a characteristic of malignant tumor tissue.

Unilocular A term used to describe a radiographic appearance of a single rounded compartment or locule.

Urticaria Multiple areas of well-demarcated swelling of the skin, usually accompanied by itching. The lesions are caused by localized areas of vascular permeability in the superficial connective tissue beneath the epithelium. Also know as *hives.*

V

Varicella-zoster virus (VZV) The virus that causes both chickenpox (varicella) and shingles (herpes zoster).

Vascular leiomyoma A benign tumor of smooth muscle that may occur in association with blood vessels. They occur occasionally in the oral cavity.

Verruca vulgaris A white, papillary, exophytic lesion caused by a human papillomavirus. It is a common skin lesion. The lips are one of the most common intraoral sites for this lesion.

Verrucous carcinoma A specific type of squamous cell carcinoma that appears as a slow-growing exophytic tumor with a pebbly white and red surface, usually in the vestibule or buccal mucosa. Often associated with the use of smokeless tobacco.

Vesicle A small, elevated, fluid-filled lesion on the epithelium that is less than 1 cm in diameter.

Vitamin B_{12} A vitamin that contains cobalt and is essential for the maturation of red blood cells.

von Willebrand disease An inherited disorder of platelet function. It is the most common hereditary coagulation anomaly in humans.

W

Well-circumscribed Used to describe the borders of a lesion that are specifically defined; one can clearly see the exact margins and extent of the lesion.

Western blot test A confirmatory test for HIV exposure that identifies antibodies to HIV proteins and glycoproteins.

Wheal A localized swelling of tissue caused by edema during inflammation; often accompanied by severe itching.

White sponge nevus An inherited disorder characterized by a white, corrugated, soft folding of the oral mucosa. The buccal mucosa is always affected, and in most patients the lesions are bilateral. A thick layer of keratin, which at times desquamates and leaves a raw mucosal surface, produces the whitening. Also called *Cannon disease* or *familial white folded mucosal dysplasia.*

Whitlow An infection involving the distal phalanx of a finger.

X

Xerophthalmia Abnormal dryness of the eyes caused by decreased lacrimal flow.

Xerostomia Dryness of the mouth caused by a decrease in salivary flow.

X-linked congenital agammaglobulinemia A type of primary immunodeficiency in which B cells do not mature. Plasma cells are deficient throughout the body; T-cells are normal. Also called *Bruton disease.*

Index

A

Note: Page numbers followed by f indicate illustrations; t, tables; and b, boxed meterial.

B

D

E

H

I

M

O

P

Q

R

S

U

V

W

X

Y

Z

TERM

This Agreement will remain in effect until terminated pursuant to the terms of this Agreement. You may terminate this Agreement at any time by removing from Your system and destroying the Electronic Media Product. Unauthorized copying of the Electronic Media Product, including without limitation, the Proprietary Material and documentation, or otherwise failing to comply with the terms and conditions of this Agreement shall result in automatic termination of this license and will make available to Elsevier legal remedies. Upon termination of this Agreement, the license granted herein will terminate and You must immediately destroy the Electronic Media Product and accompanying documentation. All provisions relating to proprietary rights shall survive termination of this Agreement.

LIMITED WARRANTY AND LIMITATION OF LIABILITY

NEITHER ELSEVIER NOR ITS LICENSORS REPRESENT OR WARRANT THAT THE INFORMATION CONTAINED IN THE PROPRIETARY MATERIAL IS COMPLETE OR FREE FROM ERROR, AND NEITHER ASSUMES, AND BOTH EXPRESSLY DISCLAIM, ANY LIABILITY TO ANY PERSON FOR ANY LOSS OR DAMAGE CAUSED BY ERRORS OR OMISSIONS IN THE PROPRIETARY MATERIAL, WHETHER SUCH ERRORS OR OMISSIONS RESULT FROM NEGLIGENCE, ACCIDENT, OR ANY OTHER CAUSE. IN ADDITION, NEITHER ELSEVIER NOR ITS LICENSORS MAKE ANY REPRESENTATIONS OR WARRANTIES, EITHER EXPRESS OR IMPLIED, REGARDING THE PERFORMANCE OF YOUR NETWORK OR COMPUTER SYSTEM WHEN USED IN CONJUNCTION WITH THE ELECTRONIC MEDIA PRODUCT.

If this Electronic Media Product is defective, Elsevier will replace it at no charge if the defective Electronic Media Product is returned to Elsevier within sixty (60) days (or the greatest period allowable by applicable law) from the date of shipment.

Elsevier warrants that the software embodied in this Electronic Media Product will perform in substantial compliance with the documentation supplied in this Electronic Media Product. If You report a significant defect in performance in writing to Elsevier, and Elsevier is not able to correct same within sixty (60) days after its receipt of Your notification, You may return this Electronic Media Product, including all copies and documentation, to Elsevier and Elsevier will refund Your money.

YOU UNDERSTAND THAT, EXCEPT FOR THE 60-DAY LIMITED WARRANTY RECITED ABOVE, ELSEVIER, ITS AFFILIATES, LICENSORS, SUPPLIERS AND AGENTS, MAKE NO WARRANTIES, EXPRESSED OR IMPLIED, WITH RESPECT TO THE ELECTRONIC MEDIA PRODUCT, INCLUDING, WITHOUT LIMITATION THE PROPRIETARY MATERIAL, AND SPECIFICALLY DISCLAIM ANY WARRANTY OF MERCHANTABILITY OR FITNESS FOR A PARTICULAR PURPOSE.

If the information provided on this Electronic Media Product contains medical or health sciences information, it is intended for professional use within the medical field. Information about medical treatment or drug dosages is intended strictly for professional use, and because of rapid advances in the medical sciences, independent verification of diagnosis and drug dosages should be made.

IN NO EVENT WILL ELSEVIER, ITS AFFILIATES, LICENSORS, SUPPLIERS OR AGENTS, BE LIABLE TO YOU FOR ANY DAMAGES, INCLUDING, WITHOUT LIMITATION, ANY LOST PROFITS, LOST SAVINGS OR OTHER INCIDENTAL OR CONSEQUENTIAL DAMAGES, ARISING OUT OF YOUR USE OR INABILITY TO USE THE ELECTRONIC MEDIA PRODUCT REGARDLESS OF WHETHER SUCH DAMAGES ARE FORESEEABLE OR WHETHER SUCH DAMAGES ARE DEEMED TO RESULT FROM THE FAILURE OR INADEQUACY OF ANY EXCLUSIVE OR OTHER REMEDY.

U.S. GOVERNMENT RESTRICTED RIGHTS

The Electronic Media Product and documentation are provided with restricted rights. Use, duplication or disclosure by the U.S. Government is subject to restrictions as set forth in subparagraphs (a) through (d) of the Commercial Computer Restricted Rights clause at FAR 52.22719 or in subparagraph (c)(1)(ii) of the Rights in Technical Data and Computer Software clause at DFARS 252.2277013, or at 252.2117015, as applicable. Contractor/Manufacturer is Elsevier Inc., 360 Park Avenue South, New York, NY 10010-5107 USA.

GOVERNING LAW

This Agreement shall be governed by the laws of the State of New York, USA. In any dispute arising out of this Agreement, you and Elsevier each consent to the exclusive personal jurisdiction and venue in the state and federal courts within New York County, New York, USA.